Advances in Prevention Science

Series editor
Zili Sloboda, Ontario, OH, USA

The emergent field of prevention science focuses on the application of theories derived from epidemiologic studies, human development, human behavior, genetics, and neuroscience to develop and evaluate cognitive and behavioral interventions. Research over the past two decades has dramatically changed the impact that preventive interventions have had on a number of problem behaviors including substance use and abuse, sexually transmitted infections including HIV and AIDS, violence and injuries, juvenile delinquency, academic failure, obesity, and even lifestyle-related diseases such as hypertension and cardiovascular disorders, cancer, and diabetes.

This book series was conceived to summarize our accumulated knowledge to date and its application to practice. In addition, the series provides suggestions for both short- and long-term research. Having moved forward knowledge about these social and health areas and how to prevent them with various degrees of success, the editors and authors of the series wish to make these findings available to researchers, practitioners, policy makers, social science students, and the public.

More information about this series at http://www.springer.com/series/8822

Zili Sloboda • Hanno Petras
Elizabeth Robertson • Ralph Hingson
Editors

Prevention of Substance Use

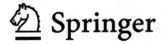

Editors
Zili Sloboda
Applied Prevention Science
International
Ontario, OH, USA

Elizabeth Robertson
University of Alabama
Tuscaloosa, AL, USA

Hanno Petras
AIR
Washington, DC, USA

Ralph Hingson
Division of Epidemiology
and Prevention Research
National Institute on Alcohol
Abuse and Alcoholism
Rockville, MD, USA

ISSN 2625-2619 ISSN 2625-2627 (electronic)
Advances in Prevention Science
ISBN 978-3-030-00625-9 ISBN 978-3-030-00627-3 (eBook)
https://doi.org/10.1007/978-3-030-00627-3

Library of Congress Control Number: 2019930840

© Springer Nature Switzerland AG 2019
This work is subject to copyright. All rights are reserved by the Publisher, whether the whole or part of the material is concerned, specifically the rights of translation, reprinting, reuse of illustrations, recitation, broadcasting, reproduction on microfilms or in any other physical way, and transmission or information storage and retrieval, electronic adaptation, computer software, or by similar or dissimilar methodology now known or hereafter developed.
The use of general descriptive names, registered names, trademarks, service marks, etc. in this publication does not imply, even in the absence of a specific statement, that such names are exempt from the relevant protective laws and regulations and therefore free for general use.
The publisher, the authors, and the editors are safe to assume that the advice and information in this book are believed to be true and accurate at the date of publication. Neither the publisher nor the authors or the editors give a warranty, express or implied, with respect to the material contained herein or for any errors or omissions that may have been made. The publisher remains neutral with regard to jurisdictional claims in published maps and institutional affiliations.

This Springer imprint is published by the registered company Springer Nature Switzerland AG
The registered company address is: Gewerbestrasse 11, 6330 Cham, Switzerland

Preface

Welcome to the "Advances in Prevention Science" series. The title of this fourth volume is *Prevention of Substance Use*. The chapters compiled herein address the state of our knowledge about the epidemiology and etiology of psychoactive substance use and abuse, effective prevention strategies and programs, the consequences of substance abuse, methodological challenges, emerging areas, and the future of substance use prevention. Prevention interventions are intended to prevent the onset of substance use and progression to abuse and thus are differentiated from treatment interventions for individuals manifesting a substance use disorder. The overarching perspective of the book is developmental within the contexts of the micro- to macro-level environments such as family, school, community, and social policy that influence our attitudes, beliefs, and behavior.

The misuse of psychoactive substances such as alcohol, tobacco, cannabis, heroin, methamphetamines, cocaine, and certain prescription medications exact a tremendous toll on individuals, families, communities, and society, for example, in the form of health problems, injuries, lost income and productivity, family and community dysfunction, and death. Importantly, due to the progress made over the past three decades in the field of prevention science, all of these negative outcomes are preventable. Prevention science is an evolving field that seeks to improve public health through identifying malleable risk and protective factors, assessing the efficacy and effectiveness of preventive interventions, and identifying optimal strategies for the implementation and adoption of evidence-based programs, policies, and practices.

Prevention science draws from diverse theoretical orientations and empirical sources. Theories of human development, encompassing physiological, genetic, psychological, behavioral, cognitive, and social perspectives, inform the design of interventions that aim to reduce risk and enhance protection at the individual, familial, peer, community, and larger environmental levels that include laws and policies related to health behaviors.

The book is divided into five parts. The first part is an introduction to the volume and provides the reader an overview of the prevention of substance use. The most current research on the nature of psychoactive substances is presented including their physiological effects and the pharmacological aspects particularly as they relate to the developing brains of children and adolescents (Chap. 1). These considerations are framed within a global perspective (Chap. 2) that views substance use as a moving target that changes across the globe and across time as patterns of substance use emerge. These trends are then considered at levels of the social ecology (Chap. 3). At the intrapersonal level, information on the roles of the brain, genetics, and epigenetics is presented (Chap. 4) again with an understanding that our knowledge in these areas is evolving at a rapid pace. The interactions between these intrapersonal developments and interpersonal dynamics through interactions both at the micro- and macro-level environments are addressed holistically from biological, psychological, and social perspectives on the initiation of substance use and progression from substance use to substance use disorders (Chap. 5). As basic science becomes more and more relevant to prevention interventions, connections are being made between basic research and prevention research that point to new opportunities for the development and testing of interventions. These connections often speak to the contents of the "Black Boxes" of theories where suspected processes become confirmed with actual physiological evidence. For example, the identification of reward centers in the brain common between food, sex, gambling, video gaming, and substance use offers new directions for interventions that target multiple problem behaviors within the same intervention or developing a "next-generation intervention" through modifications to an effective intervention for the new target(s) utilizing the theory and structure of the "parent" intervention.

The final chapters in this part tackle the sociopolitical level through discussions on societal reactions and regulations regarding both legally obtainable substances (e.g., tobacco, alcohol, and prescription drugs) and illegal drugs (Chaps. 6 and 7, respectively).

In the second part, the focus is on effective prevention interventions and strategies for substance use. Here you will encounter information on specific venues for prevention, singularly and in combination. Family (Chap. 8), school (Chap. 9), policy, and multiple component interventions (Chap. 10) are highlighted as well as specific intervention strategies such as screenings and brief interventions and referral to services where warranted (Chap. 11). In addition, the development and testing of interventions for special populations and specific examples of interventions for one type of substance are presented (Chap. 12). Although the specific focus of this volume is the prevention of psychoactive substance use, many aspects, including strategies and messages, of the interventions discussed are common to the prevention of other health-risking behaviors, disorders, and diseases.

Methodological challenges are discussed in the next part and are addressed in two ways, those related to the epidemiology of substance use (Chaps. 13 and 14, respectively) and those that relate to the evaluation of prevention interventions (Chaps. 15, 16, and 17, respectively). The emergent technologies and data collection methods and the interventions they assess raise ethical issues that require protections (Chap. 18).

Many interventions are evaluated across time, in some cases with subjects being followed into adulthood. The longitudinal nature of intervention evaluation can introduce concerns related to the overall design of the evaluation, comparability of measures across the developmental stages addressed in an intervention implementation and analysis, expected and unexpected losses from the subject pool, natural growth in the numbers of individuals using substances as they age, and the changing influence of mediating and moderating variables. These ongoing methodological challenges for intervention evaluation are complicated by the use of new technologies for intervening and collecting data (Chaps. 19, 20, and 21).

There are a number of emerging and future areas for consideration in prevention trials. Some of these are methodological in nature, for example, research employing qualitative and adaptive designs, micro-trials, and idiographic methods (Chap. 22). One question that remains largely unanswered is "What intervention works best for whom and why?" A second question is "How best to measure and present the economic value of intervening across childhood and adolescence when the true results will not be seen immediately and perhaps not for several years?"

Future challenges include how best to disseminate and sustain evidence-based interventions and policies. For much of the past 30 years, prevention science focused on the development of interventions as well as on systems for the dissemination of interventions. In recent years, prevention experts have recognized the critical importance of focusing more clearly on variables that facilitate or inhibit the uptake and adoption of prevention interventions and systems. Moreover, recent changes in health-care service delivery systems open the potential for broader adoption of prevention interventions with strong scientific support providing an unprecedented opportunity for public health benefits. In order for efforts in these areas to be fruitful in improving health, it is critical that prevention science continue to ask—and answer—the complex practice and policy questions that underlie the successful dissemination and implementation of evidence-based practices. Much progress has been made in this area with models for effective dissemination being made available to be used in diverse settings with great success (Chap. 23).

Several challenges to the support of the emergent field of prevention science and its application to the prevention of substance use and other potentially risky behaviors are international recognition and acceptance of the science foundation for prevention interventions. This recognition and support derives from the researchers and decision-makers that are involved in prevention work (Chap. 24), from the workforce (Chap. 25), and from national prevention systems (Chap. 26).

As have many other fields of scientific inquiry, prevention science has evolved over time. Indeed, over the past 30 years, there has been an explosion of research with findings from areas such as neuroscience, genetics, physiology, psychology, and sociology with relevance to prevention intervention and policies. An important distinction of prevention science is its reliance on theory and empirical evidence as foundations. New tools and technologies help us to understand both observed and theorized behavior patterns in relation to actual internal processes that our prior models only alluded to. Specific measures using technologies for genetic and physiological outcomes have been used to assess outcomes related to intervention effects and effectiveness. However, these recent advances have not been integrated into theories of human development in a way that makes them readily accessible to prevention science. The increasing precision of these tools pinpoints biological mechanisms that, in combination with environmental characteristics, are associated with behaviors that can affect life course trajectories and help in refining theories of human behavior and improving innovative prevention interventions.

There are many other areas of science and practice with relevance to or impacts on prevention science. The chapters in this volume provide an up-to-date summary on the current state of our knowledge. However, the field and associated fields are rapidly growing. Future efforts to summarize the state of knowledge will no doubt include topics not yet thought about in these chapters. Keeping up with the rapid rate of growth is difficult, but volumes such as this provide an opportunity to stay abreast of the changing landscape of science.

Ontario, OH, USA	Zili Sloboda
Washington, DC, USA	Hanno Petras
Tuscaloosa, AL, USA	Elizabeth Robertson
Rockville, MD, USA	Ralph Hingson

Contents

Part I Introduction to Substance Use

1. **A Primer on Alcohol and Adolescent Brain Development: Implications for Prevention** 3
   Aaron White and Ralph Hingson

2. **Epidemiology of Substance Use Internationally** 19
   Amy Peacock, Wayne Hall, and Louisa Degenhardt

3. **An Integrative Perspective on the Etiology of Substance Use** ... 37
   Nicole J. Roberts and Diana Fishbein

4. **Genetics and Epigenetics of Substance Use** 57
   Michael M. Vanyukov and Ralph E. Tarter

5. **Progression of Substance Use to Substance Use Disorder** 75
   Matthew R. Lee, Yoanna E. McDowell, and Kenneth J. Sher

6. **The Tobacco Control Experience: A Model for Substance Use Prevention?** 99
   Kenneth E. Warner

7. **Alcohol Marketing and Promotion** 119
   David H. Jernigan

Part II Effective Prevention Interventions and Strategies for Substance Use

8. **Family Processes and Evidence-Based Prevention** 133
   J. Douglas Coatsworth and Melissa W. George

9. **The School: A Setting for Evidence-Based Prevention Interventions and Policies** 147
   Zili Sloboda and Christopher L. Ringwalt

10. **Substance Use Policy Interventions: Intended and Unintended Consequences** 165
    Mallie J. Paschall, Rebecca Yau, and Christopher L. Ringwalt

11. **Brief Interventions as Evidence-Based Prevention Strategies** .. 181
    Emily E. Tanner-Smith and Sean P. Grant

12 ATOD Prevention in Diverse Communities:
    Research and Receptivity 193
    Anna Pagano, Raul Caetano, and Juliet P. Lee

Part III Methodological Challenges

13 Qualitative Methods in the Study of Psychoactive
    Substance Use: Origins and Contributions—Implications
    for Substance-Use Prevention 209
    J. Bryan Page and Zili Sloboda

14 Monitoring Trends: Use of Local Data 223
    Jane Mounteney and Paul Griffiths

15 The Importance of Mediation Analysis
    in Substance-Use Prevention 233
    Holly P. O'Rourke and David P. MacKinnon

16 Subgroup Analysis: "What Works Best
    for Whom and Why?" 247
    Ferdinand Keller

17 Adaptive Intervention Designs in Substance Use Prevention ... 263
    Kelly L. Hall, Inbal Nahum-Shani, Gerald J. August,
    Megan E. Patrick, Susan A. Murphy, and Daniel Almirall

18 Ethical Issues in Substance-Use Prevention Research......... 281
    Celia B. Fisher and Rimah Jaber

Part IV Emerging Areas

19 Creating Persuasive Substance-Use Prevention
    Communications: The EQUIP Model 303
    William D. Crano, Eusebio M. Alvaro, and Jason T. Siegel

20 Use of Media and Social Media in the Prevention
    of Substance Use 319
    David B. Buller, Barbara J. Walkosz, and W. Gill Woodall

21 A Role for Mindfulness and Mindfulness Training
    in Substance Use Prevention 335
    Nathaniel R. Riggs, Mark T. Greenberg,
    and Kamila Dvorakova

Part V Future Challenges

22 Bridging the Gap: Microtrials and Idiographic Designs
    for Translating Basic Science into Effective Prevention
    of Substance Use 349
    George W. Howe and Ty A. Ridenour

23	**Dissemination of Evidence-Based Prevention Interventions and Policies** 367
	Matthew Chinman, Joie Acosta, Patricia Ebener, Sarah Hunter, Pamela Imm, and Abraham Wandersman
24	**Supporting Prevention Science and Prevention Research Internationally** 385
	Jeremy Segrott
25	**The Substance-Use Prevention Workforce: An International Perspective** 395
	Harry R. Sumnall
26	**Prevention Systems: Structure and Challenges: Europe as an Example** 413
	Gregor Burkhart and Stefanie Helmer

Index 443

Contributors

Joie Acosta RAND Corporation, Arlington, VA, USA

Daniel Almirall Department of Statistics, Survey Research Center, Institute for Social Research, University of Michigan, Ann Arbor, MI, USA

Eusebio M. Alvaro Department of Psychology, Claremont Graduate University, Claremont, CA, USA

Gerald J. August Institute of Translational Science in Children's Mental Health, University of Minnesota, St. Paul, MN, USA

David B. Buller Klein Buendel, Inc., Golden, CO, USA

Gregor Burkhart European Monitoring Centre for Drugs and Drug Addiction, Lisbon, Portugal

Raul Caetano Prevention Research Center, Oakland, CA, USA

Matthew Chinman RAND Corporation, Pittsburgh, PA, USA

J. Douglas Coatsworth Human Development and Family Studies, Colorado State University, Fort Collins, CO, USA

William D. Crano Department of Psychology, Claremont Graduate University, Claremont, CA, USA

Louise Degenhardt National Drug and Alcohol Research Centre, University of New South Wales, Sydney, NSW, Australia

School of Population and Global Health, University of Melbourne, Melbourne, VIC, Australia

Department of Global Health, School of Public Health, University of Washington, Seattle, WA, USA

Kamila Dvorakova National Institute of Mental Health, Prague, Czech Republic

Patricia Ebener RAND Corporation, Santa Monica, CA, USA

Diana Fishbein Program for Translational Research on Adversity and Neurodevelopment, The Pennsylvania State University, University Park, PA, USA

Celia B. Fisher Center for Ethics Education, Fordham University, Bronx, NY, USA

Melissa W. George Colorado State University, Fort Collins, CO, USA

Sean P. Grant Indiana University, Indianapolis, IN, Indiana

Mark T. Greenberg Human Development and Family Studies, The Pennsylvania State University, University Park, PA, USA

Paul Griffiths Scientific Director, European Monitoring Centre for Drugs and Drug Addiction (EMCDDA), Lisbon, Portugal

Kelly L. Hall Yale University School of Public Health, New Haven, CT, USA

Wayne Hall University of Queensland Centre for Youth Substance Abuse Research, Herston, QLD, Australia

National Addiction Centre, Kings College London, London, UK

Stefanie Helmer Institute of Social Medicine, Epidemiology and Health Economics, Charité - Universitätsmedizin Berlin, Berlin, Germany

Ralph Hingson Division of Epidemiology and Prevention Research, National Institute on Alcohol Abuse and Alcoholism, Rockville, MD, USA

George W. Howe Department of Clinical Psychology, George Washington University, Washington, DC, USA

Sarah Hunter RAND Corporation, Santa Monica, CA, USA

Pamela Imm Private Practice, Lexington, SC, USA

Rimah Jaber Center for Ethics Education, Fordham University, Bronx, NY, USA

David H. Jernigan Department of Health Law, Policy and Management, Boston University School of Public Health, Boston, MA, USA

Ferdinand Keller Department of Child and Adolescent Psychiatry and Psychotherapy, University Hospital Ulm, Ulm, Germany

Juliet P. Lee Prevention Research Center, Pacific Institute for Research and Evaluation, Berkeley, CA, USA

Matthew R. Lee Department of Applied Psychology, Graduate School of Applied and Professional Psychology, Rutgers University, New Brunswick, NJ, USA

Department of Psychological Sciences, University of Missouri, Columbia, MO, USA

David P. MacKinnon Psychology Department, Arizona State University, Tempe, AZ, USA

Yoanna E. McDowell Department of Psychological Sciences, University of Missouri, Columbia, MO, USA

Jane Mounteney Head of Public Health Unit, European Monitoring Centre for Drugs and Drug Addiction, Lisbon, Portugal

Susan A. Murphy Department of Statistics, Radcliffe Institute, Harvard University, Cambridge, MA, USA

Department of Computer Science, Harvard John A. Paulson School of Engineering and Applied Sciences, Cambridge, MA, USA

Inbal Nahum-Shani Institute for Social Research, University of Michigan, Ann Arbor, MI, USA

Holly P. O'Rourke T. Denny Sanford School of Social and Family Dynamics, Arizona State University, Tempe, AZ, USA

Anna Pagano Prevention Research Center, Pacific Institute for Research and Evaluation (PIRE), Oakland, CA, USA

J. Bryan Page Department of Anthropology, University of Miami, Coral Gables, FL, USA

Mallie J. Paschall Prevention Research Center, Pacific Institute for Research and Evaluation, Oakland, CA, USA

Megan E. Patrick Institute for Social Research, University of Michigan, Ann Arbor, MI, USA

Amy Peacock National Drug and Alcohol Research Centre, University of New South Wales, Sydney, NSW, Australia

School of Medicine (Psychology), University of Tasmania, Hobart, TAS, Australia

Ty A. Ridenour Developmental Behavioral Epidemiologist, RTI, International, Research Triangle Park, NC, USA

Nathaniel R. Riggs Human Development and Family Studies, Colorado State University, Fort Collins, CO, USA

Christopher L. Ringwalt Injury Prevention Research Center, University of North Carolina, Chapel Hill, NC, USA

Nicole J. Roberts The Pennsylvania State University, University Park, PA, USA

Jeremy Segrott School of Social Sciences, Cardiff University, Cardiff, Wales, UK

Kenneth J. Sher Department of Psychological Sciences, University of Missouri, Columbia, MO, USA

Jason T. Siegel Department of Psychology, Claremont Graduate University, Claremont, CA, USA

Zili Sloboda Applied Prevention Science International, Ontario, OH, USA

Harry R. Sumnall Public Health Institute, Liverpool John Moores University, Liverpool, UK

Emily E. Tanner-Smith Department of Counseling Psychology and Human Services, College of Education, University of Oregon, Eugene, OR, USA

Ralph E. Tarter University of Pittsburgh, Pittsburgh, PA, USA

Michael M. Vanyukov University of Pittsburgh, Pittsburgh, PA, USA

Barbara J. Walkosz Klein Buendel, Inc., Golden, CO, USA

Abraham Wandersman Barnwell College, University of South Carolina, Columbia, SC, USA

Kenneth E. Warner Department of Health Management and Policy, University of Michigan School of Public Health, Ann Arbor, MI, USA

Aaron White National Institute on Alcohol Abuse and Alcoholism, National Institutes of Health, Bethesda, MD, USA

W. Gill Woodall Klein Buendel, Inc., Golden, CO, USA

Rebecca Yau Prevention Research Center, Pacific Institute for Research and Evaluation, Oakland, CA, USA

About the Editors

Zili Sloboda, ScD was trained in medical sociology at New York University and in mental health and epidemiology at the Johns Hopkins University Bloomberg School of Public Health. The majority of her research has been related to the delivery of health-related services to youth and adults and epidemiology. She was a founder of the Society for Prevention Research (SPR) in both the United States and Europe and is well published in the area of drug abuse epidemiology and substance use prevention. Her major books include the *Handbook of Drug Abuse Prevention*, *Epidemiology of Drug Abuse*, and *Defining Prevention Science*. She has a long-standing commitment to the dissemination of evidence-based programming and the advancement of Translation I and II research through work with SPR and with the United Nations Office on Drugs and Crime to develop international standards for substance use prevention based on research evidence. Her current work is focused on the international dissemination of the Universal Prevention Curriculum developed to build the capacity of prevention professionals worldwide to implement evidence-based prevention interventions and policies in their communities. Applied Prevention Science International, Ontario, OH, USA

Hanno Petras, PhD is a Principal Researcher at AIR where he is responsible for developing and leading rigorous research proposals in the areas of youth violence, sexual violence perpetration, substance abuse, and suicide as well as evaluating the effectiveness of research- and practice-based prevention intervention programs in school and community settings. He has over 20 years of experience designing and conducting research and evaluation of preventive interventions aimed at minimizing unhealthy and risky outcomes over the life course. His work has documented the continued vulnerability of individuals over the life course and how preventive interventions can alleviate such vulnerabilities. He has published extensively on prevention interventions related to aggressive/disruptive behavior in the classroom, mental health, tobacco use, violence against women, and HIV risk factors related to substance use. He recently co-edited together with Dr. Zili Sloboda the first book in the series entitled Advances in Prevention Science that focuses on defining prevention science, which was published by Springer Publications. Health & Social Development Program, Washington, DC, USA

Elizabeth Robertson, PhD recently retired as Professor and Associate Dean for Research in the College of Human Environmental Sciences at the University of Alabama. Prior to joining the university faculty, she was at the National Institutes of Health where she served as Chief of the Prevention Research Branch at the National Institute on Drug Abuse. Dr. Robertson has expertise in the prevention of drug use initiation and progression including a developmental focus from early childhood through adulthood and contextual foci including the family, school, the criminal justice and social welfare systems, clinical and recreational settings, and the media. In addition, she has expertise in the prevention of drug-related HIV infection and the dissemination and implementation of evidence-based practices. Her published journal articles, book chapters, and government publications focus on dissemination and implementation of evidence-based prevention interventions, inhibitory control, the effects of parental incarceration on children, the contributions of social support and economic stress to family/child dysfunction, and principles of prevention intervention. She has received awards from the Society for Prevention Research, the Secretary of the Department of Health and Human Services, and the National Institutes for Health. College of Human Environmental Sciences, University of Alabama, 207 Child Development Research Center, Tuscaloosa, AL, USA

Ralph Hingson, ScD is the Director of the Division of Epidemiology and Prevention Research at the National Institute on Alcohol Abuse and Alcoholism (NIAAA). Before joining NIAAA, he was Professor and Associate Dean for Research at the Boston University School of Public Health. He has authored or co-authored 170 research articles and book chapters on the epidemiology of alcohol-related morbidity and mortality and on the impact of environmental interventions on the these consequences of alcohol use. He has received numerous awards and recognitions for his work from such groups as Robert Wood Johnson Foundation, the International Council on Alcohol, Drugs, and Traffic Safety (ICADTS), the American Society of Addiction Medicine, and the University of Pittsburgh. In 2017, Dr. Hingson received the 2017 National Institutes of Health Director's Award for his role as a member of the Surgeon General's Report Team for the recently released Surgeon General's Report on Alcohol, Drugs, and Health. He is a Past President of ICADTS and currently serves on the World Health Organization's coordinating council to implement WHO's global strategic plan to reduce the harmful use of alcohol. Division of Epidemiology and Prevention Research, National Institute on Alcohol Abuse and Alcoholism, Rockville, MD, USA

Part I
Introduction to Substance Use

A Primer on Alcohol and Adolescent Brain Development: Implications for Prevention

Aaron White and Ralph Hingson

Introduction

Adolescence, a developmental stage observed in all mammals, is the transition from childhood dependence to the greater autonomy of young adulthood. In humans, this transition encompasses the second decade of life and perhaps longer. Adolescence brings significant improvements in cognitive skills, including problem-solving, attention, and abstract reasoning, that are needed to thrive in the complex world outside the family home. The influence of parental approval wanes and the influence of peer approval takes on increasing importance (Nelson et al., 2005). Improvements in the ability to regulate emotional expression and take the perspectives of others facilitate the development of important social skills. Friction between an adolescent's burgeoning desire for freedom and household rules can lead to conflict, which serves to facilitate the transition out of the nest. An increase in motivation to spend time with peers and a decrease in the desire to spend time with family help ensure that the march toward independence takes place.

The typical phenotypic changes that unfold during adolescence result from a combination of puberty and experience-guided neurodevelopment. For humans, the body begins the physical metamorphosis of puberty near the end of the first decade of life. While the specifics remain poorly understood, it is presumed that the early hormonal changes of puberty trigger the brain changes observed during adolescence, including sexually dimorphic patterns of development within and between several regions. In essence, puberty embodies the physical changes that prepare us to procreate and protect ourselves in the world, whereas adolescence reflects the panoply of neurological and psychological adaptations that fine-tune us to thrive in the current cultural context. Every generation goes through adolescence. Yet, because cultures change over time, the specific social skills adolescents acquire vary across generations, leading to well-known generation gaps between successive waves of parents and teens.

In this chapter, we explore the changes that unfold in the brain during adolescence and discuss the implications of these changes for both healthy and risky behavior during the second decade of life. As we will see, the changes in the brain that take place during adolescence provide incredible opportunities for personal growth and future success but also enhanced vulnerabilities to the initiation of alcohol use and the negative effects that can follow.

A. White (✉)
Office of the Director, National Institute on Alcohol Abuse and Alcoholism, National Institutes of Health, Bethesda, MD, USA
e-mail: aaron.white@nih.gov

R. Hingson
Division of Epidemiology and Prevention Research, National Institute on Alcohol Abuse and Alcoholism, National Institutes of Health, Bethesda, MD, USA
e-mail: rhingson@mail.nih.gov

Adolescent Brain Development Is a New Area Research

Until 25 years ago, it was assumed that brain development was largely completed before the age of 10. The brain is 90% of its adult size by the age of seven and existing histology on adolescent brains did not hint at the changes taking place. The moodiness and general tumult of the adolescent years were long assumed to stem from the hormone changes of puberty. Thanks to the introduction of neuroimaging techniques in the early 1990s, we now know that the organization and functioning of the brain go through complex changes during the second decade of life. Importantly, these changes appear to be unique to the adolescent years and not simply the trailing remnants of childhood brain development. In the few decades since these initial discoveries, there has been an explosion of research on the adolescent brain (see Fig. 1.1).

Our understanding of healthy and abnormal adolescent brain development should advance significantly in the years to come. In 2016, the National Institutes of Health, including the National Institute on National Institute on Alcohol Abuse and Alcohol, began to enroll subjects in a large project known as the Adolescent Brain Cognitive Development Study (ABCD), a multifaceted biobehavioral, environmental, familial, and genetic longitudinal development study of 11,500 people beginning at ages 9–10. Enrollment should be completed by the end of 2018. Participants will be followed for 10 years, during which time cognitive functioning and behavioral data, including substance use, will be assessed and neuroimaging data will be collected.

Adolescent Brain Basics

As the first decade of life comes to a close, gray matter volumes in several areas of the neocortex, including frontal lobe regions that govern important cognitive and social functions, reach their peak. Gray matter contains the cell bodies and dendrites of neurons, as well as the synapses, or points of communication, between them. The increase in gray matter sets the stage for widespread gene- and experience-driven pruning and fine-tuning of brain circuitry during adolescence. Across the second decade of life, gray matter volumes decline as lesser used synapses between cells are eliminated and the strength of often used synapses increases. It is estimated that the number of synapses in layer III of the neocortex in the frontal lobes, the layer that receives input from other areas, is reduced by 40% between the ages of 7 and 15 (Brenhouse & Andersen, 2011).

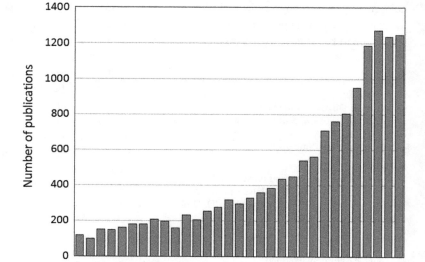

Fig. 1.1 The number of publications each year exploring adolescent brain development increased from a few dozen in the late 1980s to roughly 1200 annually in the past few years

In addition to the elimination of synapses, there is an increase in the density, or concentration, of components within the gray matter (Gennatas et al., 2017). Because these changes are strongly influenced by interactions with the world, such plasticity allows an individual to be customized to fit the demands of their particular environments (Fig. 1.2).

The decrease in gray matter volume across adolescence is accompanied by an increase in white matter volume. White matter is comprised of glial cells, which play diverse roles in brain function and health. Glial cells guide neurons to their targets during early brain development. After birth, they nurture and sustain neurons by feeding them partially metabolized glucose, fighting immune battles, cleaning up debris, and forming a key part of the blood-brain barrier that regulates the flow of molecules in and out of the brain. Glial cells play critical roles in communication between neurons. They can remove neurotransmitters from synapses and release them again when needed.

Glia are particularly important in communication between distant brain areas. To communicate with another neuron, a neuron first generates an electrochemical impulse known as an action potential, which travels down a long arm known as the axon (see Fig. 1.3). Once at the end of the axon, the action potential triggers the release of neurotransmitters into synapses with other cells. In a process called myelination, a type of glial cell known as an oligodendrocyte wraps its appendages around the axons of neurons, thereby increasing the resistance across axonal membranes and facilitating the transmission of action potentials. In this way, myelin functions much like the rubber covering around electrical wires. Some small neurons in the brain are unmyelinated but larger neurons, including those connecting distant brain areas, all contain a myelin sheath. Without myelin, action potentials would not travel as far or fast, which would severely limit communication between different brain areas. (The symptoms of multiple sclerosis, a disease in which myelin is destroyed, yield insights into just how important myelin is for brain functioning.) Myelination increases during adolescence, leading to an increase in white matter volume and improvements in the speed and efficiency of signal transmission along axonal pathways connecting circuits in the brain.

Pruning and fine-tuning of gray matter progress more quickly in areas that govern basic sensory processing and unfold more slowly in association areas that combine and process

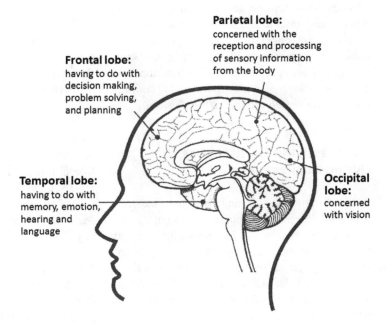

Fig. 1.2 The human brain (reproduced with permission from National Institute on Drug Abuse. Mind Over Matter, The Brain's Response to Drugs. Teacher's Guide. Bethesda, MD, National Institute on Drug Abuse; 2002, 10. Available at http://teens.drugabuse.gov/mom/teachguide/MOMTeacherGuide.pdf)

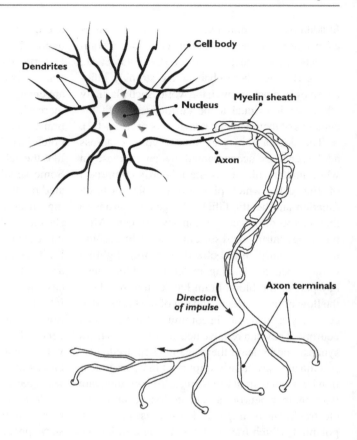

Fig. 1.3 Depiction of a neuron (reproduced with permission from National Institute on Drug Abuse. *Mind Over Matter, The Brain's Response to Drugs.* Teacher's Guide. Bethesda, MD, National Institute on Drug Abuse; 2002, 11. Available at http://teens.drugabuse.gov/mom/teachguide/MOMTeacherGuide.pdf)

information from various brain regions. The final areas to develop are those at the forward tips of the frontal lobes, known as the prefrontal cortex. In essence, the cortex develops in a back-to-front pattern, with the prefrontal cortex, which handles complex cognitive functions like decision-making and impulse control, continuing to develop into the mid-20s or beyond.

Changes in the Frontal Lobes During Adolescence

Some of the most intriguing changes in the brain during adolescence take place in the frontal lobes. These brain areas, located just behind the forehead, play critical roles in memory, voluntary movement, interpreting social cues, controlling emotional urges, making decisions, planning for the future, and other higher order cognitive functions on which adults rely for survival.

As discussed, gray matter volumes decline in the frontal lobes during adolescence while myelination of axons carrying information to and from the frontal lobes increases. This process reflects the pruning of neuronal circuits in the frontal lobes followed by the increased insulation of these circuits to ensure fast and efficient functioning. The activity of neurons requires energy and, as frontal lobe gray matter volumes fall during adolescence, a parallel decrease in overall metabolism occurs in the frontal lobes, reaching adult levels by the age of 16–18 (Chugani, 1998).

As gray matter volumes and energy needs decrease, performance on frontal lobe-dependent tasks becomes more focused and efficient, and the accuracy of performance improves (Ernst & Mueller, 2008; Schweinsburg, Nagel, & Tapert, 2005). There is a general increase in reliance on the frontal lobes to organize and control behavior as we progress through the teenage years toward young adulthood. This developmental transition toward increased reliance on the frontal lobes is known as *frontalization* (Rubia et al., 2000). Concurrent molding of circuitry as frontalization unfolds means that each individual will learn to control impulses, make plans, socialize, and regulate emotions in ways consistent with the influences of their surroundings.

The frontal lobes do not function in isolation. They gather information and exert their influences by interacting with other brain areas. In addition to revealing that changes take place within the frontal lobes during adolescence, recent research has begun to shed light on how circuits formed between the frontal lobes and other structures develop during the second decade of life. The overall picture is one of increasing specialization of function within specific subregions of the frontal lobes and increasing cohesion between these subregions and the brain areas with which they interact. For instance, in the Stroop interference task, in which subjects are shown words in different colors and must inhibit the tendency to read the words in order to name the colors, coordinated activity between the lateral prefrontal cortex and the basal ganglia, specifically the lenticular nucleus of the striatum, comes online during adolescence. Both the accuracy of performance on the task and the magnitude of activation of circuits involving the frontal lobes and basal ganglia increase throughout the adolescent years and into adulthood (Marsh et al., 2006). Similar age-related increases in activity within circuits involving the frontal lobes and basal ganglia have been observed in the tracking stop task, a response-inhibition task in which subjects must inhibit a response to a go signal if it is followed by a stop signal (Rubia, Smith, Taylor, & Brammer, 2007). Improvements in the ability to select desired responses rather than react based on initial impulses are critical for navigating the complex world of rules, laws, and social mores that awaits them when they reach adulthood.

Changes in Other Parts of the Cortex

The frontal lobes are not the only cortical areas that undergo construction during the adolescent years (Shaw et al., 2006). As with the frontal lobes, the amount of gray matter in the parietal lobes peaks at approximately age 11 and decreases throughout adolescence. Located on the sides and toward the back of the brain, the parietal lobes are involved in processing sensations from the body and understanding spatial relationships such as where the body is relative to other objects in the world. They are also important for interpreting and creating music, solving math problems, and other higher order abstract cognitive functions. In the occipital lobes, located at the back of the brain and entirely dedicated to processing visual information, gray matter volumes increase throughout adolescence and into the early 20s. The temporal lobes, which are critical for memory formation as well as processing auditory information and seeing detailed patterns and shapes, do not reach their maximum levels of gray matter until the age of 16–17, at which point they plateau. The temporal lobes contain the hippocampus, a structure that is central to creating an autobiographical record as experiences unfold.

Clearly, much of the cortex undergoes changes during adolescence, each area with its own unique progression (Ernst & Mueller, 2008; Giedd, 2004).

Structures Involved in Emotional Reactivity and Risky Behaviors

On the surface, changes in the frontal lobes and other cortical structures seem capable of explaining a wide range of typical adolescent behaviors, including difficulties inhibiting impulses and regulating emotional expression. However, Casey, Jones, and Hare (2008) asserted that changes in the frontal lobes and other cortical areas cannot explain the whole of adolescent behavior, particularly when it comes to risk-taking and strong emotional reactions. The authors argued that, similar to adolescents, children have immature frontal lobes but do not exhibit the degree of risky behavior exhibited by many teenagers. According to the authors, "[a]dolescence is a developmental period characterized by suboptimal decisions and actions that are associated with an increased incidence of unintentional injuries, violence, substance abuse, unintended pregnancy, and sexually transmitted diseases." Indeed, the National Center of Health Statistics estimates that there are roughly 16, 000 adolescent deaths per year, more than 70% of which are caused by homicides, suicides, motor vehicle crashes, and other unintentional injuries, activities that often involve problems with impulse control and emotion regulation.

Casey and colleagues concurred that immature frontal lobes certainly help explain problems regulating impulses. Maturation of the frontal lobes leads to the ability to suppress inappropriate thoughts and actions and to forego short-term satisfaction in exchange for reaching long-term goals. Immature cognitive control centers make it easier for emotional impulses to influence behavior, but what about the strong emotional impulses themselves? From where do they originate, and why are they so strong during adolescence? The authors suggested that several important emotional areas of the brain reach full operating power by mid-adolescence at a time when the frontal lobes are still in flux. Adolescents are driven by strong emotions arising from these areas and do not yet have the cognitive control necessary to regulate, consistently, these strong emotional urges. The fact that the frontal lobes are not yet working at their full potential simply makes it easier for these strong emotions to influence behavior.

The idea that adolescent risk-taking behavior reflects more than immature frontal lobe functioning has gained support from additional research. For instance, neuroimaging studies suggest that, when making risky choices and processing emotional information, adolescents exhibit larger increases in activity in the nucleus accumbens relative to the activity seen in children and adults (Ernst & Mueller, 2008). The nucleus accumbens, deep within the center of the brain, is the heart of the reward system, which provides positive reinforcement for particular behaviors. The findings suggest that engaging in risky behavior might be reinforcing for teens.

In a fascinating study, Chein, Albert, O'Brien, Uckert, and Steinberg (2011) examined brain activity and risk-taking while adolescents and adults performed a simple driving task under two conditions while brain activity was measured using fMRI. In the driving task, subjects progressed down a straight road through several intersections. As they approached the intersections, traffic lights would change color. The driver had to decide whether to proceed through the intersection or stop. In one condition, the driver was alone. In another, they were told that a peer was watching their performance on the driving task from another room. The researchers found that adults exhibited greater activity than adolescents in the left prefrontal cortex in both the alone and peer conditions. When adolescents were being observed by peers, but not when they were alone, they took more risks and exhibited significantly greater activity than adults in the ventral striatum, which contains the nucleus accumbens. These findings support the notion that frontalization leads to improved impulse control in adulthood. They also indicate that risk-taking during adolescence is influenced by social context. It appears that simply knowing that a friend is watching can lead to greater risk-taking and reward-related brain activity (Fig. 1.4).

The nucleus accumbens receives signals in the form of the neurotransmitter, dopamine, from another deep-seated structure called the ventral tegmental area (VTA). This system is strongly activated both in anticipation of reward and on the delivery of reward. Activation of this circuitry leads to both positive reinforcement (i.e., pleasure) and, via dopamine projections from the VTA to the prefrontal cortex, an increase in attention. Such activation results in learning to repeat the rewarded behavior. It also leads to the attachment of incentive salience (attraction) to stimuli associated with the reward. Animal studies suggest that the density of dopamine receptors is highest in the nucleus accumbens during adolescence, perhaps making this region particularly responsive to the rewarding signals that dopamine provides

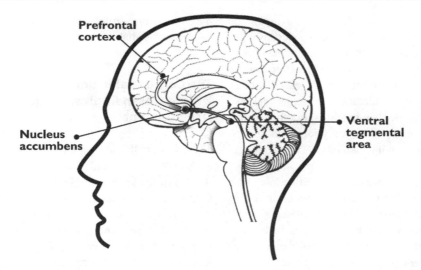

Fig. 1.4 The human brain. (Reproduced with permission from National Institute on Drug Abuse. Mind Over Matter, The Brain's Response to Drugs. Teacher's Guide. Bethesda, MD, National Institute on Drug Abuse; 2002,10. Available at, http://teens.drugabuse.gov/mom/teachguide/MOMTeacherGuide.pdf)

(Shnitko, Spear, & Robinson, 2016). In addition, the nucleus accumbens is activated more during the anticipation of reward in adolescents than in children or adults (Casey & Jones, 2010). As will be discussed in a subsequent section, these still poorly understood changes in the reward system are thought to contribute to the heightened risk of abuse and dependence when substance use begins during the adolescent years.

In addition to exhibiting differences in responsiveness to risky behaviors and rewarding stimuli, adolescents exhibit an exaggerated stress response relative to children and adults (Alloy, Abramson, Walshaw, Keyser, & Gerstein, 2006). This exaggerated stress response likely contributes to the periodic difficulties that many teenagers have regulating their emotional reactions. At the core of the stress response is the hypothalamic-pituitary-adrenal (HPA) axis. In response to stressful stimuli or events, the hypothalamus releases corticotropin-releasing hormone, which causes the pituitary to release adrenocorticotropin, which in turn triggers the cortices of the adrenal glands, located just above the kidneys, to release cortisol. Activation of the hypothalamus in response to a stressor also results in the release of epinephrine (aka, adrenaline) from the inner region, or medulla, of the adrenals.

Puberty brings increased activity in the HPA axis. Sharp increases in urine and salivary cortisol levels happen at approximately the age of 13 and remain elevated into adulthood. A little cortisol goes a long way and helps the body prepare itself to deal with stressors and form memories of stressful events. Too much cortisol is associated with the onset of depression, the death of brain cells in the hippocampus, the memory center of the brain, and weakened immune activity and cardiovascular problems down the road. Cortisol also triggers anxiety via receptors on neurons in the amygdala, discussed below, and high cortisol levels are commonly seen in adolescents, as well as children and adults, with anxiety disorders (Coplan et al., 2002). A stronger association exists between adverse life events and depression during adolescence than during adulthood, perhaps reflecting heightened reactivity to stress during the adolescent period (Walker, Sabuwalla, & Huot, 2004).

Additional evidence that adolescents are particularly reactive to stress comes from the finding that stressful stimuli cause greater skin-conductance changes in adolescents than in adults (Miller & Shields, 1980). The sympathetic nervous system activity that occurs during times of intense arousal, such as when under stress, leads to an increase in the ability of the skin to conduct electrical current. For adolescents, these changes in skin conductance are bigger and take longer to habituate than in adults. In other words, the stress response is not only larger in adolescents than adults, but it also stays activated longer once initiated.

The heightened stress response in adolescents is linked to heighted reactivity in a brain region called the amygdala. The amygdala, a small almond-shaped structure located just in front of the hippocampus in the temporal lobes on each side of the brain, plays a prominent role in assigning significance, both positive and negative, to stimuli. In the case of potentially threatening stimuli, the amygdala can trigger feelings of fear and anxiety, partly through its ability to initiate activity in the HPA axis. In a fascinating study by Yurgelon-Todd and colleagues (2002), the researchers found that, when adolescents aged 11–17 and adults were shown pictures of people with fearful facial expressions, the amygdala was more active in teens than adults and their frontal lobes were less active. Further, adolescents younger than 14 were more likely to misread the facial expressions and perceive them as reflecting anger or sadness rather than fear or anxiety. It is likely such hyper-reactivity and tendency to misread adult faces hold survival value for adolescents by facilitating their march toward independence. As adolescence unfolds, there is a shift toward relying more on the frontal lobes and less on the amygdala to interpret facial expressions. Presumably, this leads to more accurate assessments of others' emotional states with age.

As we will discuss in a later section, the amygdala is an important nexus for the negative reinforcement produced by alcohol and other drugs. Activation of the reward systems increases the odds that a behavior will be repeated due to the addition of a positive state, such as pleasure. Suppression of the amygdala increases the odds that a behavior will be repeated due to the removal of a negative state, such as fear or anxiety. Both types of reinforcement, positive and negative, play important roles in the development of substance-use habits.

The Corpus Callosum and Sex Differences in Adolescent Brain Development

The corpus callosum is a large bundle of myelinated axons that shuttles information back and forth between the two cerebral hemispheres of the brain. Several studies suggest that increases in white matter volumes in the corpus callosum during adolescence are associated with improvements in cognitive abilities. Using diffusion tensor imaging, a technique that allows researchers to assess the integrity of myelin sheaths, Fryer et al. (2008) observed that, during adolescence, the maturation of white matter in the corpus callosum is associated with improvements in vocabulary and reading abilities, visuospatial skills (such as copying complex line drawings), and psychomotor performance (such as reacting quickly and in a coordinated manner in response to stimuli). This was particularly true with regard to maturation of the splenium, which is located in the posterior (rear) portion of the corpus callosum and seems to reach full maturity later in adolescence than other regions of the corpus callosum.

Sex differences in anatomical changes in the brain during adolescence result in a larger overall brain size for males and larger corpus callosum for females. Recent studies of functional changes have revealed intriguing differences in connectivity between various areas in males and females. For example, Ingalhalikar et al. (2014) observed that, between the ages of 8 and 13, male and female brain connectivity patterns are generally similar. However, as adolescence unfolds, females develop far more connections between the two hemispheres across the corpus callosum than males, whose brains exhibit more extensive connections within individual hemispheres. Tomasi and Volkow (2012) also observed differences in the functional connectivity patterns of female and male brains and concluded, "Men's lower brain connectivity might reflect optimization of functions that require specialized processing, such as

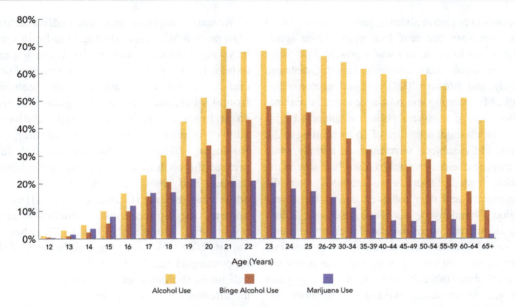

Fig. 1.5 Past month alcohol use, binge alcohol use, and marijuana use by age [source, Surgeon General report, 2017, based on data from 2015 NSDUH]

spatial orienting, whereas the women's higher brain connectivity may optimize functions that require integration and synchronization across large cortical networks such as those supporting language."

While the implications are not entirely clear, the findings of studies examining sex differences in functional connectivity during adolescence highlight the fact that male and female brains, though similar at the beginning of adolescence, differentiate considerably during the second decade of life.

Alcohol and Adolescent Brain Development

Substance use is more likely to begin during adolescence than at any other time, and the odds that such behaviors will lead to problems down the road are higher when substance use begins during adolescence relative to adulthood. Strong emotional drives that motivate adolescents to pursue positive and negative reinforcement, combined with still developing cognitive control circuits, make it easier for adolescents to head down pathways involving substance use and other risky activities. Because the brain learns so quickly during adolescence, reinforced behaviors are more likely to be repeated and develop into habits. In the case of substance use and other unhealthy rewarded behaviors, the malleability of the adolescent brain can work against us. Further, compelling evidence exists that alcohol and other substances can impede the development of cognitive skills during adolescence and alter the normal trajectory of anatomical and functional brain development (Fig. 1.5).

Of the drugs known to alter adolescent brain function and development, alcohol is the most well studied (Squeglia, Jacobus, & Tapert, 2014). Brown, Tapert, Granholm, and Delis (2000) compared 15–16-year-old adolescents in an inpatient substance-abuse treatment program to controls from the community on a battery of neuropsychological tests. Frequent drinkers (>100 total drinking sessions), particularly those who had experienced alcohol withdrawal, performed more poorly than controls on several tests, including tests of learning and memory. In a landmark longitudinal study of adolescents aged 13–19, recruited from treatment programs, Tapert and Brown (1999) observed that a return to drinking after the program led to further declines in cognitive abilities, particularly in tests of attention, over the next four years. Once again, withdrawal from alcohol was a powerful predictor of such impairments. Similarly, Tapert, Granholm, Leedy, and Brown (2002) assessed neuropsychological functioning and substance use at seven time points during an 8-year period in subjects beginning, on average, at the age of 16 and ending at 24. Many of the subjects were assessed initially while in treatment and then tracked after their stay in the facility ended. Others were recruited from the community and then followed during the 8-year period. Cumulative levels of substance use, including alcohol use, were correlated with impairments in verbal learning and memory during the final assessment. The findings suggested that heavy use of alcohol and other drugs during the teenage years predicts lower scores on tests of memory and attention when one is in their early to mid-20s and highlights the disruptive effects that substance abuse can have on healthy neuropsychological development during adolescence.

A recent study by Nguyen-Louie and colleagues (2017) examined the impact of various levels of drinking during adolescence on learning and memory function. The outcomes suggest that the amount of alcohol adolescents consume per occasion serves as an important predictor of impaired memory function across the teen years. The researchers recruited 295 adolescents between the ages of 12 and 16 years old (average age roughly 13.5) with limited experience with substances. After an average of 6.4 years, subjects were given follow-up assessments. Increasing peak estimated blood alcohol concentrations (BAC) during the previous three months predicted decreasing performance on a variety of measures of learning and memory. Similarly, when subjects were sorted into moderate (no more than 4 drinks on an occasion), binge (5–9 drinks on an occasion), and extreme binge (10+ drinks on an occasion) categories based on peak drinking in the past month, belonging in the extreme binge category was associated with learning and memory impairments. Extreme binge drinkers recalled 8–12% fewer words than moderate drinkers and 4–5% fewer than binge drinkers.

Research suggests that repeatedly reaching high peak BACs might damage the brain more in younger drinkers than adults. Exposing rats to high levels of alcohol across a period of several days causes cell death in the hippocampus, frontal lobes, and other brain regions and does so at lower levels in adolescents relative to adults (Crews, Vetreno, Broadwater, & Robinson, 2016). In addition, alcohol suppresses the birth of new neurons in the hippocampus and does so with greater ease in adolescent brains (Crews et al., 2016). In humans, the hippocampus is smaller in alcohol-abusing adolescents (Clark, Thatcher, & Tapert, 2008). Whether the smaller size of the hippocampus results from the suppression of cell birth, the death of existing cells, both, or an alternative cause is unclear but certainly warrants further exploration.

Other structures seem to suffer from the negative effects of repeated exposure to high levels of alcohol on adolescent brain development, as well. For instance, in addition to reducing frontal lobe gray matter volumes (Heikkinen et al., 2017), alcohol abuse during adolescence is associated with reduced sizes of both the amygdala and the corpus callosum (Squeglia et al., 2015). It also appears that alcohol interferes with the maturation of white matter tracts within the frontal lobes, perhaps by suppressing the activity of genes associated with the creation of the myelin sheath (Clark et al., 2008). Research with rats suggests that glial cell functioning affected by alcohol during adolescence only partially recovers with prolonged abstinence (Evrard et al., 2006).

In addition to damaging the brain, high peak levels of drinking on drinking occasions during adolescence are associated with a range of other risky behaviors and negative outcomes. Hingson and Zha (2018) reported that higher peak drinking levels in a national sample of high school students were associated with a greater likelihood of illegal drug and tobacco use, risky sexual and driving behaviors, fights, reduced sleep, and lower grades.

Differences in Sensitivity to Alcohol Between Adolescents and Adults

Several studies, primarily with rats, suggest that several initial, acute effects of alcohol differ between adolescents and adults. For instance, the hippocampus appears to be more sensitive to alcohol in adolescent rats than in adult rats. Alcohol blocks activity at the NMDA receptor, a glutamate receptor subtype central to hippocampal mediated episodic memory formation, more potently in adolescents than adults (Swartzwelder et al., 1995). Adolescent hippocampal circuits are more sensitive to the effects of alcohol on long-term potentiation, a physiological model of memory formation, than adults (Pyapali, Turner, Wilson, & Swartzwelder, 1999). Behaviorally, it appears that adolescent rats might be more sensitive to the effects of alcohol on some memory tasks than adults (Land & Spear, 2004; Markwiese, Acheson, Levin, Wilson, & Swartzwelder, 1998). In essence, less alcohol is required to disrupt the memory circuits in the adolescent, relative to adult, hippocampus (White & Swartzwelder, 2004).

The particularly negative effects of alcohol on hippocampal function in adolescent brains could help explain why memory blackouts (amnesia for events that take place while one is drinking) are so common during the adolescent years. Several studies (Wetherill & Fromme, 2016; White, 2003) suggest that 50% of college students or more have experienced at least one blackout. A survey of more than 5000 recent high school graduates during the summer before they started college revealed that more than half consumed alcohol in the two weeks before the survey and, of those who drank, 12% of males and females experienced at least one memory blackout during that two-week period (White and Swartzwelder, 2009). Similarly, in a study of 2140 older adolescents one year past high school, 20% of respondents, more females than males, who had ever consumed alcohol reported a blackout in the past 6 months (Hingson, Zha, Simons-Morton, & White, 2016). Whetherill and Fromme (2011) reported that college students with a history of blackouts exhibited larger memory impairments in laboratory tests at blood alcohol concentrations of roughly 0.08% compared to students without a history of blackouts. It remains unclear whether such outcomes reflect damage to the hippocampus and/or other brain areas as a result of prior heavy drinking or if the same mechanisms that made subjects more sensitive to the small memory impairments observed in the laboratory also predisposed them to blackouts.

In contrast to the increased sensitivity of the adolescent hippocampus to alcohol, adolescent rats are less sensitive than adults to the impact of alcohol on balance, motor coordination, and sedation. Adolescent rats are able to stay awake and maintain their balance at higher blood alcohol levels than adults (White et al., 2002). The onset of sedation after alcohol administration is slower, and the magnitude of sedation smaller, in adolescent rats than in adults (Silveri & Spear, 1998). If these differences in sensitivity to alcohol extend to humans, they could contribute to higher levels of drinking and resulting harms during adolescence. Lower levels of sensitivity to alcohol-induced motor incoordination and sedation could allow younger drinkers to stay awake longer and drink more, while greater sensitivity to the effects of alcohol on hippocampal function could contribute to larger memory impairments, including blackouts. The fact that the frontal lobes are undergoing construction during adolescence and impulse control is more challenging for teens even in a sober state could also increase the risks associated with alcohol consumption.

Interestingly, several studies suggest that alcohol exposure throughout the adolescent years prevents normal developmental changes in sensitivity to some of the effects of alcohol (see Crews et al., 2016, for review). This phenomenon, referred to as the "lock-in effect", reflects a persistent adolescent phenotype resulting from alcohol exposure (Spear & Swartzwelder, 2014). For instance, rats treated with alcohol in a binge pattern across adolescence do not show the normal increase in sensitivity to the effects of alcohol on balance and motor coordination or sedation (Matthews, Tinsley, Diaz-Granados,

Tokunaga, & Silvers, 2008; White et al., 2002). Rats exposed to alcohol during adolescence remain more sensitive than adults to alcohol-induced memory impairments (White et al., 2000). Repeated alcohol exposure during adolescence alters development of the reward system leading to greater dopamine activity, and possibly greater reinforcement, in response to alcohol during adulthood (Shnitko et al., 2016).

By preventing normal developmental changes in sensitivity to alcohol, heavy drinking during adolescence could contribute to higher levels of drinking and alcohol-related harms during adulthood, as well as increasing the likelihood of developing an alcohol-use disorder.

Age of Onset of Drinking

Considerable epidemiological evidence links early onset of alcohol use with an increased likelihood of developing an alcohol-use disorder, engaging in risky alcohol-related behaviors such as drinking and driving, and experiencing alcohol-related blackouts (Hingson & Zha, 2009; Marino & Fromme, 2016; White et al., 2002).

An early onset also increases the likelihood of alterations in adolescent neurodevelopment. Weiland et al. (2014) reported that frontal lobe gray matter volumes in subjects aged 18–23 were smaller in those subjects with early substance use and related problems, even after controlling for current substance use and family history of substance-use problems. Crews and Boettiger (2009) posited that damage to the frontal lobes due to early exposure could lead to increases in impulsivity and a higher likelihood of developing an alcohol-use disorder later in life.

Age of onset also is related to cognitive outcomes. Nguyen-Louie et al. (2017) assessed baseline neurocognitive functioning in 215 adolescents at roughly 13 years of age and then again nearly seven years later at age 20. Earlier age of drinking onset predicted worse psychomotor speed and visual attention, while an earlier age of the onset of weekly drinking predicted poorer inhibition and working memory.

Adolescent Neuroplasticity Facilitates the Learning of Both Adaptive and Maladaptive Habits

The ease with which the adolescent brain learns seems to apply to learning alcohol-related habits, as well. As mentioned above, there is a well-known relationship between earlier exposure to alcohol and risk of developing an alcohol-use disorder. It seems that the rapid learning made possible by heightened brain plasticity during the adolescent years could work against healthy development when it applies to alcohol and other substance use (Tapert et al., 2004; Carpenter-Hyland & Chandler, 2007). For instance, the initial development of tolerance to alcohol, a process that involves learning at a neurochemical level, is faster during adolescence than adulthood, and such tolerance remains evident for a much longer period of time in adolescent subjects compared with adults (White et al., 2002). The good news is that the enhanced brain plasticity of adolescence seems to lend itself to recovery and not just to the development of the initial problem. Research indicates that adolescent substance-abuse treatment works, particularly when adolescents are motivated to improve (White et al., 2004).

Implications for Prevention

The changes that occur in the adolescent brain and the resulting behavioral tendencies adolescents acquire are strongly influenced by interactions between the individual and the outside world. The risk factors for initiating alcohol use and drinking excessively during the teen years include unhealthy family dynamics, lack of healthy coping skills, and participation in peer groups that promote drinking (Rusby et al., 2018). Effective strategies for preventing alcohol use during adolescence address these issues (Das, Salam, Arshad, Finkelstein, & Bhutta, 2016; Hingson & White, 2014).

Smit, Verdurmen, Monshouwer, and Smit (2008) reviewed 18 randomized trials of family interventions to reduce adolescent drinking.

Seven reported that fewer subjects in the intervention groups initiated drinking and five reported significant reductions in past-month or past-year alcohol use. Spoth et al. (2011) assigned sixth graders and their parents in 33 schools to the Iowa Strengthening Families Program (ISFP), Preparing for the Drug Free Years (PDFY), or a control group. The ISFP sought to improve parent–child interactions, strengthen communication, and increase child coping skills through a seven-session, 13-hour, in-school intervention. The PDFY offered five weekly 2-h sessions to enhance parent–child interactions. When assessed six years later as high school seniors, one-third fewer adolescents who participated in the ISFP than the control condition reported drunkenness. At age 21, they reported significantly fewer episodes of drunkenness, alcohol problems, cigarette use, and illicit drug use. The PDFY was beneficial but the effects were smaller and no longer significant at age 21.

For many adolescents, alcohol misuse stems from difficulty coping with stress and managing mood. Schwinn, Schinke, Hopkins, Keller, and Liu (2018) examined the utility of an online prevention program for 13–14-year-old girls aimed at helping them manage stress, maintain a healthy body image, and refuse offers of alcohol and other drugs. One year later, girls who participated in the prevention program were less likely to engage in binge drinking, smoke cigarettes, and associate with peers who used drugs. Such evidence suggests that helping teens cope with stress and maintain a positive mood can reduce the likelihood of substance-use involvement.

In addition to the direct influence of peers on substance use, it is well known that many adolescents overestimate the prevalence of alcohol use among their peers. Many teens also have positive expectations regarding the effects of alcohol. Such misperceptions of norms and positive expectations regarding alcohol can motivate teens to drink and drink more heavily. Research suggests that correcting misperceptions of norms and countering positive expectations regarding the effects of drinking reduce the likelihood that adolescents with being to drink, and who already drink, reduce their levels of consumption (Hingson & White, 2014).

Collectively, research suggests that improving the quality of relationships between parents and teens, helping adolescents develop healthy coping skills, addressing faulty perceptions of normative behavior, and countering inaccurate expectations of the effects of alcohol can help protect adolescents from the deleterious effects of alcohol on short- and long-term brain development.

Conclusions

In the years that lead up to adolescence, an overabundance of synapses is created in the frontal lobes and between neurons in the frontal lobes and the brain structures with which they communicate. Early in the second decade of life, the brain simultaneously begins to shift control over behavior toward the frontal lobes and weed out less active synapses while wiring in those that are heavily utilized. Such malleability allows each successive wave of adolescents to adapt to unique and increasingly complex environments.

Once we leave adolescence and enter adulthood, the malleability of the brain decreases and it becomes increasingly difficult to make changes. That means behavioral tendencies acquired during adolescence can have a lasting impact on behavior during adulthood. The adaptive value of adolescent brain development is undeniable. However, the enhanced plasticity brings enhanced vulnerability to learning maladaptive behaviors, as well as the possibility of altering the trajectory of normal development in deleterious ways. An early onset of alcohol use is associated with an increased risk of developing an alcohol-use disorder, and heavy drinking during adolescence is associated with reductions in gray matter volumes in a variety of brain regions, as well as disruptions in the integrity of white matter tracts that allow distal brain areas to communicate with each other quickly and efficiently. As a result, young adults who drank heavily during adolescence can exhibit impairments in tasks that require attention, memory, and fast processing speeds.

The good news is that the powerful impact of experiences during adolescence on brain development and behavior can be harnessed to promote healthy choices and prevent alcohol use and related harms, including the development of alcohol-use disorder. By constructing healthy environments and contingencies, the odds that a given adolescent will make it into young adulthood cognitively and emotionally prepared for the rigors of adult life can be maximized.

References

Alloy, L. B., Abramson, L. Y., Walshaw, P. D., Keyser, J., & Gerstein, R. K. (2006). A cognitive vulnerability-stress perspective on bipolar spectrum disorders in a normative adolescence brain, cognitive, and emotional development context. *Development and Psychopathology, 18*(4), 1055–1103.

Aaron M. White, Jon G. Bae, Melanie C. Truesdale, Sukaina Ahmad, Wilkie A. Wilson, H. Scott Swartzwelder, (2002) Chronic-Intermittent Ethanol Exposure During Adolescence Prevents Normal Developmental Changes in Sensitivity to Ethanol-Induced Motor Impairments. Alcoholism: Clinical and Experimental Research 26 (7):960–968.

Brenhouse, H. C., & Andersen, S. L. (2011). Developmental trajectories during adolescence in males and females, a cross-species understanding of underlying brain changes. *Neuroscience and Biobehavioral Reviews, 35*(8), 1687–1703.

Brown, A. S., Tapert, S. F., Granholm, E., & Delis, D. C. (2000). Neurocognitive functioning of adolescents, effects of protracted alcohol use. *Alcoholism: Clinical and Experimental Research, 24*(2), 164–171.

Carpenter-Hyland, E. P., & Chandler, L. J. (2007). Adaptive plasticity of NMDA receptors and dendritic spines, implications for enhanced vulnerability of the adolescent brain to alcohol addiction. *Pharmacology, Biochemistry and Behavior, 86*(2), 200–208.

Casey, B. J., & Jones, R. M. (2010). Neurobiology of the adolescent brain and behavior, implications for substance use disorders. *Journal of the American Academy of Child and Adolescent Psychiatry, 49*(12), 1189–1201.

Casey, B. J., Jones, R. M., & Hare, T. A. (2008). The adolescent brain. *Annals of the New York Academy of Sciences, 1124*, 111–126.

Chein, J., Albert, D., O'Brien, L., Uckert, K., & Steinberg, L. (2011). Peers increase adolescent risk taking by enhancing activity in the brain's reward system. *Developmental Science, 14*(2), F1–F10.

Chugani, H. (1998). Biological basis of emotions, brain systems and brain development. *Pediatrics, 102*(5 suppl E), 1225–1229.

Clark, D. B., Thatcher, D. L., & Tapert, S. F. (2008). Alcohol, psychological dysregulation, and adolescent brain development. *Alcoholism: Clinical and Experimental Research, 32*(3), 375–385.

Coplan, J. D., Moreau, D., Chaput, F., Martinez, J. M., Hoven, C. W., Mandell, D. J., ... Pine, D. S. (2002). Salivary cortisol concentrations before and after carbon-dioxide inhalations in children. *Biological Psychiatry, 51*(4), 326–333.

Crews, F. T., & Boettiger, C. A. (2009). Impulsivity, frontal lobes and risk for addiction. *Pharmacology, Biochemistry and Behavior, 93*(3), 237–247.

Crews, F. T., Vetreno, R. P., Broadwater, M. A., & Robinson, D. L. (2016). Adolescent alcohol exposure persistently impacts adult neurobiology and behavior. *Pharmacological Reviews, 68*(4), 1074.

Das, J. K., Salam, R. A., Arshad, A., Finkelstein, Y., & Bhutta, Z. A. (2016). Interventions for adolescent substance abuse, an overview of systematic reviews. *The Journal of Adolescent Health, 59*(4 Suppl), S61–S75.

Ernst, M., & Mueller, S. C. (2008). The adolescent brain, insights from functional neuroimaging research. *Developmental Neurobiology, 68*(6), 729–743.

Evrard, S. G., Duhalde-Vega, M., Tagliaferro, P., Mirochnic, S., Caltana, L. R., & Brusco, A. (2006). A low chronic ethanol exposure induces morphological changes in the adolescent rat brain that are not fully recovered even after a long abstinence, an immunohistochemical study. *Experimental Neurology, 200*(2), 438–459.

Fryer, S. L., Frank, L. R., Spadoni, A. D., Theilmann, R. J., Nagel, B. J., Schweinsburg, A. D., & Tapert, S. F. (2008). Microstructural integrity of the corpus callosum linked with neuropsychological performance in adolescents. *Brain and Cognition, 67*(2), 225–233.

Gennatas, E. D., Avants, B. B., Wolf, D. H., Satterthwaite, T. D., Ruparel, K., Ciric, R., ... Gur, R. C. (2017). Age-related effects and sex differences in gray matter density, volume, mass, and cortical thickness from childhood to young adulthood. *Journal of Neuroscience, 37*, 5065–5073.

Giedd, J. (2004). Structural magnetic resonance imaging of the adolescent brain. *Annals of the New York Academy of Sciences, 1021*, 77–85.

Heikkinen, N., Niskanen, E., Könönen, M., Tolmunen, T., Kekkonen, V., Kivimäki, P., ... Vanninen, R. (2017). Alcohol consumption during adolescence is associated with reduced grey matter volumes. *Addiction, 112*(4), 604–613.

Hingson, R., Zha, W., Simons-Morton, B., & White, A. (2016). Alcohol-induced blackouts as predictors of other drinking related harms among emerging young adults. *Alcoholism: Clinical and Experimental Research, 40*(4), 776–784.

Hingson, R. W., & Zha, W. (2009). Age of drinking onset, alcohol use disorders, frequent heavy drinking, and unintentionally injuring oneself and others after drinking. *Pediatrics, 123*(6), 1477–1484.

Hingson, R. W., & Zha, W. (2018). Binge drinking above and below twice the adolescent thresholds and health-risk behaviors. *Alcoholism: Clinical and Experimental Research, 42*(5), 904–913.

Ingalhalikar, M., Smith, A., Parker, D., Satterthwaite, T. D., Elliott, M. A., Ruparel, K., ... Verma, R. (2014). Sex differences in the structural connectome of the human brain. *Proceedings of the National Academy of Sciences of the United States of America, 111*(2), 823–828.

Land, C., & Spear, N. E. (2004). Ethanol impairs memory of a simple discrimination in adolescent rats at doses that leave adult memory unaffected. *Neurobiology of Learning and Memory, 81*, 75–81.

Marino, E. N., & Fromme, K. (2016). Early onset drinking predicts greater level but not growth of alcohol-induced blackouts beyond the effect of binge drinking during emerging adulthood. *Alcoholism: Clinical and Experimental Research, 40*(3), 599–605.

Markwiese, B. J., Acheson, S. K., Levin, E. D., Wilson, W. A., & Swartzwelder, H. S. (1998). Differential effects of ethanol on memory in adolescent and adult rats. *Human Brain Mapping, 22*, 416–421.

Marsh, R., Zhu, H., Schultz, R. T., Quackenbush, G., Royal, J., Skudlarski, P., & Peterson, B. S. (2006). A developmental fMRI study of self-regulatory control. *Human Brain Mapping, 27*(11), 848–863.

Matthews, D. B., Tinsley, K. L., Diaz-Granados, J. L., Tokunaga, S., & Silvers, J. M. (2008). Chronic intermittent exposure to ethanol during adolescence produces tolerance to the hypnotic effects of ethanol in male rats, a dose-dependent analysis. *Alcohol, 42*, 617–621.

Miller, E. M., & Shields, S. A. (1980). Skin conductance response as a measure of adolescents' emotional reactivity. *Psychological Reports, 46*, 587–590.

Nelson, E. E., Leibenluft, E., McClure, E. B., & Pine, D. S. (2005). The social re-orientation of adolescence, a neuroscience perspective on the process and its relation to psychopathology. *Psychological Medicine, 35*(2), 163–174.

Pyapali, G. K., Turner, D. A., Wilson, W. A., & Swartzwelder, H. S. (1999). Age and dose-dependent effects of ethanol on the induction of hippocampal long-term potentiation. *Alcohol, 19*(2), 107–111.

Reagan R. Wetherill, Kim Fromme, (2011) Acute alcohol effects on narrative recall and contextual memory: An examination of fragmentary blackouts. Addictive Behaviors 36 (8):886–889.

Rubia, K., Overmeyer, S., Taylor, E., Brammer, M., Williams, S. C., Simmons, A., ... Bullmore, E. T. (2000). Functional frontalisation with age, mapping neurodevelopmental trajectories with fMRI. *Neuroscience and Biobehavioral Reviews, 24*(1), 13–19.

Rubia, K., Smith, A. B., Taylor, E., & Brammer, M. (2007). Linear age-correlated functional development of right inferior fronto-striato-cerebellar networks during response inhibition and anterior during error-related processes. *Human Brain Mapping, 28*(11), 1163–1177.

Rusby, J. C., Light, J. M., Crowley, R., & Westling, E. (2018). Influence of parent-youth relationship, parental monitoring, and parent substance use on adolescent substance use onset. *Journal of Family Psychology, 32*(3), 310–320.

Schweinsburg, A. D., Nagel, B. J., & Tapert, S. F. (2005). fMRI reveals alteration of spatial working memory networks across adolescence. *Journal of the International Neuropsychological Society, 11*(5), 631–644.

Schwinn, T. M., Schinke, S. P., Hopkins, J., Keller, B., & Liu, X. J. (2018). An online drug abuse prevention program for adolescent girls, posttest and 1-year outcomes. *Journal of Youth and Adolescence, 47*(3), 490–500.

Shaw, P., Greenstein, D., Lerch, J., Clasen, L., Lenroot, R., Gogtay, N., ... Giedd, J. (2006). Intellectual ability and cortical development in children and adolescents. *Nature, 440*(7084), 676–679.

Shnitko, T. A., Spear, L. P., & Robinson, D. L. (2016). Adolescent binge-like alcohol alters sensitivity to acute alcohol effects on dopamine release in the nucleus accumbens of adult rats. *Psychopharmacology, 233*(3), 361–371.

Silveri MM, Spear LP. (1998). Decreased sensitivity to the hypnotic effects of ethanol early in ontogeny. Alcohol Clin Exp Res 22(3):670–6.

Smit, E., Verdurmen, J., Monshouwer, K., & Smit, F. (2008). Family interventions and their effect on adolescent alcohol use in general populations; a meta-analysis of randomized controlled trials. *Drug and Alcohol Dependence, 97*(3), 195–206.

Spear, L. P., & Swartzwelder, H. S. (2014). Adolescent alcohol exposure and persistence of adolescent-typical phenotypes into adulthood, a mini-review. *Neuroscience & Biobehavioral Review, 45*, 1–8.

Spoth, R., Redmond, C., Clair, S., Shin, C., Greenberg, M., & Feinberg, M. (2011). Preventing substance misuse through community-university partnerships, randomized controlled trial outcomes 4½ years past baseline. *American Journal of Preventive Medicine, 40*(4), 440–447.

Squeglia, L. M., Jacobus, J., & Tapert, S. F. (2014). The effect of alcohol use on human adolescent brain structures and systems. *Handbook of Clinical Neurology, 125*, 501–510.

Squeglia, L. M., Tapert, S. F., Sullivan, E. V., Jacobus, J., Meloy, M. J., Rohlfing, T., & Pfefferbaum, A. (2015). Brain development in heavy-drinking adolescents. *American Journal of Psychiatry, 172*(6), 531–542.

Swartzwelder, H. S., Wilson, W. A., & Tayyeb, M. I. (1995). Differential sensitivity of NMDA receptor-mediated synaptic potentials to ethanol in immature versus mature hippocampus. *Alcoholism: Clinical and Experimental Research, 19*(2), 320–323.

Tam T. Nguyen-Louie, Georg E. Matt, Joanna Jacobus, Irene Li, Claudia Cota, Norma Castro, Susan F. Tapert, (2017) Earlier Alcohol Use Onset Predicts Poorer Neuropsychological Functioning in Young Adults. Alcoholism: Clinical and Experimental Research 41 (12):2082–2092.

Tapert, S. F., Brown, G. G., Baratta, M. V., & Brown, S. A. (2004). fMRI BOLD response to alcohol stimuli in alcohol dependent young women. *Addictive Behaviors, 29*(1), 33–50.

Tapert, S. F., & Brown, S. A. (1999). Neuropsychological correlates of adolescent substance abuse, four-year outcomes. *Journal of the International Neuropsychological Society, 5*(6), 481–493.

Tapert, S. F., Granholm, E., Leedy, N. G., & Brown, S. A. (2002). Substance use and withdrawal, neuropsychological functioning over 8 years in youth. *Journal of the International Neuropsychological Society, 8*(7), 873–883.

Tomasi, D., & Volkow, N. D. (2012). Gender differences in brain functional connectivity density. *Human Brain Mapping, 33*(4), 849–860.

Walker, E. F., Sabuwalla, Z., & Huot, R. (2004). Pubertal neuromaturation, stress sensitivity, and psychopathology. *Development and Psychopathology, 16*(4), 807–824.

Weiland, B. J., Korycinski, S. T., Soules, M., Zubieta, J. K., Zucker, R. A., & Heitzeg, M. M. (2014). Substance abuse risk in emerging adults associated with smaller frontal gray matter volumes and higher externalizing behaviors. *Drug and Alcohol Dependence, 137*(1), 68–75.

Wetherill, R. R., & Fromme, K. (2016). Alcohol-induced blackouts, a review of recent clinical research with practical implications and recommendations for future studies. *Alcoholism: Clinical and Experimental Research, 40*(5), 922–935.

White AM, Ghia AJ, Levin ED, Swartzwelder HS. (2000). Binge pattern ethanol exposure in adolescent and adult rats: differential impact on subsequent responsiveness to ethanol. Alcohol Clin Exp Res 24(8):1251–6.

White, A. M. (2003). What happened? Alcohol, memory blackouts, and the brain. *Alcohol Research and Health, 27*(2), 186–196.

White, A. M., Bae, J. G., Truesdale, M. C., Ahmad, S., Wilson, W. A., & Swartzwelder, H. S. (2002). Chronic-intermittent ethanol exposure during adolescence prevents normal developmental changes in sensitivity to ethanol-induced motor impairments. *Alcoholism: Clinical and Experimental Research, 26*(7), 960–968.

White, A. M., Jordan, J. D., Schroeder, K. M., Acheson, S., Hanusa, B., & Swartzwelder, H. S. (2004). Predictors of relapse and treatment completion among marijuana-dependent adolescents in an intensive outpatient substance abuse program. *Substance Abuse, 25*(1), 53–59.

White, A. M., & Swartzwelder, H. S. (2004). Hippocampal function during adolescence, a unique target of ethanol effects. *Annals of the New York Academy of Sciences, 1021*, 206–220.

White, A. M., & Swartzwelder, H. S. (2009). College bound students drink heavily during the summer before their freshman year. *American Journal of Health Education, 40*(2), 90–96.

White, A., & Hingson, R. (2014). The burden of alcohol use: excessive alcohol consumption and related consequences among college students. *Alcohol Research: Current Reviews, 35*(2), 201–218.

Epidemiology of Substance Use Internationally

Amy Peacock, Wayne Hall, and Louisa Degenhardt

Introduction

Quantifying the prevalence of substance use and dependence, and the extent and magnitude of associated burden, is critical to the development, implementation, and evaluation of prevention efforts. Indeed, these data often inform allocation decisions by governments, policy-makers, and funding bodies about service provision and policy. It is accordingly important that estimates of prevalence and related burden are rigorously developed, frequently updated, geographically comprehensive, and sensitive to change over time. This chapter reviews evidence on the global prevalence of substance use and dependence and the associated health burden, with comment regarding the scale and quality of the evidence.

Globally, the major drugs whose use and supply are under international drug control comprise heroin, cocaine, cannabis, and amphetamine-type stimulants (United Nations Office on Drugs and Crime UNODC, 2017b). Not all psychoactive substances are under international control; tobacco and alcohol comprise two widely used exceptions which contribute substantially to the disease burden from substance use globally. Further, various substances under international control may be legally used for medicinal purposes (e.g. pharmaceutical opioids for chronic non-cancer pain; International Narcotics Control Board, 2015). However, extra-medical use (i.e., use of pharmaceutical medicines for purposes not in line with medical advice or legal guidelines; Larance, Degenhardt, Lintzeris, Winstock, & Mattick, 2011) is typically prohibited because of the risks of dependence and related harms (Babor et al., 2010; McAllister, 2000). It should be noted that legal status of psychoactive substances for recreational use can vary within and between countries, as illustrated by recent depenalisation, decriminalisation, or legalisation of cannabis use and supply in various countries (Hall & Weier, 2015).

A. Peacock (✉)
National Drug and Alcohol Research Centre, University of New South Wales, Sydney, NSW, Australia

School of Medicine (Psychology), University of Tasmania, Hobart, TAS, Australia
e-mail: Amy.Peacock@unsw.edu.au

W. Hall
University of Queensland Centre for Youth Substance Abuse Research, Herston, QLD, Australia

National Addiction Centre, Kings College London, London, UK
e-mail: w.hall@uq.edu.au

L. Degenhardt
National Drug and Alcohol Research Centre, University of New South Wales, Sydney, NSW, Australia

School of Population and Global Health, University of Melbourne, Melbourne, VIC, Australia

Department of Global Health, School of Public Health, University of Washington, Seattle, WA, USA
e-mail: l.degenhardt@unsw.edu.au

This chapter summarises the best available evidence on the prevalence of drug use and dependence and the magnitude of health-attributable burden. Focus is restricted to alcohol, tobacco, and those substances under international drug control (i.e. opioids, cannabis, cocaine, and amphetamine-type stimulants). Discussion is also limited to use for reasons other than medical, hereafter termed 'extra-medical use' (Larance et al., 2011). New psychoactive substances (NPS; also known as emerging or novel psychoactive substances) will also be considered because of the challenges they pose to researchers, policymakers, health professionals, and consumers (Sumnall, Evans-Brown, & McVeigh, 2011). Literature on MDMA (ecstasy), hallucinogens, inhalants, steroids, and extra-medical use of other pharmaceuticals (e.g. benzodiazepines) is excluded due to a relative dearth of evidence (Charlson, Degenhardt, Mclaren, Hall, & Lynskey, 2009; Maxwell, 2005; Rogers et al., 2009; Seear, Fraser, Moore, & Murphy, 2015). We note that estimates of drug-related burden will represent an underestimate because they do not capture these substances.

Data Collections and Caveats

There are various research groups who compile estimates of the global, regional, and country-level prevalence of substance use, dependence, and related burden. Global collections are mainly held by the following organisations: the World Health Organization (WHO); United Nations Office on Drugs and Crime (UNODC); and the Institute for Health Metrics and Evaluation (IHME) Global Burden of Disease (GBD) study. These collections are regularly updated, with the most recent data available at the time of writing this chapter relating to 2015 (i.e. modelled based on the global population in that year).

It is useful to collate estimates from these collections to generate a global profile of substance use, related mortality, and burden of disease, and to highlight key gaps in evidence. Yet, these organisations have separate approaches to producing estimates that use different search processes, criteria for data inclusion, and modelling approaches. For example, crude data included in the GBD study are extracted from systematic searches of peer-reviewed scientific and medical journals, and cataloguing data from other sources (e.g. vital registration, hospital data, disease registry data, surveillance systems, censuses, and household surveys; IHME, 2015). The GBD study uses Disease Modeling – Metaregression (DisMod; Flaxman, Vos, & Murray, 2015) to check the internal consistency of existing estimates and to impute data where there are incomplete data to produce prevalence and disease burden estimates for each disease cause, age group, sex, country, and year (Barendregt, Van Oortmarssen, Vos, & Murray, 2003). Alongside point estimates, the GBD produces uncertainty intervals (UIs) which capture uncertainty from sample sizes of data sources, multiple modelling steps, and sources such as model estimation and model specification (Kassebaum et al., 2016). In contrast, the UNODC (UNODC, 2017a) primarily derives data from the Annual Reports Questionnaire (ARQ) which is completed by Governments of Member States each calendar year, supplemented by other information. Upper and lower uncertainty range estimates are calculated at a 90% confidence interval among those aged 15–64 years (see United Nations Office on Drugs and Crime UNODC, 2017a, for further details of calculation of uncertainty ranges).

There are major challenges in producing credible estimates of the prevalence of substance use, dependence, and related health burden. Certain countries and regions (e.g. Africa, Caribbean and Latin America, Asia) have limited or no data on substance use and the associated health burden (United Nations Office on Drugs and Crime UNODC, 2017b). These are typically—but not always—low- or middle-income countries. These countries often warrant monitoring because of the risk of rapid escalation in substance use and related harms with limited availability of substance treatment and harm reduction services (Degenhardt et al., 2017).

Further, quality of estimates is often poor where data are available. There is no 'gold standard' method for producing credible estimates of the number of people who make up the 'hidden population' of drug users (Hartnoll, 1997). General population surveys rely on honest self-report of substance use. Marginalised groups with high levels of problematic substance use (e.g. people who are incarcerated or homeless), or those from cultures or religions where substance use is forbidden or stigmatised (Michalak, Trocki, & Bond, 2007), are often excluded from such surveys. This leads to underestimates of the prevalence of the most stigmatised and harmful forms of substance use in ways that can vary geographically (Degenhardt & Hall, 2012). Indirect methods of estimating prevalence for more stigmatised forms of substance use (e.g. multiplier, capture-recapture, network scale-up) may be biased by data limitations (e.g. dependencies between data sources in capture-recapture studies; Jones et al., 2014). Use of multiple indirect methods to estimate a single population size may not remedy biases in individual methods, as estimates may be inconsistent, and merely averaging across estimates will not necessarily reduce bias (Wesson, Reingold, & Mcfarland, 2017). Multiparameter evidence synthesis addresses these limitations by triangulating all available evidence (including estimates of potential biases) but is technically challenging to implement (Hickman et al., 2013). Thus, no single method is ideal for all drugs or for use in all countries, and the lack of consistency in measurement and potential biases poses challenges when making cross-national comparisons (Degenhardt, Hallam, & Bewley-Taylor, 2009; Reuter & Trautmann, 2009).

Finally, there must be epidemiological evidence that alcohol, tobacco, or illicit drug exposures are causally linked to health outcomes before any injury or disease can be quantified in computing attributable burden of disease (Murray, Ezzati, Lopez, Rodgers, & Vander Hoorn, 2004). This is challenging because risk can vary according to many factors (e.g. substance type, frequency and quantity of use, route of administration, and polysubstance use). The quality of epidemiological data also varies, with stronger evidence for causal effects of alcohol and tobacco health effects than for illicit drugs.

There are a number of injury and disease categories where there is growing epidemiological evidence for causality (e.g. depression attributable to alcohol and illicit drugs; Rehm et al., 2017). These factors suggest that we underestimate the burden of alcohol, tobacco, and especially illicit drug use. Related to this, risk of harm is often increased with polysubstance use, yet estimates of polysubstance use are not systematically collected and collated across countries, nor burden from such use quantified.

For these reasons, we recommend consideration of the uncertainty range (reported in brackets) when interpreting the estimates presented below. Further discussion of measurement issues related to the epidemiology of substance use is available and discussed below.

Prevalence of Substance Use

Alcohol, Tobacco, and Illicit Drugs

Alcohol is the most widely consumed substance of those considered in this chapter. The WHO Collaborating Centre for Addiction and Mental Health[1] estimated that 6.43 (6.22, 6.63) litres of pure alcohol per capita were consumed by the adult population (aged ≥15 years) in 2015 (for further details, see Peacock et al., 2018). Approximately one-fifth (18.4%; 15.1, 21.8) of the adult population reported heavy episodic drinking (≥60 g alcohol on one occasion) in the past 30 days; this equates to two-fifths (39.6%; 32.8, 46.8) of people who consumed alcohol globally. Europe was notable for recording nearly double the global average consumption per capita. Further, nearly half of all consumers reported heavy episodic drinking that contributes substantially to acute harm (e.g. injury; World Health Organization, 2016) and risk for dependence (Rehm, Shield, Rehm, Gmel, & Frick, 2012). The

---
[1] Data were obtained from the WHO Collaborating Centre for Addiction and Mental Health for validation and later inclusion into the Global Status Report on Alcohol and Health 2018 and the Global Information System on Alcohol and Health.

lowest rates of heavy episodic drinking among the adult population were observed for North Africa and the Middle East (15.4%; 11.7, 19.8) (Fig. 2.1).

Patterns of daily tobacco smoking prevalence globally reflect those observed for alcohol, with highest rates of daily smoking observed in European and Southeast Asian regions. The GBD study 2015 (Institute for Health Metrics and Evaluation, 2016) reported that the global age-standardised prevalence of daily smoking in 2015 was 15.2% (14.7, 15.7). Across all ages globally, there were 933.1 (901.5, 966.5) million people who smoked tobacco daily. When considering absolute number of people, China (268.3 million; 263.3, 273.5), India (104.2 million; 99.2, 109.6), and Indonesia (53.7 million; 49.6, 58.3) had the largest number of daily smokers, accounting for 45.7% of all daily smokers globally. Recent reports suggest that the percentage of people who smoke daily has declined from 1990 to 2015 by 28.4% (25.8, 31.1) and 34.4% (29.4, 38.6) for men and women, respectively (GBD 2015 Tobacco Collaborators, 2017). Indeed, only four countries (Congo, Azerbaijan, Kuwait, and Timor-Leste) recorded an annual increase in tobacco smoking prevalence between 2005 and 2015 for men or women (GBD 2015 Tobacco Collaborators, 2017).

Global prevalence of illicit substance use is substantially lower. The United Nations Office on Drugs and Crime (UNODC, 2017b) estimated that 2.7–4.9% of the adult population aged 15–64 years had used cannabis in 2015 which equates to 128–238 million people. The highest levels of cannabis use were in the established market economies of North America, West and Central Africa, Western and Central Europe, and Oceania. Approximately 15–60 million people, or 0.30–1.24% of the adult population, reported using amphetamine-type stimulants, with highest rates in Oceania near major manufacturing countries. Approximately 28–43 million people, or 0.27–0.49% of the adult population, had used prescription opioids and opiates in 2015, with the highest rate in North America where the public health crisis around extra-medical pharmaceutical opioid use and heroin is burgeoning (Fischer & Rehm, 2018). Further, 13–22 million people, or 0.27–0.46% of the adult population, had used cocaine, with highest rates also in North America and Oceania.

Injecting Drug Use

A recent review showed that injecting drug use has been documented in 179 of 206 countries or territories (Degenhardt et al., 2017). This covers 99% of the population aged 15–64 years, and represents an increase of 31 countries since a 2008 review (Mathers et al., 2008). Countries for which injecting drug use was newly documented were mostly located in sub-Saharan Africa and the Pacific Island regions. Degenhardt et al. (2017) estimated that there were 15.6 million (10.2, 23.7) adults aged 15–64 years globally who inject drugs in 2015, equating to 0.33% (0.21, 0.49) of the adult population (Fig. 2.2). Nearly four times as many men (12.5 million; 7.5, 18.4) as women (3.2 million; 1.6, 5.1) were estimated to have injected drugs. Four-fifths (82.9%; 76.7, 88.9) of those (76.7, 88.9) of those who reported injecting drugs named opioids as their main drug (Fig. 2.2).

At a regional level, prevalence varied from 0.09% (0.07, 0.11) in South Asia to 1.30% (0.71, 2.15) in Eastern Europe. The percentage who were female varied substantially by region, from 30.0% (28.5, 31.5) and 33.4% (31.0, 35.6) in North America and Australasia, respectively, to 3.1% (2.1, 4.1) in South Asia. Those regions with the largest total number of people who inject drugs were East and Southeast Asia (4.0 million; 3.0–5.0), Eastern Europe (3.0 million; 1.7, 5.0), and North America (2.6 million; 1.5, 4.1). Numbers in these regions were primarily driven by the substantial population of people who inject drugs in China, Russia, and the USA, respectively.

It is important to note that various efforts are made to estimate the prevalence of injecting drug use (as well as other indicators). In the World Drug Report 2017 (United Nations Office on Drugs and Crime, 2017b) it was estimated that 0.25% (0.18, 0.36) of the adult population aged

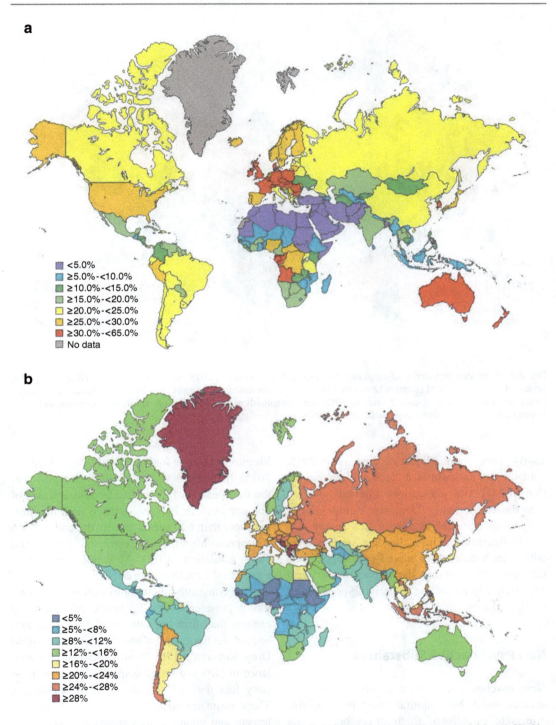

Fig. 2.1 Annual prevalence of heavy episodic alcohol use (population 10+ years old; Panel **a**) and daily tobacco smoking (age-standardised; Panel **b**), by country, 2015. *Note*: Alcohol estimates were made available by the WHO Collaborating Centre for Addiction and Mental Health; tobacco smoking estimates were made available from the GBD study 2015 (Institute for Health Metrics and Evaluation, 2016). See Peacock et al. (2018) for further details

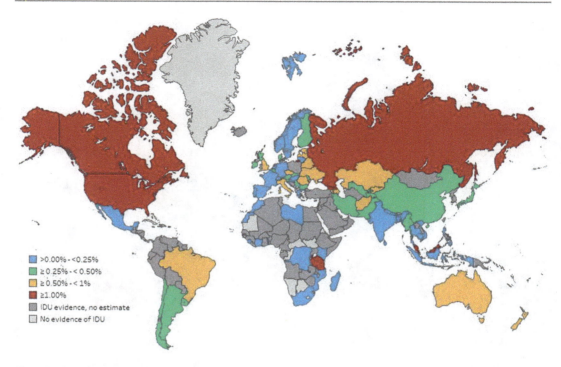

Fig. 2.2 Estimated prevalence of injecting drug use (IDU) by country, 2015. *Note*: Data are derived from a global review of the prevalence of recent (≤12 month) injecting drug use among those aged 15–64 years old based on UN population division estimates of country size in 2015 (see Degenhardt et al., 2017 for full details of estimation methods). Image reproduced here from Degenhardt et al., 2017

15–64 years reported injecting drug use in 2015, equating to an estimated 11.8 million people (8.6, 17.4). The uncertainty intervals overlap with those reported by Degenhardt et al. (2017), suggesting that the prevalence lies somewhere within this range. Often the data sources used within each country to model prevalence were the same, highlighting the impact of different approaches to modelling in deriving population-level estimates.

New Psychoactive Substances

New psychoactive substances (NPS) are substances which have similar acute psychoactive effects to established illicit drugs but are not under international control (European Monitoring Centre for Drugs and Drug Addiction, 2011). There have been unprecedented increases in the number, type, and availability of NPS (European Monitoring Centre for Drugs and Drug Addiction, 2015). Indeed, a new type of NPS was reported to the European Early Warning System at a rate of one per week in 2016, with the system monitoring more than 620 substances by the end of 2016 (European Monitoring Centre for Drugs and Drug Addiction, 2018). This rate has slowed since but the proliferation of NPS continues.

This constantly evolving market makes monitoring prevalence of NPS use challenging and ensures that there are substantial gaps in knowledge about the extent of use. The UNODC World Drug Report (2017b) listed estimates of prevalence of NPS use for 15 countries that were typically less than 1% of the sampled population. These estimates were mainly derived from adolescent and young adult samples and were typically specific to a NPS class (e.g. piperazines) or substance (e.g. mephedrone). Higher rates have been reported from the European School Survey Project on Alcohol and Other Drugs 2015 (2016), with 3% of 15–16-year-old European school students reporting NPS use at least once in the past 12 months, with the highest prevalence (8%) in Estonia and Poland. Beyond these data, we do not currently have a good understanding of the prevalence of use amongst the general population.

It is critical to have better evidence on the prevalence of NPS use given increasing reports of acute adverse effects (Logan et al., 2017) and poor understanding of the long-term effects of NPS on morbidity and mortality. Self-report data are becoming less reliable for assessing NPS because consumers may be unaware or misinformed about the substances they have consumed. Various indicators can be monitored and triangulated to quantify their use and associated harms (e.g. ambulance attendances, emergency department presentations, poisons and toxicology data, and law enforcement drug seizures; Van Buskirk, Griffiths, Farrell, & Degenhardt, 2017). Monitoring can track availability on surface and darknet websites (Roxburgh, Van Buskirk, Burns, & Bruno, 2017). Although NPS comprise a minority of the drugs listed for sale, monitoring may detect new NPS which may harm consumers, such as highly potent opioid analgesic analogues. Key to monitoring NPS is early detection of NPS entering the market that have the capacity to cause substantial harm to the consumers.

Prevalence of Substance Dependence

The health burden associated with substance use typically increases with frequency and quantity of use (Fischer, Kendall, Rehm, & Room, 1997). Those who ever use any substance and do not persist in using have, at most, a small increase in health burden that may not be detected in epidemiological studies. Consequently, it is more relevant in estimating the health burden of illicit drug use to consider substance dependence, as defined according to the Diagnostic and Statistical Manual of Mental Disorders IV (American Psychiatric Association, 2000) and the International Classification of Diseases tenth edition (World Health Organization, 1993).

Substance dependence requires the occurrence of three or more indicators for at least a month within a year. These include a strong desire to take the substance; impaired control over use; a withdrawal syndrome on ceasing or reducing use; tolerance to the effects of the drug; requiring larger doses to achieve the desired psychological effect; a disproportionate amount of time spent by the person obtaining, using and recovering from drug use; and continuing to take other drugs despite the problems that occur. A similar classification was defined by the American Psychiatric Association until the introduction of DSM-5 which introduced a dimensional definition of drug-use disorders by combining the categories of abuse and dependence and specifying the degree of severity of the disorder (mild, moderate, and severe).

According to the GBD (Institute for Health Metrics and Evaluation, 2016), alcohol dependence was the most prevalent substance of dependence in 2015, with 63.5 million (57.5, 69.9) estimated cases in 2015, equivalent to an age-standardised rate of 843.2 (763.7, 927.3) persons per 100,000 people (Table 2.1). Estimates of smoked tobacco dependence were not modelled in the GBD study, but people who smoke tobacco daily have very low probability of successful quitting in any given attempt (West, Mcewen, Bolling, & Owen, 2001) and so daily smoking (see above) can be considered indicative of a significant level of dependence.

The age-standardised rate of alcohol dependence in Eastern Europe was three times greater than the global rate (22786.7 persons per 100,000 people; 2487.3, 3109.6), with the next highest region (Caribbean) two times the global rate (1430.1 persons per 100,000 people; 1285.7, 1589.6). This reflects the high prevalence of heavy episodic use in Eastern Europe in particular, noting that prevalence varies widely between countries reflecting differences in drinking cultures and social norms (Rehm et al., 2015).

Cannabis and opioid dependence were the most common types of illicit drug dependence, with 19.8 (18.0, 21.8) and 16.7 (14.7, 19.1) million cases in 2015, respectively. This is equivalent to age-standardised rates of 259.3

Table 2.1 Modelled estimates of cases and age-standardised rates of past year substance dependence by GBD region, 2015

Region[a]	Alcohol		Amphetamines		Cannabis		Cocaine		Opioids	
	Number (95%UI)	Age SDR (95%UI)	Number (95%UI)	Age SDR (95%UI)	Number (95%UI)	Age SDR (95%UI)	Number (95%UI)	Age SDR (95%UI)	Number (95%UI)	Age SDR (95%UI)
Andean Latin America	494,000 (416,000, 570,000)	864.3 (729.3, 989.9)	67,000 (52,000, 85,000)	104.7 (82.0, 132.2)	118,000 (104,000, 132,000)	187.8 (166.3, 210.4)	56,000 (49,000, 65,000)	101.1 (88.1, 114.9)	86,000 (74,000, 101,000)	149.2 (127.8, 173.4)
Australasia	326,000 (292,000, 364,000)	1065.5 (950.8, 1203.5)	138,000 (124,000, 153,000)	491.5 (441.4, 545.5)	195,000 (182,000, 208,000)	693.7 (648.1, 744.4)	47,000 (40,000, 54,000)	160.6 (136.4, 187.1)	152,000 (135,000, 171,000)	509.9 (453.7, 577.8)
Caribbean	657,000 (589,000, 731,000)	1430.1 (1285.7, 1589.6)	7000 (5000, 8000)	14.4 (10.9, 18.2)	127,000 (112,000, 142,000)	271.6 (239.9, 305.0)	34,000 (29,000, 39,000)	74.4 (62.9, 86.3)	57,000 (49,000, 66,000)	124.5 (107.0, 144.2)
Central Asia	1,028000 (908,000, 1,163,000)	1138.7 (1011.3, 1276.8)	65,000 (51,000, 82,000)	67.1 (52.9, 83.1)	284,000 (251,000, 321,000)	300.4 (266.8, 338.2)	27,000 (22,000, 31,000)	30.2 (25.5, 34.9)	183,000 (157,000, 214,000)	196.7 (168.7, 228.4)
Central Europe	1,491,000 (1,334,000, 1,653,000)	1112.1 (992.8, 1237.6)	135,000 (111,000, 161,000)	127.7 (104.0, 154.5)	344,000 (315,000, 376,000)	324.8 (295.3, 356.5)	61,000 (54,000, 69,000)	48.7 (42.0, 55.7)	213,000 (186,000, 244,000)	168.6 (145.8, 195.5)
Central Latin America	2,694,000 (2,401,000, 3,003000)	1067.2 (957.2, 1181.6)	164,000 (126,000, 205,000)	58.8 (45.5, 73.2)	406,000 (373,000, 442,000)	148.5 (136.7, 161.4)	218,000 (187,000, 250,000)	86.8 (75.5, 98.6)	349,000 (304,000, 401,000)	135.3 (118.2, 154.3)
Central Sub-Saharan Africa	687,000 (600,000, 782,000)	796.6 (704.0, 897.4)	4000 (3000, 5000)	3.5 (2.6, 4.7)	171,000 (149,000, 199,000)	160.2 (142.0, 183.9)	9000 (7000, 11,000)	10.8 (9.0, 12.7)	81,000 (67,000, 97,000)	89.9 (75.4, 106.2)
East Asia	13,933,000 (12,723,000, 15,154,000)	839.4 (766.2, 916.4)	2,964,000 (2,350,000, 3,624,000)	205.3 (161.5, 252.9)	4,784,000 (4,280,000, 5,338,000)	330.6 (293.4, 371.2)	729,000 (633,000, 819,000)	48.2 (41.7, 54.4)	3,037000 (2,677,000, 3,435,000)	183.5 (161.5, 207.7)
Eastern Europe	6,845,000 (6,131,000, 7,585,000)	2786.7 (2487.3, 3109.6)	546,000 (444,000, 658,000)	259.7 (209.5, 313.7)	578,000 (522,000, 641,000)	294.2 (262.6, 328.7)	198,000 (168,000, 230,000)	86.4 (71.9, 102.2)	1,424,000 (1,233,000, 1,653,000)	583.7 (504.0, 680.6)
Eastern Sub-Saharan Africa	2,435,000 (2,124,000, 2,775,000)	815.6 (720.7, 915.9)	5000 (3000, 7000)	1.3 (0.9, 1.8)	651,000 (550,000, 779,000)	175.6 (151.7, 204.6)	10,000 (7000, 12,000)	3.8 (3.1, 4.6)	161,000 (136,000, 192,000)	53.7 (45.8, 63.1)
High-income Asia Pacific	960,000 (881,000, 1,046000)	500.5 (453.6, 549.8)	88,000 (71,000, 108,000)	58.8 (45.9, 72.7)	565,000 (522,000, 613,000)	379.1 (348.1, 414.8)	60,000 (53,000, 68,000)	26.8 (23.1, 30.4)	198,000 (175,000, 224,000)	104.4 (91.4, 119.4)

2 Epidemiology of Substance Use Internationally

Region	Count 1 (95% UI)	Rate 1 (95% UI)	Count 2 (95% UI)	Rate 2 (95% UI)	Count 3 (95% UI)	Rate 3 (95% UI)	Count 4 (95% UI)	Rate 4 (95% UI)	Count 5 (95% UI)	Rate 5 (95% UI)
High-income North America	4,435,000 (4,039000, 4,852,000)	1186.4 (1075.2, 1305.5)	503,000 (418,000, 599,000)	148.4 (122.0, 177.3)	2,510,000 (2,342,000, 2,705,000)	748.7 (694.8, 812.3)	1,116,000 (1,002,000, 1,229,000)	301.2 (269.3, 333.7)	2,362,000 (2,094000, 2,634,000)	650.0 (574.5, 727.3)
North Africa & Middle East	1,530,000 (1,335,000, 1,740,000)	274.2 (241.7, 309.3)	139,000 (108,000, 174,000)	22.7 (17.8, 28.1)	1,008000 (876,000, 1,168,000)	164.1 (143.7, 188.5)	92,000 (76,000, 108,000)	18.3 (15.5, 21.0)	2,691,000 (2,310,000, 3,141,000)	479.3 (412.8, 555.1)
Oceania	56,000 (49,000, 63,000)	548.9 (482.5, 618.2)	5000 (4000, 6000)	40.4 (29.9, 51.9)	46,000 (41,000, 53,000)	388.3 (345.5, 440.1)	1000 (1000, 1000)	12.4 (10.0, 14.9)	9000 (7000, 10,000)	83.5 (70.4, 98.2)
South Asia	13,085000 (11,558.000, 14,679,000)	785.7 (700.6, 873.7)	220,000 (165,000, 287,000)	11.9 (9.1, 15.4)	3,213,000 (2,896,000, 3,584,000)	173.2 (156.9, 192.4)	468,000 (385,000, 552,000)	28.9 (24.2, 33.4)	3,015000 (2,603,000, 3,475,000)	175.7 (153.3, 200.8)
Southeast Asia	3,902,000 (3,474,000, 4,374,000)	579.8 (517.3, 647.2)	824,000 (636,000, 1,046000)	117.3 (90.6, 148.9)	1,986,000 (1,652,000, 2,341,000)	284.4 (237.1, 334.7)	83,000 (70,000, 98,000)	13.6 (11.6, 15.8)	697,000 (591,000, 816,000)	102.1 (86.8, 118.9)
Southern Latin America	811,000 (729,000, 897,000)	1215.3 (1091.1, 1343.8)	85,000 (66,000, 106,000)	130.4 (101.2, 162.2)	227,000 (203,000, 254,000)	348.2 (312.2, 389.7)	29,000 (25,000, 33,000)	42.7 (37.4, 48.3)	124,000 (107,000, 143,000)	186.1 (160.0, 214.8)
Southern Sub-Saharan Africa	670,000 (592,000, 756,000)	945.1 (841.7, 1056.3)	18,000 (14,000, 23,000)	20.9 (16.4, 25.9)	167,000 (153,000, 183,000)	188.5 (172.9, 206.2)	18,000 (16,000, 21,000)	28.8 (25.0, 32.7)	159,000 (136,000, 186,000)	193.2 (167.3, 223.2)
Tropical Latin America	1,426,000 (1,284,000, 1,570,000)	617.3 (558.3, 676.6)	201,000 (155,000, 254,000)	87.2 (67.2, 110.4)	385,000 (352,000, 419,000)	167.0 (152.5, 181.6)	125,000 (107,000, 144,000)	57.0 (49.1, 65.2)	275,000 (241,000, 313,000)	119.3 (104.8, 135.8)
Western Europe	4,152,000 (3,792,000, 4,496,000)	880.7 (794.5, 965.0)	409,000 (342,000, 483,000)	112.1 (91.9, 134.3)	1,528,000 (1,432,000, 1,634,000)	424.9 (395.8, 456.0)	435,000 (388,000, 489,000)	103.4 (90.2, 118.2)	991,000 (865,000, 1,123,000)	233.4 (203.5, 265.6)
Western Sub-Saharan Africa	1,852,000 (1,617,000, 2,136,000)	584.4 (515.5, 661.9)	12,000 (9000, 16,000)	3.6 (2.8, 4.6)	472,000 (413,000, 542,000)	127.0 (112.5, 143.4)	31,000 (25,000, 37,000)	12.2 (10.4, 14.2)	482,000 (401,000, 575,000)	153.3 (129.3, 179.9)
Global	**63,469,000 (57,508,000, 69,864,000)**	**843.2 (763.7, 927.3)**	**6,600,000 (5,296,000, 8,024000)**	**86.0 (69.2, 104.6)**	**19,762,000 (17,982,000, 21,770,000)**	**259.3 (235.7, 285.5)**	**3,846,000 (3,402,000, 4,310,000)**	**52.5 (46.6, 58.7)**	**16,746,000 (14,659,000, 19,107,000)**	**220.4 (193.1, 251.0)**

Note: Data in the table above were extracted from the GBD study 2015 (Institute for Health Metrics and Evaluation, 2016). Age-standardised rates (Age SDR) is the rate per 100,000 people, estimated using the GBD world population age standard. In the GBD study, 95% uncertainty intervals (95%UI) are derived from 1000 draws from the posterior distribution of each step in the estimation process. The UIs capture uncertainty from multiple modelling steps and from sources such as model estimation and model specification

[a]Grouping of countries reflect GBD classification

(235.7, 285.5) and 220.4 (193.1, 251.0) persons per 100,000 population, respectively. Amphetamine and cocaine dependence were less prevalent, with 6.6 million (5.3, 8.0) and 3.9 million (3.4, 4.3) cases globally in 2015, corresponding to age-standardised rates of 86.0 (69.2, 104.6) and 52.5 (46.6, 58.7) persons per 100,000 population, respectively (Table 2.1).

The high prevalence of different types of substance dependence in certain regions reflected their higher prevalence of substance use. For example, the High-Income North America region had one of the most prevalent rates of cannabis (748.7 persons per 100,000 people; 694.8, 812.3), opioid (650.0; 574.5, 727.3), and cocaine (301.2; 269.3, 333.7) dependence. Australasia had the highest estimated age-standardised rates of amphetamine dependence (491.5 persons per 100,000 people; 441.4, 545.5) and high rates of cannabis (693.7; 648.1, 744.4), opioid (509.9; 453.7, 577.8), and cocaine (160.5; 136.4, 187.1) dependence. The most marked regional variation was in alcohol dependence: the highest age-standardised rate was in Eastern Europe (2786.7 per 100,000 people; 2487.3, 3109.6) and the lowest in North Africa and the Middle East (274.2; 241.7, 309.3).

Substance-Related Health Burden

Adverse health effects of substance use can be clustered into four categories (Babor et al., 2010): the *acute toxic effects* that include fatal and non-fatal overdoses; the *acute effects of intoxication*, such as unintended injury, impulsive behaviour, and violence; the risk of developing *dependence* on use of the drug; and the risk of *adverse health effects* from sustained chronic, regular use (e.g., chronic disease, blood-borne bacterial and viral infections, drug-induced psychoses, and mental disorders).

There must be evidence that exposure to alcohol, tobacco, or illicit drugs is causally linked to a health outcome before any such injury or disease is considered to be an adverse health effect that is quantified in the health burden arising from that substance (Murray et al., 2004). This relationship must be pharmacokinetically and/or pharmacodynamically biologically plausible, and alternative explanations of the association (including, but not limited to, reverse causation and confounding) improbable. Where this association can be demonstrated, it is also important to quantify the degree to which the adverse health outcome can be attributable to the use of that substance, that is, the direct burden of the substance (wholly attributable) versus substance use as a risk factor for the health outcome (partly attributable).

Various summary measures can be used to quantify health burden attributable to substance use (Gold, Stevenson, & Fryback, 2002). Mortality rates express the number within a population who have died of a cause that is wholly or partly attributable to substance use. Other indicators combine data on mortality and non-fatal health outcomes, quantifying the magnitude of diseases and injury and the fraction of the health outcome attributable to substance use. Primary amongst these are disability-adjusted life years (DALYs), an indicator that sums the years of life lost (YLL) due to premature mortality and years lost due to disability (YLD) from substance use, computed based on standard life expectancy (Murray, 1994; Murray & Acharya, 1997). The below describes the GBD study 2015 estimates of smoked tobacco, alcohol, and illicit drug all-cause attributable mortality, as well as substance use-attributable DALYs (Institute for Health Metrics and Evaluation, 2016).

Mortality

Globally, age-standardised mortality rates from the GBD study 2015 (Institute for Health Metrics and Evaluation, 2016) for smoked tobacco were 110.7 (101.0, 120.3) per 100,000 people, compared to 33.0 (28.0, 37.7), and 6.9 deaths (6.1, 7.6) per 100,000 people for alcohol and illicit drugs, respectively (Table 2.2). Alcohol- and illicit drug-attributable age-standardised mortality rates were highest in Eastern Europe (108.0 [63.5, 152.4] and 23.7 [21.0, 25.9] deaths per 100,000 people, respectively). Tobacco-

Table 2.2 Crude attributable deaths (in thousands) and age-standardised attributable death rate (per 100,000) for alcohol, tobacco and illicit drugs as risk factors for disease burden by GBD region, 2015

	Alcohol use		Tobacco smoking		Illicit drug use	
	Number (1000s; 95%UI)	Age SDR (95%UI)	Number (1000s; 95%UI)	Age SDR (95%UI)	Number (1000s; 95%UI)	Age SDR (95%UI)
Andean Latin America	13.4 (11.8, 15)	28.3 (24.7, 31.9)	18.2 (15.8, 20.9)	43.9 (37.9, 50.3)	2.1 (1.6, 2.6)	4.4 (3.4, 5.5)
Australasia	4.1 (2.2, 5.7)	12.7 (8.9, 16)	27.3 (25.7, 29.1)	64.8 (61, 68.8)	2.6 (2.3, 2.8)	7.6 (6.8, 8.4)
Caribbean	12.8 (11.1, 14.6)	28.7 (24.8, 32.7)	38.6 (35.7, 42.1)	89 (82.4, 96.9)	1.6 (1.2, 2)	3.5 (2.7, 4.4)
Central Asia	27.9 (23.8, 32)	36.2 (29.6, 42.4)	80.3 (73.6, 87.1)	125.3 (114.2, 136.4)	9.2 (8, 10.2)	12.1 (10.3, 13.7)
Central Europe	60 (52.8, 67)	37.2 (33.4, 40.7)	214.6 (203.6, 225.9)	117.3 (111.4, 123.3)	7.8 (5.9, 9.7)	5 (3.9, 6.1)
Central Latin America	70.2 (64.5, 76)	32.6 (29.6, 35.8)	90.7 (82, 98.9)	51.6 (46.6, 56.4)	15.5 (12.2, 18.5)	7.4 (5.6, 9)
Central Sub-Saharan Africa	25.5 (15.1, 41.8)	46.5 (27.8, 74.5)	42 (26.8, 65.3)	85.6 (53.7, 134.2)	3.4 (2.2, 5.3)	5.5 (3.4, 8.7)
East Asia	613.5 (557.7, 672)	38.5 (34.7, 42.6)	2045.2 (1542.5, 2588.2)	145.9 (109.4, 184.6)	89.6 (81.4, 97.7)	5.6 (5, 6.1)
Eastern Europe	313.9 (164.9, 462.2)	108 (63.5, 152.4)	451.7 (417.7, 487.2)	142.8 (132.2, 154)	61.3 (54.2, 66.7)	23.7 (21, 25.9)
Eastern Sub-Saharan Africa	92.3 (71.9, 117.5)	52.6 (40.8, 66.6)	102.7 (80.1, 131.1)	63 (49.3, 81.2)	9.7 (7.3, 12.8)	4.5 (3.2, 6.2)
High-income Asia Pacific	51.4 (43.8, 60)	17.7 (15.7, 19.9)	221.9 (203.4, 238.8)	54 (49.6, 58.2)	17.1 (11.9, 22.7)	5.3 (3.9, 6.7)
High-income North America	84.7 (74.6, 94.7)	19.6 (17.6, 21.5)	529.5 (508.8, 550.3)	101.2 (97.4, 104.9)	70.7 (65.9, 74)	16.4 (15.3, 17.2)
North Africa and Middle East	46 (39.5, 52.3)	12.3 (10.5, 14.1)	321.7 (292.7, 351.2)	94.8 (86.4, 104.1)	23.8 (18.8, 29.4)	5.5 (4.3, 7)
Oceania	1.9 (1.2, 2.8)	24.2 (16.2, 35.3)	16 (10.7, 23.7)	269.3 (184.4, 382.9)	0.2 (0.2, 0.4)	3 (2, 4.4)
South Asia	382.8 (336.5, 426.8)	29.4 (25.6, 33)	1263.6 (1123.6, 1396.5)	116.9 (103.4, 129.7)	50.7 (44.3, 59.4)	3.5 (3, 4)
Southeast Asia	163.7 (141.5, 187.8)	30.7 (26.4, 34.9)	673.9 (599.3, 753.3)	147.6 (131.7, 164.1)	40.5 (31.3, 52.7)	6.7 (5.2, 8.6)
Southern Latin America	17.5 (13.2, 21.5)	25.7 (20, 31.1)	70.4 (66, 74.9)	96.8 (91, 102.8)	5.2 (4.5, 5.8)	7.5 (6.5, 8.4)
Southern Sub-Saharan Africa	39.5 (34.1, 45.6)	68.4 (57.9, 79.6)	68.3 (59.9, 78.7)	155.9 (137.3, 177.8)	5.2 (4.5, 6.7)	7.7 (6.6, 9.7)
Tropical Latin America	84.3 (78.2, 90.1)	39.8 (36.8, 42.8)	166.2 (154.2, 178.2)	93.9 (87, 100.8)	7.9 (6.3, 9.4)	3.8 (2.9, 4.6)
Western Europe	112.9 (87.8, 137.3)	18.8 (15.9, 21.5)	632.1 (600.3, 663.6)	77.6 (73.9, 81.2)	42.8 (35.7, 49.2)	6.7 (5.8, 7.5)
Western Sub-Saharan Africa	88.4 (70.4, 117.6)	50.8 (40.9, 66.5)	89.4 (71.7, 113)	54.5 (44, 69)	21.8 (16.9, 28.2)	8.4 (6.5, 10.9)
Global	**2306.5 (1985.5, 2608.5)**	**33.0 (28, 37.7)**	**7164.5 (6544.2, 7774.8)**	**110.7 (101.0, 120.3)**	**488.8 (439.2, 537.3)**	**6.9 (6.1, 7.6)**

Note: Data in the table above were extracted from the GBD study 2015 related to deaths attributable to substance use disorders (Institute for Health Metrics and Evaluation, 2016). Age-standardised rates is the rate per 100,000 deatths, estimated using the GBD world population age standard
[a]Grouping of countries reflect GBD classification

attributable mortality rates were highest in Oceania (which includes Papua New Guinea, Kiribati, Federated States of Micronesia, Solomon Islands; 269.3 [184.4, 382.9] deaths per 100,000 people). Lowest age-standardised rates were observed for North Africa and Middle East; this finding fits with aforementioned data on estimated rates of heavy episodic alcohol consumption and alcohol dependence for these regions (Table 2.2).

Burden of Disease

Variations in burden of disease attributable to substance as the risk factor largely reflect those for mortality. The GBD study 2015 (Institute for Health Metrics and Evaluation, 2016) suggests that absolute burden in 2015 was highest for tobacco, with 170.9 million (156.2, 186.0) tobacco-attributable DALYs (Table 2.3). This was followed by 85 million (77.2, 93.0) alcohol-attributable DALYs and 27.8 million (24.4, 31.2) illicit drug-attributable DALYs.

Geographic variation in age-standardised DALYs primarily reflects variation in rates of consumption and dependence globally. The GBD study 2015 showed that alcohol-attributable burden rates were highest in the Eastern European region (4033.5 DALYs per 100,000 population; 3259.9, 4795.1) and lowest in North Africa and the Middle East region (359.3 DALYs per 100,000 population; 306.5, 407.3). Similarly, illicit drug-attributable burden was also highest in the Eastern European region (1386.5 DALYs per 100,000 population; 1229.6, 1535.4). Whilst illicit drug-attributable burden was lowest in Oceania (168.4 DALYs per 100,000 population; 127.2, 226.5), tobacco-attributable burden rates were highest in this region (7149.7 DALYs per 100,000 population; 4888.1, 10491.5) (Table 2.3).

Alcohol-attributable burden was mainly driven by cirrhosis (17.0 million DALYs; 15.6, 18.3), transport injuries (16.8 million DALYs; 14.9, 18.9), and cancers (12.1 million DALYs; 11.1, 12.9) (Institute for Health Metrics and Evaluation, 2016). The burden attributable to illicit drugs mainly comprised drug-use disorders (16.9 million DALYs; 14.0, 19.9), cirrhosis (4.7 million DALYs; 3.8, 5.5), HIV (3.0 million DALYs; 2.6, 3.6), and liver cancer (1.8 million DALYs; 1.4, 2.1) (Institute for Health Metrics and Evaluation, 2016). Much of the illicit drug burden from cirrhosis and liver cancer is attributable to hepatitis C virus (HCV).

The viruses that cause HCV are efficiently spread by contaminated blood in shared injection equipment (Donoghoe & Wodak, 1998; Macdonald, Crofts, & Kaldor, 1996). A recent global systematic review (Degenhardt et al., 2017) estimated that there were 8.2 million (4.7, 12.4) people who inject drugs who are HCV antibody positive, and that 2.8 million (1.5, 4.5) people who inject drugs are living with HIV in 2015 (Fig. 2.3). This equates to 52.3% (42.4, 62.1) and 17.8% (10.8, 24.8) of people who inject drugs globally, respectively. HIV prevalence varied substantially across geographical regions, from 1.1% (0.8, 1.4) in Australasia to 35.7% (15.0, 56.6) in Latin America. Higher estimates of HCV antibody prevalence were noted in countries within East and Southeast Asian region (e.g. Indonesia, Taiwan, Thailand).

Risk Factors for Health Harms

Risk of experiencing health harms varies according to the characteristics of the consumer, substances consumed, and patterns of consumption. For example, a history of mental disorder strongly predicts the likelihood of substance dependence (Lopez-Quintero et al., 2011); the risk of transition from use to dependence is greater for tobacco than alcohol (Lopez-Quintero et al., 2011); and the risk of opioid overdose is greater with use via injection (Degenhardt et al., 2011). However, the broader social context, and the policies implemented to discourage drug use and/or reduce drug-related harm, can also play a pivotal role in risk for health harm. People who use drugs are often stigmatised, and criminally punished in some countries, often including involuntary detention, with the purported intent of reducing drug use (Degenhardt et al., 2010). Yet, a strong body of evidence shows that compulsory

Table 2.3 Crude attributable DALYs (in thousands) and age-standardised attributable DALYs (per 100,000) for alcohol, tobacco and illicit drugs as risk factors for disease burden by GBD region, 2015

Region[a]	Alcohol use Number (1000s; 95%UI)	Alcohol use Age SDR (95%UI)	Tobacco smoking Number (1000s; 95%UI)	Tobacco smoking Age SDR (95%UI)	Illicit drug use Number (1000s; 95%UI)	Illicit drug use Age SDR (95%UI)
Andean Latin America	504.1 (451.4, 560.9)	951.3 (847.7, 1057.9)	394.6 (345.8, 450.9)	861 (755, 982.6)	135.8 (112.4, 160.8)	245.3 (202.7, 290.2)
Australasia	192.2 (170, 214.7)	610.4 (552.1, 678.8)	472.9 (443.8, 501.8)	1230.2 (1154.2, 1305.9)	205.2 (172.5, 240.5)	684.5 (571, 805.5)
Caribbean	519.8 (462.5, 582.6)	1140.2 (1013.1, 1277.2)	815.8 (755, 881.8)	1854.5 (1716, 2004.9)	90.6 (76.4, 105.9)	197.9 (166.7, 231.3)
Central Asia	1211.7 (1069.7, 1349.1)	1427.5 (1250.3, 1605.6)	2288.1 (2105.7, 2473)	3166.8 (2913.7, 3421.3)	454.9 (404.2, 506.7)	531.9 (472.2, 591.2)
Central Europe	2052.4 (1910.3, 2214.8)	1386.9 (1297.1, 1490.1)	4909.7 (4665.5, 5165.2)	2843 (2700.1, 2991.9)	395.9 (332.9, 465.7)	296.5 (250.7, 346.5)
Central Latin America	2864.7 (2673.2, 3069.3)	1186.4 (1105.4, 1274.5)	2002 (1810, 2189.8)	1021.9 (924.2, 1115)	761.6 (655.7, 862.7)	318.9 (272.2, 363.6)
Central Sub-Saharan Africa	1041.6 (641.4, 1688.4)	1506.2 (915.6, 2448.6)	1617.7 (1069.9, 2488.4)	2300.7 (1457.6, 3599.6)	185.1 (132, 266.7)	240.9 (167.1, 353.5)
East Asia	20447.6 (18657.8, 22411.1)	1221.4 (1113.4, 1339.8)	43148.3 (33306.3, 54375.7)	2730.4 (2097.5, 3428.8)	5070.5 (4355.2, 5786.7)	312.3 (266.8, 359.2)
Eastern Europe	10749.3 (8326.4, 13121.1)	4033.5 (3259.9, 4795.1)	11323.8 (10524.6, 12139.6)	3743.6 (3478.2, 4010.6)	3364.8 (2991.3, 3716.6)	1386.5 (1229.6, 1535.4)
Eastern Sub-Saharan Africa	3656.5 (2900.3, 4619)	1629.5 (1289.5, 2063.6)	3891.8 (3032.5, 4928.9)	1700 (1321.8, 2184.3)	530.7 (422.6, 654.2)	198.7 (152.8, 252.9)
High-income Asia Pacific	1463 (1300.6, 1643)	627 (569.2, 696.6)	3485.5 (3186.8, 3762.5)	1038 (943.8, 1125.6)	521.5 (420.1, 622.6)	216.4 (180.2, 250.7)
High-income North America	3498.9 (3215.9, 3787.4)	880.8 (813.8, 951.1)	10603.2 (10143.2, 11073.7)	2141.7 (2047, 2238.8)	3943.1 (3506.1, 4370.8)	1032 (911.3, 1150.2)
North Africa and Middle East	1685.8 (1459.1, 1909.4)	359.3 (306.5, 407.3)	9497.9 (8615.4, 10434.8)	2339.3 (2125.8, 2554.1)	2122.1 (1703.9, 2564.5)	395.1 (318.9, 478.9)
Oceania	85.1 (59.1, 123.9)	903.8 (625.5, 1318.8)	523.1 (353.9, 779.1)	7149.7 (4888.1, 10491.5)	16.6 (12.7, 22.2)	168.4 (127.2, 226.5)
South Asia	15654.9 (14027.2, 17410.4)	1038.8 (928.1, 1158.3)	35866.4 (31925.8, 39858.3)	2812.6 (2508.1, 3122.3)	3730.1 (3174.5, 4343)	222.2 (190.1, 257.4)
Southeast Asia	5988.3 (5255.8, 6834.3)	971.7 (854.2, 1102.7)	18138.8 (15949.6, 20408.4)	3361.3 (2971.9, 3764)	2130.2 (1740.6, 2649.9)	321.8 (263.3, 399.6)

(continued)

Table 2.3 (continued)

Region[a]	Alcohol use		Tobacco smoking		Illicit drug use	
	Number (1000s; 95%UI)	Age SDR (95%UI)	Number (1000s; 95%UI)	Age SDR (95%UI)	Number (1000s; 95%UI)	Age SDR (95%UI)
Southern Latin America	700.6 (611.5, 787.9)	1047.4 (918, 1176.8)	1412.4 (1334.9, 1496.1)	2030.9 (1915.8, 2150.6)	231.6 (200.6, 263.6)	344.3 (298, 392.5)
Southern Sub-Saharan Africa	1683.9 (1470.3, 1920.4)	2436.4 (2109.6, 2805.6)	1854.7 (1616.7, 2154.9)	3660.4 (3215.4, 4224.6)	340.3 (293.8, 424.6)	443.8 (383.9, 545.2)
Tropical Latin America	3505.7 (3276.6, 3755.6)	1561.7 (1456.8, 1672.1)	3800.6 (3523.4, 4101.4)	1931.5 (1792.8, 2080.1)	477.8 (401.4, 547.5)	211.8 (177.2, 243.6)
Western Europe	4084.1 (3633, 4554.3)	769.6 (691, 848.8)	11282.6 (10706.8, 11851.6)	1626.6 (1542.1, 1709.8)	1817 (1588.1, 2049.7)	382.2 (330.5, 431.7)
Western Sub-Saharan Africa	3400 (2779, 4468.7)	1498.9 (1215.5, 1961.9)	3558.7 (2787.4, 4480.4)	1405.8 (1141.2, 1772.9)	1305.7 (1046.1, 1637.8)	422 (338.5, 525.2)
Global	**84,990 (77180.3, 93009.8)**	**1160 (1050, 1272.1)**	**170888.6 (156215.6, 185987.6)**	**2482.8 (2269.7, 2701.2)**	**27,831 (24436.9, 31170.9)**	**372.1 (327.2, 416.3)**

Note: Data in the table above were extracted from the GBD study 2015 related to disability-adjusted life years (DALYs) attributable to substance use disorders (Institute for Health Metrics and Evaluation, 2016). Age-standardised rates is the rate per 100,000 people, estimated using the GBD world population age standard

[a]Grouping of countries reflect GBD classification

detention does not reduce relapse, injecting risk, or HIV incidence (Degenhardt et al., 2010) and increases overdose risk and blood-borne virus infection (Vescio et al., 2008). Further, it also violates drug users' human rights (Human Rights Watch, 2004; Open Society Institute International Harm Reduction Development Program, 2009; Pearshouse, 2009; Pearshouse and Canadian HIV Network, 2009; World Health Organization Western Pacific Region, 2009).

Availability of interventions and treatments to address problem drug use can also contribute to the risk of harm. This includes whether treatment is accessible; the types of treatment available; the extent of treatment coverage of all those who might need to access it; and the quality of treatment delivery. A recent review showed that, of 179 countries with evidence of injecting drug use, some level of needle-syringe exchange services was available for people who inject drugs in 93 countries, and there were 86 countries with evidence of opioid substitution therapy implementation (Larney et al., 2017). Yet, less than 1% of people who inject drugs live in countries with high coverage of both needle-syringe programmes and opioid substitution (of countries with available data on coverage of needle-syringe programmes and opioid substitution therapy; Larney et al., 2017), highlighting substantial gaps in treatment provision globally.

Conclusion

Alcohol and tobacco are commonly consumed substances globally and in most regions. Indeed, one in five adults report heavy episodic alcohol use in the past month and almost one in seven adults report daily tobacco smoking. Both high-risk consumption practices are associated with significant health harm, the latter specifically increasing the risk of various cancers, non-malignant respiratory diseases, cardiovascular disease, and many other chronic health conditions (U.S. Department of Health and Human Services, 2014). In contrast, use of illicit drugs is

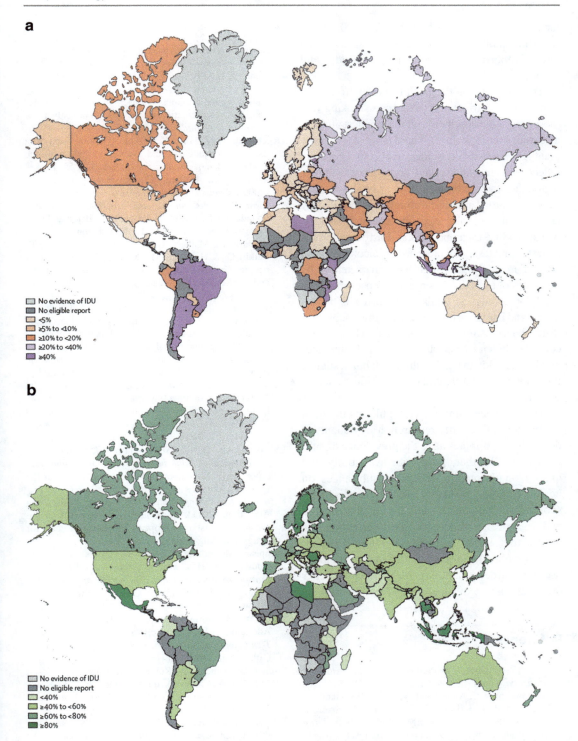

Fig. 2.3 Estimated HIV (Panel **a**) and anti-HCV (Panel **b**) prevalence among people who inject drugs by country, 2015. Images reproduced from Degenhardt et al. (2017); *IDU* = injecting drug use. (Panel **a**) HIV prevalence. (Panel **b**) HCV prevalence

far less common, with less than 1 in 20 people reporting cannabis use in the past year, and even fewer reporting amphetamine, opioid, and cocaine use.

The majority of the health burden from substance use is attributable to tobacco smoking (the most prevalent substance) and the smallest attributable to use of illicit drugs. There is substantial geographic variation in burden that unsurprisingly reflects patterns of use and dependence within a region for each substance. For example, Eastern Europe recorded amongst the highest rates of heavy episodic alcohol use, dependence, and DALYs, whilst North Africa and Middle East recorded the lowest estimates for all indicators of alcohol use and health burden. Some regions were characterised by high rates of use and burden across most substances (e.g. North America), whilst others had a high prevalence and harms associated with a single substance (e.g. tobacco estimates for Oceania). These trends could be driven by various factors, including geographic variation in legal status, availability, stigma, discrimination, and treatment availability, amongst other factors.

The evidence summarised highlights the need for further high-quality research. Many countries do not have estimates as to the prevalence of substance use. Further, poor data availability and quality on the causal effects of substances on health outcomes mean that health burden is likely substantially underestimated. Better standardised and rigorous methods for data collection are needed that would facilitate accurate assessment of geographical and temporal trends in substance use and burden, including the impact of better drug treatment provision.

References

American Psychiatric Association. (2000). *Diagnostic and statistical manual of mental disorders (DSM-IV-TR)*. Washington, DC: American Psychiatric Association.

Babor, T., caulkins, J., Edwards, G., Fischer, B., Foxcroft, D., Humphreys, K., ... Strang, J. (Eds.). (2010). *Drug policy and the public good*. Oxford: Oxford University Press.

Barendregt, J. J., Van Oortmarssen, G. J., Vos, T., & Murray, C. J. (2003). A generic model for the assessment of disease epidemiology: The computational basis of DisMod II. *Population Health Metrics, 1*, 4.

Charlson, F., Degenhardt, L., Mclaren, J., Hall, W., & Lynskey, M. (2009). A systematic review of research examining benzodiazepine-related mortality. *Pharmacoepidemiology and Drug Safety, 18*, 93–103.

Degenhardt, L., Bucello, C., Mathers, B., Briegleb, C., Ali, H., Hickman, M., & Mclaren, J. (2011). Mortality among regular or dependent users of heroin and other opioids: A systematic review and meta-analysis of cohort studies. *Addiction, 106*, 32–51.

Degenhardt, L., & Hall, W. (2012). Extent of illicit drug use and dependence, and their contribution to the global burden of disease. *The Lancet, 379*, 55–70.

Degenhardt, L., Hallam, C., & Bewley-Taylor, D. (2009). *Comparing the drug situation across countries: Problems, pitfalls and possibilities* (Beckley Foundation Drug Policy Programme Briefing Paper No. 19). London: The Beckley Foundation.

Degenhardt, L., Mathers, B., Vickerman, P., Rhodes, T., Latkin, C., & Hickman, M. (2010). HIV prevention for people who inject drugs: Why individual, structural, and combination approaches are required. *The Lancet, 376*, 285–301.

Degenhardt, L., Peacock, A., Colledge, S., Leung, J., Grebely, J., Vickerman, P., ... Larney, S. (2017). Global prevalence of injecting drug use and sociodemographic characteristics and prevalence of HIV, HBV, and HCV in people who inject drugs: A multistage systematic review. *The Lancet Global Health, 5*, e1192–e1207.

Donoghoe, M., & Wodak, A. (1998). Health and social consequences of injecting drug use. In G. Stimson, D. Des Jarlais, & A. Ball (Eds.), *Drug injecting and HIV infection: Global dimensions and local responses*. London: UCL Press.

ESPAD Group. (2016). *ESPAD report 2015: Results from the European school survey project on alcohol and other drugs*. Luxembourg: Publications Office of the European Union.

European Monitoring Centre For Drugs And Drug Addiction. (2011). *Responding to new psychoactive substances*. Lisbon: European Monitoring Centre for Drugs and Drug Addiction.

European Monitoring Centre For Drugs And Drug Addiction. (2015). *New psychoactive substances in Europe: An update from the EU early warning system*. Luxembourg: Publications Office of the European Union.

European Monitoring Centre For Drugs And Drug Addiction. (2018). *European drug report 2017: Trends and developments*. Luxembourg: Publications Office of the European Union.

Fischer, B., Kendall, P., Rehm, J., & Room, R. (1997). Charting WHO—goals for licit and illicit drugs for the year 2000: Are we 'on track'? *Public Health, 111*, 271–275.

Fischer, B., & Rehm, J. (2018). Revisiting the 'paradigm shift' in opioid use: Developments and implications 10 years later. *Drug and Alcohol Review, 37*, S199–S202.

Flaxman, A. D., Vos, T., & Murray, C. J. (2015). *An integrative metaregression framework for descriptive epidemiology*. Seattle, WA: University of Washington Press.

Global Burden of Disease Study-2015 Tobacco Collaborators. (2017). Smoking prevalence and attributable disease burden in 195 countries and territories, 1990–2015: A systematic analysis from the Global Burden of Disease Study 2015. *Lancet, 389*(10082), 1885–1906.

Gold, M. R., Stevenson, D., & Fryback, D. G. (2002). HALYS and QALYS and DALYS, Oh My: Similarities and differences in summary measures of population Health. *Annual Review of Public Health, 23*, 115–134.

Hall, W., & Weier, M. (2015). Assessing the public health impacts of legalizing recreational cannabis use in the USA. *Clinical Pharmacology & Therapeutics, 97*, 607–615.

Hartnoll, R. (1997). Cross-validating at local level. In G. V. Stimson, M. Hickman, A. Quirk, M. Frischer, & C. Taylor (Eds.), *Estimating the prevalence of problem drug use in Europe*. Luxembourg: EMCDDA.

Hickman, M., De Angelis, D., Jones, H., Harris, R., Welton, N., & Ades, A. (2013). Multiple parameter evidence synthesis—a potential solution for when information on drug use and harm is in conflict. *Addiction, 108*, 1529–1531.

Human Rights Watch. (2004). *Not enough graves: The war on drugs, HIV/AIDS, and violations of human rights*. New York: Human Rights Watch.

Institute for Health Metrics and Evaluation. (2015). *Protocol for the global burden of diseases, injuries, and risk factors study (GBD)*.

Institute for Health Metrics and Evaluation. (2016). *GBD results tool*. Seattle, WA: IHME, University of Washington.

International Narcotics Control Board. (2015). *Availability of internationally controlled drugs: Ensuring adequate access for medical and scientific purposes*. Vienna: International Narcotics Control Board.

Jones, H. E., Hickman, M., Welton, N. J., De Angelis, D., Harris, R. J., & Ades, A. (2014). Recapture or precapture? Fallibility of standard capture-recapture methods in the presence of referrals between sources. *American Journal of Epidemiology, 179*, 1383–1393.

Kassebaum, N. J., Arora, M., Barber, R. M., Bhutta, Z. A., Brown, J., Carter, A., ... Coggeshall, M. (2016). Global, regional, and national disability-adjusted life-years (DALYs) for 315 diseases and injuries and healthy life expectancy (HALE), 1990–2015: A systematic analysis for the Global Burden of Disease Study 2015. *The Lancet, 388*, 1603–1658.

Larance, B., Degenhardt, L., Lintzeris, N., Winstock, A., & Mattick, R. (2011). Definitions related to the use of pharmaceutical opioids: Extramedical use, diversion, non-adherence and aberrant medication-related behaviours. *Drug and Alcohol Review, 30*, 236–245.

Larney, S., Peacock, A., Leung, J., Colledge, S., Hickman, M., Vickerman, P., ... Degenhardt, L. (2017). Global, regional, and country-level coverage of interventions to prevent and manage HIV and hepatitis C among people who inject drugs: A systematic review. *The Lancet Global Health, 5*, e1208–e1220.

Logan, B. K., Mohr, A. L., Friscia, M., Krotulski, A. J., Papsun, D. M., Kacinko, S. L., ... Huestis, M. A. (2017). Reports of adverse events associated with use of novel psychoactive substances, 2013–2016: A review. *Journal of Analytical Toxicology, 41*, 573–610.

Lopez-Quintero, C., Cobos, J. P. D. L., Hasin, D. S., Okuda, M., Wang, S., Grant, B. F., & Blanco, C. (2011). Probability and predictors of transition from first use to dependence on nicotine, alcohol, cannabis, and cocaine: Results of the National Epidemiologic Survey on Alcohol and Related Conditions (NESARC). *Drug and Alcohol Dependence, 115*, 120–130.

Macdonald, M., Crofts, N., & Kaldor, J. (1996). Transmission of hepatitis C virus: Rates, routes, and cofactors. *Epidemiologic Reviews, 18*, 137–148.

Mathers, B., Degenhardt, L., Phillips, B., Wiessing, L., Hickman, M., Strathdee, S., ... & For The 2007 Reference Group to the UN on HIV and Injecting Drug Use. (2008). Global epidemiology of injecting drug use and HIV among people who inject drugs: A systematic review. *The Lancet, 372*, 1733–1745.

Maxwell, J. C. (2005). Party drugs: Properties, prevalence, patterns, and problems. *Substance Use & Misuse, 40*, 1203–1240.

McAllister, W. (Ed.). (2000). *Drug diplomacy in the twentieth century*. London: Routledge.

Michalak, L., Trocki, K., & Bond, J. (2007). Religion and alcohol in the US National Alcohol Survey: How important is religion for abstention and drinking? *Drug and Alcohol Dependence, 87*, 268–280.

Murray, C. J. (1994). Quantifying the burden of disease: The technical basis for disability-adjusted life years. *Bulletin of the World Health Organization, 72*, 429.

Murray, C. J., & Acharya, A. K. (1997). Understanding DALYs. *Journal of Health Economics, 16*, 703–730.

Murray, C. J. L., Ezzati, M., Lopez, A. D., Rodgers, A., & Vander Hoorn, S. (2004). Comparative quantification of health risks: Conceptual framework and methodological issues. In M. Ezzati, A. D. Lopez, A. Rodgers, & C. J. L. Murray (Eds.), *Comparative quantification of health risks: Global and regional burden of disease attributable to selected major risk factors*. Geneva: World Health Organization.

Open Society Institute International Harm Reduction Development Program. (2009). Public health fact sheet. In *Human rights abuses in the name of drug treatment: Reports from the field*. New York: Open Society Institute.

Peacock, A., Leung, J., Larney, S., Colledge, S., Hickman, M., Rehm, J., ... Degenhardt, L. (2018). Global statistics on alcohol, tobacco and illicit drug use: 2017 status report. *Addiction, 113*(10), 1905–1926.

Pearshouse, R. (2009). "Patients, not criminals"? An assessment of Thailand's compulsory drug dependence treatment system. *HIV/AIDS Policy & Law Review/Canadian HIV/AIDS Legal Network, 14*, 11–17.

Pearshouse, R., & Canadian HIV Network. (2009). *Compulsory drug treatment in Thailand: Observations* on the Narcotic Addict Rehabilitation Act BE 2545 (2002). Toronto: Canadian HIV/AIDS Legal Network.

Rehm, J., Anderson, P., Barry, J., Dimitrov, P., Elekes, Z., Feijão, F., … Kraus, L. (2015). Prevalence of and potential influencing factors for alcohol dependence in Europe. *European Addiction Research, 21*, 6–18.

Rehm, J., Gmel, G. E., Gmel, G., Hasan, O. S., Imtiaz, S., Popova, S., … Samokhvalov, A. V. (2017). The relationship between different dimensions of alcohol use and the burden of disease—an update. *Addiction, 112*(6), 968–1001.

Rehm, J., Shield, K., Rehm, M., Gmel, G., & Frick, U. (2012). *Alcohol consumption, alcohol dependence and attributable burden of disease in Europe*. Toronto: Centre for Addiction and Mental Health.

Reuter, P., & Trautmann, F. (Eds.). (2009). *A report on global illicit drugs markets 1998–2007. Full Report*. Utrecht: Trimbos Institute.

Rogers, G., Elston, J., Garside, R., Roome, C., Taylor, R. S., Younger, P., … Somerville, M. (2009). The harmful health effects of recreational ecstasy: A systematic review of observational evidence. *Health Technology Assessment, 13*, 1–315.

Roxburgh, A., Van Buskirk, J., Burns, L., & Bruno, R. (2017). *Drugs and the Internet*. Sydney: National Drug and Alcohol Research Centre.

Seear, K., Fraser, S., Moore, D., & Murphy, D. (2015). Understanding and responding to anabolic steroid injecting and hepatitis C risk in Australia: A research agenda. *Drugs: Education, Prevention and Policy, 22*, 449–455.

Sumnall, H. R., Evans-Brown, M., & McVeigh, J. (2011). Social, policy, and public health perspectives on new psychoactive substances. *Drug Testing and Analysis, 3*, 515–523.

U.S. Department OF Health and Human Services. (2014). *The health consequences of smoking. 50 years of progress. A report of the surgeon general*. Atlanta, GA: U.S. Department of Health and Human Services, Centers for Disease Control and Prevention, National Center for Chronic Disease Prevention and Health Promotion, Office on Smoking and Health.

United Nations Office on Drugs and Crime (UNODC). (2017a). *Methodology—World Drug Report 2017*. Vienna: United Nations Office on Drugs and Crime (UNODC).

United Nations Office on Drugs and Crime (UNODC). (2017b). *World Drug Report 2017*. Vienna: United Nations Office on Drugs and Crime (UNODC).

Van Buskirk, J., Griffiths, P., Farrell, M., & Degenhardt, L. (2017). Trends in new psychoactive substances from surface and "dark" net monitoring. *The Lancet Psychiatry, 4*, 16–18.

Vescio, M., Longo, B., Babudieri, S., Starnini, G., Rezza, G., & Monarca, R. (2008). Correlates of hepatitis C virus seropositivity in prison inmates: A meta-analysis. *Journal of Epidemiology and Community Health, 62*, 305–313.

Wesson, P., Reingold, A., & Mcfarland, W. (2017). Theoretical and empirical comparisons of methods to estimate the size of hard-to-reach populations: A systematic review. *AIDS and Behavior, 21*, 2188–2206.

West, R., Mcewen, A., Bolling, K., & Owen, L. (2001). Smoking cessation and smoking patterns in the general population: A 1-year follow-up. *Addiction, 96*, 891–902.

World Health Organization. (1993). *The ICD-10 classification of mental and behavioural disorders—Diagnostic criteria for research*. Geneva: World Health Organization.

World Health Organization. (2016). *Global Information System on Alcohol and Health (GISAH)* [Online]. Retrieved December 9, 2017, from http://apps.who.int/gho/data/node.gisah.GISAHhome?showonly=GISAH

World Health Organization Western Pacific Region. (2009). *Assessment of compulsory treatment of people who use drugs in Cambodia, China, Malaysia and Viet Nam: An application of selected human rights principles*. Manilla: World Health Organization.

An Integrative Perspective on the Etiology of Substance Use

Nicole J. Roberts and Diana Fishbein

Introduction to the "Ecobiodevelopmental" Framework

Persons who initiate use and later develop substance dependence transition through a number of stages, including experimental or social use, escalation, maintenance, abuse, and eventually addiction (Kandel, 2002). These pathways, however, are not without significant fluctuations in usage and desistance patterns. Subgroups of users may never escalate while maintaining moderate use for decades; others may experience intermittent periods of cessation with some abstaining permanently. And still others escalate rapidly and develop substance-abuse disorders (SUD). Determining which experimental users will continue on a path to abuse and dependence is an age-old question that has compelled researchers and practitioners to better understand, predict, and appropriately intervene in these distinct etiological pathways.

The "ecobiodevelopmental" theoretical framework, founded on an integration of behavioral science fields, is helpful in understanding variations in substance-use pathways. This model views human behavior as emerging from the biological imbedding of social and physical environmental conditions (Shonkoff et al., 2012). Individual-level characteristics, such as personality and genetics, interact with experiences and exposures to socio-environmental factors to directly affect the developing brain's structure and function (Duncan & Murnane, 2011; NRC & IOM, 2009; Yoshikawa, Aber, & Beardslee, 2012). This inherent "experience dependence" of the brain means that the nature of conditions to which individuals are exposed—optimal versus suboptimal—influences the resultant behavior. An abundance of positive experiences, such as protective factors (e.g., family support, well-equipped schools), can strengthen neural connections underlying self-regulation, impulse control, and executive decision-making. In reverse, however, negative or adverse exposures can translate to impairments in the developing child's ability to regulate behavior and emotions (Glaser, 2000; McEwen & Morrison, 2013). And importantly, exposures and experiences have differential effects on social, psychological, and neural processes contingent upon the developmental stage, which have functional and behavioral implications (Adler & Rehkopf, 2008).

N. J. Roberts (✉)
The Pennsylvania State University, University Park, PA, USA
e-mail: njr175@psu.edu

D. Fishbein
Program for Translational Research on Adversity and Neurodevelopment, The Pennsylvania State University, University Park, PA, USA
e-mail: dfishbein@psu.edu

This framework further accounts for the immediate "microlevel" (e.g., family) and surrounding "macro-level" (e.g., neighborhood) factors that influence the development and prevalence of behavior through their effects on individual functioning in multiple domains. While specific influential factors vary between individuals, and no factor alone is sufficient to lead to substance use and abuse, there is likely some critical combination of the number of risk influences present and protective influences that are absent that makes the difference between having a brain primed for substance abuse versus one that is not. Reaching this threshold can be achieved by any number of potential combinations of external and personal factors and thus will be unique for each individual. Nevertheless, brain development is so exquisitely sensitive to psychosocial experiences that their effects on the way the brain develops and functions are observable and those effects, in turn, have a direct impact on a child's ability to self-regulate and, in turn, his or her susceptibility to substance use and abuse. Prevention programming and policy have the potential to strengthen protective influences and reduce exposure to or minimize the effects of negative influences, thus redirecting development away from risky behaviors such as substance abuse.

The aim of this chapter is threefold. First, we describe the independent association of person-level, microlevel, and macro-level influences on substance use as sources of vulnerability and resilience. This evidence is then placed into the context of a developmental and integrative framework on the etiology of substance abuse (see Fig. 3.1). Finally, we discuss the translational implications of this model for identifying developmental windows of opportunity for prevention and intervention programs to curb substance use during key periods when initiation is both most common and most detrimental to development (i.e., early adolescence).

Figure 3.1 exhibits the two main categories of factors conferring risk for substance misuse, genes and the environment. Genetic variants are displayed as switches, either "on" or "off." Environmental influences are presented as dials, turned up or down depending on experience. The combination of switches and dials crosses a liability threshold priming the brain for substance misuse. As shown, the functional relationship between factors is not linear, and some environmental dials confer resiliency and may attenuate the effects of the particular genetics.

Person Level

Fundamental characteristics of individuals play a significant role in determining who will use, misuse, and, in some cases, become addicted to substances, and who will abstain or desist at points in the pathway. Consideration of these roles is important for three reasons. First, genetic variations, neurobiological integrity, personality, emerging stress, and coping responses help to determine an individual's responses to the prevailing social and environmental influences, contributing to eventual outcomes. Personal level characteristics have been shown to predict or moderate outcomes, and they interact with environmental influences in unique and complex ways. Second, knowledge regarding these characteristics is critical in helping to determine what preventive and treatment interventions may have the greatest potential to benefit any given individual or subgroup. This information can also identify opportunities during development for implementing the most effective prevention strategies. And third, we can expect to see favorable changes in these characteristics if the intervention positively influences its targets: a mediation effect. Below we describe those characteristics consistently found to be associated with risk for various substance-abuse pathways, and thus have been implicated in their etiology.

Genetic Susceptibilities and Personality Traits

Genetic susceptibility to substance use and abuse encompasses heritable factors which are believed to influence the trajectory of initiation and progression to addiction, including severity of

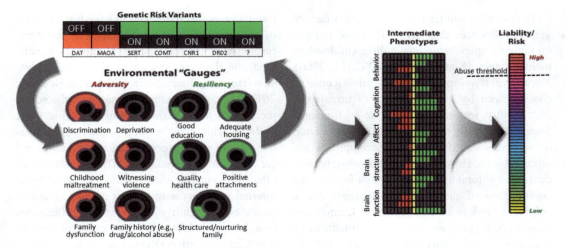

Fig. 3.1 Accumulative model of risk for substance misuse

dependence and risk of relapse (Kreek, Nielsen, Butelman, & LaForge, 2005). By identifying genetic risks that contribute to dependence, we can begin to dissect the various ways in which genes contribute to the transition from escalation to dependence in the context of environmental influences (Bierut, 2011; Vink, Willemsen, & Boomsma, 2005). Critically, studying the genetic components of substance use poses numerous challenges, such as precise phenotypic characterization of individuals, consideration of ethic/cultural backgrounds (as different backgrounds yield differences in allelic frequencies), and achieving sufficient effect sizes (Kreek et al., 2005). Thus, the findings are intriguing and provide a framework for understanding essential gene by environment interactions, but much remains to be explored.

That said, studies suggest that the search for genetic variants affecting substance use should consider the neurobiological systems and phenotypic traits they influence. Genetic variants exert a wide range of actions across multiple functions and characteristics, such as the genetic variation that leads to particular personality traits or the liability to externalizing disorders consistently implicated in the use and abuse of substances (Kendler, Prescott, Myers, & Neale, 2003). The putative role of the dopamine D_2 receptor gene, DRD2, in substance abuse and addiction susceptibility is a case in point (see Le Foll, Gallo, Le Strat, Lu, & Gorwood, 2009 for review). Single-nucleotide polymorphisms (SNPs) in DRD2, for example, have been found to predict specific behavioral traits pertaining to reward sensitivity and inhibitory control, endophenotypes implicated in addiction vulnerability (Frank, Moustafa, Haughey, Curran, & Hutchison, 2007; Klein et al., 2007). Variation in these genetically modulated personality dimensions, particularly impulsivity and novelty seeking, may contribute to the initiation of substance use as well as the transitions from initial to intermittent to regular substance use, the transition from abuse to addiction, and the propensity for repeated relapse after achieving satiety (Kreek et al., 2005). For example, cigarette smokers have been found to exhibit higher levels of novelty/sensation seeking compared to nonsmokers (Zuckerman & Kuhlman, 2000). Individuals with these traits tend to seek highly stimulating and risky situations and show less anxiety in anticipation of the consequences of their behavior (see Kreek et al., 2005). Postmortem studies of the human brain have begun to reveal the link between certain genes and these endophenotypes. Molecular characterizations reveal associations between particular SNPs, including DRD2, and expression in areas of the brain (e.g., the amygdala) linked to these endophenotypes has been implicated in increased risk for addiction (Jutras-Aswad et al., 2012).

Importantly, similar to environmental factors, genetic influences also have differential impacts on these complex behaviors at different developmental stages (Kendler et al., 2003; Li, 2006). Normative development during adolescence is characterized by increased rates of impulsivity and novelty seeking, in part due to dramatic, largely genetically modulated fluctuations in hormone levels that affect brain development and other systems. However, the subgroup of adolescents who exhibit an especially high level of any combination of these personality traits are at heightened risk to abuse substances. Lerman and Niaura (2002) propose that genetic influences on addiction susceptibility are mediated partly by individual differences in comorbid personality traits, as well as individual differences in the reinforcing effects of substances. In effect, it is critical that prevention programs are devised to specifically redirect this developmental track and identify positive outlets that are sufficiently reinforcing.

Behavioral and Mental Health

Internalizing symptoms (e.g., post-traumatic stress disorder [PTSD], depression, anxiety), externalizing behaviors (e.g., conduct disorder [CD], attention-deficit hyperactivity disorder [ADHD], oppositional defiant disorder [ODD], antisocial personality disorder [ASPD]), and mental health conditions have a significant heritable component and are strongly and consistently related to the risk of substance abuse (for review see Armstrong & Costello, 2002). Individuals with these disorders are more likely to use substances and at an earlier age than those without such disorders (De Bellis, 2002; Liddle et al., 2004). Adolescents and adults are also at heightened risk for continued substance use to manage their psychiatric symptoms and for being resistant to substance-abuse treatment (Tomlinson, Brown, & Abrantes, 2004).

The presence of mental and behavioral health disorders may exacerbate the role of poor or maladaptive stress reactivity patterns in developmental pathways to substance abuse. Individuals with internalizing disorders tend to have higher levels of arousal in brain systems responsible for stress responses which may lead to a tendency to self-medicate the symptoms of anxiety and depression (Hussong, Jones, Stein, Baucom, & Boeding, 2011). For those with externalizing disorders, there tends to be a low level of arousal in these systems, which has been associated with a relative lack of regard for consequences and a need for additional stimulation. The likelihood of effectively meeting social challenges due to these internal states is diminished as doing so requires intact neurocognitive and emotional functions (see below), which are often compromised in psychiatric disorders (Kovacs & Goldston, 1991).

Neurological Development

One pathway to substance use and abuse is believed to originate in a deviation or delay in neurological development which is thought to underlie problem (especially risky) behaviors that often precede substance use. Understanding the neurobiological contribution to the etiology of substance use involves characterization of brain maturational processes occurring during adolescence that are associated with substance use, such as reduced inhibitory control and increased reward sensitivity.

While substance abuse is the result of a developmental process beginning in the prenatal period and lasting until one's mid to late 20s, national survey data indicate that initiation is most common in mid-adolescence and that, for the subgroup that escalates, substance abuse peaks during the transition into young adulthood (SAMHSA, 2011). Critically, new social challenges (e.g., increased autonomous decision-making) facing adolescents coincide with complex changes in brain wiring and connectivity taking place throughout this time which have implications for adaptive decision-making and ability to self-regulate behavior and emotion (Giedd et al., 1999; Gogtay et al., 2004). In effect, some degree of impulsivity, risk-taking, and sensation-seeking is normative during adolescence; however, a heightened level of risk-taking may extend from a combination of social circumstances and nonnormative neurodevelopmental immaturity or dysfunction.

Neurobiological development during adolescence occurs transitionally rather than as a single snapshot in time (Casey, Jones, & Hare, 2008). The prefrontal cortex (PFC), responsible for executive cognitive functions (ECF) (e.g., decision-making, impulse control, working memory), is still under construction. A central function of ECFs is to shield long-term goals from temptations afforded by short-term benefits that often lead to negative consequences (Munakata et al., 2011). Somerville and Casey's dual-system process model (2010) demonstrates how prefrontal "top-down" cognitive regulation over subcortical regions is somewhat functionally disconnected throughout adolescence; subcortical, limbic structures which modulate affect and emotional responses to social cues mature earlier than PFC regions. As a result, adolescents are naturally biased by emotional impulses relative to cognitive control. Through both the natural course of development and environmental experience, the functional connectivity between these regions is strengthened and provides a mechanism for increasing top-down modulation of the subcortical systems (Hare et al., 2008).

In addition, ventral striatal reward processing circuits show rapid maturation during the adolescent years, reflected by an increase in the salience of a potential reward (Geier & Luna, 2009; Padmanabhan, Geier, Ordaz, Teslovich, & Luna, 2011; Somerville, Jones, & Casey, 2010). This heightening of reward sensitivity may play a unique role in substance-use initiation rates in early to mid-adolescence and may be exaggerated in the subgroup that escalates use. Subsequent use of substances may exacerbate some adolescents' already heightened ventral striatum response resulting in a strengthening of the substance's reinforcing properties (Hardin & Ernst, 2009). In line with this increase in reward sensitivity, a greater tendency to sensation/novelty seeking is typical during this developmental period (Steinberg et al., 2008). Compounding these neurological liabilities are early puberty and erratic hormone levels, as well as detrimental environmental conditions, such as stress, adversity, maltreatment, and other negative experiences that compromise neurodevelopment and can cause measurable dysfunction in these systems.

Another aspect of neurodevelopment shown to exert an influence on substance-abuse propensity is prenatal exposure to substances, considered both as a direct and mediating mechanism. Prenatal and early exposure to cigarette smoke has been shown to increase children's propensity to smoke, become dependent on nicotine, and exhibit externalizing (conduct problems such as aggression) and internalizing (e.g., depression, anxiety) symptoms (Cornelius, Goldschmidt, & Day, 2012; Piper & Corbett, 2011). Prenatal drug and alcohol exposure is associated with subsequent behavioral problems in the offspring in childhood and adolescence, including eventual substance abuse (DiNieri et al., 2011; Sithisarn, Granger, & Bada, 2012). Alterations in neurological systems associated with self-regulation, reward, and motivation in the fetus, due to the properties of the drug(s) pregnant women use, appear to be the mechanism by which prenatal drug exposure affects the child. The effects of these sorts of prenatal exposures on mental health and behavior will tend to exacerbate any preexisting susceptibilities to use, abuse, and develop addiction to a substance(s).

In sum, regardless of the source of delayed or deficient neurodevelopment, the eventual imbalance between social demands and emergent neurobiological systems during adolescence may lead to heightened vulnerability to substance use and escalation (Casey & Jones, 2010). This evidence has direct implications for the design of intervention components that target this period of development. For example, strategies that focus on incorporating risky and exciting activities (e.g., rock climbing) may provide adolescents with positive ways of obtaining needed stimulation (Perry et al., 2011). In addition, mounting evidence shows that physical activity and programs that include mindfulness have direct neurobehavioral effects; both appear to protect against PFC-mediated impulsivity and drug-use vulnerability (see Perry et al., 2011). Indeed, prevention programs are emerging that target individual-level personality and cognitive factors reflective of underlying neural mechanisms, such as impulsivity and cognitive and emotion regulatory deficits (Conrod et al., 2013).

Stress Exposures and Physiological Reactivity

Stress is a major common denominator across neurobiological, physiological, psychological, and environmental domains implicated in susceptibility to substance use, escalation, relapse, and treatment resistance. "Stress" refers to processes involving perception, appraisal, and response to harmful, threatening, or challenging external events or conditions, known as "stressors," such as poverty, prenatal exposures, child maltreatment, divorce, and bereavement (Pechmann, Levine, Loughlin, & Leslie, 2005). Numerous studies have demonstrated associations between increasing levels of emotional and physiological stress and decreases in behavioral control, higher levels of impulsivity, and high levels of maladaptive behaviors, including substance use (e.g., Hayaki, Stein, Lassor, Herman, & Anderson, 2005; Greco & Carli, 2006; Fishbein et al., 2006; Hatzinger et al., 2007). There is also substantial evidence to support the role of stress in substance-use pathways (e.g., Fishbein et al., 2006; Lee, Neighbors, & Woods, 2007; Simons-Morton & Chen, 2006). Early-life adversity, in particular, is markedly associated with increased risk for substance use, abuse, and dependence (Dube et al., 2003). This fundamental relationship is clearly demonstrated by results of the Adverse Childhood Experiences (ACE) study; results claimed that population-attributable substance-use risk associated with early-life adversity was 50% for substance abuse, 65% for alcoholism, and 78% for intravenous drug use (Chapman et al., 2004; Dube et al., 2003), suggesting that very early development sets the stage for response to initiation by primary biological, psychological, and social responses to initiation.

Similar to all other risk factors, exposure to stress has differential effects on social, psychological, and neural functioning, contingent upon the developmental stage of exposure (Adler & Rehkopf, 2008). In fact, repeated and/or severe exposure to stressors compromises the development of neural systems that underlie social, behavioral, cognitive, and emotional functioning in profound and enduring ways (Davidson, 1994; Pechtel & Pizzagalli, 2011). Andersen and Teicher (2008) argue that early-life stress predisposes individuals to abuse substances via alterations in immature neurophysiological systems that have yet to come on board. Then later in adolescence, when these emergent systems become increasingly functional, the damage is expressed in heightened risk for psychopathology. With greater levels of stress, changes in brain circuitry—which largely occur in the prefrontal cortex (Teicher et al., 2010)—lower behavioral and cognitive control, demonstrating that regulatory brain pathways are targets of brain stress chemicals (see Sinha, 2001 for a review).

More specifically, stress exposures disrupt hormonal systems (e.g., cortisol) that regulate these functions (Huether, 1998); chronically elevated levels of stress hormones can impair learning, memory, decision-making, and other functions that normally support self-regulation of behavior (Nelson & Carver, 1998). Studies also show effects of stress on physiological responses such as heart rate and skin conductance that, when disrupted, are associated with poor behavioral and emotional regulation and cognitive and coping skill deficits (Lovallo, 2012). These physiological and behavioral stress responses activate the same neural systems underlying the positive reinforcing effect of drugs (Koob & Le Moal, 1997), potentially reinforcing drug-taking behaviors. As a result, when an individual experiences a great deal of stress or adversity, these neurologically based processes are affected and lead to poor ability to cope with stress, both behaviorally and physiologically. In these cases, there is often impaired coordination between social, cognitive, psychological, emotional, and biological responses; such impairments have been found to increase drug-seeking behavior (Robinson & Berridge, 2000). As a result, drug taking may occur as a maladaptive response to stressful experiences.

In sum, the changes in biological and psychological processes induced by stress are strongly related to early onset of substance use (Sinha, 2001) and may predict the escalation of drug use, relapse, and intractability. Recognizing the increased risk for substance use in people who have experienced early-life stressors is critical to guide prevention efforts designed to both prevent the exposure and counteract the potential subsequent negative consequences by teaching children ways in which to cope with early-life stress in healthy ways.

Microlevel Influences

Substance use cannot be understood or addressed without understanding the social context within which individuals grow, develop, and interact. This section considers not only liability factors that influence problem behavior, but also environmental conditions that may insulate individuals from negative outcomes.

Parenting and Family Functioning

The home environment is the single most profound influence on early child development in multiple domains of functioning (NRC & IOM, 2013). Parenting and family continue to be important through adolescence when youth begin to have more autonomy and opportunities for either prosocial or risky behaviors (Ernst & Mueller, 2008). The effects of a chaotic home environment, ineffective parenting, and lack of mutual attachment are particularly impactful on overall child outcomes (Springer, Sheridan, Kuo, & Carnes, 2007). The regulatory skills children need to resist substance use and other problem behaviors are instilled early in life, suggesting that a favorable home environment may confer protection against negative outcomes.

The strength of parental influence on substance use has been well documented (e.g., Lippold, Greenberg, Graham, & Feinberg, 2014; Wood, Read, Mitchell, & Brand, 2004). The quality of parenting has been found to interact with factors such as psychological well-being, exposure to stress, and social support in predicting general antisocial behavior, as well as substance use (NIDA No. 94-4212, 1997). Parenting techniques that foster healthy development (e.g., appropriate discipline practices, warmth, affection, secure attachment, involvement, limit setting, and monitoring) are protective (Mayberry, Espelage, & Koenig, 2009; Velleman, Templeton, & Copello, 2005). For example, Lippold et al.'s (2014) results demonstrated that parent efforts to monitor youth in Grade 6 predicted substance use in Grade 8. In addition, their findings suggest that the monitoring process may be influenced by the quality of the parent-youth relationship; within warmer relationships, parent attempts to solicit information from youth may be perceived more positively by youth.

Conversely, parenting behaviors that are harsh, restrictive, inconsistent, hostile, and/or high in conflict can often lead to negative behavioral outcomes in children (Barrett & Turner, 2005). Among children exposed to these negative parenting qualities, there is a 2–4 times higher likelihood of mental and physical health issues compared to national norms (Herrenkohl, Lee, Kosterman, & Hawkins, 2012). At the extreme of parenting behavior, abuse, neglect, and domestic violence, in particular, threaten every aspect of children's development. Additionally, parental substance abuse, which is often associated with poorer quality of parenting, has repeatedly been a strong predictor of substance use in adolescence (e.g., De Micheli & Formigoni, 2002; Madu & Matla, 2003). In addition to parenting, various aspects of the family environment can influence the child's subsequent substance-use behavior, including structure, family cohesion, family communication, and family management (see Velleman et al., 2005). Family processes that tend to be most effective are those with limited levels of stress exposure and coercion (Barrett & Turner, 2006). Additionally, higher levels of substance use have been found in adolescents from single-parent families, consistent with studies reporting that dual-parent families afford protection against substance use (e.g., Adlaf, Ivis, Smart, & Walsh, 1996). This finding could be due to the lack of a protective presence of an additional person in the home which can buffer the child from stress exposure and lack of monitoring.

In response to these reports, family-based preventive interventions recognize that many aspects of the family context play an important part in socializing children to adjust to the demands and pressures of the social environment. Preventing poor outcomes (e.g., mental, emotional, and behavioral problems, substance use) in children often involves parent skill training, relieving the stressors and mental health problems of caregivers, and trauma prevention and trauma-informed treatment strategies (Shay & Knutson, 2008).

A needs assessment of 129 parents discovered that parents did not know how to identify "teachable moments," and they lacked the appropriate requisite language when trying to speak about substance issues with their children (Velleman, Templeton, & Copello, 2005). The National Survey of Children's Health (2003) reported that there is a significant relationship between parental communication of their disapproval of substance use and less subsequent use by their child. Together, these findings suggest that prevention programs should incorporate an educational component which teaches parents the extent to which their own behavior influences young people's use of substances, and ways in which they can initiate and carry out conversations with their child about substance use. Indeed, prevention programs (e.g., "Preparing for the Drug Free Years") have begun to incorporate such educational components (Kosterman, Hawkins, Haggerty, Spoth, & Redmond, 2001).

Schools and Educational Opportunities

The quality of the school environment, its teachers, curriculum, and students' social networks in school are major socializing influences on student learning and behavior (Bond et al., 2007; Cleveland, Feinberg, Bontempo, & Greenberg, 2008). At a very basic level, attendance in school protects against poor outcomes on multiple levels, and may exert a particularly powerful effect for children with self-regulatory problems (Christle, Jolivette, & Nelson, 2005). In addition, unqualified teachers, ineffective teaching practices, and low-quality curricula confer significant additional risks, leading to academic failure (Christle et al., 2005; Darling-Hamond, 2000). Lack of a good education and poor classroom management set the stage for lower levels of cognitive functioning, poor social skills, high levels of stress, and perceptions of inadequacy and failure (Engle & Black, 2008), each of which is implicated in risk for substance abuse. And eventually, a poor-quality education results in an inability to compete in the workforce and obtain jobs that pay a good wage (Campbell, Ramey, Pungello, Sparling, & Miller-Johnson, 2002), factors also associated with substance abuse.

Effectively teaching students the academic and social skills necessary to succeed in school and in life requires that schools also address the special needs of children with social, learning, mental health, and emotional issues that could interfere with success in the classroom (Adelman & Taylor, 1999). Lack of support within the schools for these children often means that disadvantaged or special-needs youth fail to receive the attention they require to overcome their challenges. Absent adequate educational support and/or targeted school programs, learning disabilities, and mental health problems increase the risk for substance abuse (Mason et al., 2010).

Another aspect of school influences is the important role of school connectedness. Research suggests that youth are more likely to have mental health problems and an increased likelihood to use substances in their later years of schooling when they report low school connectedness and interpersonal conflict in early secondary school (Bond et al., 2004; Catalano, Oesterle, Fleming, & Hawkins, 2004). Bond et al. (2007) found that young people in grade 8 who were socially connected, but not connected with school, were more likely to become regular smokers and use marijuana 2 years later, suggesting that students who do not have good school connectedness, regardless of their social relationships, are at greater risk for engaging in subsequent substance-use behaviors. A child's attachment to school appears to be a component of resilience, indicating that effective and responsive teachers, evidence-based curriculum, and classroom reinforcements may play an important role in substance-abuse prevention.

Peer Influences

There is a strong association between adolescent substance use and contact with drug-using peers. Research suggests that there may be social aspects of adolescent substance use in that other adolescents provide a unique source of access, reinforcement, and opportunity to use drugs (Kirke, 2004; Simons-Morton & Farhat, 2010). Urberg, Luo, Pilgrim, and Degirmencioglu (2003) and others have questioned the extent to which peer influence is responsible for adolescent substance use, claiming that there is a difference between *selection* and *influence* of friends. Adolescents tend to be similar to their friends with respect to behaviors, attitudes, and personality traits (Urberg, Değirmencioğlu, Tolson, & Halliday-Scher, 1995; Urberg et al., 2003), and similarities appear to be present even before friendships are established. Studies have proposed models suggesting that adolescents who choose substance-using friends may differ from those who do not. The quality of the friendship seems to also be a factor in determining the extent an individual may be influenced by a friend; a high-quality relationship may be more valued by the adolescent, who then may be more likely to change their behavior to please the friend. Better friends also may spend more time together, resulting in more modeling and emulation of deviant behavior. Additionally, the weight of their influence may be a function of other factors, such as parental monitoring, school rules regarding off-campus access during school hours, and so forth. Regardless of the difference between *selection* and *influence* of a friend, a more complete understanding of these complementary processes will greatly assist prevention science in developing ways to decrease the risk factors associated with acquiring and having substance-using friends (Prinstein & Wang, 2005; Tragesser, Aloise-Young, & Swaim, 2006).

Interestingly, one of the ways in which peers *appear* to influence one another is through the idea of "pluralistic ignorance" (Prentice & Miller, 1993). In other words, a subgroup of adolescents have a general belief that more individuals are engaging in substance use than actually are and, in turn, they themselves are more likely to then use substances (Prinstein & Wang, 2005; Tragesser, Aloise-Young, & Swaim, 2006). Conversely, those who believe that substance use will have harmful consequences are less likely to use. For example, a survey conducted by the Center of Addiction and Substance Abuse found that teens who viewed substance use favorably in terms of the benefits of substance use (e.g., popularity, weight control, self-medication, stress relief) were more likely to smoke, drink, and use other drugs than those who perceived use less favorable or had stronger perceptions of risk (CASA, 2011).

Understanding the contextual factors that increase or attenuate susceptibility to peer influence is crucial for the development of prevention and intervention programs. Research on the role of peers suggests that programs need to focus their efforts broadly on the multiple social contexts in which adolescents behave, and not just on peer influence, to be most successful.

Macro-Level Influences

The Neighborhood and Physical Environment

Social conditions in neighborhoods have important implications for risk for substance use; they shape social norms, enforce patterns of social control, influence perception of the risk of substance use, and effect psychological and physiological stress responses (Shonkoff & Phillips, 2000). Informal social controls and norms are vital and embraced for maintaining neighborhood viability, including issues such as observable violence, child maltreatment, and public consumption of illegal drugs, among other risky behaviors. In particular, decades of research have demonstrated that the risk for substance use is related to the prevailing norm toward substance use in the social environment (Elek, Miller-Day, & Hecht, 2006).

One aspect of neighborhood influence is the perception of social cohesion—an indicator of attachment to and satisfaction with the neighborhood and its residents and, thus, involves trust and support for one another in a community. Socially cohesive neighborhoods allow parents to depend on each other for help when needed to maintain norms for positive social behavior and communication in the neighborhood, and support each other in guiding children and adolescents. High social cohesion has been suggested to be associated with lower substance use among adolescents (Winstanley et al., 2008), fewer perceived youth drug problems (Duncan, Duncan, & Strycker, 2002), and lower drug-related mortalities (Anderson & Baumberg, 2006a, 2006b).

Another influential factor is the extent to which the neighborhood is perceived as disorganized or disordered—an area characterized by vandalism, abandoned buildings and lots, graffiti, noise, and dirt. The neighborhood context has been found to be particularly influential for low-income urban youth due to the high level of exposure to drug activity, disorder, and violence in their neighborhoods, all of which may influence substance use (Furr-Holden et al., 2011). Indeed, Lambert, Brown, Phillips, & Ialongo (2004) found that perceptions of neighborhood disorganization in grade 7 predicted increased tobacco, alcohol, and marijuana use in grade 9 among urban black youths. Additionally, Buu et al. (2009) reported that children whose neighborhoods became more stable from early childhood to adolescence tended to develop fewer alcohol-use disorder symptoms relative to children who remained in disorganized neighborhoods. Many aspects of the physical design of the environment can also harm young people's overall development (Leventhal & Brooks-Gunn, 2000; Shonkoff & Phillips, 2000), social relations, and crime, all of which have implications for substance use.

Decayed and abandoned buildings, ready access to alcohol and drugs, urbanization of the area, and neighborhood deprivation are associated with drugs, crime, violence, and accidents. High level of exposure to toxic substances (e.g., heavy metals, in utero alcohol, lead, cadmium, mercury, manganese, arsenic) is another aspect of the physical environment that can harm overall development. During the prenatal period and early childhood, such exposures have been strongly and consistently linked to functional deficits (e.g., cognitive dysfunction and psychological disorders; Bellinger, 2012), and later risk for substance abuse, as well as other forms of psychopathology. Lead exposure, in particular, at even only moderately elevated levels, has been shown to lead to mental retardation, and lower levels have been related to hyperactivity and violence in children. Although the research is scant with respect to their direct association with substance use, exposures are more definitively related to personal characteristics (e.g., psychiatric disorders, lack of impulse control, cognitive deficits) that are known to increase the risk for substance abuse (Andrade et al., 2014).

The media is one of the most insidious influences on social norms and other messages that are favorable toward substance use (Feinstein, Richter, & Foster, 2012). Adolescents in particular spend a great deal of time being entertained by television, movies, radio, the Internet, magazines, smartphones, and social media cites. In essence, these messages can make substance use appear to be normative behavior and can alter attitudes about the safety of substance use. As such, social media has been repeatedly linked to initiation of substance use (see Feinstein et al., 2012).

Income/Resources

Over the past few decades, a growing body of evidence has been amassed to help us better understand how overall conditions in impoverished communities lead to considerable delays or deficits in child and adolescent development (see Blair, 2010). Impoverished neighborhoods with a high rate of single-parent families, racial segregation, inequality (based on race, sex, or other characteristics), homelessness, transiency, and poorly equipped school and teachers are profound risk factors for substance use, along with high levels of child abuse, infant mortality, school dropout, academic failure, crime, delinquency, and mental illness.

On an individual level, poverty's influence on families and parenting can lead to harmful effects on child and youth development by increasing stress among parents and caregivers, by reducing their ability to invest in learning and educational opportunities, and by compromising their ability to be involved, patient, responsive, and nurturing parents to their children (Ginsburg, 2007). As previously described, all of these conditions—both individually and through their interaction—are risk factors for substance use. Indeed, many studies have demonstrated that economic adversity is associated with disruptions in parenting behaviors and that psychological distress in parents is linked to substance abuse in children (e.g., Jackson, Brooks-Gunn, Huang, & Glassman, 2000). Furthermore, the caregiving environment for low-income children is more likely to be disorganized and lacking in appropriate stimulation and support, thereby creating conditions that are stressful for children (Evans, 2004; Repetti, Taylor, & Seeman, 2002). And stress, in the context of an impoverished, unsupportive environment, impedes growth, leads to dysregulated physiological responses to stressful situations, increases risk for psychological disorders (e.g., depression, anxiety, and traumatic stress disorders), and compromises development of self-regulatory skills, key vulnerability factors in substance use.

Youth who experience poverty and/or a lack of resources are subject to a host of environmental and health factors including homelessness, street involvement, exposure to toxic substances, and work at a young age. As a result, there is a high incidence of behavioral and psychological problems, including use and abuse of substances, in these youth (Meltzer, Ford, Bebbington, & Vostanis, 2012; Nada & El Daw, 2010). In each of these scenarios, there is a lack of available services or supports (starting with assessments to identify and address particular needs) to lift children out of these circumstances (Marshall & Hadland, 2012). With increased availability of badly needed services for these children, plus political and healthcare involvement, there is potential for them to develop skills that would improve their chances of success in school and life, combatting many of the risk factors for substance abuse (Hudson & Nandy, 2012).

Public Policy/Government Influence

Despite governments' attempts to reduce disparity, certain racial, ethnic, income, and gender groups continue to receive differential treatment and have restricted access to the goods and services available in their society. Research has focused on understanding discrimination both as involving social processes that impact identifiable groups and as social acts experienced by individual members of that group. Discriminatory attitudes, policies, and practices limit the power, status, and wealth of these groups which contributes to patterns of social isolation and concentrated poverty (see Thompson, 2016). In turn, residents in these poor neighborhoods often tend to experience lower levels of physical and mental health, educational attainment, and employment, and exhibit higher levels of risk behaviors such as substance abuse compared to residents residing in more advantaged neighborhoods (Small & Newman, 2001).

The implications of discrimination and social exclusion for child development arise from both a structural and cultural perspective. Structural inequalities lead to adverse educational, health, and behavioral outcomes, and are largely due to differential access to material needs, such as adequate nutrition, quality housing and schools, as well as increased exposure to environmental toxins and hazards. Poor access to services and social supports and a lack of collective neighborhood efficacy compound the problem (Chou, 2012; Odgers et al., 2009; Saechao et al., 2012). Adding to the challenge is the lack of effective coping strategies that often characterize disadvantaged children. These problems tend to be compounded in individuals with an immigrant status. Cumulative adversity in immigrants, including language and legal status barriers (Perreira & Ornelas, 2013), perceived discrimination (Tran, Lee, & Burgess, 2010), and acculturation issues have all been related to risk for substance abuse and mental health problems.

An Integrative Perspective of the Etiology of Substance Use

Both Shonkoff's et al. (2012) and Bronfenbrenner's (1997) seminal works were instrumental in developing an initial framework for conceptualizing contextual influences on development. They propose that development is shaped by a range of nested, contextual systems whose joint impact is remarkably influential in healthy development. A clear demonstration of this (Mayberry, Espelage, & Koenig, 2009) found that adolescents' views of their school and community were associated with the amount of substance use they report. Moreover, these contextual systems acted as protective factors in relation to negative peer pressure and negative parenting attitudes and behavior. Prevention practices and interventions that focus on the *interaction* of communities, school, peers, parents, and individual development, and how they can influence each other as protective or risk factors for substance use, abuse, and addiction, are most powerful (see Brody et al., 2006; Hecht et al., 2003; Pantin et al., 2003). Programs need to train socialization agents to be better at what they do (e.g., parenting, teaching) as socialization defines the interaction between an individual, micro- and macroenvironments, and final outcomes.

In addition, preventive programs and interventions would benefit from integrative services that simultaneously consider various contexts of development, and the complex interrelated needs of individuals. Protective factors need to be developed and honed in the individual's peer group and family, and in the communities and schools. To truly understand the etiology of substance use with the critical mindset of prevention, one must understand developmental sequencing and how the aforementioned factors interact during distinct stages of development. Several important differences across stages of development influence outcomes in individuals who are exposed to the abovementioned factors and who exhibit the personal characteristics that have been related to propensity to experiment, use, and abuse substances. Each stage of development, from prenatal to early adulthood, is associated with a certain expected range of intellectual ability; language development; cognitive, emotional, and psychological functioning; and social competency skills that need attention to prevent the onset of substance abuse. Effective interventions that focus on these developmental milestones have been mapped to each stage as described in the foregoing.

In infancy, responsiveness to the environment and caregivers' interactions, and vice versa, and learning how to be effective in having needs met are of great importance for successful outcomes (Mullany et al., 2012—Family Spirit and Nurse-Family Partnership). Later, in early childhood, language, cooperation, control of emotions, collective conscience (cooperation), social and emotional skills, and problem-solving begin to develop and predict later social competence (Dishion et al., 2008—Early Steps Family Check-Up). Maintaining attention, controlling emotions, social inclusivity, effective communication, and reception emerge in middle childhood (Riggs, Greenberg, Kusché, & Pentz, 2006—Promoting Alternative Thinking Styles and Good Behavior Game). And in adolescence, social and emotional skills to establish stable relationships, sensitivity to needs of others, conflict resolution, prosocial skills, and impulse control are integral to self-regulation of emotion and behavior, which are predictive of favorable outcomes in early adulthood (Botvin & Griffin, 2004—Life Skills Training). Relatedly, delaying initiation of substance use in adolescence can be considered a goal for prevention policy. Each factor described above has an impact on the tendency to begin using substances early in adolescence, which has been repeatedly associated with risk for escalation and eventual abuse and addiction (e.g.,

McCabe, West, Morales, Cranford, & Boyd, 2007).

Given these differential levels of competency throughout childhood and adolescence, the social and physical environmental factors outlined above are expected to have different effects on the individual depending upon their developmental stage. Similarly, the phase of development must be considered when targeting interventions to particular risk factors, populations, and settings, as the programs themselves will be received and processed differently given the level of maturity in these processes. For example, the development of ECFs is a multistage process starting in early childhood when the building blocks for these higher order cognitive functions begin to form, followed by a period of complex refinement in adolescence (Zelazo & Carlson, 2012). The more complex features of executive cognitive functions (ECF) such as problem-solving, goal-setting, impulse control, and working memory only begin to surface in adolescence and do not coalesce until early adulthood (Geier & Luna, 2009). During adolescence, demands for coping with competing social, cognitive, biological, and academic changes are high and have important long-term implications for the emergence of risk behaviors (Petersen, Leffert, & Graham, 1995; Pope et al., 2003; Thadani, 2002). Taking into account the level of development of ECFs along with prevailing social demands of the individual helps to determine what type of interventions will work best—in terms of being understandable and executable—during adolescence as opposed to early stages when ECFs are much less developed. Given the prominent role of ECF deficits as an etiological factor in substance abuse, these are important considerations. The same issues are relevant for social and physical environmental risk factors which will exert different effects from a risk standpoint depending on the developmental period of exposure, as well as personal characteristics such as psychological disorders which develop and evolve over time.

Research has begun to explore the interactions of many of these influences in an effort to understand how they interact, shape, and affect each other. There is evidence that peers moderate neighborhood effects, such that high levels of positive peer support lead to a decrease in deviant behavior for children who live in impoverished neighborhoods. And community/school contexts have been found to moderate the association between parent/peer factors and adolescent substance use even after taking into account the variance that parents, peers, school, and community have individually on substance use (Mayberry, Espelage, & Koenig, 2009). In sum, the earlier and the more multifaceted the intervention is, the more effectively we can redirect behavioral pathways, increase resiliency, and reduce exposure to the potentially long-term adverse effects of the above etiological conditions, including the early use of drugs itself. In all cases, an enriched environment, external supports, and high-quality education are essential at all ages.

Crucially, sustaining the effort over time is critical to exert positive effects into late adolescence and early adulthood with appropriately different goals and approaches. Adolescence and early adulthood are not too late for intervention given the tremendous amount of brain plasticity and maturation of cognitive and emotional regulatory functions that are taking place, providing a window of opportunity to improve outcomes, such as substance use, abuse, and addiction. Many mental health, emotional, and behavioral problems result from impulsive, sensation-seeking activities among teenagers. And in adulthood, influences on these behaviors persist and require ongoing attention to prevent further escalation of use, addiction, and relapse.

Translational Implications of Etiological Research

Considerable evidence indicates that the myriad of behavioral problems are preventable; based on that knowledge, several evidence-based programs (EBPs) have emerged from various disciplinary perspectives. EBPs that focus on socio-emotional and cognitive functioning, development of which is particularly vulnerable to adverse psychosocial and environmental influences, may redirect and possibly normalize specific dimensions of a child's developmental pathway in behavioral, emotional, mental, and physical (e.g., brain function) domains. The effects of appropriately targeted interventions, even those that are universally implemented, may be particularly remarkable for children who are disadvantaged by poverty and other social ills. Research that integrates multiple disciplines to better understand influences and outcomes related to substance abuse have directed us toward solutions for these problems that target underlying mechanisms and not solely substance abuse, per se. It is vital that we address the factors that eventually lead to substance abuse prior to its development, the key behind prevention science.

Taking all the evidence together, the integrity of the way the brain develops from gestation through adolescence is a significant prerequisite for adaptive responses to socio-environmental challenges. Thanks to vast brain plasticity throughout childhood there is a great deal of variability in the way children develop in response to environmental inputs. This scenario throughout development provides an optimal window of opportunity for intervention. When neurodevelopment is on course or shows a trend toward improvement, overall intervention outcomes are likely to be favorable. In contrast, existing or emergent neurodevelopmental deficits or delays may compromise intervention effects, potentially explaining differential outcomes in response to even the most highly regarded and efficacious programs. A comprehensive evidence-based set of solutions (programs and policies) to prevent psychopathology and eventually substance abuse operate to enhance developmental indicators of brain function in multiple domains. This approach will, in turn, improve the ability to self-regulate behavior and reduce the risk for developing substance abuse.

Applying this integrative and developmental perspective will lead to significant advancements in our ability to prevent substance use and eventuality of abuse and addiction for some. Indeed, researchers have begun to incorporate cognitive training, mindfulness approaches, behavioral and environmental modifications, and other innovative strategies that target neurodevelopmental processes that contribute to substance abuse (Bryck & Fisher, 2012; Twamley, Narvaez, Becker, Bartels, & Jeste, 2008). There are many outstanding questions in this line of research; however, we do know enough about prevailing conditions that influence the risk for substance abuse to exert a positive impact now.

References

Adelman, H. S., & Taylor, L. (1999). Mental health in schools and system restructuring. *Clinical Psychology Review, 19*, 137–163.

Adlaf, E. M., Ivis, F. J., Smart, R. G., & Walsh, G. W. (1996). Enduring resurgence or statistical blip? Recent trends from the Ontario Student Drug Use Survey. *Canadian Journal of Public Health, 87*(3), 189–192.

Adler, N. E., & Rehkopf, D. H. (2008). US disparities in health: Descriptions, causes, and mechanisms. *Annual Review of Public Health, 29*, 235–252.

Andersen, S. L., & Teicher, M. H. (2008). Stress, sensitive periods and maturational events in adolescent depression. *Trends in Neurosciences, 31*(4), 183–191.

Anderson, P., & Baumberg, B. (2006a). Stakeholders' views of alcohol policy. Nordic Studies on Alcohol and Drugs, 23(6), 393-414.

Anderson, P., & Baumberg, B. (2006b). *Alcohol in Europe: A public health perspective*. A report for the European Commission.

Andrade, L. H., Alonso, J., Mneimneh, Z., Wells, J. E., Al-Hamzawi, A., Borges, G., ... Florescu, S. (2014). Barriers to mental health treatment: Results from the WHO World Mental Health surveys. *Psychological Medicine, 44*(6), 1303–1317.

Armstrong, T. D., & Costello, E. J. (2002). Community studies on adolescent substance use, abuse, or dependence and psychiatric comorbidity. *Journal of Consulting and Clinical Psychology, 70*(6), 1224.

Barrett, A. E., & Turner, R. J. (2005). Family structure and mental health: The mediating effects of socioeconomic status, family process, and social stress. *Journal of Health and Social Behaviors, 46*(2), 156–169.

Barrett, A. E., & Turner, R. J. (2006). Family structure and substance use problems in adolescence and early adulthood: Examining explanations for the relationship. *Addiction, 101*(1), 109–120.

Bellinger, D. C. (2012). Comparing the population neurodevelopmental burdens associated with children's exposures to environmental chemicals and other risk factors. *Neurotoxicology, 33*, 641–643.

Bierut, L. J. (2011). Genetic vulnerability and susceptibility to substance dependence. *Neuron, 69*(4), 618–627.

Blair, C. (2010). Stress and the development of self-regulation in context. *Child Development Perspectives, 4*, 181–188.

Bond, L., Butler, H., Thomas, L., Carlin, J., Glover, S., Bowes, G., & Patton, G. (2007). Social and school connectedness in early secondary school as predictors of late teenage substance use, mental health, and academic outcomes. *Journal of Adolescent Health, 40*(4), 357–3e9.

Bond, L., Patton, G., Glover, S., Carlin, J. B., Butler, H., Thomas, L., & Bowes, G. (2004). The Gatehouse Project: Can a multilevel school intervention affect emotional wellbeing and health risk behaviours? *Journal of Epidemiology and Community Health, 58*(12), 997–1003.

Botvin, G. J., & Griffin, K. W. (2004). Life skills training: Empirical findings and future directions. *Journal of Primary Prevention, 25*(2), 211–232.

Brody, G. H., Murry, V. M., Kogan, S. M., Gerrard, M., Gibbons, F. X., Molgaard, V., ... Wills, T. A. (2006). The Strong African American families program: A cluster-randomized prevention trial of long-term effects and a mediational model. *Journal of Consulting and Clinical Psychology, 74*(2), 356.

Bronfenbrenner, U. (1997). *The ecology of cognitive development: Research models and fugitive findings. College student development and academic life: Psychological, intellectual, social and moral issues.* New York: Garland.

Bryck, R. L., & Fisher, P. A. (2012). Training the brain: Practical applications of neural plasticity from the intersection of cognitive neuroscience, developmental psychology, and prevention science. *American Psychologist, 67*(2), 87.

Buu, A., Dipiazza, C., Wang, J., Puttler, L. I., Fitzgerald, H. E., & Zucker, R. A. (2009). Parent, family, and neighborhood effects on the development of child substance use and other psychopathology from preschool to the start of adulthood. *Journal of Studies on Alcohol and Drugs, 70*(4), 489–498.

Campbell, F. A., Ramey, C. T., Pungello, E., Sparling, J., & Miller-Johnson, S. (2002). Early childhood education: Young adult outcomes from the Abecedarian Project. *Applied Developmental Science, 6*(1), 42–57.

Casey, B. J., & Jones, R. M. (2010). Neurobiology of the adolescent brain and behavior: Implications for substance use disorders. *Journal of the American Academy of Child & Adolescent Psychiatry, 49*(12), 1189–1201.

Casey, B. J., Jones, R. M., & Hare, T. A. (2008). The adolescent brain. *Annals of the New York Academy of Sciences, 1124*(1), 111–126.

Catalano, R. F., Oesterle, S., Fleming, C. B., & Hawkins, J. D. (2004). The importance of bonding to school for healthy development: Findings from the Social Development Research Group. *Journal of School Health, 74*(7), 252–261.

Chapman, D. P., Whitfield, C. L., Felitti, V. J., Dube, S. R., Edwards, V. J., & Anda, R. F. (2004). Adverse childhood experiences and the risk of depressive disorders in adulthood. *Journal of Affective Disorders, 82*(2), 217–225.

Chou, K. L. (2012). Perceived discrimination and depression among new migrants to Hong Kong: The moderating role of social support and neighborhood collective efficacy. *Journal of Affective Disorders, 138*, 63–70.

Child and Adolescent Health Measurement Initiative (2005). National Survey of Children's Health, 2003. Data Resource Center on Child and Adolescent Health Web site. Available at: www.childhealthdata.org.

Christle, C. A., Jolivette, K., & Nelson, C. M. (2005). Breaking the school to prison pipeline: Identifying school risk and protective factors for youth delinquency. *Exceptionality, 13*(2), 69–88.

Cleveland, M. J., Feinberg, M. E., Bontempo, D. E., & Greenberg, M. T. (2008). The role of risk and protective factors in substance use across adolescence. *Journal of Adolescent Health, 43*(2), 157–164.

Conrod, P. J., O'Leary-Barrett, M., Newton, N., Topper, L., Castellanos-Ryan, N., Mackie, C., & Girard, A. (2013). Effectiveness of a selective, personality-targeted prevention program for adolescent alcohol use and misuse: A cluster randomized controlled trial. *JAMA Psychiatry, 70*(3), 334–342.

Cornelius, M. D., Goldschmidt, L., & Day, N. L. (2012). Prenatal cigarette smoking: Long-term effects on young adult behavior problems and smoking behavior. *Neurotoxicology and Teratology, 34*, 554–559.

Darling-Hamond, L. (2000). Teacher quality and student academic achievement: A review of state policy evidence. *Education Policy Archives, 8*, 1–44.

Davidson, R. J. (1994). Asymmetric brain function, affective style and psychopathology: The role of early experience and plasticity. *Development and Psychopathology, 6*, 741–758.

De Bellis, M. D. (2002). Developmental traumatology: A contributory mechanism for alcohol and substance use disorders. *Psychoneuroendocrinology, 27*, 155–170.

De Micheli, D., & Formigoni, M. L. O. (2002). Are reasons for the first use of drugs and family circumstances predictors of future use patterns? *Addictive Behaviors, 27*(1), 87–100.

DiNieri, J. A., Wang, X., Szutorisz, H., Spano, S. M., Kaur, J., Casaccia, P., ... Hurd, Y. L. (2011). Maternal cannabis use alters ventral striatal dopamine D2 gene regulation in the offspring. *Biological Psychiatry, 70*, 763–769.

Dishion, T. J., Shaw, D., Connell, A., Gardner, F., Weaver, C., & Wilson, M. (2008). The family check-up With high-risk indigent families: Preventing problem behavior by increasing parents' positive behavior support in early childhood. *Child Development, 79*(5), 1395–1414.

Dube, S. R., Felitti, V. J., Dong, M., Chapman, D. P., Giles, W. H., & Anda, R. F. (2003). Childhood abuse, neglect, and household dysfunction and the risk of illicit drug use: The adverse childhood experiences study. *Pediatrics, 111*(3), 564–572.

Duncan, G. J., & Murnane, R. J. (Eds.). (2011). *Whither opportunity?: Rising inequality, schools, and children's life chances.* New York: Russell Sage Foundation.

Duncan, S. C., Duncan, T. E., & Strycker, L. A. (2002). A multilevel analysis of neighborhood context and youth alcohol and drug problems. *Prevention Science, 3*, 125–133.

Elek, E., Miller-Day, M., & Hecht, M. L. (2006). Influences of personal, injunctive, and descriptive norms on early adolescent substance use. *Journal of Drug Issues, 36*, 147–172.

Engle, P. L., & Black, M. M. (2008). The effect of poverty on child development and educational outcomes. *Annals of the New York Academy of Sciences, 1136*(1), 243–256.

Ernst, M., & Mueller, S. C. (2008). The adolescent brain: Insights from functional neuroimaging research. *Developmental Neurobiology, 68*, 729–743.

Evans, G. W. (2004). The environment of childhood poverty. *American Psychologist, 59*, 77–92.

Feinstein, E. C., Richter, L., & Foster, S. E. (2012). Addressing the critical health problem of adolescent substance use through health care, research, and public policy. *Journal of Adolescent Health, 50*, 431–436.

Fishbein, D. H., Herman-Stahl, M., Eldreth, D., Paschall, M. J., Hyde, C., Hubal, R., ... Ialongo, N. (2006). Mediators of the stress–substance–use relationship in urban male adolescents. *Prevention Science, 7*(2), 113–126.

Frank, M. J., Moustafa, A. A., Haughey, H. M., Curran, T., & Hutchison, K. E. (2007). Genetic triple dissociation reveals multiple roles for dopamine in reinforcement learning. *Proceedings of the National Academy of Sciences, 104*(41), 16311–16316.

Furr-Holden, C. D. M., Lee, M. H., Milam, A. J., Johnson, R. M., Lee, K. S., & Ialongo, N. S. (2011). The growth of neighborhood disorder and marijuana use among urban adolescents: A case for policy and environmental interventions. *Journal of Studies on Alcohol and Drugs, 72*, 371–379.

Geier, C., & Luna, B. (2009). The maturation of incentive processing and cognitive control. *Pharmacology Biochemistry and Behavior, 93*(3), 212–221.

Giedd, J. N., Blumenthal, J., Jeffries, N. O., Castellanos, F. X., Liu, H., Zijdenbos, A., ... Rapoport, J. L. (1999). Brain development during childhood and adolescence: A longitudinal MRI study. *Nature Neuroscience, 2*(10), 861.

Ginsburg, K. R. (2007). The importance of play in promoting healthy child development and maintaining strong parent-child bonds. *Pediatrics, 119*(1), 182–191.

Glaser, D. (2000). Child abuse and neglect and the brain—a review. *The Journal of Child Psychology and Psychiatry and Allied Disciplines, 41*(1), 97–116.

Gogtay, N., Giedd, J. N., Lusk, L., Hayashi, K. M., Greenstein, D., Vaituzis, A. C., ... Rapoport, J. L. (2004). Dynamic mapping of human cortical development during childhood through early adulthood. *Proceedings of the National Academy of Sciences, 101*(21), 8174–8179.

Greco, B., & Carli, M. (2006). Reduced attention and increased impulsivity in mice lacking NPY Y2 receptors: Relation to anxiolytic-like phenotype. *Behavioural Brain Research, 169*(2), 325–334.

Hardin, M. G., & Ernst, M. (2009). Functional brain imaging of development-related risk and vulnerability for substance use in adolescents. *Journal of Addiction Medicine, 3*(2), 47.

Hare, T. A., O'Doherty, J., Camerer, C. F., Schultz, W., & Rangel, A. (2008). Dissociating the role of the orbitofrontal cortex and the striatum in the computation of goal values and prediction errors. *Journal of Neuroscience, 28*(22), 5623–5630.

Hatzinger, M., Brand, S., Perren, S., von Wyl, A., von Klitzing, K., & Holsboer-Trachsler, E. (2007). Hypothalamic–pituitary–adrenocortical (HPA) activity in kindergarten children: Importance of gender and associations with behavioral/emotional difficulties. *Journal of Psychiatric Research, 41*(10), 861–870.

Hayaki, J., Stein, M. D., Lassor, J. A., Herman, D. S., & Anderson, B. J. (2005). Adversity among drug users: Relationship to impulsivity. *Drug and Alcohol Dependence, 78*(1), 65.

Hecht, M. L., Marsiglia, F. F., Elek, E., Wagstaff, D. A., Kulis, S., Dustman, P., & Miller-Day, M. (2003). Culturally grounded substance use prevention: An evaluation of the keepin' it REAL curriculum. *Prevention Science, 4*(4), 233–248.

Herrenkohl, T. I., Lee, J. O., Kosterman, R., & Hawkins, J. D. (2012). Family influences related to adult substance use and mental health problems: A developmental analysis of child and adolescent predictors. *Journal of Adolescent Health, 51*, 129–135.

Hudson, A. L., & Nandy, K. (2012). Comparisons of substance abuse, high-risk sexual behavior and depressive symptoms among homeless youth with and without a history of foster care placement. *Contemporary Nurse, 42*, 178–186.

Huether, G. (1998). Stress and the adaptive self-organization of neuronal connectivity during early childhood. *International Journal of Neuroscience, 16*, 297–306.

Hussong, A. M., Jones, D. J., Stein, G. L., Baucom, D. H., & Boeding, S. (2011). An internalizing pathway to alcohol use and disorder. *Psychology of Addictive Behaviors, 25*(3), 390.

Jackson, A. P., Brooks-Gunn, J., Huang, C. C., & Glassman, M. (2000). Single mothers in low-wage jobs: Financial strain, parenting, and preschoolers' outcomes. *Child Development, 71*, 1409–1423.

Jutras-Aswad, D., Jacobs, M. M., Yiannoulos, G., Roussos, P., Bitsios, P., Nomura, Y., ... Hurd, Y. L. (2012). Cannabis-dependence risk relates to synergism between neuroticism and proenkephalin SNPs associated with amygdala gene expression: Case-control study. *PLoS One, 7*(6), e39243.

Kandel, D. B. (2002). *Stages and pathways of drug involvement: Examining the gateway hypothesis*. Cambridge: Cambridge University Press.

Kendler, K. S., Prescott, C. A., Myers, J., & Neale, M. C. (2003). The structure of genetic and environmental risk factors for common psychiatric and substance use disorders in men and women. *Archives of General Psychiatry, 60*(9), 929–937.

Kirke, D. M. (2004). Chain reactions in adolescents' cigarette, alcohol, and drug use: Similarity through peer influence or the patterning of ties in peer networks. *Social Networks, 26,* 3–28.

Klein, T. A., Neumann, J., Reuter, M., Hennig, J., von Cramon, D. Y., & Ullsperger, M. (2007). Genetically determined differences in learning from errors. *Science, 318*(5856), 1642–1645.

Koob, G. F., & Le Moal, M. (1997). Substance abuse: Hedonic homeostatic dysregulation. *Science, 278,* 52–58.

Kosterman, R., Hawkins, J. D., Haggerty, K. P., Spoth, R., & Redmond, C. (2001). Preparing for the drug free years: Session-specific effects of a universal parent-training intervention with rural families. *Journal of Drug Education, 31*(1), 47–68.

Kovacs, M., & Goldston, D. (1991). Cognitive and social cognitive development of depressed children and adolescents. *Journal of the American Academy of Child & Adolescent Psychiatry, 30,* 388–392.

Kreek, M. J., Nielsen, D. A., Butelman, E. R., & LaForge, K. S. (2005). Genetic influences on impulsivity, risk taking, stress responsivity and vulnerability to substance abuse and addiction. *Nature Neuroscience, 8,* 1450–1457.

Lambert, S. F., Brown, T. L., Phillips, C. M., & Ialongo, N. S. (2004). The relationship between perceptions of neighborhood characteristics and substance use among urban African American adolescents. *American Journal of Community Psychology, 34*(3-4), 205.

Le Foll, B., Gallo, A., Le Strat, Y., Lu, L., & Gorwood, P. (2009). Genetics of dopamine receptors and drug addiction: A comprehensive review. *Behavioral Pharmacology, 20,* 1–17.

Lee, C. M., Neighbors, C., & Woods, B. A. (2007). Marijuana motives: Young adults' reasons for using marijuana. *Addictive Behaviors, 32*(7), 1384–1394.

Lerman, C., & Niaura, R. (2002). Applying genetic approaches to the treatment of nicotine dependence. *Oncogene, 21*(48), 7412.

Leventhal, T., & Brooks-Gunn, J. (2000). The neighborhoods they live in: The effects of neighborhood residence on child and adolescent outcomes. *Psychological Bulletin, 126,* 309–337.

Li, M. D. (2006). The genetics of nicotine dependence. *Current Psychiatry Reports, 8*(2), 158–164.

Liddle, H. A., Rowe, C. L., Dakof, G. A., Ungaro, R. A., & Henderson, C. E. (2004). Early intervention for adolescent substance abuse: Pretreatment to posttreatment outcomes of a randomized clinical trial comparing multidimensional family therapy and peer group treatment. *Journal of Psychoactive Drugs, 36*(1), 49–63.

Lippold, M. A., Greenberg, M. T., Graham, J. W., & Feinberg, M. E. (2014). Unpacking the effect of parental monitoring on early adolescent problem behavior mediation by parental knowledge and moderation by parent–youth warmth. *Journal of Family Issues, 35*(13), 1800–1823.

Lovallo, W. R. (2012). Early life adversity reduces stress reactivity and enhances impulsive behavior: Implications for health behaviors. *International Journal of Psychophysiology, S0167-8760*(12), 00622–00628.

Madu, S. N., & Matla, M. Q. P. (2003). Illicit drug use, cigarette smoking and alcohol drinking behaviour among a sample of high school adolescents in the Pietersburg area of the Northern Province, South Africa. *Journal of Adolescence, 26*(1), 121–136.

Marshall, B. D., & Hadland, S. E. (2012). The immediate and lasting effects of adolescent homelessness on suicidal ideation and behavior. *Journal of Adolescent Health, 51,* 407–408.

Mason, M. J., Valente, T. W., Coatsworth, J. D., Mennis, J., Lawrence, F., & Zelenak, P. (2010). Place-based social network quality and correlates of substance use among urban adolescents. *Journal of Adolescence, 33,* 419–427.

Mayberry, M. L., Espelage, D. L., & Koenig, B. (2009). Multilevel modeling of direct effects and interactions of peers, parents, school, and community influences on adolescent substance use. *Journal of Youth and Adolescence, 38*(8), 1038–1049.

McCabe, S. E., West, B. T., Morales, M., Cranford, J. A., & Boyd, C. J. (2007). Does early onset of non-medical use of prescription drugs predict subsequent prescription drug abuse and dependence? Results from a national study. *Addiction, 102*(12), 1920–1930.

McEwen, B. S., & Morrison, J. H. (2013). The brain on stress: Vulnerability and plasticity of the prefrontal cortex over the life course. *Neuron, 79*(1), 16–29.

Meltzer, H., Ford, T., Bebbington, P., & Vostanis, P. (2012). Children who run away from home: Risks for suicidal behavior and substance misuse. *Journal of Adolescent Health, 51,* 415–421.

Mullany, B., Barlow, A., Neault, N., Billy, T., Jones, T., Tortice, I., … Walkup, J. (2012). The family spirit trial for American Indian teen mothers and their children: CBPR rationale, design, methods and baseline characteristics. *Prevention Science, 13*(5), 504–518.

Munakata, Y., Herd, S. A., Chatham, C. H., Depue, B. E., Banich, M. T., & O'Reilly, R. C. (2011). A unified framework for inhibitory control. *Trends in Cognitive Sciences, 15*(10), 453–459.

Nada, K. H., & El Daw, A. S. (2010). Violence, abuse, alcohol and drug use, and sexual behaviors in street children of Greater Cairo and Alexandria, Egypt. *AIDS, 24,* S39–S44.

Nelson, C. A., & Carver, L. J. (1998). The effects of stress and trauma on brain and memory: A view from developmental cognitive neuroscience. *Development and Psychopathology, 10*(4), 793–809.

Nehring, I., Lehmann, S., & Von Kries, R. (2013). Gestational weight gain in accordance to the IOM/NRC criteria and the risk for childhood overweight: a meta-analysis. *Pediatric obesity, 8*(3), 218–224.

Odgers, C. L., Moffitt, T. E., Tach, L. M., Sampson, R. J., Taylor, A., Matthews, C. L., & Caspi, A. (2009). The protective effects of neighborhood collective efficacy on British children growing up in deprivation: A developmental analysis. *Developmental Psychology, 45*, 942.

Padmanabhan, A., Geier, C. F., Ordaz, S. J., Teslovich, T., & Luna, B. (2011). Developmental changes in brain function underlying the influence of reward processing on inhibitory control. *Developmental Cognitive Neuroscience, 1*(4), 517–529.

Pantin, H., Coatsworth, J. D., Feaster, D. J., Newman, F. L., Briones, E., Prado, G., … Szapocznik, J. (2003). Familias Unidas: The efficacy of an intervention to promote parental investment in Hispanic immigrant families. *Prevention Science, 4*(3), 189–201.

Pechmann, C., Levine, L., Loughlin, S., & Leslie, F. (2005). Impulsive and self-conscious: Adolescents' vulnerability to advertising and promotion. *Journal of Public Policy & Marketing, 24*(2), 202–221.

Pechtel, P., & Pizzagalli, D. A. (2011). Effects of early life stress on cognitive and affective function: An integrated review of human literature. *Psychopharmacology, 214*(1), 55–70.

Perreira, K. M., & Ornelas, I. (2013). Painful passages: Traumatic experiences and post-traumatic stress among US Immigrant Latino adolescents and their primary caregivers. *International Migration Review, 47*(4), 976–1005.

Perry, J. L., Joseph, J. E., Jiang, Y., Zimmerman, R. S., Kelly, T. H., Darna, M., … Bardo, M. T. (2011). Prefrontal cortex and drug abuse vulnerability: Translation to prevention and treatment interventions. *Brain Research Reviews, 65*(2), 124–149.

Petersen, A. C., Leffert, N., & Graham, B. L. (1995). Adolescent development and the emergence of sexuality. *Suicide and Life-Threatening Behavior, 25*, 4–17.

Piper, B. J., & Corbett, S. M. (2011). Executive function profile in the offspring of women that smoked during pregnancy. *Nicotine & Tobacco Research, 14*(2), 191–199.

Pope, H. G., Jr., Gruber, A. J., Hudson, J. I., Cohane, G., Huestis, M. A., & Yurgelun-Todd, D. (2003). Early-onset cannabis use and cognitive deficits: What is the nature of the association? *Drug and Alcohol Dependence, 69*(3), 303–310.

Prentice, D. A., & Miller, D. T. (1993). Pluralistic ignorance and alcohol use on campus: Some consequences of misperceiving the social norm. *Journal of Personality and Social Psychology, 64*(2), 243.

Prinstein, M. J., & Wang, S. S. (2005). False consensus and adolescent peer contagion: Examining discrepancies between perceptions and actual reported levels of friends' deviant and health risk behaviors. *Journal of Abnormal Child Psychology, 33*(3), 293–306.

Repetti, R. L., Taylor, S. E., & Seeman, T. E. (2002). Risky families: Family social environments and the mental and physical health of offspring. *Psychological Bulletin, 128*(2), 330.

Riggs, N. R., Greenberg, M. T., Kusché, C. A., & Pentz, M. A. (2006). The mediational role of neurocognition in the behavioral outcomes of a social-emotional prevention program in elementary school students: Effects of the PATHS curriculum. *Prevention Science, 7*(1), 91–102.

Robinson, T. E., & Berridge, K. C. (2000). The psychology and neurobiology of addiction: An incentive–sensitization view. *Addiction, 95*, 91–117.

Saechao, F., Sharrock, S., Reicherter, D., Livingston, J. D., Aylward, A., Whisnant, J., … Kohli, S. (2012). Stressors and barriers to using mental health services among diverse groups of first-generation immigrants to the United States. *Community Mental Health Journal, 48*, 98–106.

Shay, N. L., & Knutson, J. F. (2008). Maternal depression and trait anger as risk factors for escalated physical discipline. *Child Maltreatment, 13*, 39–49.

Shonkoff, J. P., Garner, A. S., Siegel, B. S., Dobbins, M. I., Earls, M. F., McGuinn, L., … Committee on Early Childhood, Adoption, and Dependent Care. (2012). The lifelong effects of early childhood adversity and toxic stress. *Pediatrics, 129*(1), e232–e246.

Shonkoff, J. P., & Phillips, D. A. (2000). *From neurons to neighborhoods: The science of early childhood development*. Washington, DC: National Academy Press.

Simons-Morton, B., & Chen, R. S. (2006). Over time relationships between early adolescent and peer substance use. *Addictive Behaviors, 31*(7), 1211–1223.

Simons-Morton, B. G., & Farhat, T. (2010). Recent findings on peer group influences on adolescent smoking. *The Journal of Primary Prevention, 31*(4), 191–208.

Sinha, R. (2001). How does stress increase risk of substance abuse and relapse? *Psychopharmacology, 158*, 343–359.

Sithisarn, T., Granger, D. T., & Bada, H. S. (2012). Consequences of prenatal substance use. *International Journal of Adolescent Medicine and Health, 24*, 105–112.

Small, M. L., & Newman, K. (2001). Urban poverty after the truly disadvantaged: The rediscovery of the family, the neighborhood, and culture. *Annual Review of Sociology, 27*, 23–45.

Somerville, L. H., Jones, R. M., & Casey, B. J. (2010). A time of change: Behavioral and neural correlates of adolescent sensitivity to appetitive and aversive environmental cues. *Brain and Cognition, 72*(1), 124–133.

Springer, K. W., Sheridan, J., Kuo, D., & Carnes, M. (2007). Long-term physical and mental health consequences of childhood physical abuse: Results from a large population-based sample of men and women. *Child Abuse & Neglect, 31*, 517–530.

Steinberg, L., Albert, D., Cauffman, E., Banich, M., Graham, S., & Woolard, J. (2008). Age differences in sensation seeking and impulsivity as indexed by behavior and self-report: Evidence for a dual systems model. *Developmental Psychology, 44*(6), 1764.

Substance Abuse and Mental Health Services Administration (SAMHSA) (2011) *Results from the 2010 National Survey on Drug use and Health: Summary of national findings* (NSDUH Series H-41, HHS Publication No. (SMA) 11-4658). Rockville, MD: Office of Applied Studies.

Teicher, M. H., Rabi, K., Sheu, Y. S., Seraphin, S. B., Andersen, S. L., Anderson, C. M., & Tomoda, A. (2010). Neurobiology of childhood trauma and adversity. In R. A. Lanius & E. Vermetten (Eds.), *The impact of early life trauma on health and disease: The hidden epidemic* (pp. 112–122). Cambridge: Cambridge University Press.

Thadani, P. V. (2002). The intersection of stress, substance abuse and development. *Psychoneuroendocrinology, 27*, 221–230.

The National Center on Addiction and Substance Abuse (CASA) at Columbia University. (2011). *Adolescent substance use: America's #1 public health problem* (p. 406). New York: CASA.

Thompson, N. (2016). *Anti-discriminatory practice: Equality, diversity and social justice*. Basingstoke: Palgrave Macmillan.

Tomlinson, K. L., Brown, S. A., & Abrantes, A. (2004). Psychiatric comorbidity and substance use treatment outcomes of adolescents. *Psychology of Addictive Behaviors, 18*, 160–169.

Tragesser, S. L., Aloise-Young, P. A., & Swaim, R. C. (2006). Peer influence, images of smokers, and beliefs about smoking among preadolescent nonsmokers. *Social Development, 15*(2), 311–325.

Tran, A. G., Lee, R. M., & Burgess, D. J. (2010). Perceived discrimination and substance use in Hispanic/Latino, African-born Black, and Southeast Asian immigrants. *Cultural Diversity and Ethnic Minority Psychology, 16*(2), 226.

Twamley, E. W., Narvaez, J. M., Becker, D. R., Bartels, S. J., & Jeste, D. V. (2008). Supported employment for middle-aged and older people with schizophrenia. *American Journal of Psychiatric Rehabilitation, 11*(1), 76–89.

Urberg, K. A., Değirmencioğlu, S. M., Tolson, J. M., & Halliday-Scher, K. (1995). The structure of adolescent peer networks. *Developmental Psychology, 31*(4), 540.

Urberg, K. A., Luo, Q., Pilgrim, C., & Degirmencioglu, S. M. (2003). A two-stage model of peer influence in adolescent substance use: Individual and relationship-specific differences in susceptibility to influence. *Addictive Behaviors, 28*(7), 1243–1256.

Velleman, R. D., Templeton, L. J., & Copello, A. G. (2005). The role of the family in preventing and intervening with substance use and misuse: A comprehensive review of family interventions, with a focus on young people. *Drug and Alcohol Review, 24*(2), 93–109.

Vink, J. M., Willemsen, G., & Boomsma, D. I. (2005). Heritability of smoking initiation and nicotine dependence. *Behavior Genetics, 35*(4), 397–406.

Winstanley, E. L., Steinwachs, D. M., Ensminger, M. E., Latkin, C. A., Stitzer, M. L., & Olsen, Y. (2008). The association of self-reported neighborhood disorganization and social capital with adolescent alcohol and drug use, dependence, and access to treatment. *Drug and Alcohol Dependence, 92*, 173–182.

Wood, M. D., Read, J. P., Mitchell, R. E., & Brand, N. H. (2004). Do parents still matter? Parent and peer influences on alcohol involvement among recent high school graduates. *Psychology of Addictive Behaviors, 18*(1), 19.

Yoshikawa, H., Aber, J. L., & Beardslee, W. R. (2012). The effects of poverty on the mental, emotional, and behavioral health of children and youth: Implications for prevention. *American Psychologist, 67*(4), 272.

Zelazo, P. D., & Carlson, S. M. (2012). Hot and cool executive function in childhood and adolescence: Development and plasticity. *Child Development Perspectives, 6*(4), 354–360.

Zuckerman, M., & Kuhlman, D. M. (2000). Personality and risk-taking: Common biosical factors. *Journal of Personality, 68*(6), 999–1029.

Genetics and Epigenetics of Substance Use

Michael M. Vanyukov and Ralph E. Tarter

Introduction

Psychoactive substance use is a behavior that occurs in various contexts, therapeutic and recreational. It is mainly the latter that is under review herein, considered from the standpoint that the existence of the human organism is impossible without, and thus is fully determined by, both its genome and its environment. No research in biological systems would be complete without studying what controls development and function, i.e., the genetic program and the epigenetic mechanisms[1] that regulate its unfolding. It would be equally limiting not to consider the circumstances under which these systems develop and function, i.e., the environment.

Despite its name, genetic research addresses both genetics and the environment—from two general causal perspectives. One perspective considers *mechanistic* causes of individual development and function, relating the structure and function of genetic material as such (genome and epigenome) and the structure and function of the enzymes and polypeptides of metabolic and neurobiological paths that comprise the organism's response to psychoactive substances. The other perspective addresses causes of *individual phenotypic variation* and has two complementary aspects. One of them, biometric genetics, deals with the quantitative evaluation of genetic contribution to individual differences in the population, known as heritability—along with the contributions of nongenetic (environmental) causes of variation. The other aspect, molecular genetic, addresses the material content of these statistical variance components. This content is variation in the chemical structure of specific genes and in concrete environmental factors that could account for individual variation in the probability of behaviors such as psychoactive substance use (herein termed substance use).

Both mechanistic and variation perspectives inform each other. For instance, the search for genetic variations (polymorphisms[2]) contributing

---

[1] Broadly, epigenetic mechanisms are those that influence gene expression (see the *Epigenetics* section below). Although some epigenetic changes are due to changes in the DNA structure, those changes are dynamic modifications (methylation and demethylation), rather than stable mutations, of one of the four of DNA-building blocks (cytosine). Other epigenetic changes occur in proteins surrounding DNA, histones, reversibly enabling or disabling DNA transcription into RNA. Yet other epigenetic mechanisms are due to modulation of DNA transcription (or RNA translation into peptides and proteins) by microRNAs (miRNAs).

[2] The presence in the population of more than one structural variant (allele) at a particular location (locus) of the DNA molecule comprises a polymorphism.

M. M. Vanyukov (✉) · R. E. Tarter
University of Pittsburgh, Pittsburgh, PA, USA
e-mail: mmv@pitt.edu

to substance use-related phenotypic variation began from the genes known to be involved in addictive substances' metabolism and neurobiological mechanisms of action. An as-yet unknown mechanism may be suggested by a finding of a genetic association obtained in a genome-wide association study (GWAS). Significant heritability as estimated in biometric genetic studies is often a precondition for attempting to find genetic polymorphisms contributing to phenotypic variation. For traits whose heritability is (very) low, searching for genetic variation that determines that heritability may be less practical than focusing on other, e.g., environmental, causes of individual differences.

Both biometric and molecular genetic aspects of variation pertaining to substance use, abuse, and addiction have been accorded considerable attention. Albeit relatively recent, epigenetic data have also been accumulating. Despite these successes, there are also continuing conceptual and methodological problems that both hinder discovery in these areas and hamper translation of the results into practice. While not purporting to be exhaustive in covering this large area of research, this chapter critically reviews relevant literature, focusing on human studies, and suggests possible directions to expanding its progress with a special focus on etiological implications for prevention.

The Trait and the Phenotypes in Substance (Ab)use

Ever since Mendel's discoveries over 150 years ago, it has been known that the trait and its definition (along with, in his case, the experimental object) are critically important for genetic research. Indeed, Mendel's experiments with asexually reproducing hawkweed (*Hieracium*) questioned the generalizability of his foundational findings with peas. Even after the rediscovery of Mendel's laws, scientists thought for some time that there existed another set of laws, the "Hieracium type of inheritance" as opposed to the "Pisum type of inheritance" (Nogler, 2006). Nevertheless, Mendelian inheritance was confirmed not only for plants but also for many human characteristics, including some diseases, representing the so-called monogenic or Mendelian traits. Unfortunately, the traits that are under study in human behavior, and in substance use in particular, are much more complex in both their mechanisms and the causes of their variation than the traits that Mendel dealt with in peas and hawkweed. Mendelian inheritance is due to a trait's (almost) perfect covariation with a single gene (the discrete phenotypes correspond to the genotypes for that gene). Variation in the traits related to substance use behavior is not determined entirely by genes, let alone by any single gene. Nor is this behavior fully determined by its apparent direct cause, drugs of abuse, and their availability, because drugs' ending up in a human organism most often results from a willful act and active drug procurement.

Substance abuse costs society over $600 billion a year (Volkow, 2012), which is still not an adequate reflection of the human cost of substance abuse. Although this estimate is over five years old, it is unlikely that the cost has diminished, considering that there has been no decrease in addiction prevalence over the years: for example, past month illicit drug use among people aged 18–25 was 19.4% in 2004, and 22.0% ten years later (SAMHSA, 2015). Interestingly, in the 12–17 age group, past month illicit drug use did not appreciably change, but the use of licit substances (which are not legal at this age range), tobacco and alcohol, declined by half. The illicit drug use statistics also contrast with another behavior-related problem, HIV infection, for which the annual number of new diagnoses declined by 19% during the same period (CDC, 2016).

The persistence of substance abuse and addiction despite the enormous resources expended on controlling drug supply and exposure suggests the continued inadequacy of the preventive measures applied. A former "drug czar" (the director of the White House Office of National Drug Control Policy) has suggested that the "old war on drugs" was wrong because of the prior lack of "scientific understanding" of addiction (CBS News, 2015). Nevertheless, there has been substantial progress in research—unsurprisingly, considering that substance-use problems are directly dealt with by two NIH institutes, National Institute on Drug Abuse and National Institute on Alcohol Abuse and Alcoholism, as well as by other governmental organizations and private foundations. Wars—on drugs or otherwise,—however, have not necessarily been waged scientifically. Moreover, the application of research findings to prevention and treatment may have been hindered not only by their shortage or by resistance to change, but also by objective difficulties, many of which are the same as those complicating research and related to the nature of the traits under study.

For instance, in contrast to other psychiatric disorders, addiction is commonly recognized as largely a direct natural outcome of *voluntary* substance use. The perception that substance use is a voluntary behavior is inevitably followed by stigmatization regardless of how it is labeled medically (Vanyukov et al., 2012). Stigmatization is also related to criminalization, which is stigmatization's legal form, although the image of an addict in any event has never been attractive or even neutral (smoking is an exception that proves the rule). Stigmatization is a term that is used indiscriminately, to denote what may be viewed as prejudice as well as what is shunned as harmful behavior. In the latter case, however, stigmatization, an ancient social mechanism of behavior regulation, which has often evolved—for better or worse—into legal constraints on behavior, may have positive impact: the societal stigmata may prevent engaging in that behavior. In contrast, legalization (e.g., of cannabis use) may achieve the opposite: unjustified decrease in risk and harm perception (e.g., Mandelbaum & de la Monte, 2017). The social and legal status of a substance is a potent environmental factor having numerous points of influence—from forming the individual threshold to substance experimentation and use to determining the composition of phenotypic variance. This influence is mediated by the differential availability of substances but also by the individual response to the societal restrictions on substance use. Moreover, liabilities to addictions to licit and illicit substances comprise two respective genetically related but distinct groups (Kendler, Myers, & Prescott, 2007).

Another problem is that, as is usual with distinction between the norm and the pathology in psychiatry, there is also no clear distinction between the clinically significant phenotypes—addicted and nonaddicted. The term "addiction" that we use here interchangeably with "substance use disorder" (SUD) stands for compulsive pursuit of drugs. This differs from "substance dependence," which is a normal physiological response to chronic drug exposure that may or may not be present in addiction and does not necessarily connote addiction, and whose adoption in clinical classification has been called "a serious mistake" (O'Brien, Volkow, & Li, 2006). The DSM-5 (American Psychiatric Association, 2013) SUD symptoms almost exclusively describe behaviors (e.g., "Taking the substance in larger amounts or for longer than the you meant to"; "Using substances again and again, even when it puts the you in danger"). Addiction is therefore defined as a behavioral phenotype reflecting impaired control, social impairment, risky use, and, to a lesser degree, physiological status (withdrawal and tolerance). Since there are hundreds of combinations of the 11 DSM-5 SUD symptoms, any two of which sufficing for a positive diagnosis, this phenotype is clinically heterogeneous even for a specific substance. Whereas substance use disorders have a physiological component, they significantly differ from other psychiatric disorders in that they mostly result from voluntary deliberate behavioral choices with likely pathological outcomes that are well known beforehand. As such, these complex phenomena present numerous obstacles for genetic studies.

As for many other psychiatric disorders, the disease phenotype in addiction research can be viewed as located in the upper portion of the distribution of the continuous latent (unobservable) trait of liability[3] (Falconer, 1965) to addiction.

---

[3]Liability as a human genetics term (approximately synonymous with sometimes used but less well defined "vulnerability," "diathesis," and "susceptibility") can be confused with what is called "drug addiction liability" as a property of chemical compound, relating risk for addiction to classes of substances.

The disease phenotypes are generally located beyond the threshold, a certain point on the liability scale. Liability's variation in the population results from the entire complex of numerous factors related to the probability of the disorder. In this sense, addiction liability is a *multifactorial (complex)* trait. According to the central limit theorem of statistics, a sum of a large number of variables is normally distributed, which allows inferring a likely approximately normal distribution for liability to addiction in the population (similar to the distributions of other multifactorial traits such as IQ or stature). The genetic component of its variation is likely polygenic, that is, due to an unknown number of polymorphic (existing in different variants) genes, each of which contributes a small proportion to overall variation in liability. When the continuous liability distribution is dichotomized by the binary diagnosis, genetic analysis deals with genes' contribution to the (average) differences between affected (SUD; addicted) and unaffected (no-SUD; normal) individuals. Thus, it is the genetics of liability to addiction that is studied, even when the shorthand and imprecise expressions like "genetics of addiction" or "genetic influence on (risk for) addiction," or "heritability of addiction", or "genetic contribution to the development of addiction," or "genetic contribution to initiation of substance use" are used. *More precisely, most of this genetic research is focused on finding the genetic mechanisms of variation in liability to SUD.* While influencing the probability of the disorder, these mechanisms, strictly speaking, are not necessarily the direct cause of SUD or even etiological at all.

While genetic research in addiction includes experimental models, we focus here on human research—for several reasons. One is related to limitations of animal models of addiction. Humans, to a great degree, do share neurobiological mechanisms of drug response with other animals (Darwin discussed the commonality of tastes for the same stimulants as evidence of common evolutionary origin (Darwin, 1871)), and our knowledge of these mechanisms—neurobiological pathways involved, drug metabolism—is substantially contributed by experimental research. Nevertheless, addiction, as noted, is a *human behavioral* phenotype, not synonymous with physiological dependence. Moreover, even if drug-related behaviors in experimental animals and humans were identical, the mechanisms of their variation—both genetic and environmental—would not be. Genetic polymorphisms contributing to phenotypic variation differ even among human populations, and variation in the human family and social environments is difficult to model in animals. Finally, a considerable literature has been accumulated to justify in this brief review a discussion of problems, methods, and data that are specific to human research.

Genetic Studies of Addiction

Biometric Genetic Studies

Human genetics must limit itself to observational studies as experimental manipulation would be unethical. Nevertheless, observations have long established the familiality of SUD, with risk for the offspring of addicts being higher than for children of nonaddicts. To determine the proportion of these differences that is contributed by genetic variation in a population, genetics often uses a natural experiment, the genetic differences between monozygotic (MZ; "identical") and dizygotic (DZ; fraternal) twins. Briefly, twins within MZ pairs, which develop from the same fertilized egg cell, a zygote, are assumed to be genetically identical (they are to a large degree, except for the events that occur after fertilization). In DZ pairs, in which twins develop from two different zygotes, they are as genetically similar as regular siblings, sharing on average only 50% of their segregating genes.

Given that MZ twins are genetically identical, all phenotypic differences between twins within MZ pairs are assumed to be due to nongenetic, i.e., environmental, sources of variation that are unique to each twin, including the omnipresent error of measurement, which together form the unique (or nonshared) environmental variance component (within-family nongenetic variance).

In addition to identical genetics, phenotypic similarity within MZ pairs is ascribed to the environmental factors that act on both twins in pairs in the same manner, the so-called common (or shared) environmental component (it also corresponds to between-family nongenetic variance). The environmental components are assumed to be the same in MZ and DZ twins—the "equal environment" assumption. This assumption appears to hold for SUD—at least to the degree that the self-perception of twins' similarity does not influence their similarity for the diagnosis (Kendler, Neale, Kessler, Heath, & Eaves, 1993; Xian et al., 2000).

Human genetic program is recorded in 46 paired chromosomes, present in almost all cell nuclei of the body. A chromosome, a complex of DNA and proteins that envelope it, contains a set of instructions specific to the chromosome pair, in the form of the genes, stretches of a DNA molecule that are blueprints for the construction of a structural or functional element of the cell and the organism, such as proteins and peptide neurotransmitters. Each of the approximately 20,000 genes comprising the human genome is thus present in two copies (except for those genes that are contained in the sex chromosomes in males, which are different, X and Y, whereas the females have a pair of X chromosomes). The two gene copies could be either the same variant (allele), forming a homozygous genotype, or different alleles, in a heterozygous genotype. Polymorphisms contributing to phenotypic variation may exist in numerous locations (loci) within a gene as well as in DNA loci that are not genes themselves but, e.g., influence genes' expression.

When DNA variation is related to variation in a trait under study, the homozygotes for alternative alleles have different mean values (phenotypes) of the trait. The sum of these differences originating from different loci forms the additive genetic component of phenotypic variance in the trait, a measure of the influence of genetic differences between individuals on their phenotypic differences, such as differences in liability to addiction in the population. The means of the heterozygotes may differ from the averages of the means of the alternative homozygotes, thereby giving rise to the dominance (nonadditive) genetic component of variance. The proportions of these components in the phenotypic variance, again, are assumed to be identical in the twins of MZ pairs, who share 100% of both additive and dominance genetic variance components. In DZ pairs, it is established that 50% of the additive genetic variance and 25% of the dominance variance are shared. Because only the genetic similarity of twins within MZ and DZ pairs presumably differs, it is possible to relate that difference to differences in phenotypic similarity between twins in pairs, and test alternative models for sources of these differences. The models traditionally focus mainly on narrow sense heritability, the proportion of the additive genetic component in the phenotypic variance, usually denoted h^2.

As follows from this discussion, the h^2 statistic pertains to the population rather than individuals, and to trait variation rather than to the trait itself or to its variant (phenotype). A heritability estimate in biometric genetic studies of addiction gives a proportion of genetic variation's contribution to the variance (measure of variation) of liability (trait) to addiction (phenotype), rather than genetic contribution to liability, or to addiction, or to addiction's etiology/development. This obviates the erroneous interpretation of heritability for the notorious "nature or nurture" conundrum, which is particularly meaningless when dealing with what is clearly impossible without an environmental agent (drugs) regardless of heritability. In addition to twins, adoptions too provide an opportunity to assess phenotypic variance components: adopted-away children's similarity with their biological parents is assumed to be only due to their genetic sharing.

These methodology and concepts are obviously not applicable to the traits that are uniform, lacking variation—like the normal number of hands in humans—while there can be no doubt that genetics plays a role in the formation of the hands. Heritability can vary from 0 to 100%, with the latter's being a likely value, for instance, for Mendelian (monogenic) traits. A heritability of 0 is not an indicator of the absent contribution of genetics to the trait. For instance, the heritability of the number of hands in general is likely zero, as only traumas/absence thereof contribute to its variation. As with other similar cases, this trait, however, is under strict genetic control at the mechanistic level.

Heritability of the same trait can differ in different populations, including between sexes, depending on the population's genetic structure and environmental conditions, the sources of variation. For instance, whereas heritability of liability to alcoholism in populations of European origin has been estimated to be close to 50% (Verhulst, Neale, & Kendler, 2015), it is possible that in the East Asian populations it is much higher. This is because a large proportion of East Asians (e.g., Japanese) possess the ALDH2*2 allele of an aldehyde dehydrogenase gene, which is virtually absent in other populations, encoding the inactivated enzyme form that confers elevated resistance to alcoholism due to the disulfiram-like noxious effect of unmetabolized acetaldehyde (Goedde et al., 1983; Harada, Agarwal, & Goedde, 1985; Harada, Agarwal, Goedde, Tagaki, & Ishikawa, 1982). Indeed, this genetic contribution to variation, when present in the population, may render liability closer to Mendelian than to other multifactorial traits, and would make the ALDH2 deficiency a "genetic disorder" if, to the contrary, it did not help to maintain health. The *ALDH2* gene in some populations thus can be a "major" gene, a rare occurrence in behavior and psychiatric disorders, where commonly numerous genes of small effect are known to contribute to variation in liability (e.g., Terwilliger & Goring, 2009). The rest of ALDH2 variation only weakly, if at all, influences alcoholism risk (Macgregor et al., 2009). It is also possible that heritability of alcoholism liability among individuals of African ancestry differs from that in the European extraction populations, but the sample sizes of the former have been too small to determine that (Dick, Barr, Guy, Nasim, & Scott, 2017).

Heritability estimates also depend on trait definition and measurement. For instance, in a study that focused on data for four substances (alcohol, cannabis, cocaine, and opioids), the binary trait definition (endorsement of at least one of the diagnostic criteria) had a heritability estimate of 54%, while the heritability of a continuous index, derived from a factor analysis of DSM-IV dependence symptoms for those substances, was estimated to be 86% (Wetherill et al., 2015).

Importantly, while heritabilities for disorders related to specific substances vary from ~20% to over 70% (e.g., Kendler, Jacobson, Prescott, & Neale, 2003), liabilities to SUD related to various substances have been shown to share virtually the entirety of the genetic sources of variation (Karkowski, Prescott, & Kendler, 2000; Kendler, Jacobson, et al., 2003; Tsuang et al., 1998) despite the differences between chemical structures, routes of administration, and pharmacological properties. This finding supports the concept of general (common) liability to addiction, GLA (Vanyukov et al., 2003; Vanyukov et al., 2012), the trait that likely underlies the high comorbidity of drug-specific addictions. Substance users usually do not restrict their consumption to one primary drug, displaying a pattern of polydrug use (Darke & Hall, 1995). That, in addition to other evidence, may make studying GLA both more promising and feasible than research in specific addictions. This trait also appears to have significant genetic continuity from childhood to adulthood, based on the genetic correlation between the childhood index of addiction liability and the adult SUD diagnosis (Vanyukov et al., 2015). That allows early quantitative estimation of addiction liability, applicable in prevention targeting.

The concept of GLA as a behavioral trait rather than, more narrowly, a pharmacological response to psychoactive substances is also supported by the high correlations, including genetic correlations, between liabilities to addiction and to behavioral disorders (Kendler, Prescott, Myers, & Neale, 2003; Krueger et al., 2002) usually grouped as "externalizing," such as attention-deficit hyperactivity, conduct, and antisocial personality disorders. These disorders can be viewed as pertaining to the violations of social behavior conventions, as is substance abuse itself. This is consistent with the finding of two highly correlated but distinct genetic factors accounting for genetic variation in liabilities to addiction to licit and illicit substances (Kendler et al., 2007). It is clearly not the pharmacologic properties of the substances that genetically separate the respective disorder groups, but the barrier of social norms. The genetic overlaps between drug-specific liabilities are not surprising, considering that a substantial genetic commonality underlies a much wider if not the entire range of psychiatric taxonomy (Khanzada, Butler, & Manzardo, 2017; Lee et al., 2013).

Psychometric analysis of the symptoms of substance use disorders supports a model that incorporates both significant proportions of GLA and drug-specific liabilities in symptom endorsement (Kirisci, Tarter, Reynolds, & Vanyukov, 2016). As noted, the role of GLA suggests both potential benefits and effectiveness of searching for factors, including genetic, that are not substance-specific. This is also supported by genetic association findings discussed below. At the neurobiological level, these phenotypic and genetic associations likely reflect the common mechanisms of drug action and genetic variation that affect organismic response to virtually all psychoactive substances. In particular, these shared mechanisms have long been known to include the dopaminergic mesocorticolimbic system but also involve the neuroregulation of other consummatory behaviors (nutrition, sex), social behavior, stress, and physiological maturation, having deep evolutionary connections (rev. in Vanyukov et al., 2012). It is these connections that likely result, for instance, in the developmental relationships between the rate of sexual maturation, adiposity, and peer delinquency in mediating the parent-child transmission of SUD risk in girls (Kirillova et al., 2014).

GLA also explains the so-called gateway sequence—frequently (but not always) from "softer" to "hard" drugs. According to the GLA concept, this sequence is opportunistic, and depends on the availability of and social attitudes to particular substances. Importantly, what is presented as "gateway" by the proponents of this concept pertains to substance use initiation only (Kandel & Jessor, 2002) rather than to addiction development. In the GLA framework, and consistent with the data, any abusable substance can serve as a "gateway" drug—if the individual's liability is sufficiently high to progress beyond its use,—annulling the "gateway" drug's specificity and rendering the term redundant. Liability to addiction, in contrast to relatively stable traits like eye color but similar to traits like body mass, is labile and changes during lifetime due to biological ontogenesis (which in part determines access to psychoactive substances), exposure to these substances (which is often active and intentionally sought or not objected to strenuously enough), as well as other age-related organismic and environmental changes, some of which reciprocally influence each other (Tarter & Vanyukov, 1994; Vanyukov & Tarter, 2000). It is, therefore, not a "gateway drug" but gateway behavior that determines the initiation, as well as continuation, of the development of addiction.

The estimated GLA heritability of ~50% notwithstanding (the actual estimates fluctuate for different drugs, populations, and age groups), the measures that could be proposed to prevent or treat a disorder may have little to do with the natural mechanisms of liability variation, but would interfere with etiopathogenic mechanisms.

Considering the ubiquity of psychoactive compounds in the human environment, addiction is the price humans currently pay for behavior variation, part genetic, part environmental. This is not to say, to be sure, that the problem cannot in principle be fixed, but if substance users' prevalence starts diminishing (hence, the threshold moving up the liability scale), it can be expected that the individuals who become affected will be more deviant phenotypically, and thus genetically and/or environmentally, and perhaps more difficult to impact with universal or even selective prevention interventions. Indeed, while the prevalence of smoking has decreased, its association with psychopathology has increased (Talati et al., 2013). If social attitudes toward smoking remain relatively uniformly negative, at least within the mainstream society, and price for purchasing cigarettes is not a substantially limiting factor, it may be expected that the heritability of liability to tobacco addiction will increase as its frequency further decreases. Any such possible changes in smoking heritability would not, however, necessarily entail that the measures that may result in the eradication of this habit should become genetic, just as the decrease in smoking—by 50% since 1965—could not have been due to any genetic causes and hence is due to environmental changes.

Molecular Genetic Causes of Variation

There are two approaches commonly employed to determine the DNA-level causes of variation in liability to a disorder, a.k.a. "gene mapping": linkage and association (linkage disequilibrium mapping). The term "linkage" refers to genetic loci's behaving nonindependently of each other during meiosis[4] due to their location on the same chromosome—their greater than 50% chance to be inherited together—rather than due to the coinheritance of a marker with a presence/absence of a disease. In practice, however, in linkage analysis dealing with disorders, it is assumed that the phenotype (affected or unaffected) reflects the genotype for an unknown "disease" locus, and the family data (parents and children; affected siblings) on marker polymorphisms and the disorder are used to evaluate the strength of linkage evidence. These methods are effective in the presence of a "major" gene, accounting for a substantial proportion of liability variation (Carey & Williamson, 1991; Risch & Merikangas, 1996), in the absence of substantial genetic heterogeneity of the disorder. Neither of these conditions is the case with addiction.

Association approaches, population- and family-based, rely on detecting a statistical association of a genetic locus with disorder liability in the population. The population-based approach aims to establish a higher frequency of an allele of a genetic marker polymorphism in unrelated affected individuals in a case-control design. The family-based approach, usually applying the transmission-disequilibrium test, TDT (Spielman, McGinnis, & Ewens, 1993), allows for simultaneously testing for linkage and association, the "overtransmission" (over 50% of the time) of certain alleles from heterozygous parents to affected offspring. In the latter design, the control consists of nontransmitted alleles, while cases are the transmitted alleles.

Association studies in general and in addiction have initially dealt with concrete single "candidate" genes, selected based on their mechanistic relationships with the processes involved in the pathogenesis of the disorder—e.g., for substance addictions, the genes involved in the dopaminergic system, or in the relevant neurobiological system (like opiate receptors for opioid addictions), or in the metabolism of the substance (like alcohol dehydrogenase and aldehyde dehydrogenase genes). Moreover, single, presumably functional, polymorphisms within or at that gene have been selected for genotyping. A higher efficiency of population-based, as compared with family-based, approaches, combined with the ability to densely cover the genome with marker polymorphisms, eventually typing the complete genomic sequence, has established the current predominance of the genome-wide association scans (GWAS). These studies are not hypothesis-driven, in contrast to those with mechanism-based gene selection, and in the pre-GWAS era would be considered the epitome of a "fishing expedition" or "exploratory." While candidate gene studies have been accused of producing too many false positives because of a large number of statistical tests involved, this problem is much greater in the GWAS, with the increasingly denser genotyping (Martin & Schmidt, 2008; Zaykin & Zhivotovsky, 2005). This approach assumes that an allele of a single-nucleotide polymorphism (SNP) causally related to the risk for the disorder is common, thus conveying large attributable risk in the population, even if of small effect statistically (Risch & Merikangas, 1996). This common allele assumption has been questioned based on both human evolutionary history and empirical data (Terwilliger & Goring, 2000, 2009; Weiss, 2010). Such attributable risks are rare. Also, because the marker loci are not (necessarily) functional but rather must have a

---

[4] The two-stage cell division process that results in the formation of sex cells (gametes), eggs, and sperm, which have only one set of chromosomes instead of two as in body cells.

strong connection (linkage disequilibrium, LD) with a functional ("disease") locus for an association to be detected (LD is complete when the marker *is* the "disease" locus), "a substantial proportion of the affected individuals must have inherited the same disease allele identical by descent from a common ancestor" for it to be discoverable by LD methods (Terwilliger & Goring, 2000). Variation may exist in numerous nucleotides, i.e., in the form of numerous SNPs, with similar effects of their alleles, each related to a very small attributable risk fraction. Although GWAS is usually viewed as an alternative to "candidate gene" studies, it is in fact an alternative to selection of candidate genes by their mechanistic involvement: the associations resulting from a GWAS are supposed to be then assigned to some meaningful variable element, i.e., to a gene or a regulatory DNA element.

Although there have been GWAS discoveries of "novel" genes (i.e., previously not known/suspected to be mechanistically involved), the most compelling and replicated GWAS finding in addiction to date pertains to the gene long known to be involved in response to nicotine, coding for an acetylcholine nicotinic receptor subunit (Bierut et al., 2007). Tellingly, this was simultaneously a successfully acquired target of the parallel candidate gene study by the same team that conducted the GWAS (Saccone et al., 2007). This association finding was soon extended to other subunits encoded in the same *CHRNA5/A3/B4* gene cluster. Interestingly, the positive findings for the same loci were obtained not only for nicotine but also for alcohol—particularly for the age of use initiation (Schlaepfer et al., 2008). That variable could be interpreted as suggestive of behavioral deviance contributing to general addiction liability, considering that both are illegal in adolescence when the majority of users in the sample initiated use. Prior to that, the only known valid addiction-related associations were for alcoholism, with genes known to be involved in alcohol metabolism, whose variants cause elevated alcohol toxicity and consequent natural aversion to alcohol: those encoding alcohol dehydrogenases contributing to the production of toxic acetaldehyde from ethanol, and aldehyde dehydrogenases contributing to its catabolism to acetate. These variants, as mentioned above, are largely found in East Asian populations. Unsurprisingly, the only replicated GWAS result for alcoholism in a US population was that with a SNP in an alcohol dehydrogenase gene, *ADH1C* (Biernacka et al., 2013).

Another genetic association confirmed for addiction is that for a functional (resulting in amino acid sequence differences) polymorphism in the opioid receptor μ1 gene, *OPRM1* (Schwantes-An et al., 2016), implicated in addiction-related phenomena based on its mechanistic involvement. Notably, while originally studied in relation to opiate addiction, the association confirmed in this meta-analytic study was with nonspecific, general liability to addiction. A genome-wide analysis showed that common SNPs account for over 30% of the variance in symptom-based indices of nonspecific severity of drug problems/addiction across substances (Palmer et al., 2015), in essence, quantitative GLA indices.

Similarly, an association between GLA and the arginine-vasopressin receptor 1A gene, *AVPR1A*, also with a likely functional SNP, has been detected in males and confirmed in independent samples (Maher et al., 2011). Supporting the study's hypothesis based on the gene's known participation in the mechanisms of formation of social/affiliative behaviors, that relationship was mediated by a variable reflecting spousal bonding. It is important that the association was not detected in females, consistent with sex-specific roles of vasopressin and oxytocin.

The approach used in the Maher et al. study presents an alternative to GWAS. The set of genes whose associations were tested in the study had been selected based on the prior knowledge of their involvement in the CNS function and drug response, and represented major neurobiological systems. The mediation analysis serves as both an internal control and the mechanistic model test, illustrating a possibility of return to hypothesis-driven research in addiction liability genetics. It provides an empirical implementation of the concept of endophenotype (Gottesman & Gould, 2003; Gottesman & Shields, 1967), an intermediate trait that is closer to a biological mechanism(s) of behavior variation. Being nonspecific not only to a drug but also to addiction in general, this mechanism points to a potentially malleable area of behavior regulation.

Attaining power to detect ever smaller genetic effects with samples growing into tens if not hundreds of thousands and genome coverage expanding ultimately to the complete DNA sequence, it may be interesting to evaluate how much the discovered associations account for estimated heritability. So far, the proportion of genetic variance in liability to addiction accounted for by SNPs is small, a situation similar to other psychiatric disorders and behavioral and other complex traits— the so-called missing heritability (Maher, 2008). There are several explanations for that. One is the above-discussed trait/phenotype definition difficulties. Findings may also be nonreplicated because the populations differ in their genetic structure (cf. the *ALDH2* situation). Apart from errors in the measurement of the trait, violations of statistical assumptions, and restrictive significance requirements to control for false positives, there are many factors that in principle prevent matching biometric and SNP heritability estimates. They include non-SNP genetic variation (e.g., repeated elements in DNA, inversions, deletions). The genes are largely treated as independent of each other, while their products frequently comprise complex cascades, with each subsequent reaction dependent on the outcome of the previous one(s), thus forming functional gene-gene as well as genotype-environment interactions.

It is questionable, however, that the goal of accounting for heritability is of much heuristic value *per se*. There is no indication that even if 100% of heritability is accounted for, we will be closer to understanding how addiction develops or what is needed to prevent it, unless genetic findings point to malleable etiologic biological mechanisms. Prevention or treatment of behavioral disorders cannot yet and hopefully never will involve manipulations with genetic material such as gene editing, which is becoming available for Mendelian disorders (Tang et al., 2017). Moreover, biological mechanisms in general may be less actionable than nonbiological factors that might be applied to modify behavior.

Epigenetics

One of the important factors that preclude measured genetic variation's matching estimated heritability is epigenetic modifications of the chromosomal material, chromatin, both DNA and its protein (histone) envelope. Phenotypic changes in the course of biological development and in response to environmental events are regulated by the dynamic system of transcription factors and epigenetic control determining gene expression. The transcription factors must access DNA to act, resulting in the production of mRNA that is translated into proteins. This access is selectively controlled by two main epigenetic mechanisms: DNA methylation, apparently irreversibly inactivating specific parts of the genome (Bestor, Edwards, & Boulard, 2015), and histone modification (acetylation, methylation, ubiquitination, and phosphorylation) (Sweatt, 2009). The importance of epigenetic processes in general is well illustrated by ontogenetic cell differentiation (Maze & Nestler, 2011), which progresses from toti- to pluripotency,[5] largely via DNA methylation, without changes in the cell genotype (Surani, Hayashi, & Hajkova, 2007).

DNA methylation is catalyzed by DNA methytransferases (DNMT). DNA methylation profiles vary considerably among healthy individuals, which may be related to variations in the DNMT activities (Bock et al., 2008). This epigenetic variation appears to be related to genetic differences: DZ twins demonstrated higher intrapair differences in methylation profiles than MZ twins (Kaminsky et al., 2009; Ollikainen et al., 2010). It has been shown that DNA methylation is highly dependent on the genotype and has substantial familiality (Gertz et al., 2011). While these latter data pertain to DNA as a substrate, the enzymatic component of the methylation process is also likely to be genetically variable.

---

[5]The ability of an undifferentiated cell to develop into any or many of the tissue-specific cell varieties.

Epigenetic modifications play a significant role in drug response, both acute exposure and perhaps accounting for the long-lasting effects of drugs, including addiction phenomena (Berkel & Pandey, 2017; Cadet, 2016; Massart et al., 2015; Szyf, Tang, Hill, & Musci, 2016). For instance, DNA methylation has been found to be changed in heroin addicts in the *OPRM1* gene (Nielsen et al., 2009), thus perhaps indicating a mechanism of dependence. Moreover, and perhaps of greater interest from the standpoint of GLA, the entire process of behavioral phenotype development is influenced by epigenetic modifications that occur in response to the environmental conditions, translating, for instance, child maltreatment into not only long-lasting individual effects on the victim but also behavioral changes that possibly cross into the next generation (Szyf et al., 2016).

Dynamic changes in addiction liability in response to drug consumption can also be caused by histone modification. These changes too are not substance-specific (Sanchis-Segura, Lopez-Atalaya, & Barco, 2009). The coordinated activity of acetylation and deacetylation, as well as other histone-modifying mechanisms in the brain, correlates with and perhaps controls changes in gene expression, neuroadaptations, and ultimately behavior, including addiction-related behaviors (Feng & Nestler, 2013; Renthal et al., 2009; Renthal & Nestler, 2009). Therefore, genetic polymorphism of the enzymes regulating these modifications, e.g., histone acetyltransferases and deacetylases, HATs and HDACs, may influence individual variation in GLA and its development. The activators of epigenetic response to drugs include not only events related to drugs *per se* but also any salient environmental stimuli that induce epigenetic modifications preceding and contemporaneous with drug use. For instance, the influences unfolding during social development necessarily involve epigenetic modifications, including histone (de)acetylation. Hence, variation in the (de)acetylation status may precede drug exposure, be related to behaviors influencing the risk for drug exposure and addiction development such as impulsivity and antisociality, and be, at least in part, genetic in origin.

The histone acetylation-related processes are intimately involved in long-term memory formation (Haettig et al., 2011; Korzus, Rosenfeld, & Mayford, 2004; McQuown et al., 2011). Changes in expression of HDAC3, −4, and −10 are coordinated and likely to contribute to gene expression related to feeding behavior (Funato, Oda, Yokofujita, Igarashi, & Kuroda, 2011). Importantly, acetylation-related processes are more relevant in the development of long-lasting effects maintaining addictive behavior than in drug-specific mechanisms of tolerance and dependence (Sanchis-Segura et al., 2009). Moreover, HDAC inhibitors (HDACi) modify effects of drugs belonging to different pharmacologic families, such as cocaine, ethanol, and morphine. HDACi influences expression of genes that are nonspecific to particular drugs or psychoactive substances in general, such as circadian clock genes, BDNF, c-Fos, and FosB. Similar nonspecific roles may be played by other histone-modifying enzymes as well as DNA methylation/demethylation enzymes.

Modifications may increase estimated heritability of liability—e.g., due to heritability of epigenetic modifications (Kaminsky et al., 2009). Epigenetics-related decrease in heritability, contributing to estimates of environmental variance, is also possible—e.g., due to divergence in epigenetic patterns in monozygotic twins over time (Fraga et al., 2005). Importantly, however, estimated heritability of behavioral traits, particularly of externalizing behavior that is strongly associated with GLA, grows rather than decreases with age (Bergen, Gardner, & Kendler, 2007), and so does heritability of liability to addiction itself (Gillespie et al., 2007; Tully, Iacono, & McGue, 2010). While that growth may be contributed to by active genotype-environment correlation (due to genetically biased active choice of the environment (Scarr & McCartney, 1983)), rendering environment part of the extended phenotype, heritability of epigenetic contributions to intra-pair differences is also a plausible explanation, particularly considering the long process of behavior phenotype development. Such contribution could be possible due to genetic polymorphisms in the enzymes involved in epigenetic modifications (e.g., HATs and HDACs) and influencing the organism's response to the environment. In other words, genetic differences between the two classes of twins likely involve not only DNA coding but also epigenetic mechanisms operating on DNA and histones and mediating as well as moderating the role of environment.

Disruptions in epigenetic processes are related not only to the environmental impacts but also to genetic variation, as is prominently displayed in Prader-Willi and fragile X syndromes (Mann & Bartolomei, 1999; Walter, Mazaika, & Reiss, 2009). It is thus possible that genetic variation may also result in less dramatic changes in epigenetic events, and potentially provide biomarkers of addiction risk. Epigenetic factors by their nature may combine the effects of, and mediate, genetic and environmental sources of variation in GLA, and could thus be targets for developing prevention and treatment interventions. The applicability of these factors by manipulations directly at the chromatin level, however, is dubious: such an intervention would be comparable to a genetic change (and even possibly inherited, if causing DNA methylation), with the same objections that could be applied to that.

Some Possible Future Directions

Any health-related research has practical application as its desired and oft-stated goal. It is not immediately clear, however, how genetic and epigenetic findings can be applied in prevention or treatment. Even among those optimists who, related to the Human Genome Project, promised optimization of treatment of complex diseases based on genetic findings (Bell, 1998), that initial excitement has given way to a more sober understanding that "[c]linical genetics ... will soon have to move onto aspects of genetics that are less 'deterministic' for a particular disease" (Bell, 2004).

One reason for the overestimation of the practical potential of genetic (and epigenetic) research is the above-cited conflation of the causes of the disorder and the sources/causes of liability variation, sometimes hiding behind vague expressions like "genes implicated in addiction." Indeed, with a rare exception of the *ALDH2* gene in East Asians, no gene with its polymorphisms has been shown to contribute such a significant amount of variance that it could be categorized as a *cause of addiction*, and then the *ALDH2* finding pertains to the causes of health rather than disease, an important distinction (Maher, Latendresse, & Vanyukov, 2016; Vanyukov et al., 2016a, b). Indeed, behavioral variation is contributed by numerous variables at the psychological phenotypic level, including differences in cognitive and affective control. Going deeper—into the mechanisms of behavior and decisions in regard to substances, and macro- and microenvironment that influences those decisions; effects of substances; metabolic, neurochemical, and neuroanatomical pathways that determine those effects and the response to the environment; and polymorphic proteins (enzymatic and structural), neuropeptides, hormones, and other molecules that compose and regulate those pathways, interacting at both functional and statistical levels and contingent on the prior processes in the mechanistic chains—it becomes clear that polymorphic genes that encode those molecular components and regulate their synthesis and catabolism, as well as the regulatory epigenetic mechanisms, are very far from the ultimate behavioral phenotype.

Despite attempts, based on the addictions' known straightforward "preventable environmental cause," to downgrade addiction compared to other psychiatric disorders when defining funding priorities in genetic research (Merikangas & Risch, 2003), the situation is hardly different for disorders where such causes are unknown. The same arguments (e.g., "literally thousands of genes will be involved") can be applied to all complex psychiatric disorders (Berrettini et al., 2004), and response to that article). Moreover, the real cause of addiction is not the substance as such but the complex behavior resulting in its consumption. The relationship between the beginning and the end of the mechanistic chains in psychiatric etiopathogenesis, even if strong between the adjacent links, is likely to erode into nonsignificance when assessed by association strength and variance accounted for, belying the importance of the outset cause.

The *ALDH2* story also points to another reason why genetic findings have so far not contributed to solving the addiction or other psychiatric problems. As discussed in detail in Vanyukov et al. (2016b), etiology research has historically been conducted in search of "risk factors," associated with disease rather than absence thereof, with the intent of elimination or neutralization of those factors. Discoveries of factors that increase *resistance* to disease (Vanyukov et al., 2016b), which is the liability aspect symmetric to risk, have largely been inadvertent, such as findings of "protective" alleles (i.e., present at lower frequencies among affected individuals) while looking for risk factors (e.g., Enoch et al., 2016). Turning the research perspective 180°—from risk to resistance—may allow adaptation of genetic and epigenetic research away from the monogenic-like paradigm of complex disorders including addiction (Vanyukov et al., 2016b). It is the resistance-raising factors that may have the greatest translation potential, prevention value, and health impact.

The ALDH2 finding could be an example of genetic research that resulted in disorder treatment—if the known-mechanism-based disulfiram effect that mimics the *ALDH2*2*-inactivated enzymes had not been discovered before that. The ALDH2 history, therefore, can serve as an illustration of the resistance-oriented genetic approach (rev. in Maher et al., 2016). First, a high-resistance population—one in which high sensitivity to alcohol effect ("flushing") was prevalent, combined with low alcoholism frequency—was identified in comparing the Japanese with Caucasians. Then, flushing was related to ALDH deficiency, and, finally, traced to the *ALDH2*2* allele absent in Caucasians.

The identification of high-resistance—as opposed to high-risk—populations is the critical difference between the resistance approach and the forms of risk/disease-oriented research, whereby high-risk (e.g., affected or children of affected individuals) "cases" are compared with "controls." While risk and resistance are the symmetric aspects of liability, the sampling approaches are asymmetric. Whereas cases are sampled from the high end of the liability distribution (top 10-5%) and are thus enriched with "risk" factors, the controls are usually sampled from virtually the entire distribution, having, on average, average liability. The resistance factors under the common case-control/high-risk paradigm are thus even less discoverable than the notoriously rare reliable risk factors. High-resistance sampling, such as using tools allowing quantitative measurement of liability and identification of low-addiction-liability individuals (Kirisci et al., 2009; Vanyukov et al., 2003; Vanyukov et al., 2009; Vanyukov et al., 2015), would increase the power for discovery of genetic factors that confer elevated resistance to the disorder (Maher et al., 2016). Notably, however, the resistance factors thus potentially discoverable do not need to be limited to the genetic ones. Indeed, the malleable resistance factors will be likely environmental rather than genetic. For instance, there are data that potentially preventable childhood herpesvirus infections may be related to psychological effects in adulthood, including elevated SUD risk (Vanyukov et al., 2018). It is thus desirable to include a wide range of candidate environmental variables into genetic and epigenetic research.

Conclusions

Individual variation in liability to addiction is significantly contributed by genetic differences and epigenetic mechanisms influencing gene expression. Analysis of molecular genetic and epigenetic studies in addiction suggests, however, that positive findings are scarce and often limited to known nonspecific neurobiological mechanisms of behavior and response to substances. Moreover, the utility of these findings in practice is unclear. It is possible, however, that the reversal of the research perspective from risk/disease to resistance/health could improve practical significance of genetic and epigenetic research. The high-resistance paradigm may allow detection of malleable environmental factors that can offset even high genetic predisposition to the disorder, and be extended to the rest of the population.

References

American Psychiatric Association. (2013). *DSM-5 task force. Diagnostic and statistical manual of mental disorders: DSM-5* (5th ed.). Washington, D.C: American Psychiatric Association.

Bell, J. (1998). The new genetics in clinical practice. *British Medical Journal, 316*, 618–620.

Bell, J. (2004). Predicting disease using genomics. *Nature, 429*, 453–456. https://doi.org/10.1038/nature02624

Bergen, S. E., Gardner, C. O., & Kendler, K. S. (2007). Age-related changes in heritability of behavioral phenotypes over adolescence and young adulthood: A meta-analysis. *Twin Research and Human Genetics, 10*, 423–433. https://doi.org/10.1375/twin.10.3.423

Berkel, T. D., & Pandey, S. C. (2017). Emerging role of epigenetic mechanisms in alcohol addiction. *Alcoholism: Clinical and Experimental Research, 41*, 666–680. https://doi.org/10.1111/acer.13338

Berrettini, W., Bierut, L., Crowley, T. J., Cubells, J. F., Frascella, J., Gelernter, J., … Wanke, K. (2004). Setting priorities for genomic research. *Science, 304*, 445–1447; author reply 1445–1447. https://doi.org/10.1126/Science.304.5676.1445c

Bestor, T. H., Edwards, J. R., & Boulard, M. (2015). Notes on the role of dynamic DNA methylation in mammalian development. *Proceedings of the National Academy of Sciences, 112*, 6796–6799. https://doi.org/10.1073/pnas.1415301111

Biernacka, J. M., Geske, J. R., Schneekloth, T. D., Frye, M. A., Cunningham, J. M., Choi, D. S., … Karpyak, V. M. (2013). Replication of genome wide association studies of alcohol dependence: Support for association with variation in ADH1C. *PLoS One, 8*(3), e58798. https://doi.org/10.1371/journal.pone.005879

Bierut, L. J., Madden, P. A., Breslau, N., Johnson, E. O., Hatsukami, D., Pomerleau, O. F., … Ballinger, D. G. (2007). Novel genes identified in a high-density genome wide association study for nicotine dependence. *Human Molecular Genetics, 16*, 24–35. https://doi.org/10.1093/hmg/ddl441

Bock, C., Walter, J., Paulsen, M., & Lengauer, T. (2008). Inter-individual variation of DNA methylation and its implications for large-scale epigenome mapping. *Nucleic Acids Research, 36*, e55.

Cadet, J. L. (2016). Epigenetics of stress, addiction, and resilience: Therapeutic implications. *Molecular Neurobiology, 53*, 545–560. https://doi.org/10.1007/s12035-014-9040-y

Carey, G., & Williamson, J. (1991). Linkage analysis of quantitative traits: Increased power by using selected samples. *American Journal of Human Genetics, 49*, 786–796.

CBS News. (2015). *60 minutes: A new direction on drugs. CBS News, December 13, 2015*. Retrieved August 22, 2017, from http://www.cbsnews.com/news/60-minutes-a-new-direction-on-drugs/.

Centers for Disease Control and Prevention. (2016). *HIV in the United States: At A Glance. Division of HIV/AIDS Prevention, National Center for HIV/AIDS, Viral Hepatitis, Sexual Transmitted Diseases and Tuberculosis Prevention,* Centers for Disease Control and Prevention. Retrieved February 2, 2017, from https://www.cdc.gov/hiv/statistics/overview/ataglance.html.

Darke, S., & Hall, W. (1995). Levels and correlates of polydrug use among heroin users and regular amphetamine users. *Drug and Alcohol Dependence, 39*, 231–235.

Darwin, C. (1871). *The Descent of Man, and Selection in Relation to Sex*. London: John Murray.

Dick, D. M., Barr, P., Guy, M., Nasim, A., & Scott, D. (2017). (Invited review) Genetic research on alcohol use outcomes in African American populations: A review of the literature, associated challenges, and implications. *American Journal of Addiction, 26*, 486–493. https://doi.org/10.1111/ajad.12495

Enoch, M. A., Hodgkinson, C. A., Shen, P. H., Gorodetsky, E., Marietta, C. A., Roy, A., & Goldman, D. (2016). GABBR1 and SLC6A1, Two genes involved in modulation of GABA synaptic transmission, influence risk for alcoholism: Results from three ethnically diverse populations. *Alcoholism: Clinical and Experimental Research, 40*, 93–101. https://doi.org/10.1111/acer.12929

Falconer, D. S. (1965). The inheritance of liability to certain diseases, estimated from the incidence among relatives. *Annals of Human Genetics, 29*, 51–76.

Feng, J., & Nestler, E. J. (2013). Epigenetic mechanisms of drug addiction. *Current Opinion in Neurobiology, 23*(4), 521–528. https://doi.org/10.1016/j.conb.2013.01.001

Fraga, M. F., Ballestar, E., Paz, M. F., Ropero, S., Setien, F., Ballestar, M. L., … Esteller, M. (2005). Epigenetic differences arise during the lifetime of monozygotic twins. *Proceedings of the National Academy of Sciences U S A, 102*(30), 10604–10609. https://doi.org/10.1073/pnas.0500398102

Funato, H., Oda, S., Yokofujita, J., Igarashi, H., & Kuroda, M. (2011). Fasting and high-fat diet alter histone deacetylase expression in the medial hypothalamus. *PLoS One, 6*(4), e18950. https://doi.org/10.1371/journal.pone.0018950

Gertz, J., Varley, K. E., Reddy, T. E., Bowling, K. M., Pauli, F., Parker, S. L., … Myers, R. M. (2011). Analysis of DNA methylation in a three-generation family reveals widespread genetic influence on epigenetic regulation. *PLoS Genetics, 7*, 1–10.

Gillespie, N. A., Kendler, K. S., Prescott, C. A., Aggen, S. H., Gardner, C. O., Jr., Jacobson, K., & Neale, M. C. (2007). Longitudinal modeling of genetic and environmental influences on self-reported availability of psychoactive substances: Alcohol, cigarettes, marijuana, cocaine and stimulants. *Psychological Medicine, 37*(7), 947–959. https://doi.org/10.1017/S0033291707009920

Goedde, H. W., Agarwal, D. P., Harada, S., Meier-Tackmann, D., Ruofu, D., Bienzle, U., … Hussein, L. (1983). Population genetic studies on aldehyde dehydrogenase isozyme deficiency and alcohol sensitivity. *American Journal of Human Genetics, 35*(4), 769–772.

Gottesman, I. I., & Gould, T. D. (2003). The endophenotype concept in psychiatry: Etymology and strategic intentions. *American Journal of Psychiatry, 160*(4), 636–645. https://doi.org/10.1176/appi.ajp.160.4.636

Gottesman, I. I., & Shields, J. (1967). A polygenic theory of schizophrenia. *Proceedings of the National Academy of Sciences U S A, 58*(1), 199–205.

Haettig, J., Stefanko, D. P., Multani, M. L., Figueroa, D. X., McQuown, S. C., & Wood, M. A. (2011). HDAC inhibition modulates hippocampus-dependent long-term memory for object location in a CBP-dependent manner. *Learning and Memory, 18*(2), 71–79. https://doi.org/10.1101/lm.1986911

Harada, S., Agarwal, D. P., & Goedde, H. W. (1985). Aldehyde dehydrogenase polymorphism and alcohol metabolism in alcoholics. *Alcohol, 2*(3), 391–392.

Harada, S., Agarwal, D. P., Goedde, H. W., Tagaki, S., & Ishikawa, B. (1982). Possible protective role against alcoholism for aldehyde dehydrogenase isozyme deficiency in Japan. *Lancet, 2*(8302), 827.

Kaminsky, Z. A., Tang, T., Wang, S. C., Ptak, C., Oh, G. H., Wong, A. H., ... Petronis, A. (2009). DNA methylation profiles in monozygotic and dizygotic twins. *Nature Genetics, 41*(2), 240–245. https://doi.org/10.1038/ng.286

Kandel, D., & Jessor, R. (2002). The gateway hypothesis revisited. In D. B. Kandel (Ed.), *Stages and pathways of drug involvement: Examining the gateway hypothesis* (pp. 365–372). Cambridge, MA: Cambridge University Press.

Karkowski, L. M., Prescott, C. A., & Kendler, K. S. (2000). Multivariate assessment of factors influencing illicit substance use in twins from female-female pairs. *American Journal of Medical Genetics, 96*(5), 665–670. https://doi.org/10.1002/1096-8628(20001009)96:5<665::AID-AJMG13>3.0.CO;2-O

Kendler, K. S., Jacobson, K. C., Prescott, C. A., & Neale, M. C. (2003). Specificity of genetic and environmental risk factors for use and abuse/dependence of cannabis, cocaine, hallucinogens, sedatives, stimulants, and opiates in male twins. *American Journal of Psychiatry, 160*(4), 687–695.

Kendler, K. S., Myers, J., & Prescott, C. A. (2007). Specificity of genetic and environmental risk factors for symptoms of cannabis, cocaine, alcohol, caffeine, and nicotine dependence. *Archives of General Psychiatry, 64*(11), 1313–1320. https://doi.org/10.1001/archpsyc.64.11.1313

Kendler, K. S., Neale, M. C., Kessler, R. C., Heath, A. C., & Eaves, L. J. (1993). A test of the equal-environment assumption in twin studies of psychiatric illness. *Behavioral Genetics, 23*(1), 21–27.

Kendler, K. S., Prescott, C. A., Myers, J., & Neale, M. C. (2003). The structure of genetic and environmental risk factors for common psychiatric and substance use disorders in men and women. *Archives of General Psychiatry, 60*(9), 929–937. https://doi.org/10.1001/archpsyc.60.9.92960/9/929

Khanzada, N. S., Butler, M. G., & Manzardo, A. M. (2017). GeneAnalytics pathway analysis and genetic overlap among autism spectrum disorder, bipolar disorder and schizophrenia. *International Journal of Molecular Sciences, 18*(3), 527. https://doi.org/10.3390/ijms18030527

Kirillova, G., Reynolds, M., Kirisci, L., Mosovsky, S., Ridenour, T., Tarter, R., & Vanyukov, M. (2014). Familiality of addiction and its developmental mechanisms in girls. *Drug Alcohol Dependence, 143*, 213–218. https://doi.org/10.1016/j.drugalcdep.2014.07.032

Kirisci, L., Tarter, R., Mezzich, A., Ridenour, T., Reynolds, M., & Vanyukov, M. (2009). Prediction of cannabis use disorder between boyhood and young adulthood: Clarifying the phenotype and environ type. *American Journal of Addictions, 18*(1), 36–47. https://doi.org/10.1080/10550490802408829

Kirisci, L., Tarter, R. E., Reynolds, M., & Vanyukov, M. M. (2016). Item response theory analysis to assess dimensionality of substance use disorder abuse and dependence symptoms. *International Journal of Person Centered Medicine, 6*(4), 260–273.

Korzus, E., Rosenfeld, M. G., & Mayford, M. (2004). CBP histone acetyltransferase activity is a critical component of memory consolidation. *Neuron, 42*(6), 961–972. https://doi.org/10.1016/j.neuron.2004.06.002

Krueger, R. F., Hicks, B. M., Patrick, C. J., Carlson, S. R., Iacono, W. G., & McGue, M. (2002). Etiologic connections among substance dependence, antisocial behavior, and personality: Modeling the externalizing spectrum. *Journal of Abnormal Psychology, 111*(3), 411–424.

Lee, S. H., Ripke, S., Neale, B. M., Faraone, S. V., Purcell, S. M., Perlis, R. H., ... Cross-Disorder Group of the Psychiatric Genomics Consortium, International Inflammatory Bowel Disease Genetics C. (2013). Genetic relationship between five psychiatric disorders estimated from genome-wide SNPs. *Nature Genetics, 45*, 984–994. https://doi.org/10.1038/ng.2711

Macgregor, S., Lind, P. A., Bucholz, K. K., Hansell, N. K., Madden, P. A., Richter, M. M., ... Whitfield, J. B. (2009). Associations of ADH and ALDH2 gene variation with self-report alcohol reactions, consumption and dependence: An integrated analysis. *Human Molecular Genetics, 18*(3), 580–593. https://doi.org/10.1093/hmg/ddn372

Maher, B. (2008). Personal genomes: The case of the missing heritability. *Nature, 456*(7218), 18–21. https://doi.org/10.1038/456018a

Maher, B. S., Latendresse, S., & Vanyukov, M. M. (2016). Informing prevention and intervention policy using genetic studies of resistance. *Prevention Science, 19*, 49–57. https://doi.org/10.1007/s11121-016-0730-8

Maher, B. S., Vladimirov, V. I., Latendresse, S. J., Thiselton, D. L., McNamee, R., Kang, M., ... Vanyukov, M. M. (2011). The AVPR1A gene and substance use disorders: Association, replication, and functional evidence. *Biological Psychiatry, 70*(6), 519–527. https://doi.org/10.1016/j.biopsych.2011.02.023

Mandelbaum, D. E., & de la Monte, S. M. (2017). Adverse Structural and Functional Effects of Marijuana on the Brain: Evidence Reviewed. *Pediatric Neurology, 66*, 12–20. https://doi.org/10.1016/j.pediatrneurol.2016.09.004

Mann, M. R., & Bartolomei, M. S. (1999). Towards a molecular understanding of Prader-Willi and Angelman syndromes. *Human Molecular Genetics, 8*(10), 1867–1873.

Martin, E. R., & Schmidt, M. A. (2008). The future is now—will the real disease gene please stand up? *Human Heredity, 66*(2), 127–135. https://doi.org/10.1159/000119112

Massart, R., Barnea, R., Dikshtein, Y., Suderman, M., Meir, O., Hallett, M., ... Yadid, G. (2015). Role of DNA methylation in the nucleus accumbens in incubation of cocaine craving. *The Journal of Neuroscience, 35*(21), 8042–8058. https://doi.org/10.1523/JNEUROSCI.3053-14.2015

Maze, I., & Nestler, E. J. (2011). The epigenetic landscape of addiction. *Annals of the New York Academy of Sciences, 1216*, 99–113. https://doi.org/10.1111/j.1749-6632.2010.05893.x

McQuown, S. C., Barrett, R. M., Matheos, D. P., Post, R. J., Rogge, G. A., Alenghat, T., ... Wood, M. A. (2011). HDAC3 is a critical negative regulator of long-term memory formation. *The Journal of Neuroscience, 31*(2), 764–774. https://doi.org/10.1523/JNEUROSCI.5052-10.2011

Merikangas, K. R., & Risch, N. (2003). Genomic priorities and public health. *Science, 302*(5645), 599–601. https://doi.org/10.1126/science.1091468

Nielsen, D. A., Yuferov, V., Ho, A., Chen, A., Levran, O., Ott, S., & Kreek, M. J. (2009). Increased OPRM1 DNA methylation in lymphocytes of methadone-maintained former heroin addicts. *Neuropsychopharmacology, 34*, 867–873.

Nogler, G. A. (2006). The lesser-known Mendel: His experiments on Hieracium. *Genetics, 172*(1), 1–6.

O'Brien, C. P., Volkow, N., & Li, T. K. (2006). What's in a word? Addiction versus dependence in DSM-V. *The American Journal of Psychiatry, 163*(5), 764–765. https://doi.org/10.1176/appi.ajp.163.5.764

Ollikainen, M., Smith, K. R., Joo, E. J., Ng, H. K., Andronikos, R., Novakovic, B., ... Craig, J. M. (2010). DNA methylation analysis of multiple tissues from newborn twins reveals both genetic and intrauterine components to variation in the human neonatal epigenome. *Human Molecular Genetics, 19*, 4176–4188.

Palmer, R. H., Brick, L., Nugent, N. R., Bidwell, L. C., McGeary, J. E., Knopik, V. S., & Keller, M. C. (2015). Examining the role of common genetic variants on alcohol, tobacco, cannabis and illicit drug dependence: Genetics of vulnerability to drug dependence. *Addiction, 110*(3), 530–537. https://doi.org/10.1111/add.12815

Renthal, W., Kumar, A., Xiao, G., Wilkinson, M., Covington, H. E., 3rd, Maze, I., ... Nestler, E. J. (2009). Genome-wide analysis of chromatin regulation by cocaine reveals a role for sirtuins. *Neuron, 62*(3), 335–348. https://doi.org/10.1016/j.neuron.2009.03.026

Renthal, W., & Nestler, E. J. (2009). Histone acetylation in drug addiction. *Seminars in Cell & Developmental Biology, 20*(4), 387–394. https://doi.org/10.1016/j.semcdb.2009.01.005

Risch, N., & Merikangas, K. (1996). The future of genetic studies of complex human diseases. *Science, 273*(5281), 1516–1517.

Saccone, S. F., Hinrichs, A. L., Saccone, N. L., Chase, G. A., Konvicka, K., Madden, P. A., ... Bierut, L. J. (2007). Cholinergic nicotinic receptor genes implicated in a nicotine dependence association study targeting 348 candidate genes with 3713 SNPs. *Human Molecular Genetics, 16*(1), 36–49. https://doi.org/10.1093/hmg/ddl438

SAMHSA. (2015). Behavioral health barometer: United States, 2015. HHS Publication No. SMA–16–Baro–2015. Center for behavioral health statistics and quality, substance abuse and mental health services administration. http://www.samhsa.gov/data/sites/default/files/2015_National_Barometer.pdf.

Sanchis-Segura, C., Lopez-Atalaya, J. P., & Barco, A. (2009). Selective boosting of transcriptional and behavioral responses to drugs of abuse by histone deacetylase inhibition. *Neuropsychopharmacology, 34*(13), 2642–2654. https://doi.org/10.1038/npp.2009.125

Scarr, S., & McCartney, K. (1983). How people make their own environments: A theory of genotype greater than environment effects. *Child Development, 54*(2), 424–435.

Schlaepfer, I. R., Hoft, N. R., Collins, A. C., Corley, R. P., Hewitt, J. K., Hopfer, C. J., ... Ehringer, M. A. (2008). The CHRNA5/A3/B4 gene cluster variability as an important determinant of early alcohol and tobacco initiation in young adults. *Biological Psychiatry, 63*(11), 1039–1046. https://doi.org/10.1016/j.biopsych.2007.10.024

Schwantes-An, T. H., Zhang, J., Chen, L. S., Hartz, S. M., Culverhouse, R. C., Chen, X., ... Saccone, N. L. (2016). Association of the OPRM1 variant rs1799971 (A118G) with non-specific liability to substance dependence in a collaborative de novo meta-analysis of European-ancestry cohorts. *Behavior Genetics, 46*(2), 151–169. https://doi.org/10.1007/s10519-015-9737-3

Spielman, R. S., McGinnis, R. E., & Ewens, W. J. (1993). Transmission test for linkage disequilibrium: The insulin gene region and insulin-dependent diabetes mellitus (IDDM). *American Journal of Human Genetics, 52*(3), 506–516.

Surani, M. A., Hayashi, K., & Hajkova, P. (2007). Genetic and epigenetic regulators of pluripotency. *Cell, 128*(4), 747–762. https://doi.org/10.1016/j.cell.2007.02.010

Sweatt, J. D. (2009). Experience-dependent epigenetic modifications in the central nervous system. *Biological Psychiatry, 65*(3), 191–197. https://doi.org/10.1016/j.biopsych.2008.09.002

Szyf, M., Tang, Y. Y., Hill, K. G., & Musci, R. (2016). The dynamic epigenome and its implications for behavioral interventions: A role for epigenetics to inform disorder prevention and health promotion. *Translational Behavioral Medicine, 6*(1), 55–62. https://doi.org/10.1007/s13142-016-0387-7

Talati, A., Wickramaratne, P. J., Keyes, K. M., Hasin, D. S., Levin, F. R., & Weissman, M. M. (2013). Smoking and psychopathology increasingly associated in recent birth cohorts. *Drug and Alcohol Dependence, 133*(2), 724–732. https://doi.org/10.1016/j.drugalcdep.2013.08.025

Tang, L., Zeng, Y., Du, H., Gong, M., Peng, J., Zhang, B., ... Liu, J. (2017). CRISPR/Cas9-mediated gene editing in human zygotes using Cas9 protein. *Molecular Genetics and Genomics, 292*, 525–533. https://doi.org/10.1007/s00438-017-1299-z

Tarter, R. E., & Vanyukov, M. (1994). Alcoholism: A developmental disorder. *Journal of Consulting and Clinical Psychology, 62*(6), 1096–1107.

Terwilliger, J. D., & Goring, H. H. (2000). Gene mapping in the 20th and 21st centuries: Statistical methods, data analysis, and experimental design. *Human Biology, 72*(1), 63–132.

Terwilliger, J. D., & Goring, H. H. (2009). Update to Terwilliger and Goring's "Gene mapping in the 20th and 21st centuries" (2000): Gene mapping when rare variants are common and common variants are rare. *Human Biology, 81*(5–6), 729–733. https://doi.org/10.3378/027.081.0617

Tsuang, M. T., Lyons, M. J., Meyer, J. M., Doyle, T., Eisen, S. A., Goldberg, J., ... Eaves, L. (1998). Co-occurrence of abuse of different drugs in men: The role of drug-specific and shared vulnerabilities. *Archives of General Psychiatry, 55*(11), 967–972.

Tully, E. C., Iacono, W. G., & McGue, M. (2010). Changes in genetic and environmental influences on the development of nicotine dependence and major depressive disorder from middle adolescence to early adulthood. *Development and Psychopathology, 22*(4), 831–848. https://doi.org/10.1017/S0954579410000490

Vanyukov, M., Kim, K., Irons, D., Kirisci, L., Neale, M., Ridenour, T., ... Iacono, W. (2015). Genetic relationship between the addiction diagnosis in adults and their childhood measure of addiction liability. *Behavior Genetics, 45*(1), 1–11. https://doi.org/10.1007/s10519-014-9684-4

Vanyukov, M. M., Cornelius, M. D., De Genna, N. M., Reynolds, M. D., Kirillova, G. P., Maher, B. S., & Kirisci, L. (2016a). Measurement of liability to addiction: Dimensional approaches. *International Journal of Person Centered Medicine, 6*, 250–259.

Vanyukov, M. M., Kirisci, L., Moss, L., Tarter, R. E., Reynolds, M. D., Maher, B. S., ... Clark, D. B. (2009). Measurement of the risk for substance use disorders: Phenotypic and genetic analysis of an index of common liability. *Behavior Genetics, 39*(3), 233–244. https://doi.org/10.1007/s10519-009-9269-9

Vanyukov, M. M., Kirisci, L., Tarter, R. E., Simkevitz, H. F., Kirillova, G. P., Maher, B. S., & Clark, D. B. (2003). Liability to substance use disorders: 2. A measurement approach. *Neuroscience and Biobehavioral Reviews, 27*(6), 517–526.

Vanyukov, M. M., Nimgaonkar, V. L., Kirisci, L., Kirillova, G. P., Reynolds, M. D., Prasad, K., ... Yolken, R. H. (2018). Association of cognitive function and liability to addiction with childhood herpesvirus infections: A prospective cohort study. *Development and Psychopathology, 30*, 143–152.

Vanyukov, M. M., & Tarter, R. E. (2000). Genetic studies of substance abuse. *Drug and Alcohol Dependence, 59*(2), 101–123.

Vanyukov, M. M., Tarter, R. E., Conway, K. P., Kirillova, G. P., Chandler, R. K., & Daley, D. C. (2016b). Risk and resistance perspectives in translation-oriented etiology research. *Translational Behavioral Medicine, 6*(1), 44–54. https://doi.org/10.1007/s13142-015-0355-7

Vanyukov, M. M., Tarter, R. E., Kirillova, G. P., Kirisci, L., Reynolds, M. D., Kreek, M. J., ... Ridenour, T. A. (2012). Common liability to addiction and gateway hypothesis: Theoretical, empirical and evolutionary perspective. *Drug and Alcohol Dependence, 123*(Suppl 1), S3–S17. https://doi.org/10.1016/j.drugalcdep.2011.12.018

Vanyukov, M. M., Tarter, R. E., Kirisci, L., Kirillova, G. P., Maher, B. S., & Clark, D. B. (2003). Liability to substance use disorders: 1. Common mechanisms and manifestations. *Neuroscience and Biobehavioral Reviews, 27*(6), 507–515.

Verhulst, B., Neale, M. C., & Kendler, K. S. (2015). The heritability of alcohol use disorders: A meta-analysis of twin and adoption studies. *Psychological Medicine, 45*(5), 1061–1072. https://doi.org/10.1017/S0033291714002165

Volkow, N.D. (2012). *Fiscal year 2013 budget request. Testimony before the house subcommittee on labor-HHS-education appropriations. National Institute on Drug Abuse*. Retrieved October 6, 2015, from http://www.drugabuse.gov/about-nida/legislative-activities/testimony-to-congress/2012/03/fiscal-year-2013-budget-request

Walter, E., Mazaika, P. K., & Reiss, A. L. (2009). Insights into brain development from neurogenetic syndromes: Evidence from fragile X syndrome, Williams syndrome, Turner syndrome and velocardiofacial syndrome. *Neuroscience, 164*(1), 257–271. https://doi.org/10.1016/j.neuroscience.2009.04.033

Weiss, K. M. (2010). Seeing the forest through the gene-trees. *Evolutionary Anthropology: Issues, News, and Reviews, 19*(6), 210–221. https://doi.org/10.1002/evan.20286

Wetherill, L., Agrawal, A., Kapoor, M., Bertelsen, S., Bierut, L. J., Brooks, A., ... Foroud, T. (2015). Association of substance dependence phenotypes in the COGA sample. *Addiction Biology, 20*(3), 617–627. https://doi.org/10.1111/adb.12153

Xian, H., Scherrer, J. F., Eisen, S. A., True, W. R., Heath, A. C., Goldberg, J., ... Tsuang, M. T. (2000). Self-Reported zygosity and the equal-environments assumption for psychiatric disorders in the Vietnam Era Twin Registry. *Behavior Genetics, 30*(4), 303–310.

Zaykin, D. V., & Zhivotovsky, L. A. (2005). Ranks of genuine associations in whole-genome scans. *Genetics, 171*(2), 813–823. https://doi.org/10.1534/genetics.105.044206

Progression of Substance Use to Substance Use Disorder

Matthew R. Lee, Yoanna E. McDowell, and Kenneth J. Sher

Introduction

Substance use disorders (SUDs) are among the most prevalent mental illnesses in the USA, with an estimated 21.5 million (8.1%) of Americans over age 12 warranting a past-year SUD diagnosis (Center for Behavioral Health Statistics and Quality [CBHSQ], 2015). This is of great public health concern, as problematic substance use costs the USA an estimated $700 billion per year (National Institute on Drug Abuse, 2015). Further, tobacco, alcohol, and illicit drugs represent the nation's first, third, and ninth leading causes of preventable mortality (respectively; Mokdad, Marks, Stroup, & Gerberding, 2004).

This chapter focuses on understanding SUD and other forms of problematic substance use (as opposed to substance use per se; see Defining Problematic Substance Use). Problematic substance use can occur with a variety of psychoactive substances including illegal substances, legal substances, and even pharmaceutical medications. This chapter is written primarily from a developmental perspective. Thus, when reviewing epidemiology, in addition to characterizing SUD prevalence rates and recent historic changes in these rates, we also emphasize the marked age-prevalence gradient in SUD rates that likely reflects changes in risk over the course of development. Age-prevalence gradients for various substances reveal a robust pattern of increasing SUD prevalence during adolescence and emerging adulthood, followed by reductions beginning in young adulthood and continuing throughout later developmental periods. This developmental pattern also informs our later reviews of research on SUD etiology and SUD desistance. In discussing etiology, we emphasize factors that can contribute to adolescent and emerging adult escalation of problematic substance use. In discussing desistance, we emphasize factors that contribute to age-related reductions in problematic substance use in young adulthood and later developmental periods. Indeed, both an understanding of how SUDs develop and an understanding of how natural desistance occurs can offer key insights toward informing prevention and treatment intervention efforts.

Writing of this chapter was supported by National Institute on Alcohol Abuse and Alcoholism grants K99-AA024236 to Matthew R. Lee and K05-AA017242 to Kenneth J. Sher.

M. R. Lee (✉)
Department of Applied Psychology, Graduate School of Applied and Professional Psychology, Rutgers University, New Brunswick, NJ, USA

Department of Psychological Sciences, University of Missouri, Columbia, MO, USA
e-mail: matthew.r.lee@rutgers.edu

Y. E. McDowell · K. J. Sher
Department of Psychological Sciences, University of Missouri, Columbia, MO, USA
e-mail: yem7c9@mail.missouri.edu; sherk@missouri.edu

Defining Problematic Substance Use

Clinical SUD Diagnosis

The current diagnostic system of the fifth edition of the American Psychiatric Association's (APA) *Diagnostic and Statistical Manual of Mental Disorders* (*DSM-5*) operationalizes pathological substance use through a diagnosis of Substance Use Disorder (SUD; APA, 2013). The *DSM-5* defines SUD as "a cluster of cognitive, behavioral, and physiological symptoms indicating that the individual continues using the substance despite significant substance-related problems" (APA, 2013, p. 483). An SUD diagnosis is made by assessing eleven criteria viewed as reflecting four different domains of symptomatology: (1) impaired control (e.g., unsuccessful efforts to control use), (2) social problems (e.g., failures in major obligations), (3) risky use (e.g., in hazardous situations), and (4) physiologic dependence (e.g., withdrawal). An SUD diagnosis is given if two or more of the eleven criteria are met, with severity specified as mild for 2–3 criteria, moderate for 4–5 criteria, and severe for 6 or more criteria.

The *DSM-5* diagnostic system differs substantially from those preceding it, as *DSM* editions dating back to the *DSM-III* (APA, 1980) distinguished between two disorders termed substance abuse and substance dependence. However, the same criteria were largely retained in the transition from *DSM-IV* to *DSM-5*, with the exception that the *DSM-5* dropped the *DSM-IV* "legal problems" criterion and added a "craving" criterion (for more *DSM* history, see Martin, Chung, & Langenbucher, 2016).

Although it is beyond this chapter's scope to further review the advances made in the *DSM-5* and remaining issues that have been raised (see Hasin, 2015; Martin et al., 2016; Wakefield, 2015), it is important to note that such issues are highly pertinent to etiologic and applied research aiming to inform or evaluate prevention and prevention intervention strategies. For instance, from a developmental standpoint, possible biases in some criteria that may inflate false-positive diagnoses at earlier ages should be understood as a possible source of age-related artifactual bias in research on SUD etiology, prevention, and treatment (Boness, Lane, & Sher, 2016).

Other Indices of Problematic Use

In addition to clinical diagnosis, pathological substance use can be indexed by a variety of other measures of substance-related problems and/or excessive consumption (see Del Boca, Darkes, & McRee, 2016). For assessing problematic/risky substance involvement, there exists a wide variety of surveys (e.g., the Rutgers Alcohol Problem Index; Neal, Corbin, & Fromme, 2006) and screening instruments (e.g., the Alcohol Use Disorders Identification Test; Allen, Litten, Fertig, & Babor, 1997), often assessing content that overlaps substantially with diagnostic criteria. Some such measures can be useful for prevention research purposes in providing relatively dimensional indices that capture variability at subdiagnostic levels of problematic use.

For assessing excessive consumption, the clearest definitions exist for alcohol. The National Institute on Alcohol Abuse and Alcoholism (NIAAA, 2004) defines binge drinking as reaching a blood alcohol concentration of 0.08% or above. This corresponds roughly to consuming five or more drinks in two hours for the average man and four or more drinks in two hours for the average women, so research often uses this definition to approximate binge drinking. For other substances, it is more difficult to quantify consumption, let alone establish definitions of excessive use. For nicotine, variations in smoking behavior lead to substantial variability in nicotine intake that is not captured by an assessment of cigarette use quantity (Hammond, Fong, Cummings, & Hyland, 2005). For illicit drugs, there is substantial variability in potency and purity (e.g., Parrott, 2004). Thus, assessments of illicit drug consumption often focus on frequency of use, for instance, with daily use reflecting a relatively severe pattern of consumption.

Epidemiology of SUDs

Prevalence Rates and Historic Trends

The US National Survey on Drug Use and Health (NSDUH) reports yearly SUD prevalence rates since 2002 (CBHSQ, 2015). A rougher picture over a longer historic period can be gleaned by contrasting data from the 1991 National Longitudinal Alcohol Epidemiologic Survey (NLAES) and the 2001 and 2012 National Epidemiologic Survey on Alcohol and Related Conditions (NESARC; Grant, Peterson, Dawson, & Chou, 1994; Grant, Moore, Shepard, & Kaplan, 2003; Grant et al., 2014). Other national studies such as Monitoring the Future (MTF) provide rich data on substance *use* but not SUD (Miech, Johnston, O'Malley, Bachman, & Schulenberg, 2015).

Based on 2014 NSDUH data (see Fig. 5.1), among the 8.1% of the US population with some type of SUD, 67% had alcohol use disorder only, 21% had drug use disorder only, and 12% had both. However, NSDUH did not consider nicotine use disorder, which exceeds the prevalence of alcohol use disorder in the USA, according to NESARC data (e.g., 12.8% vs. 8.5% in 2001; Grant, Hasin, Chou, Stinson, & Dawson, 2004). Among SUDs with illicit substances, marijuana use disorder is by far most common. In 2014, US SUD prevalence rates were 1.6% for marijuana, 0.3% for cocaine, and 0.2% for heroin (see Fig. 5.1). A recent concern has been the abuse of pharmaceutical medications, with an SUD prevalence rate of 0.9% in 2014, thus surpassing SUD prevalence rates for both cocaine (0.3%) and heroin (0.2%).

While risky/problematic use is especially common for alcohol and nicotine, there have been relatively dramatic recent historic decreases associated with these substances, as described below.

Alcohol

As depicted in Fig. 5.1, NSDUH showed that alcohol use disorder prevalence rates dropped from 7.7% in 2002 to 6.4% in 2014. Further, more marked reductions over this period were shown for adolescents (ages 12–17; 5.9% to 2.7%) and young adults (ages 18–25; 17.7% to 12.3%). This is mirrored by MTF data showing reductions in heavy drinking over recent decades, but with far more pronounced reductions for adolescents than for college students or other young adults (Miech et al., 2015).

Smoking and Nicotine Use

Both MTF and NSDUH show substantial smoking reductions over recent years. MTF data on high schoolers and young adults shows that, since a peak in daily smoking rates of around 20–25% in the late 1990s, rates dropped to a historic low of around 5–10% by 2015 (Miech et al., 2015). NSDUH data also shows that smoking reductions since 2002 were especially pronounced for adolescents and young adults compared to those over age 26 (CBHSQ, 2015). However, a recent concern is nicotine use via e-cigarettes and vaporizers, with MTF data showing that this has grown even more common than traditional smoking among high schoolers (Miech et al., 2015). This appears partially attributable to perceived risk, as less than 20% of 2015 high schoolers perceived great risk in regular vaporizer use, while over 40% perceived great risk in smoking 1–5 cigarettes per day (Miech et al., 2015).

Illicit Drugs

The MTF data tell an interesting story regarding historic trends in the use of marijuana and other illicit drugs among US high schoolers. Miech et al. (2015) describe a 1990s "relapse" characterized by spiking rates of illicit drug use. They argue that public policy reactions since then have succeeded in bringing these rates back down, with the exception that marijuana use has remained relatively elevated. This may reflect increased public permissiveness regarding marijuana, consistent with MTF data showing relatively low perceived harm of marijuana use (Miech et al., 2015).

Pharmaceuticals

Recent concerns about pharmaceutical medications are consistent with NSDUH data showing gradual increases in SUD prevalence rates for

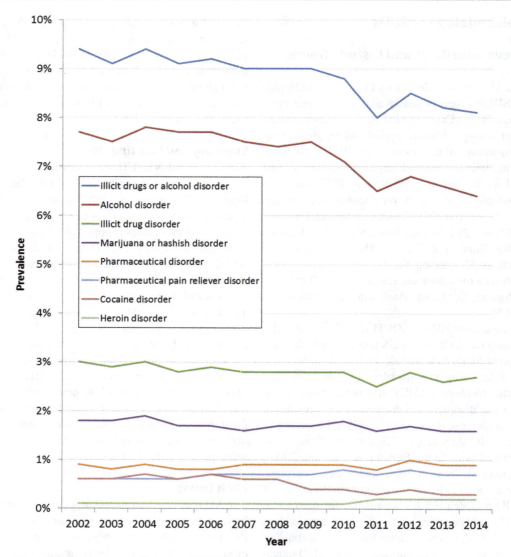

Note. Prevalence rates are based on NSDUH data (CBHSQ, 2015) on rates of DSM-IV abuse or dependence (APA, 1994) among individuals aged 12 or older in the U.S.

Fig. 5.1 US Yearly Trends in Past-Year Substance Disorder Prevalence Rates for Different Specific Substances

these substances since 2002, especially for pharmaceutical pain relievers (see Fig. 5.1). MTF data also raise concerns about rising rates of abuse of Adderall and other pharmaceutical stimulants (Miech et al., 2015).

The Developmental Age Gradient of SUD Prevalence

Perhaps the most striking demographic feature of SUD is the age-prevalence gradient characterized by increasing SUD rates during adolescence, peaks around ages 18–22, and reductions beginning in young adulthood and continuing throughout later developmental periods (see Jackson & Sartor, 2016). However, studies showing age differences in SUD rates for epidemiologic purposes tend to contrast relatively broad age groups, and a finer-grained depiction is informative from a developmental standpoint. Thus, as shown in Fig. 5.2, we conducted our own descriptive analyses of SUD prevalence rates as a function of age using NSDUH and NESARC data.

While Fig. 5.2 generally illustrates that some form of age-prevalence gradient is observed across a variety of substances, it also suggests a unique developmental stability of nicotine use disorder relative to other SUDs. That is, while rates of other SUDs show rapid declines beginning around the 20s, rates of nicotine use disorder remain relatively elevated throughout the 20s, 30s, and 40s, with dramatic declines beginning only around the 50s. This is consistent with MTF data showing relative developmental stability in rates of daily smoking rates throughout the 20s–30s (Johnston, O'Malley, Bachman, Schulenberg, & Miech, 2015). Also noteworthy in Fig. 5.2 are contrasts between illicit drugs and alcohol that are facilitated by our relatively fine-grained age grouping. SUDs rates for marijuana and other drugs show a relatively early downturn in the *early* 20s, whereas rates of alcohol use disorder begin to decline slightly later in the *late* 20s. This is consistent with MTF data showing that daily marijuana use declines rapidly throughout the 20s, whereas heavy drinking declines only gradually in the 20s and more rapidly from the late 20s to mid-30s (Johnston et al., 2015).

Of course, caution is warranted in interpreting cross-sectional age differences as reflecting patterns of developmental change. Indeed, the appearance of a developmental age gradient could be artifactually produced by factors such as differential mortality of those with SUDs and secular changes in prevalence rates. However, it

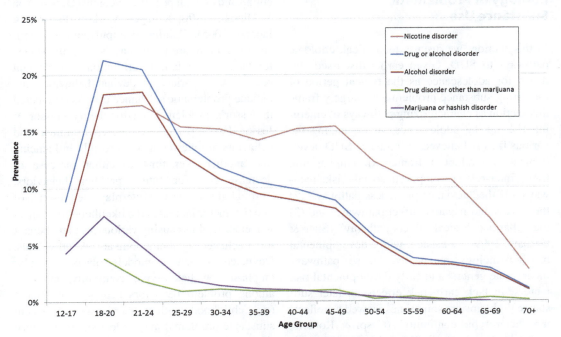

Note. Prevalence rates for ages 12 to 17 are based on U.S. 2002 NSDUH data (CBHSQ, 2015). Prevalence rates for ages 18 to 70+ are based on U.S. 2001-2002 NESARC data (Grant et al., 2014). Disorder rates reflect DSM-IV abuse or dependence except for nicotine disorder which reflects DSM-IV nicotine dependence (APA, 1994).

Fig. 5.2 The Age-Prevalence Gradient: US Past-Year Substance Disorder Rates Across Age Groups for Different Specific Substances

is unlikely that these other factors could plausibly explain the magnitude of age variability that is observed, given the somewhat limited extent of overall mortality and secular variation. Further, the age-prevalence gradient has also been observed in a number of longitudinal studies that can assess how prevalence rates change as a sample ages (e.g., Chen & Jacobson, 2012).

The robust evidence for an age-prevalence gradient motivates and informs the conceptualization of SUD from a developmental psychopathology standpoint (Chassin, Colder, Hussong, & Sher, 2016; Sher & Gotham, 1999). In particular, it motivates an emphasis on developmental factors that contribute to the escalation of problematic substance use leading up to the early 20s, as well as an emphasis on developmental factors that contribute to the later reductions beginning in young adulthood. These are the two primary topics covered throughout the remainder of this chapter.

Etiology of Problematic Substance Use

In this section, we discuss theoretical, etiologic pathways to SUD. Given earlier-discussed evidence for adolescence as the typical period of escalating substance problems, we largely frame this section as characterizing pathways of emerging risk during adolescence. In organizing the various factors believed to influence SUD development, we adopt a framework emphasizing three inter-related biopsychosocial risk pathways: (1) the "deviance proneness pathway," (2) the "stress and negative affect pathway," and (3) the "pharmacological effects pathway" (Sher & Gotham, 1999). Consistent with a developmental psychopathology perspective, these pathways incorporate genetic and early developmental risk factors. In fact, early risk effects on later substance problems are sometimes viewed as reflecting "heterotypic continuity" (Caspi & Roberts, 1999), with stable underlying risk merely manifesting differently in different developmental periods. The three etiologic pathways are not viewed as competing nor mutually exclusive. Rather, reflecting the principle of equifinality, different pathways may best explain SUD for different individuals, and many individuals may be influenced by multiple pathways. Indeed, our review below emphasizes findings suggesting ways that these pathways may be more interrelated than previously recognized. Our review also emphasizes potential prevention/intervention targets stemming from research on these pathways (for a more comprehensive review, see Chassin et al., 2016).

The Deviance Proneness Pathway

Deviance proneness models view problematic substance use as part of a broader "externalizing spectrum" that includes other problem behaviors (e.g., conduct disorder, antisociality). Developmentally speaking, these externalizing behaviors are viewed as generally originating from genetic risk and early impulsivity, in combination with contextual risk factors like poor parenting and deviant peer involvement (Gottfredson & Hirschi, 1990; Krueger, Markon, Patrick, & Iacono, 2005). Childhood impulsivity and deficient parenting are viewed as "setting the stage" for later school failure, affiliation with deviant peers, and a variety of deviant behaviors that include problematic substance use. As articulated in Jessor's problem behavior theory (Jessor & Jessor, 1977), personality, the environment, and behaviors are viewed as reciprocally influencing one another over time to either increase or decrease risk for future problem behaviors. Through this reciprocal interplay, the presence of one risk factor increases the likelihood that others will emerge, thus causing various problem behaviors to cluster together among at-risk individuals. Deviance proneness models place particular emphasis on heterotypic continuity, as links among problem behaviors across development (e.g., childhood conduct disorder and adolescent substance problems) may reflect stable deviance proneness risk (e.g., impulsivity) that manifests differently as development progresses (Schulenberg, Maggs, & O'Malley, 2003).

There is a great deal of empirical support for deviance proneness models, including prediction of SUDs by a number of early childhood externalizing behaviors like aggression, defiance, achievement problems, and poor peer relations (King, Iacono, & McGue, 2004). Further, there is particularly marked comorbidity of SUDs with other externalizing disorders (e.g., conduct disorder, antisociality), along with factor analytic evidence that externalizing disorders can be viewed as facets of a broader externalizing spectrum of psychopathology (Cooper, Wood, Orcutt, & Albino, 2003). These factor analytic studies also confirm impulsivity as a key predictor of the externalizing spectrum, complementing other evidence for impulsivity as a predictor of SUDs, more specifically (Sher, Littlefield, & Lee, 2017).

Regarding contextual factors believed to influence deviance proneness, it is important to rule out the possibility that these are mere correlated contextual markers of more causal intraindividual risk processes. For instance, because parenting is genetically influenced, it is noteworthy that research has found poor parenting to predict adolescent substance problems even when controlling for genetic risk (e.g., Dick et al., 2007; Miles, Silberg, Pickens, & Eaves, 2005). Further, because parenting can be influenced by impulsivity of the child, it is noteworthy that research has shown bidirectionality of effects between parenting and impulsivity (Ge et al., 1996) and unique effects of both on later substance problems (Brody & Ge, 2001). Similar findings exist for contextual effects of deviant peer affiliation, with unique effects of peers on substance problems even when controlling for gene- and impulsivity-related peer selection (e.g., Burk, Van Der Vorst, Kerr, & Stattin, 2012; Chassin et al., 2012). Further highlighting the importance of contextual factors like parents and peers, there is evidence that positive contextual influences can buffer effects of intrapersonal risk factors, thereby reducing risk for substance problems among otherwise high-risk individuals (Dick et al., 2007; Miles et al., 2005).

Practical Implications

A key practical implication of research on the deviance proneness pathway is that contextual factors indeed appear capable of buffering risk for adolescent substance problems, as is also indicated by evidence that parenting changes can mediate intervention effects (e.g., Sandler, Schoenfelder, Wolchik, & MacKinnon, 2011). Thus, while deviance proneness models emphasize the developmental continuity of risk that can result from reciprocal effects between individual and context (as described above), it is critical to also note that exposures to positive contexts can create developmentally discontinuous turning points, diverting individuals off of a high-risk trajectory (Rutter, 1996; Schulenberg et al., 2003). Further, the concept of heterotypic continuity highlights that, even in early prevention among youth with no substance use experience, prevention of initiation among high-risk individuals can require disruption of an ongoing risk trajectory characterized not by substance involvement but by other earlier developmental manifestations of deviance proneness (e.g., externalizing behaviors, impulsivity).

Regarding the central role of impulsivity in deviance proneness models, it is noteworthy that there has been increased recent attention to the idea of clinically targeted personality change (including impulsivity reduction; Magidson, Roberts, Collado-Rodriguez, & Lejuez, 2014). Further, it has been argued that universal prevention programs fostering early self-control could confer substantial benefits to most individuals and the population as a whole (Moffitt et al., 2011). Among clinical strategies for adolescent impulsivity reduction, family interventions should emphasize this as a goal of parenting skills training.

The Stress and Negative Affect Pathway

Stress and negative affect models have emphasized the role that substance use can play in alleviating negative emotions, with negative emotionality viewed as sometimes stemming from early stress and traumatic life events (Cappell & Herman, 1972; Greeley & Oei, 1999). However, while a role of affect in SUD etiology is suggested by comorbidity of affective and substance problems, past research has often found weak or null effects of negative affect on substance problems, especially when tested prospectively or with key covariates (e.g., externalizing; Colder et al., 2013; Hussong, Ennett, Cox, & Haroon, 2017). Further, it has been noted that covariation between affective and substance problems could reflect affective consequences of substance use and the related role of affect in maintaining an existing substance problem (Sher & Grekin, 2007).

However, research has shown clearer effects of daily fluctuations in negative affect on daily fluctuations in problematic substance use. This research supports the notion that, on a day-to-day basis, at least some individuals use substances to cope with negative affect (Epstein et al., 2009; Hussong, Galloway, & Feagans, 2005; Hussong, Gould, & Hersh, 2008). Further, moderated effects show that those most prone to problematic substance use in response to negative affect are those high on impulsivity, externalizing behaviors, and coping-related drinking motives (Hussong et al., 2005; Hussong et al., 2008; Menary et al., 2015). Importantly, by incorporating impulsivity and externalizing behaviors, these findings represent a potential point of synthesis between the deviance proneness and negative affect pathways. This potential synthesis is also reflected in recent evidence for the important etiologic role of "negative urgency" (Settles et al., 2012), a facet of disinhibition characterized by *impulsivity* under conditions of *negative affect* (Cyders & Smith, 2008).

Regarding the stress/trauma component of negative affect models, there is consistent evidence, especially among females, that substance problem development is influenced by early stressful events (e.g., conflict/violence exposure, parental neglect/abuse; Kristman-Valente & Wells, 2013; Sartor et al., 2013; Young-Wolff, Kendler, Ericson, & Prescott, 2011). However, the prediction that this relationship is mediated by negative affect has not been supported. It is therefore noteworthy that early stress/trauma may also impede normal development of behavior and emotion regulation capabilities, and it may be through these mechanisms that early stress/trauma influences substance problem development (Andersen & Teicher, 2009). This represents another potential point of synthesis between the deviance proneness and negative affect pathways, suggesting that risk conferred by early trauma may be partially mediated by impulsivity, including impulsivity in response to negative affect (i.e., negative urgency). This is consistent with evidence that early stress effects on later substance problems are mediated by externalizing but not internalizing symptomatology (Haller & Chassin, 2013; King & Chassin, 2008). Reflecting these empirical advances, more recent articulations of stress and negative affect models have placed greater emphasis on etiologic risk from emotional and behavioral dysregulation, rather than from negative affect per se (e.g., Hussong, Jones, Stein, Baucom, & Boeding, 2011).

Practical Implications

A key practical implication of research on the stress/negative affect pathway stems from the robust evidence for contextual influences of early stress and trauma, which highlights the need for policy, prevention, and treatment intervention strategies to reduce childhood stress/trauma exposure. Further, the potential points of overlap between deviance proneness and stress/negative affect models highlight early stress/trauma exposure as an early risk factor that may have broader effects on a wider variety of later risk processes than has been previously recognized.

Regarding the apparent etiologic importance of negative urgency, in addition to evidence for its broad effects on various forms of psychopathology (Settles et al., 2012), our review highlights its potential role as a common mechanism that could help bridge deviance proneness and stress/negative affect models. Further, in line with our earlier discussion of the movement toward personality-targeting interventions, negative urgency may hold particular promise as a powerful mediator of change in such programs.

The Pharmacological Effects Pathway

Pharmacological effects models focus on individual differences in sensitivity to psychoactive substance effects, with individual differences in sensitivity believed to confer differential risk for SUD development (Newlin & Thomson, 1990; Schuckit, 1987; Wise & Bozarth, 1987). Interestingly, two competing theories make two different partially conflicting sets of predictions regarding how substance-effect sensitivity relates to etiologic risk. The low level of response (LLR) model suggests that high-risk individuals have an overall lower sensitivity to substance effects, with insensitivity viewed as conveying risk in part because greater quantities must be used to achieve desired effects (Schuckit, 1987). In contrast, the differentiator model suggests that the relationship between substance-effect sensitivity and risk varies across types of substance effects (Newlin & Thomson, 1990). While agreeing with the LLR model in predicting that high-risk individuals will be less sensitive to sedating or unpleasant effects, the differentiator model disagrees with the LLR model in predicting that high-risk individuals will be *more* sensitive to stimulating or rewarding effects (de Wit & Phillips, 2012; Quinn & Fromme, 2011). Despite a vast body of past research, inconsistencies between these models remain largely unresolved (de Wit & Phillips, 2012; Morean & Corbin, 2010; Quinn & Fromme, 2011).

However, it can be generally stated that there is evidence across various substances that substance-effect sensitivity relates to risk for future use and related problems. For alcohol, there is particularly clear evidence for risk associated with low sensitivity, especially for more sedating or unpleasant effects (de Wit & Phillips, 2012; Quinn & Fromme, 2011). Indeed, low response to alcohol is viewed as a key alcohol use disorder endophenotype for genetic research, with evidence that it is heritable, predicted by familial alcohol use disorder, and prospectively predictive of alcohol use disorder development (Ray, Mackillop, & Monti, 2010). However, an empirical challenge in human research has been disentangling inborn insensitivity (existing prior to substance initiation) from acquired tolerance to the substance, thus leaving questions regarding directionality of effects between insensitivity and substance problems. Nonetheless, animal research provides evidence for inborn insensitivity effects on substance problem development (de Wit & Phillips, 2012). Regarding nicotine and other drugs (e.g., marijuana, opiates, cocaine), research is generally sparser and extant findings are mixed. However, when effects are detected, they generally show risk associated with *higher* sensitivity to stimulating or rewarding effects and risk associated with *lower* sensitivity to sedating or unpleasant effects (de Wit & Phillips, 2012).

The alcohol literature provides prospective research characterizing a number of mechanisms that may mediate risk originating from substance insensitivity. Based on this research, such mechanisms may include (1) use of greater quantities of the substance to achieve desired effects, (2) selection of heavier substance-using peers, and (3) pro-substance changes in substance-related social norms, substance-effect expectancies, and motives for substance use (e.g., Schuckit et al., 2011; Schuckit, Smith, Trim, Tolentino, & Hall, 2010). The role of deviant peer group affiliation in these processes suggests a potential point of synthesis between deviance proneness and pharmacological effects models. Further, potential overlap between these two pathways is reflected by evidence for associations between impulsivity and substance-effect insensitivity (e.g., Kirkpatrick, Johanson, & de Wit, 2013; Scott & Corbin, 2014).

Arguably, these pathways can "set the stage" for escalation to more severe problematic substance use characterized by what is often termed "addiction." Although there is no precise agreed-upon definition of addiction, most models of addiction are based upon the notion that, with sufficient substance exposure, relatively durable changes in brain circuitry lead to compulsive patterns of use characterized by drug seeking even in the face of punishment. These changes are sometimes described as reflecting a shift from "liking" to "wanting" of a substance (e.g., as in incentive-sensitization theory; Robinson & Berridge, 2008), a shift from instrumental behavior to a compulsive habit (e.g., Everitt & Robbins, 2005), or an "allostatic" shift in hedonic set-point (sparking a cycle of compensatory substance use and further deviations in the hedonic set-point; Volkow, Koob, & McLellan, 2016). Importantly, these changes suggest that early interventions that precede progression to addiction should perhaps be designed very differently than those targeting individuals exhibiting clear signs of addiction.

Desistance from Problematic Substance Use

As described earlier, epidemiologic data show dramatic age-related reductions in problematic substance use beginning in young adulthood, thus motivating empirical efforts to understand SUD desistance from a developmental perspective. Knowledge of naturally occurring factors that drive desistance can offer unique insights into the nature of SUD and inform public health and clinical interventions (NIAAA, 2008). The following sections review evidence for different possible mechanisms of desistance, beginning with effects of young adult role transitions (e.g., marriage, parenthood) and personality maturation (e.g., decreased impulsivity and neuroticism). Further sections then discuss the need for more lifespan developmental research to explain the later substance-related reductions observed in developmental periods beyond young adulthood, noting some mechanisms that may be particularly relevant to desistance in these periods (e.g., problem recognition, substance-related health concerns).

A key point pertaining to all mechanisms reviewed here is that more research is needed on possible historic changes in how these mechanisms have operated. Preliminary descriptive evidence suggests historic differences across cohorts in the age-related trend of adolescent/emerging-adult escalation and subsequent young adult reduction of substance involvement (e.g., see Fig. 5-18d in Johnston et al., 2015). Key public policy insights could be gleaned from in-depth analyses of such cohort changes in age trends and how they may relate to cohort changes in desistance mechanisms (e.g., the prevalence, life course timing, and impact of adult role transitions). It is also noteworthy that evidence exists for gender, racial, and ethnic differences in both patterns and mechanisms of age-related drinking reductions (e.g., see Chassin et al., 2016). Although discussion of such differences is largely beyond the scope of the current chapter, this should be noted as another important topic in need of further exploration in future research.

Young Adult Maturing Out

Particular attention has been paid in past research to explaining the normative reductions in problematic substance use that occur in young adulthood (Winick, 1962). Speaking to the substantial nature of these reductions, in addition to the fact that declines are observed even in rates of syndromal SUDs (as opposed to less severe indices of problem use; see Fig. 5.2), there is even evidence that the majority of declines in this period occur among individuals with relatively severe pre-young adult patterns of problematic use (Jackson, Sher, Gotham, & Wood, 2001; Lee, Chassin, & Villalta, 2013). These findings indicate a clinical relevance of young adult maturing out, suggesting that efforts to understand this phenomenon could provide key insights guiding the design and improvement of prevention and treatment intervention efforts.

Effects of Young Adult Contextual Transitions

In explaining the reductions in problematic substance use that occur in young adulthood, much attention has been paid to the rapid contextual change that occurs in this developmental period. Of course, when considering possible contextual effects, it is important to bear in mind the distinction between socialization and selection effects (per role incompatibility theory; Yamaguchi & Kandel, 1985). That is, while a changing context *may* influence individuals' behaviors (i.e., socialization), apparent effects of context may instead reflect individuals' entry into contexts that are fitting with their pre-existing individual characteristics (i.e., selection).

In conceptualizing how contextual change may influence young adult reductions in problematic substance use, it is relevant to consider not only transitions into low-risk environments (e.g., marriage, parenthood) but also contextual transitions out of high-risk environments (e.g., college graduation). For instance, prior to young adulthood, there is evidence for socialization effects of college attendance on increased substance involvement (Bachman, Wadsworth, O'Malley, & Johnston, 1997), as well as other socialization effects of more specific high-risk contexts within the college environment (e.g., fraternity/sorority affiliation; Park, Sher, & Krull, 2008). Thus, as may be expected, there is also evidence that transitions out of high-risk (e.g., college-related) environments may partially explain the subsequent reductions in problematic substance use observed to occur around young adulthood (Bartholow, Sher, & Krull, 2003; Sher, Bartholow, & Nanda, 2001). It is important to bear this in mind in addition to the more common explanation of young adult substance-related reductions as occurring due to normative transitions into lower-risk environments.

Indeed, most past research on young adult "maturing out" has focused on developmental transitions into relatively low-risk adult roles such as marriage, parenthood, and full-time employment. Young adulthood is marked by widespread adoption of such roles (Bachman et al., 1997), and well-established developmental theory views these transitions as key young adult developmental tasks (Erikson, 1968). In studies accounting for role selection as a potential alternative explanation, both young adult marriage and parenthood have generally been shown to convey role socialization effects on reduced substance use and related problems (e.g., Bachman et al., 1997; Curran, Muthen, & Harford, 1998; Flora & Chassin, 2005; Gotham, Sher, & Wood, 2003; Lee, Chassin, & MacKinnon, 2010; Warr, 1998). In contrast, previous research has often failed to show socialization effects of young adult employment on substance-related reductions (e.g., Bachman et al., 1997; Gotham et al., 2003; Warr, 1998), although with some evidence for certain specific occupational categories (e.g., "professional" employment; Staff et al., 2010).

Practical Implications of Effects of Young Adult Contextual Transitions

Supporting the practical (e.g., clinical) relevance of these young adult role effects, in addition to evidence that family roles can spur SUD desistance (e.g., Gotham et al., 2003), there is even evidence that family role effects may be strongest among those with relatively severe pre-role problematic substance use. As depicted in Fig. 5.3, Lee, Chassin, and MacKinnon (2015) found that young adult marriage spurred an especially large drinking trajectory downturn for those with particularly severe problem drinking symptomatology prior to marriage. It is also noteworthy that, beyond family role effects on substance-related maturing out, there is a growing consensus across diverse literatures that family roles (and marriage in particular) can convey various wide-ranging benefits, both catalyzing adaptation and mitigating psychopathology (Derrick & Leonard, 2016; Roberts, Wood, & Smith, 2005; Sampson, Laub, & Wimer, 2006; Walters, 2000).

However, despite the potential importance of family roles from a public health standpoint, surprisingly little is currently known about processes explaining their effects on substance-related maturing out. Existing mediation findings show the most robust support for mediation of family role effects via decreased socializing with peers, with additional mixed evidence for mediation via changes in drinking-related attitudes and increased religiosity (Bachman et al. 2002; Lee et al., 2010; Staff et al., 2010; Warr, 1998). Mediation via reduced socializing with peers is particularly consistent with a role incompatibility explanation, which emphasizes how demands of new family roles can restrict opportunities for substance involvement. However, as articulated in Platt's (1964) commentary on ways to achieve "strong inference," future studies should conduct "riskier" tests of the role incompatibility explanation. This means testing hypotheses that could

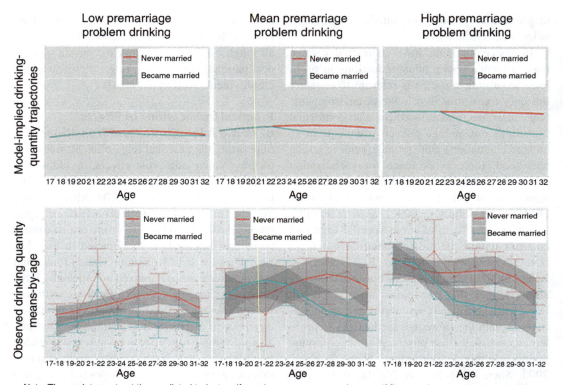

Note. These plots contrast the predicted trajectory if marriage never occurred versus if first marriage occurred at age 23, although age 23 is arbitrary, as the model estimates a uniform marriage effect across ages. Plots of observed means-by-age show triangles for means (with connecting lines), color-coded dots for individual data points, bars two standard deviations from means, ans smoothes loess lines with shaded 95% confidence regions.

Fig. 5.3 Problem drinking severity moderates marriage effects on drinking trajectories: Marriage effects on drinking quantity trajectories at three different levels of premarriage problem drinking

provide discriminating support for this over other plausible explanations, and testing hypotheses that could disconfirm this in favor of other plausible explanations. For instance, an explicit assessment of conflict between drinking and family role demands could provide discriminating support for the role incompatibility explanation (Lee, Chassin, & MacKinnon, 2015). Further, this should be tested against other plausible explanations including those emphasizing possible role-driven personality maturation (Lee, Ellingson, & Sher, 2015) and the relational bonds that family roles can forge (e.g., Roberts & Chapman, 2000; Sampson et al., 2006).

Effects of Young Adult Personality Development

Despite a vast, longstanding literature linking personality to substance use and related pathology (Sher et al., 2017), research has only recently considered how personality may relate to maturing out of problematic substance use. This may be due to the traditional view of personality emphasizing stability of personality traits, with research only recently attending to the ways that personality traits change across the lifespan. For instance, Fig. 5.4 depicts meta-analytic evidence for lifespan increases in conscientiousness and emotional stability (akin to lack of neuroticism) (Roberts, Walton, & Viechtbauer, 2006). Perhaps motivated by this work on personality maturation, a subsequent series of studies showed that problem drinking reductions from age 18 to 35 were correlated with decreasing impulsivity, increasing conscientiousness, and decreasing neuroticism across the same age span (Littlefield, Sher, & Wood, 2009, 2010a). A follow-up study using the same data (Littlefield, Sher, & Wood,

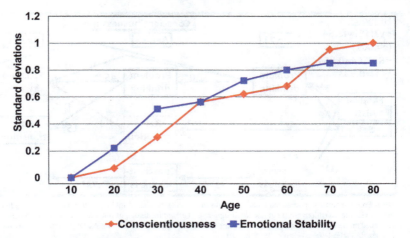

Fig. 5.4 Developmental personality maturation across the lifespan

Note. This figure was adapted from Roberts et al. (2006). It depicts results from their meta-analysis characterizing developmental changes in personality across the lifespan.

2010b) also showed that the correlated change between personality maturation and problem drinking reductions was mediated by reductions in coping-related drinking motives. Although most research on this topic has focused on problem drinking, similar evidence for correlated change has also been found linking developmental impulsivity reductions with reductions in marijuana and cigarette use (Quinn, & Harden, 2013; Littlefield & Sher, 2012).

The above studies of correlated change between personality and substance problems have forged an entirely new avenue for maturing out research, with an important next step being the investigation of different possible directions of effects. Toward this objective, Lee, Ellingson, and Sher (2015) estimated cross-lag models testing bidirectional effects between personality and problem drinking across four waves spanning ages 21–35. As depicted in Fig. 5.5, results showed prospective effects where both lower impulsivity and higher conscientiousness predicted lower subsequent problem drinking. This evidence for prospective effects complements earlier evidence for correlated change, thereby bolstering confidence in effects of impulsivity and conscientiousness maturation on substance-related maturing out. In contrast, results did not show prospective effects between neuroticism and problem drinking in either direction.

Past studies of correlated change between personality and problem drinking controlled for effects of family roles (Littlefield et al., 2009, 2010a), but beyond this, little else has been done to establish an integrated model of adult role and personality effects on maturing out. Toward this objective, Lee, Ellingson, and Sher's (2015) cross-lag models (described above) included family role transitions (marriage *or* parenthood) at each wave to test mediation between roles and personality in predicting problem drinking. As shown in Fig. 5.5, personality effects were mediated by family role transitions. Specifically, higher conscientiousness and lower impulsivity at age 21 predicted transitions to a family role by age 25, which in turn predicted lower problem drinking at age 29. In contrast, role effects were not mediated by personality, as prospective role effects on personality were not found at any age (see Fig. 5.5).

Practical Implications of Effects of Young Adult Personality Development

In line with our earlier discussion of the movement toward personality-targeting interventions, the above research on personality and maturing out further highlights the likely utility of intervention programs aimed at reducing impulsivity and increasing conscientiousness. Littlefield et al. (2009) speculated that such programs could

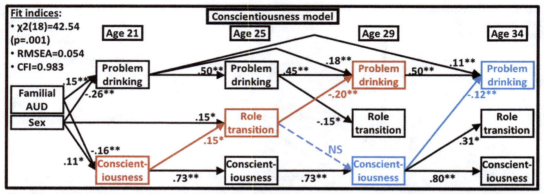

Fig. 5.5 An integrative model of role and personality effects on maturing out of problem drinking: Results of a cross-lagged panel model of problem drinking, familial role transitions (marriage or parenthood), and conscientiousness across four longitudinal time points

perhaps cause relatively durable changes in drinking behavior by addressing a relatively "deep" underlying component of susceptibility. Consistent with this notion, a recent review concluded that brief cognitive-behavioral treatments for substance use often have enduring effects on personality (Roberts et al., 2017). Further, Lee, Ellingson, and Sher (2015) noted based on their mediational findings that early impulsivity- and conscientiousness-targeting programs could convey protective effects in part by aiding successful subsequent transitions into young adult family roles.

Maturing Out of Substance Problems beyond Young Adulthood

As discussed earlier, epidemiologic data shows that age-related reductions in problematic substance use are not confined to young adulthood, but rather begin in young adulthood and continue throughout the adult lifespan. Beyond this epidemiologic evidence, some additional research exists offering a more precise account of changes in problematic substance use across the adult lifespan. Vergés et al. (2012, 2013) assessed changes across the lifespan in rates of SUD persistence, onset, and recurrence to understand their unique contributions to overall age-related reductions in SUD rates. As depicted in Fig. 5.6, results showed especially marked age reductions in new onsets (Fig. 5.6, middle panel). Thus, although the term "maturing out" may be taken to imply age increases in *desistance*, the continual declines in SUD rates observed throughout the lifespan instead appear largely attributable to age reductions in *new onsets*. In contrast, although not emphasized by Vergés et al., rates of desistance appeared to peak in young adulthood. For instance, based on their alcohol dependence persistence rates (Fig. 5.6, upper panel), it can be inferred that the rate of desistance peaked at 72% by ages 28–32, then declined to a low of 55% by ages 43–52, and then remained somewhat low thereafter. Thus, an interesting possibility is that risk for SUD onset may continually decline throughout the lifespan, whereas potential for desistance from an existing SUD may peak in young adulthood. Perhaps confirming and extending the latter notion, a recent study by this chapter's authors (Lee et al., 2018) investigated desistance across the lifespan while differentiating mild, moderate, and severe alcohol use disorder (per *DSM-5*; APA, 2013). Results showed that, for those with a *severe* alcohol use disorder, desistance rates were substantially higher in young adulthood than in later developmental

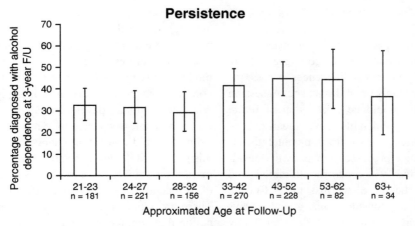
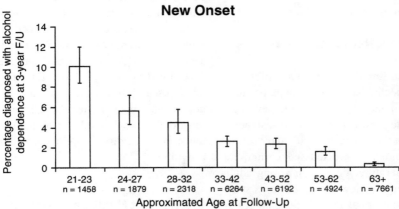
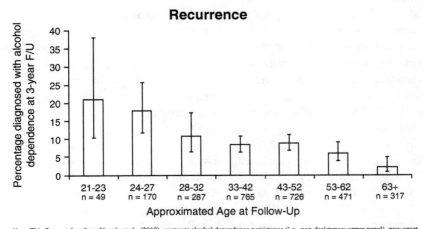

Note. This figure, taken from Vergés et al., (2012), contrasts alcohol dependence persistence (i.e., non-desistance; upper panel), new onset (middle panel), and recurrence (lower panel) as three distinct contributors to age differences in overall alcohol dependence prevalence rates. Rates of persistence, new onset, and recurrence over a three-year period are depicted within different age groups of the NESARC sample (Grant et al., 2014). Persistence rate was defined as the percentage of participants with a past-year alcohol dependence diagnosis at the baseline wave who also had a past-year alcohol dependence diagnosis at the three-year follow-up wave. New onset rate was defined as the percentage of participants with no lifetime history of alcohol dependence at baseline who had a diagnosis of past-year alcohol dependence at the three-year follow-up wave. Recurrence rate was defined as the percentage of participants with lifetime but not past-year alcohol dependence at the baseline wave who had a diagnosis of past-year alcohol dependence by the three-year follow-up wave. Brackets show the 95% confidence intervals around means,

Fig. 5.6 Deconstructing the age-prevalence gradient: Rates of longitudinal alcohol dependence persistence, onset, and recurrence within different age groups

periods (e.g., 46–49% at ages 25–34 vs. 25–29% at ages 35–55).

The above evidence for differences across the lifespan in patterns of desistance suggests there may also be important differences across the lifespan in mechanisms of desistance. Assessing this possibility should be a key goal of future research, as key insights have clearly been gleaned by attending to developmental differences in etiologic processes across earlier developmental periods (i.e., across childhood and adolescence; Chassin, Sher, Hussong, & Curran, 2013). Below we consider some specific ways that the mechanisms influencing desistance may vary across periods of the adult lifespan.

Maturing Out vs. Natural Recovery Models

Predictions regarding developmental differences in desistance mechanisms can perhaps be made based on Watson and Sher's (1998) review highlighting dramatic differences in how desistance is viewed between the "maturing out" and "natural recovery" literatures. As discussed earlier, the maturing out literature focuses on young adulthood and has largely viewed desistance as stemming from maturational contextual changes in this developmental period (e.g., marriage; Bachman et al., 1997) and accompanying role demands that conflict with substance involvement (Yamaguchi & Kandel, 1985). Importantly, these processes are rarely conceptualized as involving acknowledgement or concern regarding one's substance use (Jackson & Sartor, 2016; Watson & Sher, 1998). A starkly different view of desistance comes from the "natural recovery" literature, which has investigated precursors of desistance, mostly in midlife samples (e.g., mean age = 41 [SD = 9.1] in a review by Sobell, Ellingstad, & Sobell, 2000). Informed in part by stage models of behavior change, this literature often views desistance as stemming from an accumulation of consequences that can prompt (1) deliberate reappraisals of one's substance use, followed by (2) self-recognition of a substance problem, and then (3) targeted efforts to change substance use behaviors (Klingemann & Sobell, 2007).

Predictions can perhaps stem from an overarching premise that the maturing out and natural recovery literatures may both offer valid conceptualizations of desistance, but with maturing out models applying predominantly to young adulthood and natural recovery models applying predominantly to later developmental periods. That is, young adult desistance may more often stem from the rapid contextual changes occurring in this period, while desistance in later periods may more often stem from more deliberate processes of problem recognition and effortful change. These predictions are consistent with the general notion that contextual effects on behavioral outcomes may decrease with age as individuals increasingly exert control over their environments (Kendler et al., 2007; Scarr & McCartney, 1983). Although quite speculative, these predictions illustrate the potential for lifespan desistance research to reconcile ostensibly discrepant conceptual models, thereby advance the field toward a more unified understanding of desistance and guiding developmentally informed programs.

Older Adult Health and Desistance

Older adulthood brings various health-related physical and cognitive challenges that may increase in importance as possible desistance mechanisms in this late developmental period (White, 2006). For instance, there is evidence that over 50% of US seniors drink alcohol at levels deemed risky in the context of co-occurring medical conditions (Moore et al., 2006). Further, along with these health issues comes increased use of medications that could interact harmfully with alcohol or other substances, with a striking 76% of US seniors using multiple prescription medications (Gu, Dillon, & Burt, 2010). Of the small extant literature on older adult substance use, health issues are among the most commonly reported reasons for desistance (e.g., Schutte, Moos, & Brennan, 2006). However, studies of prospective effects of health problems on substance-related reductions are more equivocal (e.g., Moos, Brennan, Schutte, & Moos, 2010;

Schutte et al., 2006), perhaps owing to the complex relevance of affect- and coping-related issues to older adult substance use (Schulte & Hser, 2014). For instance, there is evidence that health problems can spur substance use reductions, but can also have the opposite effect for those who use substances to cope (Moos et al., 2010).

An important objective should be to expand upon existing research in this area. This should include further study of how affect- and coping-related factors may impede adaptive responding to substance-related health issues, as well as how these processes are influenced by aging-related substance-effect sensitivity (Heuberger, 2009) and changing social support systems (White, 2006). This is particularly important given the increases in older adult substance problems that are projected to coincide with the aging of the "baby boomer" generation (Han, Gfroerer, Colliver, & Penne, 2009), thus suggesting a great future need for empirically informed substance use interventions for older adults.

Concluding Comments

Substance use and SUDs are among the most common risky behaviors and mental health issues in the developed world, creating considerable burden to society and suffering of individuals and their loved ones. Studying the course of substance use and SUDs in the general population reveals a marked age gradient characterized by escalation during adolescence and peaks around ages 18–22. This developmental escalation of risk, and individual differences in this escalation, can be understood to occur through multiple etiologic risk pathways. Broadly speaking, key pathways to SUD include (1) a "deviance proneness pathway" involving an impulsivity-based general tendency toward risky/deviant behaviors; (2) a "stress/negative affect pathway" involving early stress/trauma exposure, negative emotionality, and emotional/behavioral dysregulation; and (3) a "pharmacological effects pathway" involving individual differences in sensitivity to substance effects. Each risk pathway is distally influenced by genetic and early developmental risk factors, and also mediated and moderated by contextual influences. Our review highlights research indicating points of potential overlap among these three pathways that should be further investigated toward advancing a more unified understanding of SUD etiology.

Following the peak developmental period of SUD risk around ages 18–22, the modal course beginning in young adulthood is characterized by desistance and reduced risk for onset or relapse. The shift toward "maturing out" in young adulthood has long been recognized as owing to developmental transitions into adult roles (e.g., marriage, parenthood), although closer examination is needed to better understand the mechanisms of these role effects. Recent research shows that psychosocial maturation is another key contributor to young adult substance-related maturing out, with particularly strong evidence for effects of age-related decreases in impulsivity and increases in conscientiousness. More research is needed to establish an integrated model of adult role and personality effects on young adult maturing out.

Recent findings also highlight that developmental reductions in substance-related risk continue throughout the adult lifespan. Future research should investigate the possibility that certain desistance mechanisms may operate predominantly in young adulthood (e.g., family role effects), while others may become more important in later developmental periods (e.g., "problem recognition" and effortful change, substance-related health concerns). Such work may help reconcile diverse conceptual models of desistance and thereby advance the field toward a more unified understanding of how desistance occurs.

Practical Implications

As discussed throughout this chapter, key insights guiding prevention and treatment intervention efforts can be gleaned from research on problematic substance use epidemiology, etiologic risk pathways, and desistance mechanisms.

Epidemiologic data on age differences identifies periods of normative escalation and normative peaks in risk, thereby guiding decisions about optimal developmental timing for implementing different levels of prevention and treatment intervention programs. An understanding of the etiologic pathways through which problematic substance use develops can assist intervention efforts by (1) informing strategies for early identification of at-risk individuals (e.g., for selective prevention), (2) indicating modifiable risk factors that should be targeted for clinical change, and (3) suggesting ways that other (e.g., nonmodifiable) risk factors may moderate program effects. An understanding of naturally occurring processes of desistance from problematic substance use can inform interventions aimed at goading similar changes.

A key conclusion that should be drawn from our review is the substantial impact that contextual factors can have on substance problem trajectories. For instance, this is reflected in the potential for positive parenting and peer influences to buffer risk for substance problem development in deviance proneness models, as well as the potential for adult role transitions to spur maturing out of problematic substance use. This evidence that positive contextual influences can create turning points that disrupt established high-risk trajectories should motivate continual efforts to improve public policy and clinical programs aimed at early intervention with high-risk individuals. In addition, the influence of context highlights the importance of programs preventing exposure to high-risk environments, as is illustrated by the evidence for various mechanisms of risk that can stem from early stress and trauma.

Our review also highlights that certain dispositional characteristics (e.g., impulsivity) track the modal rise and fall of substance-related risk across the entire lifespan. This holds broad practical relevance, as there are likely various applications for interventions targeting such dispositional characteristics, ranging from early prevention to adult SUD intervention. This is particularly noteworthy in light of recent attention to impulsivity reduction as a target for programs ranging from childhood universal prevention to adult clinical treatment.

Regarding mechanisms of desistance, a richer understanding of the specific processes through which normative young adult role transitions (e.g., marriage, parenthood) spur maturing out may reveal ways that these naturally occurring processes can be leveraged in a clinical setting. For young adult problematic substance users, an efficient clinical strategy may be to emphasize anticipated or ongoing adult role transitions in order to initiate or amplify potentially ongoing normative processes of adult role preparation and adaptation. Further, it may be possible for prevention programs to spur earlier initiation of these maturational processes and thereby prevent onset or escalation of substance problems during the critical risk period around ages 18–22. Regarding desistance in later developmental periods, greater empirical attention to possible developmental differences in mechanisms of desistance could help guide lifespan developmental tailoring of prevention and treatment intervention programs.

Limitations

This review is restricted in that the developmental course described here, although characterizing modal trends in the USA and other developed countries, might not be universal. Caution is therefore warranted in generalizing to other cultures (Jackson & Sartor, 2016). Even within the USA, there is evidence for differences among non-Hispanic Caucasians, Hispanics, and African-Americans in age gradients of problematic substance use (see Chassin et al., 2016), perhaps reflecting differences in the timing and nature of adult role transitions and employment opportunities. Also, most empirical knowledge on this subject is based on alcohol research. Although the age-prevalence curve for most other drug use disorders appears largely similar to that of alcohol use disorder (Vergés et al. 2012; Vergés et al. 2013), we noted earlier that this is not true for smoking and tobacco use disorder. This may be one relatively clear example of a broader issue: that developmental patterns can vary across drugs as a function of factors such as intrinsic addiction potential and/or social acceptability. Thus, greater attention to commonalities and differences across cultures, ethnicities, and substance types is needed to establish an accurate developmental account of problematic substance use.

References

Allen, J. P., Litten, R. Z., Fertig, J. B., & Babor, T. (1997). A review of research on the Alcohol Use Disorders Identification Test (AUDIT). *Alcoholism: Clinical and Experimental Research, 21*(4), 613–619.

American Psychiatric Association. (1980). *Diagnostic and statistical manual of mental disorders: DSM-III* (3rd ed.). Washington, DC: American Psychiatric Association.

American Psychiatric Association. (1994). *Diagnostic and statistical manual of mental disorders: DSM-IV* (4th ed.). Washington, DC: American Psychiatric Association.

American Psychiatric Association. (2013). *Diagnostic and statistical manual of mental disorders: DSM-5* (5th ed.). Washington, DC: American Psychiatric Association.

Andersen, S., & Teicher, M. (2009). Desperately driven and no brakes: Developmental stress exposure and subsequent risk for substance abuse. *Neuroscience and Biobehavioral Reviews, 33*, 516–524.

Bachman, J. G., O'Malley, P. M., Schulenberg, J. E., Johnston, L. D., Bryant, A. L., Merline, A. C. (2002) Why substance use declines in young adulthood: Changes in social activities, roles, and beliefs. Mahwah, NJ: Lawrence Erlbaum Associates.

Bachman, J. G., Wadsworth, K. N., O'Malley, P. M., & Johnston, L. D. (1997). *Smoking, drinking, and drug use in young adulthood: The impacts of new freedoms and new responsibilities.* Hillsdale, NJ: Lawrence Erlbaum Associates, Inc.

Bartholow, B. D., Sher, K. J., & Krull, J. L. (2003). Changes in heavy drinking over the third decade of life as a function of collegiate fraternity and sorority involvement: A prospective, multilevel analysis. *Health Psychology, 22*(6), 616.

Boness, C. L., Lane, S. P., & Sher, K. J. (2016). Assessment of withdrawal and hangover are confounded in the AUDADIS: Withdrawal prevalence is likely inflated. *Alcoholism: Clinical and Experimental Research, 40*(8), 1691–1699.

Brody, G. H., & Ge, X. (2001). Linking parenting processes and self-regulation to psychological functioning and alcohol use during early adolescence. *Journal of Family Psychology, 15*, 82–94.

Burk, W. J., Van Der Vorst, H., Kerr, M., & Stattin, H. (2012). Alcohol use and friendship dynamics: Selection and socialization in early-, middle-, and late-adolescent peer networks. *Journal of Studies on Alcohol and Drugs, 73*(1), 89–98.

Cappell, H., & Herman, C. P. (1972). Alcohol and tension reduction: A review. *Quarterly Journal of Studies on Alcohol, 33*, 33–64.

Caspi, A., & Roberts, B. W. (1999). Personality change and continuity across the life course. In L. A. Pervin & O. P. John (Eds.), *Handbook of personality theory and research* (Vol. 2, pp. 300–326). New York: Guilford.

Center for Behavioral Health Statistics and Quality [CBHSQ]. (2015). *Behavioral health trends in the United States: Results from the 2014 National Survey on Drug Use and Health (HHS Publication No. SMA 15-4927, NSDUH Series H-50).* Retrieved from http://www.samhsa.gov/data/

Chassin, L., Colder, C. R., Hussong, A., & Sher, K. J. (2016). Substance use and substance use disorders. In D. Cicchetti (Ed.), *Developmental psychopathology* (Vol. 3, pp. 1–65).

Chassin, L., Lee, M. R., Cho, Y. I., Wang, F. L., Agrawal, A., Sher, K. J., & Lynskey, M. T. (2012). Testing multiple levels of influence in the intergenerational transmission of alcohol disorders from a developmental perspective: The example of alcohol use promoting peers and μ-opioid receptor M1 variation. *Development and Psychopathology, 24*(3), 953–967.

Chassin, L., Sher, K. J., Hussong, A., & Curran, P. (2013). The developmental psychopathology of alcohol use and alcohol disorders: Research achievements and future directions. *Development and Psychopathology, 25*(4pt2), 1567–1584.

Chen, P., & Jacobson, K. C. (2012). Developmental trajectories of substance use from early adolescence to young adulthood: gender and racial/ethnic differences. *Journal of Adolescent Health, 50*(2), 154–163.

Colder, C. R., Scalco, M., Trucco, E. M., Read, J. P., Lengua, L. J., Wieczorek, W. F., & Hawk, L. W., Jr. (2013). Prospective associations of internalizing and externalizing problems and their co-occurrence with early adolescent substance use. *Journal of Abnormal Child Psychology, 41*(4), 667–677.

Cooper, M. L., Wood, P. K., Orcutt, H. K., & Albino, A. (2003). Personality and the predisposition to engage in risky or problem behaviors during adolescence. *Journal of Personality and Social Psychology, 84*, 390–410.

Curran, P. J., Muthen, B. O., & Harford, T. C. (1998). The influence of changes in marital status on developmental trajectories of alcohol use in young adults. *Journal of Studies on Alcohol, 59*, 647–658.

Cyders, M. A., & Smith, G. T. (2008). Emotion-based dispositions to rash action: positive and negative urgency. *Psychological Bulletin, 134*(6), 807–828.

De Wit, H., & Phillips, T. J. (2012). Do initial responses to drugs predict future use or abuse? *Neuroscience & Biobehavioral Reviews, 36*(6), 1565–1576.

Del Boca, F., Darkes, J., & McRee, B. (2016). Self-report assessments of psychoactive substance use and dependence. In K. J. Sher (Ed.), *Oxford handbook of substance use disorders*. New York, NY: Oxford University Press.

Derrick, J. L., & Leonard, K. E. (2016). Substance use in committed relationships. In K. J. Sher (Ed.), *Oxford handbook of substance use disorders*. New York, NY: Oxford University Press.

Dick, D. M., Viken, R., Purcell, S., Kaprio, J., Pulkkinen, L., & Rose, R. J. (2007). Parental monitoring moderates the importance of genetic and environmental influences on adolescent smoking. *Journal of Abnormal Psychology, 116*, 213–218.

Epstein, D. H., Willner-Reid, J., Vahabzadeh, M., Mezghanni, M., Lin, J. L., & Preston, K. L. (2009). Real-time electronic diary reports of cue exposure and mood in the hours before cocaine and heroin craving and use. *Archives of General Psychiatry, 66*(1), 88–94.

Erikson, E. H. (1968). *Identity: Youth and crisis*. Oxford, England: Norton & Co.

Everitt, B. J., & Robbins, T. W. (2005). Neural systems of reinforcement for drug addiction: From actions to habits to compulsion. *Nature Neuroscience, 8*(11), 1481–1489.

Flora, D. B., & Chassin, L. (2005). Changes in drug use during young adulthood: The effects of parent alcoholism and transition into marriage. *Psychology of Addictive Behaviors, 19*(4), 352–362.

Ge, X., Conger, R., Cadoret, R., Neiderheiser, J., Yates, W., Troughton, E., & Stewart, M. (1996). The developmental interface between nature and nurture: A mutual influence model of child antisocial behavior and parent behavior. *Developmental Psychology, 32*, 574–589.

Gotham, H. J., Sher, K. J., & Wood, P. K. (2003). Alcohol involvement and developmental task completion during young adulthood. *Journal of Studies on Alcohol, 64*, 32–42.

Gottfredson, M., & Hirschi, T. (1990). *A general theory of crime*. Stanford, CA: Stanford University Press.

Grant, B. F., Amsbary, M., Chu, A., Sigman, R., Kali, J., Sugawana, Y., ... Chou, P. (2014). *Source and accuracy statement: national epidemiologic survey on alcohol and related conditions-III*. Rockville, MD: National Institute on Alcohol Abuse and Alcoholism.

Grant, B. F., Hasin, D. S., Chou, S. P., Stinson, F. S., & Dawson, D. A. (2004). Nicotine dependence and psychiatric disorders in the United States: Results from the national epidemiologic survey on alcohol and related conditions. *Archives of General Psychiatry, 61*(11), 1107–1115.

Grant, B. F., Moore, T. C., Shepard, J., & Kaplan, K. (2003). *Source and accuracy statement: Wave 1 National epidemiologic survey on alcohol and related conditions (NESARC)*. Bethesda, MD: National Institute on Alcohol Abuse and Alcoholism.

Grant, B. F., Peterson, A., Dawson, D. A., & Chou, P. S. (1994). *Source and accuracy statement for the National longitudinal alcohol epidemiologic survey (NLAES)*. Bethesda, MD: National Institute on Alcohol Abuse and Alcoholism.

Greeley, J., & Oei, T. (1999). Alcohol and tension reduction. In K. Leonard & H. Blane (Eds.), *Psychological theories of drinking and alcoholism* (2nd ed., pp. 14–53). New York, NY: Guilford Press.

Gu, Q., Dillon, C. F., & Burt, V. L. (2010). Prescription drug use continues to increase: US prescription drug data for 2007–2008. *NCHS Data Brief, 42*, 1–8.

Haller, M., & Chassin, L. (2013). The influence of PTSD symptoms on alcohol and drug problems: Internalizing and externalizing pathways. *Psychological Trauma: Theory, Research, Practice, and Policy, 5*(5), 484.

Hammond, D., Fong, G. T., Cummings, K. M., & Hyland, A. (2005). Smoking topography, brand switching, and nicotine delivery: Results from an in vivo study. *Cancer Epidemiology Biomarkers & Prevention, 14*(6), 1370–1375.

Han, B., Gfroerer, J. C., Colliver, J. D., & Penne, M. A. (2009). Substance use disorder among older adults in the United States in 2020. *Addiction, 104*(1), 88–96.

Hasin, D. (2015). DSM-5 SUD diagnoses: changes, reactions, remaining open questions. *Drug and Alcohol Dependence, 148*, 226.

Heuberger, R. A. (2009). Alcohol and the older adult: A comprehensive review. *Journal of Nutrition for the Elderly, 28*(3), 203–235.

Hussong, A., Jones, D., Stein, G., Baucom, D., & Boeding, S. (2011). An internalizing pathway to alcohol use and disorder. *Psychology of Addictive Behaviors, 25*, 390–404.

Hussong, A. M., Ennett, S. T., Cox, M. J., & Haroon, M. (2017). A systematic review of the unique prospective association of negative affect symptoms and adolescent substance use controlling for externalizing symptoms. *Psychology of Addictive Behaviors, 31*(2), 137.

Hussong, A. M., Galloway, C. A., & Feagans, L. A. (2005). Coping motives as a moderator of daily mood-drinking covariation. *Journal of Studies on Alcohol, 66*(3), 344–353.

Hussong, A. M., Gould, L. F., & Hersh, M. A. (2008). Conduct problems moderate self-medication and mood-related drinking consequences in adolescents. *Journal of Studies on Alcohol and Drugs, 69*(2), 296.

Jackson, K., & Sartor, C. (2016). The natural course of substance use and dependence. In K. J. Sher (Ed.), *Oxford handbook of substance use disorders*. New York, NY: Oxford University Press.

Jackson, K. M., Sher, K. J., Gotham, H. J., & Wood, P. K. (2001). Transitioning into and out of large-effect drinking in young adulthood. *Journal of Abnormal Psychology, 110*, 378–391.

Jessor, R., & Jessor, S. L. (1977). *Problem behavior and psychosocial development: A longitudinal study of youth*. San Diego, CA: Academic Press.

Johnston, L. D., O'Malley, P. M., Bachman, J. G., Schulenberg, J. E., & Miech, R. A. (2015). *Monitoring the Future national survey results on drug use, 1975–2014: Volume 2, College students and adults ages*

19–55. Ann Arbor: Institute for Social Research, The University of Michigan.

Kendler, K. S., Jacobson, K. C., Gardner, C. O., Gillespie, N., Aggen, S. A., & Prescott, C. A. (2007). Creating a social world: A developmental twin study of peer-group deviance. *Archives of General Psychiatry, 64*, 958.

King, K. M., & Chassin, L. (2008). Adolescent stressors, psychopathology, and young adult substance dependence: A prospective study. *Journal of Studies on Alcohol and Drugs, 69*(5), 629–638.

King, S. M., Iacono, W. G., & McGue, M. (2004). Childhood externalizing and internalizing psychopathology in the prediction of early substance use. *Addiction, 99*(12), 1548–1559.

Kirkpatrick, M. G., Johanson, C. E., & de Wit, H. (2013). Personality and the acute subjective effects of d-amphetamine in humans. *Journal of Psychopharmacology, 27*(3), 256–264.

Klingemann, H. K., & Sobell, L. C. (2007). *Promoting self-change from addictive behaviors: Practical implications for policy, prevention, and treatment.* New York, NY: Springer.

Kristman-Valente, A., & Wells, E. A. (2013). The role of gender in the association between child maltreatment and substance use behavior: A systematic review of longitudinal research from 1995 to 2011. *Substance Use & Misuse, 48*(8), 645–660.

Krueger, R. F., Markon, K. E., Patrick, C. J., & Iacono, W. G. (2005). Externalizing psychopathology in adulthood: A dimensional-spectrum conceptualization and its implications for DSM-V. *Journal of Abnormal Psychology, 114*, 537–550.

Lee, M. R., Chassin, L., & MacKinnon, D. (2010). The effect of marriage on young adult heavy drinking and its mediators: results from two methods of adjusting for selection into marriage. *Psychology of Addictive Behaviors, 24*(4), 712–718. PMID: 21198229; PMCID: PMC3058715.

Lee, M. R., Chassin, L., & MacKinnon, D. (2015). Role transitions and young adult maturing out of heavy drinking: Evidence for larger effects of marriage among more severe pre-marriage problem drinkers. *Alcoholism: Clinical and Experimental Research, 39*(6), 1064–1074. https://doi.org/10.1111/acer.12715

Lee, M. R., Chassin, L., & Villalta, I. K. (2013). Maturing out of alcohol involvement: Transitions in latent drinking statuses from late adolescence to adulthood. *Development and Psychopathology, 25*, 1137–1153.

Lee, M. R., Ellingson, J. M., & Sher, K. J. (2015). Integrating social-contextual and intrapersonal mechanisms of "maturing out": Joint influences of familial role transitions and personality maturation on problem drinking reductions. *Alcoholism: Clinical and Experimental Research, 39*(9), 1775–1787.

Lee, M. R., Marshall, C. L., McDowell, Y. E., Vergés, A., Steinley, D. L., & Sher, K. J. (2018). Desistance and severity of alcohol use disorder: A lifespan-developmental analysis. *Clinical Psychological Science, 6*, 90–105.

Littlefield, A. K., & Sher, K. J. (2012). Smoking desistance and personality change in emerging and young adulthood. *Nicotine & Tobacco Research, 14*(3), 338–342. https://doi.org/10.1093/ntr/ntr219

Littlefield, A. K., Sher, K. J., & Wood, P. K. (2009). Is 'maturing out' of problematic alcohol involvement related to personality change? *Journal of Abnormal Psychology, 118*, 360–374.

Littlefield, A. K., Sher, K. J., & Wood, P. K. (2010a). A personality-based description of maturing out of alcohol problems: Extension with a five-factor model and robustness to modeling challenges. *Addictive Behaviors, 35*, 948–954.

Littlefield, A. K., Sher, K. J., & Wood, P. K. (2010b). Do changes in drinking motives mediate the relation between personality change and "maturing out" of problem drinking? *Journal of Abnormal Psychology, 119*, 93–105.

Magidson, J. F., Roberts, B. W., Collado-Rodriguez, A., & Lejuez, C. W. (2014). Theory-driven intervention for changing personality: Expectancy value theory, behavioral activation, and conscientiousness. *Developmental Psychology, 50*(5), 1442–1450.

Martin, C. S., Chung, T., & Langenbucher, J. (2016). Historical and cultural perspectives on substance use and substance use disorders. In K. J. Sher (Ed.), *Oxford handbook of substance use disorders*. New York, NY: Oxford University Press.

Menary, K. R., Corbin, W. R., Leeman, R. F., Fucito, L. M., Toll, B. A., DeMartini, K., & O'Malley, S. S. (2015). Interactive and indirect effects of anxiety and negative urgency on alcohol-related problems. *Alcoholism: Clinical and Experimental Research, 39*(7), 1267–1274.

Miech, R. A., Johnston, L. D., O'Malley, P. M., Bachman, J. G., & Schulenberg, J. E. (2015). *Monitoring the Future national survey results on drug use, 1975–2014: Volume I, Secondary school students.* Ann Arbor: Institute for Social Research, The University of Michigan http://monitoringthefuture.org/pubs.html#monographs

Miles, D. R., Silberg, J. L., Pickens, R. W., & Eaves, L. J. (2005). Familial influences on alcohol use in adolescent female twins: Testing for genetic and environmental interactions. *Journal of Studies on Alcohol, 66*, 445–451.

Moffitt, T. E., Arseneault, L., Belsky, D., Dickson, N., Hancox, R. J., Harrington, H., … Caspi, A. (2011). A gradient of childhood self-control predicts health, wealth, and public safety. *Proceedings of the National Academy of Sciences, 108*(7), 2693–2698.

Mokdad, A. H., Marks, J. S., Stroup, D. F., & Gerberding, J. L. (2004). Actual causes of death in the United States, 2000. *Journal of the American Medical Association, 291*(10), 1238–1245.

Moore, A. A., Giuli, L., Gould, R., Hu, P., Zhou, K., Reuben, D., … Karlamangla, A. (2006). Alcohol use, comorbidity, and mortality. *Journal of the American Geriatrics Society, 54*(5), 757–762.

Moos, R. H., Brennan, P. L., Schutte, K. K., & Moos, B. S. (2010). Older adults' health and late-life drinking patterns: A 20-year perspective. *Aging and Mental Health, 14*(1), 33–43.

Morean, M. E., & Corbin, W. R. (2010). Subjective response to alcohol: A critical review of the literature. *Alcoholism: Clinical and Experimental Research, 34*(3), 385–395.

National Institute on Alcohol Abuse and Alcoholism. (2004). *NIAAA council approves definition of binge drinking, NIAAA Newsletter, No. 3*. Bethesda, MD: National Institute on Alcohol Abuse and Alcoholism.

National Institute on Alcohol Abuse and Alcoholism. (2008). *The National Institute on Alcohol Abuse and Alcoholism Five Year Strategic Plan: FY09–14 "Alcohol Across the Lifespan"*. 2008.

National Institute on Drug Abuse. (2015). *Trends & Statistics*. Retrieved from https://www.drugabuse.gov/related-topics/trends-statistics

Neal, D. J., Corbin, W. R., & Fromme, K. (2006). Measurement of alcohol-related consequences among high school and college students: Application of item response models to the Rutgers alcohol problem index. *Psychological Assessment, 18*(4), 402.

Newlin, D. B., & Thomson, J. B. (1990). Alcohol challenge with sons of alcoholics: A critical review and analysis. *Psychological Bulletin, 108*(3), 383–402.

Park, A., Sher, K. J., & Krull, J. L. (2008). Risky drinking in college changes as fraternity/sorority affiliation changes: a person-environment perspective. *Psychology of Addictive Behaviors, 22*(2), 219.

Parrott, A. C. (2004). Is ecstasy MDMA? A review of the proportion of ecstasy tablets containing MDMA, their dosage levels, and the changing perceptions of purity. *Psychopharmacology, 173*, 234–241.

Platt, J. R. (1964). Strong inference. *Science, 146*(3642), 347–353.

Quinn, P. D., & Fromme, K. (2011). Subjective response to alcohol challenge: A quantitative review. *Alcoholism: Clinical and Experimental Research, 35*(10), 1759–1770.

Quinn, P., & Harden, K. (2013). Differential changes in impulsivity and sensation seeking and the escalation of substance use from adolescence to early adulthood. *Development and Psychopathology, 25*(1), 223–239.

Ray, L. A., Mackillop, J., & Monti, P. M. (2010). Subjective responses to alcohol consumption as endophenotypes: Advancing behavioral genetics in etiological and treatment models of alcoholism. *Substance Use & Misuse, 45*(11), 1742–1765.

Roberts, B. W., & Chapman, C. N. (2000). Change in dispositional well-being and its relation to role quality: A 30-year longitudinal study. *Journal of Research in Personality, 34*, 26–41.

Roberts, B. W., Luo, J., Briley, D. A., Chow, P. I., Su, R., & Hill, P. L. (2017). A systematic review of personality trait change through intervention. *Psychological Bulletin, 143*(2), 117–141.

Roberts, B. W., Walton, K. E., & Viechtbauer, W. (2006). Patterns of mean-level change in personality traits across the life course: a meta-analysis of longitudinal studies. *Psychological Bulletin, 132*(1), 1–25.

Roberts, B. W., Wood, D., & Smith, J. L. (2005). Evaluating five factor theory and social investment perspectives on personality trait development. *Journal of Research in Personality, 39*(1), 166–184.

Robinson, T. E., & Berridge, K. C. (2008). The incentive sensitization theory of addiction: some current issues. *Philosophical Transactions of the Royal Society of London B: Biological Sciences, 363*(1507), 3137–3146.

Rutter, M. (1996). Transitions and turning points in developmental psychopathology: As applied to the age span between childhood and mid-adulthood. *International Journal of Behavioral Development, 19*, 603–626.

Sampson, R. J., Laub, J. H., & Wimer, C. (2006). Does marriage reduce crime? A counterfactual approach to within-individual causal effects. *Criminology, 44*, 465–508.

Sandler, I., Schoenfelder, E., Wolchik, S., & MacKinnon, D. (2011). Long-term impact of prevention programs to promote effective parenting: lasting effects but uncertain processes. *Annual Review of Psychology, 62*, 299.

Sartor, C. E., Waldron, M., Duncan, A. E., Grant, J. D., McCutcheon, V. V., Nelson, E. C., … Heath, A. C. (2013). Childhood sexual abuse and early substance use in adolescent girls: The role of familial influences. *Addiction, 108*, 993–1000.

Scarr, S., & McCartney, K. (1983). How people make their own environments: A theory of genotype→ environment effects. *Child Development, 54*, 424–435.

Schuckit, M. A. (1987). Biological vulnerability to alcoholism. *Journal of Consulting and Clinical Psychology, 55*(3), 301–309.

Schuckit, M. A., Smith, T. L., Trim, R. S., Allen, R. C., Fukukura, T., Knight, E. E., … Kreikebaum, S. A. (2011). A prospective evaluation of how a low level of response to alcohol predicts later heavy drinking and alcohol problems. *The American Journal of Drug and Alcohol Abuse, 37*(6), 479–486.

Schuckit, M. A., Smith, T. L., Trim, R. S., Tolentino, N. J., & Hall, S. A. (2010). Comparing structural equation models that use different measures of the level of response to alcohol. *Alcoholism: Clinical and Experimental Research, 34*(5), 861–868.

Schulenberg, J., Maggs, J. L., & O'Malley, P. M. (2003). How and why the understanding of developmental continuity and discontinuity is important: The sample case of long-term consequences of adolescent substance use. In J. T. Mortimer & M. Shanahan (Eds.), *Handbook of the life course* (pp. 413–436). New York: Kluwer Academic/Plenum Publishers.

Schulte, M. T., & Hser, Y. I. (2014). Substance use and associated health conditions throughout the lifespan. *Public Health Reviews, 35*(2), 1–27.

Schutte, K. K., Moos, R. H., & Brennan, P. L. (2006). Predictors of untreated remission from late-life drinking problems. *Journal of Studies on Alcohol, 67*(3), 354–362.

Scott, C., & Corbin, W. R. (2014). Influence of sensation seeking on response to alcohol versus placebo: Implications for the acquired preparedness model. *Journal of Studies on Alcohol and Drugs, 75*(1), 136.

Settles, R. E., Fischer, S., Cyders, M. A., Combs, J. L., Gunn, R. L., & Smith, G. T. (2012). Negative urgency: A personality predictor of externalizing behavior characterized by neuroticism, low conscientiousness, and disagreeableness. *Journal of Abnormal Psychology, 121*(1), 160.

Sher, K. J., Bartholow, B. D., & Nanda, S. (2001). Short- and long-term effects of fraternity and sorority membership on heavy drinking: A social norms perspective. *Psychology of Addictive Behaviors, 15*(1), 42.

Sher, K. J., & Gotham, H. J. (1999). Pathological alcohol involvement: A developmental disorder of young adulthood. *Development and Psychopathology, 11*(04), 933–956.

Sher, K. J., & Grekin, E. R. (2007). Alcohol and affect regulation. In J. J. Gross (Ed.), *Handbook of emotion regulation* (pp. 560–580). New York, NY: Guilford Press.

Sher, K. J., Littlefield, A. K., & Lee, M. R. (2017). Personality processes related to the development and resolution of alcohol use disorders. In H. E. Fitzgerald & L. I. Puttler (Eds.), *Developmental psychopathology of alcohol use disorders*. New York, NY: Oxford University Press.

Sobell, L. C., Ellingstad, T. P., & Sobell, M. B. (2000). Natural recovery from alcohol and drug problems: Methodological review of the research with suggestions for future directions. *Addiction, 95*(5), 749–764.

Staff, J., Schulenberg, J. E., Maslowsky, J., Bachman, J. G., O'Malley, P. M., Maggs, J. L., & Johnston, L. D. (2010). Substance use changes and social role transitions: Proximal developmental effects on ongoing trajectories from late adolescence through early adulthood. *Development and Psychopathology, 22*, 917–932.

Vergés, A., Haeny, A. M., Jackson, K. M., Bucholz, K. K., Grant, J. D., Trull, T. J., … Sher, K. J. (2013). Refining the notion of maturing out: Results from the national epidemiologic survey on alcohol and related conditions. *American Journal of Public Health, 103*(12), e67–e73.

Vergés, A., Jackson, K. M., Bucholz, K. K., Grant, J. D., Trull, T. J., Wood, P. K., & Sher, K. J. (2012). Deconstructing the age-prevalence curve of alcohol dependence: Why "maturing out" is only a small piece of the puzzle. *Journal of Abnormal Psychology, 121*(2), 511–523.

Volkow, N. D., Koob, G. F., & McLellan, A. T. (2016). Neurobiologic advances from the brain disease model of addiction. *New England Journal of Medicine, 374*(4), 363–371.

Wakefield, J. C. (2015). DSM-5 substance use disorder: how conceptual missteps weakened the foundations of the addictive disorders field. *Acta Psychiatrica Scandinavica, 132*(5), 327–334.

Walters, G. D. (2000). Spontaneous remission from alcohol, tobacco, and other drug abuse: Seeking quantitative answers to qualitative questions 1. *The American Journal of Drug and Alcohol Abuse, 26*, 443–460.

Warr, M. (1998). Life-course transitions and desistance from crime. *Criminology, 36*, 183–216.

Watson, A. L., & Sher, K. J. (1998). Resolution of alcohol problems without treatment: Methodological issues and future directions of natural recovery research. *Clinical Psychology: Science and Practice, 5*, 1–18.

White, W. (2006). Recovery across the life cycle. *Alcoholism Treatment Quarterly, 24*(1–2), 185–201.

Winick, C. (1962). Maturing out of narcotic addiction. *Bulletin on Narcotics, 14*(1), 1–7.

Wise, R., & Bozarth, M. (1987). A psychomotor stimulant theory of addiction. *Psychological Review, 94*, 469–492.

Yamaguchi, K., & Kandel, D. B. (1985). On the resolution of role incompatibility: A life event history analysis of family roles and marijuana use. *American Journal of Sociology, 90*(6), 1284–1325.

Young-Wolff, K. C., Kendler, K. S., Ericson, M. L., & Prescott, C. A. (2011). Accounting for the association between childhood maltreatment and alcohol-use disorders in males: A twin study. *Psychological Medicine, 41*(1), 59–70.

The Tobacco Control Experience: A Model for Substance Use Prevention?

Kenneth E. Warner

Introduction and Overview

In terms of "body count"—the number of deaths it causes—tobacco use, and cigarette smoking in particular, is the world's most important form of substance abuse. According to the World Health Organization, in the twentieth century tobacco caused the deaths of 100 million people worldwide. If current tobacco use trends persist, tobacco will kill a billion of the globe's citizens in the twenty-first century (Eriksen, Mackay, & Ross, 2015). In the USA alone, smoking claims nearly 500,000 lives every year, accounting for a fifth of all deaths (CDC, 2016a). Smoking kills far more Americans than all other substances of abuse combined. And increasingly, the victims of smoking come from society's marginalized populations. Rates of smoking—and deaths from smoking—are far higher among the poor and less educated. For example, 43% of Americans with a GED certificate are smokers today. Among individuals with a postgraduate degree, only 5.4% smoke (Jamal et al., 2015).

That's the bad news. The good news is that tobacco control, the admixture of public and private sector efforts to diminish the toll of tobacco, has dramatically reduced smoking and its burden of preventable, premature disease and death. In the USA (the focus of this chapter), over the past half century tobacco control has reduced the prevalence of smoking by about two-thirds and prevented more than eight million premature deaths that would have occurred in its absence. Each of those deaths would have cost its victim on average nearly 20 years of life (Holford et al., 2014). Social norms concerning smoking have shifted 180°: In the 1950s, smoking was considered a sign of sophistication, sex appeal, sociability, and even athleticism. Today, fairly or not, smokers are viewed as weak-willed objects of scorn (Proctor, 2012).

Progress against smoking appears to have accelerated in the most recent years. According to the National Health Interview Survey, from 2014 to 2015 age-adjusted adult smoking prevalence fell by a tenth, to 15.1%, the largest single-year drop in history. And that followed a 5% decline the preceding year (CDC, 2016b). Students' 30-day smoking prevalence is the lowest it has been in the 40 years such data have been collected. In 1976, 38.8% of high school seniors had smoked in the past 30 days. In 2015, that figure had fallen to 11.4%, and the intensity of smoking (number of days during the month) had declined dramatically as well. The percentage declines in 30-day smoking prevalence in 2014–2015 were the largest ever (Monitoring the Future, 2015).

K. E. Warner (✉)
Department of Health Management and Policy,
University of Michigan School of Public Health,
Ann Arbor, MI, USA
e-mail: kwarner@umich.edu

In this chapter we examine applicable lessons deriving from the tobacco control experience for dealing with other substance abuse issues. First, however, we describe the history of tobacco control policy and drill down into its component parts, reviewing the evidence base as it applies to traditional tobacco control interventions and identifying novel possible directions for tobacco control, themselves presently the subject of much controversy. With regard to at least one of these novel directions, harm reduction, the field of tobacco control has much to learn from experience dealing with other substance abuse problems.

Tobacco Control Policies and Their Impacts

For the first six decades of the twentieth century until 1963, cigarette smoking followed a nearly relentless upward path, increasing annually except for brief interruptions occasioned by the Great Depression, World War II, and a smoking-and-cancer scare sparked by the first scientific evidence strongly linking smoking to lung cancer (Wynder & Graham, 1950; Doll and Hill, 1950). The release of the first Surgeon General's report on smoking and health on January 11, 1964 (USDHEW, 1964), proved to be the turning point for smoking. Adult per capita cigarette consumption (total cigarette consumption divided by the population age ≥ 18) began a period of annual declines (see Fig. 6.1). Release of the report was one of the biggest news items of the year. Smoking fell by 15% in the three months following the release. By the end of the year, recidivism had caused the overall decline to fall to 5%. But 1963 marked the high point for smoking in America, never to be seen again (USDHHS, 2014).

The policy response to the report was swift. From 1964 to 1971, states adopted an unusually large number of cigarette excise tax increases, raising the real price of cigarettes (the price relative to inflation) and thereby depressing cigarette sales. A large body of research demonstrates that a 10% increase in the price of cigarettes decreases adult cigarette consumption by 2.5–5%. Approximately half of that decline is associated with reductions in the number of cigarettes continuing smokers consume, while the other half reflects price-induced quitting. Tax increases are perceived to be particularly effective tools for discouraging smoking among young people who are two to three times more price responsive than adults (Chaloupka, Yurekli, & Fong, 2012).

Upping a state's cigarette tax allowed the legislature to do good—decreasing smoking—while also doing well—increasing revenues (Warner, 1984). However, because some states chose not to raise their tax rates, particularly the southeastern tobacco states, price differences among states led to significant interstate cigarette smuggling. This in turn slowed the rate of adoption of new tax increases for a decade, and the real price of cigarettes fell from 1971 to 1981 (Warner, 1982). A slowing of smuggling led to reduced concerns about it, and a new spate of state tax increases followed (U.S. Department of Health and Human Services, 1989).

Federal Policies

The Surgeon General's 1964 report called for "appropriate remedial action." The first federal government response was passage of the Federal Cigarette Labeling and Advertising Act of 1965. The act required a warning label on cigarette packages reading "Caution: Cigarette Smoking May Be Hazardous to Your Health." The warning was the first of its kind in the world. The act also required an annual report to Congress on the health consequences of smoking (the Surgeon General's reports on smoking and health), with the Secretary of Health's recommending needed legislation. At the same time, however, the act prohibited the Federal Trade Commission from adopting any regulations on cigarette advertising for four years. The tobacco industry had successfully pressured Congress to produce a weak bill with a warning label substantially watered down from that which the FTC had originally desired (Brandt, 2007). This was the first instance, of many, in which the tobacco industry lobbying

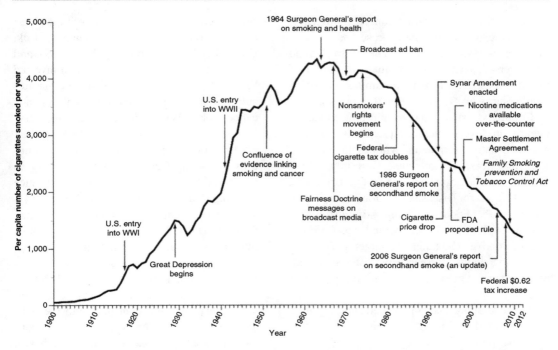

Fig. 6.1 Adult per capita cigarette consumption and major events, 1900–2012. Source: USDHHS, 2014, Figure 2.1, page 18

succeeded in blocking or minimizing the impact of federal legislation on smoking and health.

Although symbolically important, the warning labels had no demonstrable impact on smoking, especially after their novelty wore off. In part this was attributable to the weak wording; in part it reflected the obscure placement of the warnings (on the sides of cigarette packs), their small font, and often their hard-to-see color (e.g., gold-leaf text on a white background).

The second major federal "remedial action" occurred shortly thereafter. The Federal Communications Commission ruled that its Fairness Doctrine applied to the issue of smoking and health. The doctrine was originally adopted to ensure balanced coverage of controversial political issues in the nation's broadcast media. Its principal application had been to require TV and radio stations to donate airtime to political viewpoints opposite those for which airtime had been purchased. A young attorney, John Banzhaf, convinced the Commission that smoking and health fell under the doctrine, as only one side of the "controversial issue" was then being represented on the broadcast media, namely through cigarette companies' substantial investment in TV and radio cigarette advertising.

The novel antismoking ads aired during 1967–1970. Their effect was dramatic: While adult per capita cigarette consumption had risen modestly in 1965–1966, following its sizable decline in 1964, it fell all four of the years the policy was in effect, the first time that per capita consumption had declined more than two consecutive years (see Fig. 6.1).

Ironically (although intentionally), the highly effective Fairness Doctrine ads (per capita consumption declined >5%) were removed from the media following Congress's passage of the Public Health Cigarette Smoking Act of 1969 which banned broadcast advertising of cigarettes. While eliminating cigarette ads was initially considered a public health triumph, in fact the law was adopted in direct response to behind-the-scene lobbying by the cigarette companies. Ending cigarette advertising would eliminate the requirement for the Fairness Doctrine ads. The act thus freed the companies from the deleterious effect of the Fairness Doctrine ads on cigarette sales; adult per capita consumption rose for the next three years (Warner, 1979). The upward trend was reversed, permanently, from the beginning of the state-based movement to limit smoking in public places in 1973 (more on this below).

Counteradvertising has been produced subsequently in several states, including California, Massachusetts, Florida, and Minnesota, and, in a few instances, nationwide. Currently, three national media campaigns are in operation, one by the Centers for Disease Control and Prevention, one from the Food and Drug Administration's Center for Tobacco Products, and one from the Truth Initiative. The latter two target adolescents and young adults. Research indicates that both past and current media campaigns have depressed smoking.

The federal presence in tobacco control policy has been modest. In part this reflects an assessment that policy should be largely at the discretion of the states, excepting issues of interstate commerce. In part, it represents the oppressive influence of the tobacco industry on Congress, acting primarily through Representatives and Senators from the six major tobacco-producing states, but also, directly, through substantial campaign contributions to individual legislators (Saloojee & Dagli, 2000). The industry has prevented or diminished policies at the state and local levels too, but even the resources of the tobacco industry are not unlimited. As such, it has proven easier to adopt smoking-restriction policies at the state and local levels.

Federal involvement in tobacco control has included the following:

- Congress has strengthened package warning labels over the years. The 1969 act strengthened the wording. The Comprehensive Smoking Education Act of 1984 introduced the nation's first rotating labels. Rotating labels were mandated on smokeless tobacco products in 1986.
- While the USA led the world by introducing pack warnings, the country now lags the international standard: graphic warning labels (GWLs), depicting the damage inflicted by smoking, in most instances covering at least half the front and back of the cigarette pack. Under the Family Smoking Prevention and Tobacco Control Act of 2009, which invested FDA with the authority to regulate cigarettes and certain other tobacco products, the agency called for GWLs. However, an industry-initiated lawsuit succeeded in blocking their implementation. Evidence from other countries, including Canada, the first country to adopt GWLs, suggests that they can reduce smoking (Huang, Chaloupka, & Fong, 2014).
- The Department of Health and Human Services (DHHS) has continued to publish Surgeon General's reports. Some have captured a great deal of media and public attention. In particular, the 1986 report (USDHHS, 1986) covering the then-emerging science on involuntary smoking contributed to the public's increasing understanding that environmental tobacco smoke constituted a health hazard for nonsmokers. Scientific interest in the subject was sparked by a study published five years earlier in which Hirayama (1981) demonstrated that in Japan the nonsmoking wives of smoking husbands had an elevated risk of lung cancer. The report reinforced the state-level movement, under way since 1973, to restrict or ban smoking in public places. A 1992 ruling by the Environmental Protection Agency labeled cigarette smoke a human carcinogen, providing additional authoritative basis for laws and policies restricting smoking in public places, although only a handful of the ensuing restrictions have come from the federal government.
- Another especially influential Surgeon General's report, released in 1988 (USDHHS, 1988), definitively identified smoking as an addiction. The report awakened the public to the notion that smoking was not simply a "habit."
- Congress has raised cigarette (and other tobacco products) taxes on several occasions. The 1952 federal cigarette excise tax of 8 cents per pack was doubled 31 years later, and then raised to 20 cents in 1991, 24 cents two years thereafter, 34 cents in 2000, 39 cents in

2002, and $1.01 in 2009. A marked decline in smoking in 2010 followed the particularly large 2009 increase.
- Congress and federal agencies have restricted smoking in public places. In 1973 the Civil Aeronautics Board required separate seating for smokers on domestic flights. A year later the Interstate Commerce Commission restricted smoking to the back 20% of seats on interstate buses. In 1987, DHHS itself went smoke-free, prohibiting smoking in any of its facilities.
- The following year Congress banned smoking on domestic flights of $\leq$2 h, extending the ban to $\leq$6 h in 1990, thereby *de facto* banning smoking on all domestic flights. The airplane ban is instructive, given that it is one of few substantial congressionally mandated tobacco control policies. While it passed in response to highly effective lobbying led by flight attendants, the fact that industry opposition did not prevent the ban reflected a unique situation: Congressional representatives and Senators constitute perhaps the nation's premier "frequent flier club," in many instances flying weekly between Washington and their home state. Most were not smokers. They did not want to have to breathe the smoke of their fellow fliers. As well, because fliers are on average more educated and affluent than those who do not fly, the proportion of the flying public who would object was relatively small (Holm & Davis, 2004).
- Recently, through the Affordable Care Act, Congress required states to provide smoking cessation support through their Medicaid programs. Previously, state coverage was highly variable (Schauffler, Barker, & Orleans, 2001). Evidence clearly indicates that, administered properly, particularly with good clinical support, FDA-approved cessation pharmaceuticals can double or triple the odds of quitting compared to unsupported cessation attempts (Fiore et al., 2008). The evidence is less clear, however, that use of nicotine replacement products bought over the counter (e.g., nicotine gum and patches) increases the odds of successful quitting (Hughes, Peters, & Naud, 2011).

Policies that have *not* been adopted through federal channels are as notable as those that have. The 1989 Surgeon General's report (USDHHS, 1989) identified a dozen or more federal policies that, had they simply been applied to smoking, would have required the government to ban cigarettes. In all instances the responsible government agencies chose not to apply the policies to cigarettes or were mandated by Congress to exempt cigarettes. A prominent example of the latter was a proposed investigation of the safety of cigarettes by the Consumer Products Safety Commission. Congress specifically amended CPSC's charter to prohibit it from regulating tobacco products. Ironically, cigarettes kill far more Americans than all of the products CPSC has ever investigated.

Another example of a failure to regulate smoking is an exception that proves the rule. In the 1990s, then commissioner of the FDA, David Kessler, pursued an investigation of cigarette smoking, concluding that it was a "pediatric disease" because nearly all smoking, and hence nicotine addiction, was initiated during childhood. Kessler proposed a number of regulatory measures that were stopped by an industry lawsuit, which eventually reached the Supreme Court. The court ruled that FDA did not have the authority to regulate cigarettes because Congress had never intended the agency to include cigarettes in the Food, Drug, and Cosmetics Law (Kessler, 2001).

A third and final example of Congress's failure to regulate tobacco products occurred in the mid- to late 1990s. A series of lawsuits by the states against the tobacco industry, seeking compensation for smoking-related Medicaid costs, were culminating in the possibility of a 46-state settlement (the other states having already won their individual lawsuits). Congress contemplated legislation that effectively would have mooted the idea of a settlement. In a fierce debate (Pertschuk, 2001), the legislation ultimately failed. Instead, the states settled with the industry. In addition to restricting industry marketing and funding a youth smoking prevention foundation (now the Truth Initiative), the Master Settlement Agreement (as it was called) required the participating manufacturers (including all of the major companies) to pay billions of dollars to the states annually in perpetuity. This increased the price of cigarettes, as the industry passed on the penalty to their consumers. The states' attorneys general missed an opportunity to maximize the impact of the settlement by failing to require that any of the states' funds be devoted to tobacco control, or even to public health more generally. As a consequence, only a handful of states have ever devoted to tobacco control a CDC-recommended minimum expenditure (Huang, Walton, Gerzoff, King, & Chaloupka, 2015).

As noted above, FDA has finally acquired regulatory authority regarding tobacco products (FDA, 2016a). The authority is broad and substantial, now covering virtually all tobacco products and novel nicotine-yielding products. In concept the agency could use its new authority to require the reduction of toxins in cigarettes, including reducing nicotine yields of combusted tobacco products to levels unlikely to sustain addiction. To date, however, the agency has been able to implement only a few modest regulations. Notably, FDA has required the elimination of all characterizing flavors from cigarettes, with the exception of one of the most pervasive and quite possibly the most dangerous: menthol. The agency recently announced limited regulations on novel products such as electronic or e-cigarettes (FDA, 2016b).

The agency faces an extraordinary challenge to implementing meaningful regulations, reflecting the legislated need for convincing proof of public health benefit, the enormity of the bureaucratic process required to propose and ultimately implement a regulation, the extremely challenging political environment in which the agency must operate, and the certainty of industry lawsuits of any proposed regulations that might adversely affect the sale of tobacco products.

State and Local Policies

As noted above, much of formal tobacco control policy has emanated from the states and, in some instances, local units of government. This is certainly the case with cigarette taxation, with each year's seeing multiple states raising their tax rates. As well, and as previously mentioned, states were the locus of media counteradvertising campaigns following the Fairness Doctrine ads and preceding the national truth campaign.

Possibly the states' greatest contribution has been in the area of mandating clean indoor air, or smoke-free environments. In 1973 Arizona adopted the first state-level restrictions in some public places. The following year, Connecticut enacted the first restrictions on smoking in restaurants. In 1975 Minnesota adopted what was then widely considered the model state clean indoor air law. It required no-smoking areas in buildings open to the public. Other states followed in reasonably rapid succession, and over time states that had already adopted laws strengthened them. The state laws moved from partial restrictions to complete bans beginning with Delaware's 2002 law, the first state law to completely prohibit smoking in all workplaces, restaurants, and bars (USDHHS, 2014). Currently about half the states have adopted comprehensive smoke-free workplace laws (Americans Nonsmokers' Rights Foundation, 2018).

Evidence demonstrates that smoke-free workplace laws protect workers from second-hand smoke. Further, smoke-free policies reduce smoking, with one prominent study estimating an impact comparable to that of a moderate-sized excise tax increase (Fichtenberg & Glantz, 2002). Smoke-free policies thereby directly improve the public's health. Several studies have found a reduction in hospitalizations for myocardial infarctions in jurisdictions that have adopted smoke-free laws. Research also demonstrates that smoke-free policies in restaurants and bars do not reduce spending in such establishments. This is particularly important in that restaurant and bar associations, often backed by tobacco industry money, lobby against adoption of smoke-free workplace laws based on the argument that they will harm business (Warner, 2006).

States have adopted a number of policies that, thus far, show limited evidence of affecting smoking. Laws prohibiting sales to minors, as well as possession, use, and purchase of tobacco products by minors ("PUP" laws), have had little demonstrable impact on young people's smoking (Lantz et al., 2000). This said, there is a movement afoot to raise the minimum age of purchase and possession of tobacco products to 21. Bolstered by good theory and some empirical evidence, this twist on the minimum age policy might reduce smoking among young people (Bonnie, Stratton, & Kwan, 2015). As of this writing, Hawaii is the only state to have adopted this policy, but it is under consideration in others. A few cities have also adopted the policy.

State and local policies mandating school health education on smoking similarly have had little impact. While model health education programs can reduce smoking among school children, as implemented in practice the programs have little effect. They receive limited resources and, frankly, do not rank high among school boards' and hence principals' and teachers' priorities. Nor are teachers well prepared to present them (Lantz et al., 2000).

Policies Regarding Novel Products

While the FDA now has the authority to regulate novel nicotine and tobacco products, the states have taken the lead on developing policies regarding such products, especially e-cigarettes. Nearly all states prohibit sale of e-cigarettes to minors. As of this writing, ten states explicitly prohibit the use of vapor products in areas in which smoking is not permitted; other state laws may have that effect as well (American Nonsmokers' Rights Foundation, 2018). Currently, two states have imposed excise taxes on vapor products (NCSL, 2016). Additional legislative activity can be expected in the coming months and years.

A fractious debate divides public health supporters and opponents of the novel products. The former argue that, with their rapid delivery of nicotine and simulation of the smoking experience, e-cigarettes can help adult smokers to quit the far more hazardous combusted products. Opponents worry that the novel products will addict a new generation of kids to nicotine and reverse progress in preventing the initiation of smoking. They fret, as well, that for many smokers dual use of cigarettes and e-cigarettes will replace quitting.

As yet there is insufficient evidence to resolve the conflicting views (Belluz, 2016). Ironically, by the time such evidence is developed, if ever, e-cigarettes may be passé. Major cigarette companies are test-marketing a new generation of "heat-not-burn" cigarettes outside the USA. The companies claim that heat-not-burn products simulate the smoking experience better than e-cigarettes while also substantially reducing the hazards associated with combusted tobacco products (PMI Science, 2015).

Non-policy Interventions

As with other forms of substance abuse, treatment, intended to help smokers quit, is a significant enterprise. Counseling efforts range from formal counseling sessions with healthcare professionals to online tailored cessation programs to telephone quit lines. Counseling is often supplemented with, or replaced by, use of nicotine cessation pharmaceuticals (nicotine replacement products, including nicotine gum, patch, lozenge, and inhaler, bupropion, and varenicline). As noted above, clinical trials have demonstrated that each of these interventions can increase the cessation rate two- to threefold (Fiore et al., 2008). However, evidence for the effectiveness of over-the-counter nicotine replacement products is questionable (Hughes et al., 2011).

While treatment per se is not policy, policies about treatment influence its availability and utilization. As mentioned previously, for example, for years states have varied in the amount of coverage they offer in their Medicaid programs. The Affordable Care Act extended coverage to all.

Individual and class action lawsuits against the tobacco industry have played a significant role in influencing cigarette price and marketing practices and in developing detailed understanding of industry behavior (USDHHS, 2014). Almost certainly the most impactful lawsuits were those that culminated in the multistate settlement with the industry in 1998. In addition to those mentioned previously, one provision was to force the companies to make millions of pages of internal documents public. These documents are now available through the Truth Tobacco Industry Documents Library at the University of California, San Francisco (UCSF, 2016).

Last but not least have been the efforts of nongovernmental organizations to discourage children and adolescents from starting to smoke and to encourage adults to quit. These organizations include both the major disease-specific voluntaries (American Cancer Society, American Heart Association, American Lung Association) and tobacco control-specific organizations (including the Campaign for Tobacco-free Kids, Americans for Non-Smokers' Rights, Action on Smoking and Health, and the settlement-funded Truth Initiative). These organizations' efforts have ranged from offering cessation services to running media campaigns, from presenting detailed information on tobacco control laws and policies to lobbying state legislatures and Congress to support tobacco control policy.

Lessons from Tobacco Control Relevant to Other Forms of Substance Abuse

A Policy Typology

The tobacco control experience lends itself most naturally, and most broadly, to addressing substance abuse regarding legally sold products, specifically alcohol abuse and what might be labeled "food abuse," particularly overeating and otherwise unhealthy eating. This said, there are lessons that are clearly applicable to illicit substance abuse. With the movement toward the legalization of marijuana, we observe the permeability of the line between illegal and legal. With that permeability, variations in the applicability of lessons from tobacco control become clear. And, of course, there are significant societal abuse problems associated with prescribed pharmaceuticals, with the problems involving both licit and illicit use and product distribution. Some tobacco control lessons apply here, while others may not.

All of the tobacco control policies described in the preceding section fit neatly into three categories of policies. Indeed, policies with regard to any behavior-related societal concern fall into the three domains of a policy typology (Warner et al., 1990). They are the following:

1. *Information and education.* In the case of tobacco control, notable examples of policy information and education interventions include publication of the Surgeon General's reports, warning labels on cigarette packs and advertisements, media campaigns, and school health education on tobacco and health. Government has a long history of policy-making in this domain, including, with regard to other substances, required warning labels on alcoholic beverages and nutrition labeling of manufactured foods in interstate commerce. Information and education policies can be directed simply at informing the public about facts that can assist them in their behavioral decision-making. On occasion, such interventions can use emotive themes in an effort to exhort people to avoid deleterious behaviors. Or they can attempt to educate citizens in a more profound manner, attempting to improve their ability to process new information.

2. *Incentives.* The principal forms of policy incentives relate to product pricing. The obvious example from the tobacco control experience is excise taxation on cigarettes and other tobacco products. Like tobacco, alcoholic beverages are also subject to excise taxation at the federal and state levels. In the past few years, several jurisdictions have introduced "snack" taxes, excises placed on processed snack foods high in sugar and/or salt. In June 2016 Philadelphia adopted a sugary beverage tax. The intent of all such excise taxes, once labeled "sin" taxes, is to discourage their use by effectively raising the price of the product above that of the unfettered market.

   Differential life insurance premiums based on smoking status constitute another price-based incentive to avoid smoking, although most such policies are dictated by the insurer, rather than a governmental policy. An important exception lies in the Affordable Care Act which permits states to charge a penalty, in the form of a higher insurance premium, for smokers. Ironically, intended to encourage smokers to quit (with the act's now requiring coverage of cessation services), this policy may have discouraged smokers from enrolling for insurance (Friedman, Schpero, & Busch, 2016).

Recently a few jurisdictions have adopted minimum price policies for cigarettes, another incentive policy. New York City, for example, requires that no cigarettes be sold at less than $10.50 per pack.

3. *Laws and regulations*. Perhaps the most recognized category of policies, laws, and regulations dictates what individuals or organizations must or must not do, generally specifying penalties for violation. In the case of cigarette smoking, the laws of half the states, and of many communities within the other states, prohibit smoking in workplaces and public places. Tobacco products cannot be sold to anyone under the age of 18 in most states (with a new movement to raise the minimum age of purchase to 21). Cigarettes can no longer be advertised on the broadcast media, nor in publications with sizable youth readerships. Some jurisdictions prohibit tobacco advertising within a specified distance of schools.

Laws and regulations play significant roles in other areas of substance abuse prevention. Alcohol, the other major psychoactive licit substance, is subject to many of the same kinds of laws and regulations. All jurisdictions have minimum age of purchase and possession laws. Many restrict the sale of alcohol to specified times and places. Sellers typically have to be licensed.

Among the illicit substances, the most important, if obvious, law or regulation is the prohibition of possession, sale, or use of the substance. What makes marijuana so interesting at present is its transition from an illicit to a licit substance in a few cities and states. In those cases, laws prohibiting sale or possession have been altered to define the parameters of sale or use (time, place, etc.) and marketing. Note, incidentally, that cigarettes have run the gamut of legal to illegal to legal again. From 1890 to 1927, 15 states banned the sale of cigarettes. All of these laws were repealed shortly thereafter. But states and most communities still possess the legal authority to ban the sale of cigarettes (Proctor, 2013).

A policy can fall into one category of this typology from the perspective of the individual consumer or citizen and another from the perspective of a business or governmental organization. For example, consider warning labels on cigarettes and alcoholic beverages. For manufacturers, including these labels on product packages is a legal requirement. From the perspective of the consumer, the labels constitute an information or education intervention. The manufacturer that failed to comply with the requirement to include the labels would be subject to significant financial penalties. For the consumer, the label forces no behavior change, nor does it increase the cost of consumption (except, possibly, psychologically).

Information and Education Policies

Attempts to inform, exhort, and educate the public constitute a core set of policies with regard to all forms of substance abuse. A principal lesson deriving from the tobacco experience is that it is important to focus on those interventions that evidence finds most likely to reduce substance abuse. Identifying these is not always easy. For example, research has found little association between cigarette and alcohol package warning labels (or nutrition labels) and behavior change. But that may reflect the nature of the warnings (more on this below). Specific information dissemination efforts have been effective (e.g., the first Surgeon General's report on smoking), the result of intensive media coverage, while most have achieved little impact. Many counteradvertising media campaigns have been documented to work, while others have failed dismally. In general, school health education efforts appear not to have impacted young people's behavior, at least during the years of research follow-up. But it is possible that all such efforts have contributed to changing social norms around substance use. While we can point to specific tobacco control interventions that have reduced smoking—taxation and smoke-free laws being notable examples—it seems likely that the single biggest factor in the change in smoking is the intangible but critical change in social norms. Likely all of the policies reviewed have contributed to that important outcome.

Norm changes attributable to information and educational campaigns have occurred regarding other forms of substance use. A great example is the highly successful campaign to have a designated driver in a group (often of young people) that consumes alcohol. One of the intriguing tools for this effort involved enlisting producers of television shows to build the idea of the designated driver into their show plot lines (Powell, 2010). More recently, the multifaceted but largely informational focus on obesity appears to be working with regard to young children, whose obesity rates have fallen significantly, although the same does not hold for older children and adults (Ogden, Carroll, Kit, & Flegal, 2014). It is possible that parental concern is modifying the diets of younger children, but older children and indeed the parents themselves have a more difficult time changing long-established dietary behaviors.

School Health Education

The motherhood-and-apple-pie of information and education policies has been school health education programs. As noted above, the empirical evidence indicates that smoking prevention programs, documented to work in optimal research settings, have not affected smoking rates in those school systems that provide health education on smoking (Lantz et al., 2000). Similarly, perhaps the nation's largest ever attempt to educate elementary school children about substance abuse, the original DARE program, failed dismally. A review of multiple studies found no impact of DARE on reducing substance use by children (West & O'Neal, 2004). Ironically, the only study that found a statistically significant impact reported that DARE graduates experimented with drugs at an earlier age. Despite this evidence, the program persisted for years until the management of DARE acknowledged the program's ineffectiveness and redesigned it (Nordrum, 2014). The new program for middle school kids, Keepin' it REAL, has demonstrated success.

Product Warning Labels

Tobacco control is in the process of learning a lesson that may have widespread implications for dealing with other forms of substance abuse. Graphic cigarette package warnings are now encouraged by the Framework Convention on Tobacco Control, the world's first global health treaty (ratified by 180 of the 196 member countries of the World Health Assembly; the USA is one of the three large nations not to have joined). Graphic warning labels include large photos (occasionally drawings) depicting the damage inflicted by tobacco. To date, approximately 90 countries have required graphic warning labels, with Uruguay and Australia as exemplars in the extent to which such warnings cover the cigarette pack (Campaign for Tobacco-Free Kids, 2016). Early evidence suggests that graphic warning labels do encourage smokers to make quit attempts and, in the process, reduce smoking (Huang et al., 2014). This is in stark contrast to the conventional print-only messages long required on cigarette packs in the USA, for which there is no evidence of impact.

The applicability of this lesson begins with cigarettes themselves. The FDA's Center for Tobacco Products announced a requirement for graphic warning labels, which were to be on packs by September 2012, but industry legal action blocked its implementation. Alcoholic beverages, too, could have much more noticeable warnings than they do at present. In dealing with obesity and quality of diets, standard package nutrition labeling has limited effect on behavior, particularly within populations most in need of dietary change (Soederberg Miller & Cassady, 2015). A relatively new "traffic light" system employed in the UK is much simpler, clearer, and, importantly, noticeable. Using green, yellow, and red to indicate whether a product's fat content, calories, salt, and sugar are okay, the system better informs consumers as to the nutritional value of what they are purchasing. The UK planned to require the system for all processed foods but was stopped by industry legal action. As such, the system is employed only on a voluntary basis for now.

One can readily imagine creative, attention-getting labeling of prescription drugs, alcoholic beverages, and marijuana products available in jurisdictions in which recreational marijuana use has been legalized. Current labels on food products (nutrition labels), alcohol, prescription drugs, and cigarettes were all designed to fail. Labels on food products and pharmaceuticals are so dense as to be almost unreadable, except for the highly educated consumer who "works" to read and understand them. Warning labels on cigarettes and alcoholic beverages are small and inconspicuous and, in the instance of alcohol, far too wordy. In summary, conventional warning labels appear to have little if any impact on product utilization. Large graphic warnings, in contrast, hold promise, with potential applicability to all legal substances of abuse.

Media Campaigns

The history of substance abuse media campaigns reveals a mixed bag of success. The "Just Say No" campaign had little observable impact on illicit drug use. In contrast, several media campaigns regarding smoking have been documented to have worked well. The most notable evidence-based campaigns include the Fairness Doctrine anti-smoking ads in the late 1960s, state-based campaigns in California and Massachusetts, the Truth campaign, and, most recently, CDC's Tips from Former Smokers campaign (DHHS, 2014). The hallmarks of the successful campaigns included:

- Substantial funding, sustained over a significant period of time.
- Highly creative and attention-getting ads.
- Professionally designed ads, based on empirical evidence as to what themes and approaches work (and which do not).
- Ads tailored to specific groups of smokers (varying by age, race/ethnicity, socioeconomic status, etc.)
- Ads periodically refreshed to maintain interest.

Media campaigns to address both licit and illicit substance abuse will require each of the defining characteristics noted above. Finding a source of funding to mount and sustain an effective campaign is exceedingly difficult, however. This is unfortunate as well-designed campaigns tend to be quite cost-effective interventions, the result of their very wide reach (Xu et al., 2015).

Incentives

One of the most important lessons from tobacco control reflects a centuries-old conventional wisdom in economics: price matters. The law of demand—demand for a product decreases when its price increases—turns out to be not only a universal human response but also even a universal trans-species law. Laboratory animals that are so addicted to drugs that they will choose their drug over lifesaving food or water are also "price responsive." Raise the "price" of a dose of drug to a laboratory animal—for example, increase the number of lever pushes they must make to get a dose—and they reduce the amount of the drug they consume. The response-cost curve in studies of laboratory animal drug self-administration looks suspiciously like the demand curves of humans for cigarettes (Griffiths, Bigelow, & Henningfield, 1980).

The relationship between cigarette price and consumption is likely the best established evidence base in the field of tobacco control, and it has led taxation to become a first principle of tobacco control. Raising the price of tobacco products was included in the Framework

Convention on Tobacco Control as an essential ingredient in all nations' efforts to reduce tobacco use.

The tobacco control experience offers lessons for dealing with other forms of substance abuse. In some instances the lessons are quite direct. If one wishes to reduce alcohol abuse, increased product prices, typically through increased taxation, will help. If one wants to limit the use of legal marijuana by young people, imposing taxes at the retail level will support that policy objective. (Recreational marijuana is not legally available to minors. However, minors acquiring marijuana will often have to pay for it. If they buy from sources who have purchased the marijuana legally, the price will reflect taxation.)

The impact of price applies to illicit substances too. Raise the price of heroin on the street and consumption will decline. The problem, of course, is how to increase the price, since tax is not an option. Efforts to reduce the supply of illicit drugs at their source have not translated into substantial increases in street-level price (Boyum & Reuter, 2005).

Misuse of prescription drugs reflects both misuse by those for whom the drugs are prescribed and abuse through a secondary market. Here too price can matter. The challenge, however, is that one does not want to increase price for legitimate users of the drugs.

When thinking about "price," the term logically should be construed broadly. Anything that makes a substance more difficult to obtain can be thought of as a "price" increase. For example, law enforcement targeting the distribution of illicit drugs in a community can make users' search for supplies more time consuming and challenging in other ways. These barriers to easy access can and should be thought of as similar to price increases.

While the principal lesson from taxing tobacco is a simple one, subtleties abound and warrant careful consideration. Part of the reaction to higher cigarette taxes has been for a subset of consumers to switch from more expensive brand-name cigarettes to less expensive generic cigarettes or to other tobacco products. The taxes in question reduced smoking overall, but this subset of smokers changed the nature of their consumption but not its fact (Chaloupka et al., 2012). One can readily imagine parallels with regard to other drugs. For example, if the street price of heroin rises, one would expect more diluted (impure) product to gain in popularity. Conversely, when the street price moderates, more pure heroin will be sold, possibly contributing to more overdoses by naïve consumers (Boyum & Reuter, 2005).

Although the threat is often exaggerated, typically by opponents of a tax, if tax-induced prices in one jurisdiction rise too much, the policy opens the door to increased smuggling. Above we noted the experience with state cigarette tax increases. This risk would apply to snack or sugary beverage taxes, alcohol products, and legal marijuana.

Research on tobacco price response includes relatively few studies of the price elasticity of demand of tobacco products other than cigarettes, and only a handful of cross-elasticity studies (Chaloupka et al., 2012). Cross-elasticity of demand measures how the demand for product A changes in response to a change in the price of product B. If A and B are substitutes, one expects an increase in the price of B to lead to increased demand for A. Other things being equal, an increase in the price of coffee would be expected to increase the demand for tea. In contrast, if A and B are complementary products, an increase in the price of B would be expected to decrease the demand for A. Coffee and cream illustrate the case of complements. If A and B are neither complements nor substitutes, a change in the price of B should not affect the demand for A. For example, an increase in the price of sugar would not affect the demand for calculators.

The limited literature regarding tobacco products suggests that increases in the price of cigarettes will increase the demand for other tobacco products and for smoking cessation pharmaceuticals, both of which are substitutes for cigarette smoking (Chaloupka et al., 2012). The theoretical implications of cross-elasticity for other forms of substance abuse are obvious, but the specific impacts will depend on the degree of complementarity or substitutability. For example, raising the price of alcohol through taxation could affect the demand for marijuana (legal or otherwise), but in which direction? Are alcohol and marijuana complements or substitutes, or is the demand for one independent of the price of the other?

Cross-elasticity of demand should always be considered in making drug policy and can be exploited through tax policy. In the case of tobacco, most of the public health "Establishment" has long supported harmonizing taxes on different kinds of tobacco products, primarily to reduce substitution of other tobacco products (OTPs) for cigarettes when cigarette taxes are increased.

Decades ago, New York City experimented briefly with a differential cigarette tax based on the tar and nicotine content of different brands, to get smokers to substitute lower taxed low-tar and nicotine cigarettes for the conventional higher tar product. Differential taxation had a theoretical basis (Harris, 1980). The differential tax failed, however, in part because it turned out that the machine-measured differences in tar and nicotine had little to do with human consumption patterns. As the industry knew at the time, and as research later confirmed, smokers smoked the low-tar products more intensively (harder drags, more frequent puffs, smoking further toward the butt end of the cigarette) and smoked more of them. This made the low-tar and nicotine cigarette a boon for the industry. Later research demonstrated that cotinine (a derivative of nicotine) in the blood of low-tar smokers varied much less, compared to that of smokers of high-tar cigarettes, than did the brands' machine measurements of nicotine. The net effect: low-tar smokers ended up developing lung cancers further down into the lung, reflecting their deeper drags to extract nicotine from their low-tar brands, and smoking-related death rates did not decline among low-tar smokers (USDHHS, 2014).

The idea of differential taxation has been resurrected recently, however. With the raging debate over harm reduction in tobacco control (Belluz, 2016), the result primarily of the success of electronic (e-) cigarettes, much of the tobacco control community has come to appreciate that there are big differences in the toxicities of different kinds of nicotine and tobacco products. At one end of the spectrum, by far the most dangerous product is the cigarette. Next come other combusted forms of tobacco (cigars, cigarillos, pipes, water pipes). Next are a variety of high-nitrosamine smokeless products, followed by low-nitrosamine smokeless. At the lowest risk end of the spectrum are nicotine replacement therapy (NRT) products. E-cigarettes fit somewhere on the low end of the risk spectrum. The Surgeon General has stated that combusted products, and particularly cigarettes, are the source of the vast majority of diseases and deaths attributable to tobacco products (USDHHS, 2014).

Recognizing the large differences in risk to health, Chaloupka, Sweanor, and Warner (2015) recently called for consideration of differential taxes based on the degree of risk. The authors proposed that very large taxes be placed on cigarettes and other combustible tobacco products, with correspondingly lower taxes on lower risk products, including no tax on NRTs. They noted that a modest tax could be placed on e-cigarettes, with the objective of discouraging their uptake, and addiction, by the most price-sensitive consumers—kids. By creating a large price gap between heavily taxed cigarettes and low-taxed e-cigarettes, smokers would have an incentive to switch to the much less risky product.

Differential taxation or its opposite, harmonization of taxes across variants in a product category, certainly has a role to play in the domain of alcohol policy. If a legislature wishes to curtail binge drinking among college students, it could increase the state tax on beer. By so doing, the legislature would decrease the quantity of beer consumed. However, if comparable tax increases were not imposed on wine and spirits, there is a risk, indeed likelihood, that the policy might have the unintended consequence of increasing their consumption as beer drinking declined. On balance, the beer tax should reduce total alcohol consumption, but not by the amount that it decreases beer consumption.

One area of substance use in which the tobacco tax experience is being actively explored today is food, with differential taxation at the core of the idea. Nutrition activists have called for taxes on calorie-dense (but nutrition limited) snack foods and sugary beverages. The notion is that by raising the products' retail prices, the taxes will reduce consumer demand for them. Limited evidence supports this expectation (Thow, Downs, & Jan, 2014). An interesting subsidiary question is whether other, healthier foods might see an increase in demand for them, depending on whether consumers perceive them to be substitutes. While a significant number of local jurisdictions have adopted such taxes, most have been withdrawn in response to strong public opposition. Philadelphia's 2016 tax will be watched with great interest by food activists and the food industry.

As noted above, "price" to a consumer can include a number of factors besides the monetary cost. In applying the experience with taxation of tobacco products to illicit forms of substance abuse, this is a crucial message. Anything that increases the potential consumer's inconvenience (or risk, etc.) in acquiring his or her drug will, like a price increase, decrease the overall demand for the drug. While many drug control policies have sought to achieve this effect, through greater law enforcement, for example, few have been motivated by the conscious understanding that what they were doing was increasing the "price" or cost of the drug to the consumer.

Laws and Regulations

As noted above, all licit potential psychoactive substances of abuse are subject to any number of laws and regulations. Alcoholic beverages, and now marijuana in select jurisdictions, cannot be sold to minors and cannot be used in particular settings. Prescription drugs are, by their very name, limited for legal sale to individuals who have a doctor's prescription. Food products in interstate commerce are subject to FDA rules regarding their contents. For example, additives must meet the GRAS standard (Generally Regarded as Safe). A few jurisdictions now require restaurants to post the caloric content of their offerings.

Restrictions on Substance Use in Public

The most significant law/regulation contribution to tobacco control likely derives from the requirement that public places and workplaces be smoke free. Completely smoke-free workplaces, including restaurants and bars, are now mandated in half the US states, with cities and towns in other states also prohibiting smoking in such locations. The behavioral and health impacts were noted above.

Today's smoke-free workplace laws follow in a long-standing (40-year) tradition of increasingly strong restrictions on smoking in public places (USDHHS, 2014). These laws and regulations have undoubtedly derived from and subsequently reinforced the growing nonsmoking norm of the past half century. The origins of the policies lay in the increasing belief, later confirmed by extensive research, that second-hand smoke endangered nonsmokers. As well, many people felt that, regardless of the health effects of second-hand smoke, smokers did not have the right to foul the air being breathed by nonsmokers.

Smoke-free workplaces and public places constitute the heart of tobacco control. As such, their applicability to other substances of abuse, or lack thereof, seems particularly important. In at least one instance, the applicability seems self-evident. For example—and for the same reasons—a prohibition on smoking legal marijuana in public settings and workplaces seems only logical, and policies in relevant jurisdictions include such prohibitions. A related logic applies to prohibitions on drinking alcoholic beverages in many public and work settings. Although inebriated individuals may not foul the air as do smokers, they create distinctly unpleasant negative externalities (in the economist's jargon), potentially disturbing both adults and children.

When contemplating the relevance of smoke-free environment-like policy options, perhaps the most interesting case of licit substance use is the abuse of food, particularly in the form of overeating. There really is no useful analogy to second-hand smoke. As such, the battle against obesity suffers from the lack of a highly visible, galvanizing, norm-changing policy comparable to smoke-free laws. By itself, this is likely to retard progress against obesity.

The very illegality of the illicit substances means that their use is not permitted in public places (or any place).

Restrictions on Advertising and Promotion

Until fairly recently, alcoholic beverages other than beer and wine made a practice of not advertising on the broadcast media. Expansion of the media, via cable, the Internet, and other modes, has produced numerous exceptions to the practice. The ban on TV and radio advertising of cigarettes likely has had beneficial effects on smoking, perhaps especially among youth, although there is no definitive study to that effect. The most authoritative study on the impact of a complete ban on all forms of advertising and promotion of cigarettes concluded that complete bans reduce smoking on the order of 6% (Saffer & Chaloupka, 2000), a relatively modest share of the problem but, given the size of the problem, a significant public health benefit. As such, reinstating the *de facto* ban on advertising of spirits is an obvious policy opportunity.

A similar switch in practice has witnessed the emergence of an enormous broadcast media market for advertising of pharmaceuticals, which previously were never advertised on TV and radio. It is plausible that advertising of pharmaceuticals has contributed to the abuse of prescription drugs that has become so prevalent, although evidence to that effect is not abundant. A legal return to an era without broadcast advertising of pharmaceuticals might diminish the abuse of pharmaceuticals (and almost certainly would reduce their use, abusive or otherwise).

In the new era of legal recreational marijuana, one presumes that states and maybe eventually the federal government will develop policies limiting or prohibiting advertising and possibly many other forms of promotion of marijuana products. In the absence of such restrictions, one can readily envision a world in which advertising of marijuana on TV and radio is pervasive, with themes of sophistication, sex appeal, and adventure mirroring those of cigarette advertising in the period prior to the broadcast media ban in 1971. The glamorization of marijuana could well contribute to the normalization of the use of pot in much the same manner it did for cigarettes in the 1950s–1960s.

Concerns about obesity and other unhealthy eating practices have led activists to campaign for legal restrictions on what food products can be advertised on TV shows directed at children (World Health Organization, 2014).

The principal lesson that emerges from the tobacco control experience is the obvious one: Restrictions or prohibitions on advertising and promotion of substances can diminish their abuse.

Treatment

It is not at all clear that tobacco control offers meaningful lessons for dealing with other forms of substance abuse through treatment. The tobacco control experience does not provide an especially encouraging model. A number of smoking cessation pharmaceuticals have been developed and marketed, and a wide variety of counseling practices are available to smokers, individually and in groups, in-person and online. Until recently, coverage of formal medical treatment of smoking varied from state to state. Research has demonstrated that FDA-approved pharmaceuticals are efficacious (Fiore et al., 2008). Less clear is whether they are effective in everyday circumstances (Hughes et al., 2011). Under best practice conditions, supervised use of nicotine pharmaceuticals can double or triple the rate of quitting of smoking compared to placebo. However, as many of the drugs are used, especially the over-the-counter nicotine replacement therapy products, there is limited evidence of any population impact on quitting. The majority of smokers who quit continue to do so without the use of pharmaceutical aids or counseling (Centers for Disease Control and Prevention, 2017).

The limited success of treatment in the world of smoking cessation is not, therefore, an area ripe for lessons for dealing with the use of other substances, except to understand the limits of treatment. This said, tobacco control might well learn lessons from the treatment of other substances, including the treatment of illicit drug use. All such substances, however, share the inadequacies of treatment that, if overcome, might reduce substance abuse significantly. The medical profession's sensitivity to dealing with substance abuse, from heroin to obesity, appears to be growing.

Harm Reduction

Medical treatment of heroin, especially with substitution of methadone, is relevant in contemplating an important issue for tobacco control: harm reduction. The notion of tobacco harm reduction is the most controversial and indeed challenging issue in tobacco control in decades. The controversy has grown since the emergence of electronic or e-cigarettes, products that both young people and many adult smokers have found attractive. E-cigarettes have bifurcated the tobacco control community into two camps. One, including much of the public health "Establishment" (e.g., CDC and state health departments), opposes the promotion of novel nicotine and tobacco products, even those that are clearly less hazardous than smoking, for fear that they will lead to increases in nicotine addiction and eventually smoking, and the renormalization of smoking. The other camp, whose leading voices come from a subset of academics and activists, believes that alternative nicotine delivery systems, including e-cigarettes, hold the potential to assist large numbers of smokers to quit smoking. The latter group believes that market forces stand a much better chance of reducing tobacco's damage than does a thus-far ineffective regulatory regime (Belluz, 2016).

Harm reduction has an illustrious history in public health, including not only methadone treatment of heroin addiction, but also dealing with such public health problems as teenage pregnancy (e.g., making condoms available in schools), the spread of HIV/AIDS (e.g., clean needle distribution programs), and the decriminalization of marijuana. In all of these areas, harm reduction methods have diminished the problems (references). The potential applicability of this experience to tobacco control is clear, at least to supporters of tobacco harm reduction.

One of the best examples of harm reduction in public health comes from tobacco control. In the only major natural experiment with tobacco harm reduction, Sweden decades ago transitioned a large proportion of Swedish males from cigarette smoking to the use of snus, a low-nitrosamine form of smokeless tobacco, primarily by imposing far higher taxes on cigarettes than on snus. Today 19% of Swedish males are daily snus users (another 6% use snus occasionally), while only 9% smoke cigarettes daily (and 12% smoke occasionally) (Public Health Agency of Sweden, 2016). All told, the prevalence of tobacco use among Swedish males is higher than the average of European countries, but the prevalence of male cigarette smoking is the lowest of all European nations. Correspondingly, rates of tobacco-related diseases are far lower among Swedish males than among the men of all other European countries. Females in Sweden, few of whom use snus, have smoking rates more typical of European women and higher than average rates of lung cancer and other smoking-related diseases (Ramstrom & Wikmans, 2014). Despite what appears to be the self-evident success of this natural experiment, many public health authorities, including officials in Sweden, do not accept that the shift from smoking to snus has produced substantial public health gains (Bolinder, 2003).

The battle over tobacco harm reduction will continue for the foreseeable future. Lessons are as likely to be learned *for* tobacco control as *from* it. One area of very likely experimentation with harm reduction is diet and obesity, focusing on the substitution of healthier options for eating and drinking for the carbohydrate-loaded foods that dominate so much of the nation's diet.

Conclusion

Much remains to be learned about how we can share evidence-based insights across the areas of the use of psychoactive substances. All too often, as is emblematic of public health more generally (and indeed public policy in all domains), we treat each problem as unique, failing to contemplate and benefit from experiences in related areas. Simply opening the exploration of potential lessons can be helpful. As noted above, a rich research literature on the effects of taxation on cigarette smoking and disease is being employed in discussions about taxing sugary beverages and fat- and salt-intensive snack foods. Policy experimentation has occurred and is likely to be repeated and possibly expand in the coming years. But as successful as tobacco control has been over the past half century, the toll of smoking remains enormous. The tobacco control community must seek lessons from experiences dealing with other legal substances of abuse and with illicit drugs. All domains of substance abuse will benefit from the exchange.

References

American Nonsmokers' Rights Foundation (2018). *States, commonwealths, and territories with 100% smoke-free laws in all non-hospitality workplaces, restaurants, or bars*. Retrieved November 29, 2018, from https://no-smoke.org/wp-content/uploads/pdf/100ordlist.pdf.

Belluz, J. (2016). *E-cigarettes and health: Here's what the evidence actually says*. Retrieved August 21, 2016, from http://www.vox.com/2015/6/26/8832337/e-cigarette-health-fda-smoking-safety.

Bolinder, G. (2003). Swedish snuff: A hazardous experiment when interpreting scientific data into public health ethics. *Addiction, 98*, 1201–1203.

Bonnie, R. J., Stratton, K., & Kwan, L. Y. (Eds.). (2015). *Public health implications of raising the minimum age of legal access to tobacco products*. Washington D.C.: National Academies Press.

Boyum, D., & Reuter, P. (2005). *An analytic assessment of U.S. Drug Policy*. Washington, D.C.: AEI Press.

Brandt, A. M. (2007). *The cigarette century: The rise, fall, and deadly persistence of the product that defined America*. New York: Basic Books.

Campaign for Tobacco-Free Kids. (2016). *Warning labels*. Retrieved August 21, 2016, from http://global.tobaccofreekids.org/en/solutions/international_issues/warning_labels/.

Centers for Disease Control and Prevention. (2016a). *Smoking & tobacco use*. Retrieved August 20, 2016, from http://www.cdc.gov/tobacco/data_statistics/fact_sheets/fast_facts/index.htm#toll.

Centers for Disease Control and Prevention. (2016b). *Early release of selected estimates based on data from the national health interview survey, 2015*. Retrieved August 20, 2016, from http://www.cdc.gov/nchs/data/nhis/earlyrelease/earlyrelease201605_08.pdf.

Centers for Disease Control and Prevention. (2017). Quitting smoking among adults—United States, 2000–2015. *The Morbidity and Mortality Weekly Report, 65*(52), 1457–1464. Retrieved January 24, 2017.

Chaloupka, F. J., Sweanor, D., & Warner, K. E. (2015). Differential taxes for differential risks—Toward reduced harm from nicotine-yielding products. *New England Journal of Medicine, 373*, 594–597. https://doi.org/10.1056/NEJMp1505710

Chaloupka, F. J., Yurekli, A., & Fong, G. T. (2012). Tobacco taxes as a tobacco control strategy. *Tobacco Control, 21*, 172–180. https://doi.org/10.1136/tobaccocontrol-2011-050417

Doll, R., & Hill, A. B. (1950). Smoking and carcinoma of the lung. *British Medical Journal, 2*(4682), 739–748.

Eriksen, M., Mackay, J., & Ross, H. (2015). Tobacco atlas, 5th ed. American Cancer Society, Atlanta. Retrieved August 20, 2016, from http://www.tobaccoatlas.org/topic/smokings-death-toll/.

Fichtenberg, C. M., & Glantz, S. A. (2002). Effect of smoke-free workplaces on smoking behaviour: Systematic review. *British Medical Journal, 325*, 188–195.

Fiore, M. C., Jaén, C. R., Baker, T. B., Bailey, W. C., Benowitz, N. L., Curry, S. J., … Wewers, M. E. (2008). *Treating tobacco use and dependence: 2008 update. Clinical practice guideline*. Rockville: U.S. Department of Health and Human Services.

Food and Drug Administration. (2016a). *Family smoking prevention and tobacco control act*. Retrieved August 20, 2016, from http://www.fda.gov/TobaccoProducts/GuidanceComplianceRegulatoryInformation/ucm237092.htm.

Food and Drug Administration. (2016b). *Vaporizers, e-cigarettes, and other electronic nicotine delivery systems (ENDS)*. Retrieved August 20, 2016, from http://www.fda.gov/tobaccoproducts/labeling/productsingredientscomponents/ucm456610.htm#regulation.

Friedman, A. S., Schpero, W. L., & Busch, S. H. (2016). Evidence suggests that the aca's tobacco surcharges reduced insurance take-up and did not increase smoking cessation. *Health Affairs, 35*, 1176–1183. https://doi.org/10.1377/hlthaff.2015.1540

Griffiths, R. R., Bigelow, G. E., & Henningfield, J. E. (1980). Similarities in animal and human drug taking behavior. *Advances in Substance Abuse: Behavioral and Biological Research, 1*, 1–90.

Harris, J. E. (1980). Taxing tar and nicotine. *American Economic Review, 70*, 300–311.

Holford, T. R., Meza, R., Warner, K. E., Meernik, C., Jeon, J., Moolgavkar, S. H., & Levy, D. T. (2014). Tobacco control and the reduction of smoking-related premature deaths in the United States, 1964–2012. *Journal of the American Medical Association, 311*, 164–171.

Holm, A. L., & Davis, R. M. (2004). Clearing the airways: Advocacy and regulation for smoke-free airlines. *Tobacco Control, 13*, 30–i36. https://doi.org/10.1136/tc.2003.005686

Huang, J., Chaloupka, F. J., & Fong, G. T. (2014). Cigarette graphic warning labels and smoking prevalence in Canada: A critical examination and reformulation of the FDA regulatory impact analysis. *Tobacco Control, 23*(Suppl. 1). https://doi.org/10.1136/tobaccocontrol-2013-051170

Huang, J., Walton, K., Gerzoff, R. B., King, B. A., & Chaloupka, F. J. (2015). State tobacco control program spending—United States, 2011. *The Morbidity and Mortality Weekly Report, 64*, 673–678.

Hughes, J. R., Peters, E. N., & Naud, S. (2011). Effectiveness of over-the-counter nicotine replacement therapy: A qualitative review of nonrandomized trials. *Nicotine and Tobacco Research, 13*, 512–522. https://doi.org/10.1093/ntr/ntr055

Jamal, A., Homa, D. M., O'Connor, E., Babb, S. D., Caraballo, R. S., Singh, T., … King, B. A. (2015). Current cigarette smoking among adults—United States, 2005–2014. *Morbidity and Mortality Weekly Report, 64*, 1233–1240. Retrieved August 20, 2016, from http://www.cdc.gov/mmwr/preview/mmwrhtml/mm6444a2.htm?s_cid=mm6444a2_w.

Kessler, D. (2001). *A question of intent: A great American battle with a deadly industry*. New York: Public Affairs.

Lantz, P. M., Jacobson, P. D., Warner, K. E., Wasserman, J., Pollack, H. A., Berson, J., & Ahlstrom, A. (2000). Investing in youth tobacco control: A review of smoking prevention and control strategies. *Tobacco Control, 9*, 47–63.

Monitoring the Future. (2015). *Trends in prevalence of use of cigarettes in grades 8, 10, and 12*. Retrieved August 20, 2016, from http://www.monitoringthefuture.org/data/15data/15cigtbl1.pdf.

National Conference of State Legislatures. (2016). *Alternative nicotine products|Electronic cigarettes*. Retrieved August 21, 2016, from http://www.ncsl.org/research/health/alternative-nicotine-products-e-cigarettes.aspx.

Nordrum, A. (2014). *The new D.A.R.E. program—This one works. Scientific American*. Retrieved August 21, 2016, from http://www.scientificamerican.com/article/the-new-d-a-r-e-program-this-one-works/.

Ogden, C. L., Carroll, M. D., Kit, B. K., & Flegal, K. M. (2014). Prevalence of childhood and adult obesity in the United States, 2011–2012. *Journal of the American Medical Association, 311*, 806–814. https://doi.org/10.1001/jama.2014.732

Pertschuk, M. (2001). *Smoke in their eyes: Lessons in movement leadership from the tobacco wars*. Nashville: Vanderbilt University Press.

PMI Science. (2015). *Heat-not-burn*. Retrieved August 21, 2016, from https://www.pmiscience.com/platform-development/platform-portfolio/heat-not-burn.

Powell, A. (2010). *Designated driver campaign: Harvard center helped to popularize solution to a national problem*. Retrieved August 21, 2016, from https://www.hsph.harvard.edu/news/features/harvard-center-helped-to-popularize-solution-to-a-national-problem/.

Proctor, R. N. (2012). *Golden holocaust—origins of the cigarette catastrophe and the case for abolition*. Oakland: University of California Press.

Proctor, R. N. (2013). Why ban the sale of cigarettes? The case for abolition. *Tobacco Control, 22*, i27–i30. https://doi.org/10.1136/tobaccocontrol-2012-050811

Public Health Agency of Sweden. (2016). *Public health reporting and statistics*. Retrieved August 21, 2016, from https://www.folkhalsomyndigheten.se/about-folkhalsomyndigheten-the-public-health-agency-of-sweden/.

Ramstrom, L. & Wikmans, T. (2014). Mortality attributable to tobacco among men in Sweden and other European countries: An analysis of data in a WHO report. Tobacco Induced Diseases, 12, 1–4. Retrieved August 22, 2016, from http://download.springer.com/static/pdf/321/art%253A10.1186%252F1617-9625-12-14.pdf?originUrl=http%3A%2F%2Ftobaccoinduceddiseases.biomedcentral.com%2Farticle%2F10.1186%2F1617-9625-12-14&token2=exp=1471906757~acl=%2Fstatic%2Fpdf%2F321%2Fart%25253A10.1186%25252F1617-9625-12-14.pdf*~hmac=0f38223344988 49e6b8d267bd481a1df51e3983853e58ec02bce7e0 51ad83712.

Saffer, H., & Chaloupka, F. (2000). The effect of tobacco advertising bans on tobacco consumption. *Journal of Health Economics, 19*, 1117–1137.

Saloojee, Y., & Dagli, E. (2000). Tobacco industry tactics for resisting public policy on health. *Bulletin of the World Health Organization, 78*, 902–910. https://doi.org/10.1590/S0042-96862000000700007

Schauffler, H. H., Barker, D. C., & Orleans, C. T. (2001). Medicaid coverage for tobacco dependence. *Health Affairs, 20*, 298–303. https://doi.org/10.1377/hlthaff.20.1.298

Soederberg Miller, L. M., & Cassady, D. L. (2015). The effects of nutrition knowledge on food label use. A review of the literature. *Appetite, 92*, 207–216.

Thow, A. M., Downs, S., & Jan, S. (2014). A systematic review of the effectiveness of food taxes and subsidies to improve diets: Understanding the recent evidence. *Nutrition Reviews, 72*, 551–565. https://doi.org/10.1111/nure.12123

University of California—San Francisco. (2016). *Truth tobacco industry documents*. Retrieved June 26, 2016, from https://www.industrydocumentslibrary.ucsf.edu/tobacco/.

U.S. Department of Health and Human Services. (1986). *The health consequences of involuntary smoking*.

A report of the surgeon general. Washington: U.S. Government Printing Office.

U.S. Department of Health and Human Services. (1988). *The health consequences of smoking: Nicotine addiction. A report of the surgeon general.* Washington: U.S. Government Printing Office.

U.S. Department of Health and Human Services. (1989). *Reducing the health consequences of smoking: 25 years of progress. A Report of the Surgeon General. DHHS Publication No. (CDC) 89–8411.* Rockville: Public Health Service.

U.S. Department of Health and Human Services. (2014). *The health consequences of smoking: 50 years of progress. A report of the Surgeon General.* Atlanta: USDHHS.

U.S. Department of Health, Education, and Welfare. (1964). *Smoking and health. Report of the Advisory Committee to the Surgeon General of the Public Health Service. Public Health Service Publication No. 1103.* Washington: U.S. Government Printing Office.

Warner, K. E. (1979). Clearing the airwaves: The cigarette ad ban revisited. *Policy Analysis, 5*, 435–450.

Warner, K. E. (1982). Cigarette excise taxation and interstate smuggling: An assessment of recent activity. *National Tax Journal, 35*, 483–490.

Warner, K. E. (1984). Cigarette taxation: Doing good by doing well. *Journal of Public Health Policy, 5*, 312–319.

Warner, K. E. (2006). Tobacco policy research: Insights and contributions to public health policy. In K. E. Warner (Ed.), *Tobacco control policy.* San Francisco: Jossey-Bass.

Warner, K. E., Citrin, T., Pickett, G., Rabe, B. G., Wagenaar, A., & Stryker, J. (1990). Licit and illicit drug policies: A typology. *British Journal of Addiction, 85*, 255–262.

West, S. L., & O'Neal, K. K. (2004). Project D.A.R.E. outcome effectiveness revisited. *American Journal of Public Health, 94*, 1027–1029.

World Health Organization. (2014). *Protecting children from the harmful effects of food and drink marketing.* Retrieved August, 21, 2016, from http://www.who.int/features/2014/uk-food-drink-marketing/en/.

Wynder, E. L., & Graham, E. A. (1950). Tobacco smoking as a possible etiologic factor in bronchiogenic carcinoma; a study of 684 proved cases. *Journal of the American Medical Association, 143*, 329–336.

Xu, X., Alexander, R. L., Jr., Simpson, S. A., Goates, S., Nonnemaker, J. M., Davis, K. C., & McAfee, T. (2015). A cost-effectiveness analysis of the first federally funded antismoking campaign. *American Journal of Preventive Medicine, 48*, 318–325.

Alcohol Marketing and Promotion

David H. Jernigan

Introduction

Alcohol use is responsible for 3.3 million deaths per year worldwide (World Health Organization, 2014). It is the leading cause of death and disability of young men aged 15–24 in all regions of the world except the Eastern Mediterranean, and of young women in that age group in the wealthy countries and Latin America (Gore et al., 2011). In the USA, alcohol is responsible for 4300 deaths per year among persons under the age of 21 (Center for Disease Control and Prevention, 2013), and is the leading drug among high school students (Miech et al., 2017). Binge drinking (more than four drinks on an occasion for young women, or five for young men) among young people in the USA is associated with increased risk of riding with a drinking driver, being currently sexually active, smoking tobacco or using illegal drugs, suicide, and being a victim of dating violence (Miller, Naimi, Brewer, & Jones, 2007). Compared to those who wait until the legal purchase age of 21, young people who begin drinking at earlier ages are more likely to become alcohol dependent (Grant & Dawson, 1997) and suffer from alcohol-related injuries, motor vehicle crashes, and fights after drinking (Hingson, Edwards, Heeren, & Rosenbloom, 2009).

Substantial progress has been made in reducing underage drinking among high school students (roughly ages 13–18) in the USA since the turn of the century: by 2016, binge drinking participation among 8th, 10th, and 12th grades had fallen 68%, 59%, and 45% in the three grades, respectively, although one in six 12th graders still reported binge drinking in the past two weeks (Miech et al., 2017). However, in contrast relatively little progress has been made among college students and young women (Grucza, Norberg, & Bierut, 2009), and national surveys of young people aged 12–20, including those not currently in school, find smaller gains: a drop of 45% for males since 2000, and only 19% for females (Substance Abuse and Mental Health Services Administration, 2017). Change among young adults as a group (ages 19–30) was even smaller: a 10% decline from 2000 to 2016 (Schulenberg et al., 2017). As of 2016, 7.4 million US young people ages 12–20 reported drinking in the past month, and 4.5 million reported binge drinking (Substance Abuse and Mental Health Services Administration, 2016).

Because the younger the age of initiation, the greater risks alcohol use holds for young people, delaying initiation into alcohol use is a public health goal. A constellation of factors influences young people's decisions to drink. At the state level, greater prevalence of adult drinking is a powerful predictor of increased college drinking

D. H. Jernigan (✉)
Department of Health Law, Policy and Management,
Boston University School of Public Health,
Boston, MA, USA
e-mail: dhjern@bu.edu

prevalence, while more restrictive state-level alcohol policies are a protective factor (Nelson, Naimi, Brewer, & Wechsler, 2005). Alcohol taxes in particular influence both youth and adult consumption through their effects on alcohol prices (Elder et al., 2010; Hollingworth et al., 2006; Xuan et al., 2013). Throughout the world, religious and cultural values and beliefs are important factors influencing young people's drinking (Room et al., 2002).

However, another macro-level factor that appears to influence youth drinking is exposure to alcohol marketing. Alcohol companies spend heavily on such marketing: in 2016, they paid an estimated $2.1 billion to advertise in the USA in the traditional media of television, radio, print, and outdoors (World Health Organization, 2014). This total leaves out the single largest category of spending, which in 2011 according to the Federal Trade Commission was point of purchase and Internet advertising; it also does not include other "below-the-line" spending such as sponsorships and promotional allowances. Were these to be included, the total would be at least double what was spent on traditional media (Federal Trade Commission, 2014). In addition, globally the alcohol industry was estimated to have spent $3.5 billion on social media advertising alone in 2013 (Berey, Loparco, Leeman, & Grube, 2017).

Young People and Alcohol Marketing

That young people see, hear, and read this alcohol advertising is undisputed. That they see more of it per person than adults of the legal purchase age in the USA has been demonstrated repeatedly in the work of the Center on Alcohol Marketing and Youth (CAMY). On radio, in 2011 CAMY used Arbitron data to assess youth and adult exposure in 75 markets in the USA, and found that 32% of alcohol ads played on programming were more likely to be heard by youth per capita than adults (Center on Alcohol Marketing and Youth, 2011b). In magazines, more than 70% of youth exposure has consistently come from advertising youth were more likely per person to view than adults of legal purchase age (Center on Alcohol Marketing and Youth, 2011b). On broadcast network and cable television, more than one in five advertisements were more likely to have been viewed by youth than adults (Center on Alcohol Marketing and Youth, 2010); individual television market data reveal that the youthful skew of audience for alcohol advertising is even greater (Jernigan, Ross, Ostroff, McKnight-Ely, & Brewer, 2013). According to a recent survey of youth and adult exposure to advertising in digital and social media, youth are nearly twice as likely to report exposure to alcohol marketing as adults (29.4% vs. 16.6%), and were also more likely, in social media, to have "shared" those advertisements (Jernigan, Padon, Ross, & Borzekowski, 2017).

Alcohol marketing also abounds in other media likely to be seen or heard by youth. For instance, alcohol brand appearances in films trended steadily upwards from 1996 to 2009, with a rise in appearances of youth-rated films (that is, films rated G or PG) responsible for the increase (Bergamini, Demidenko, & Sargent, 2013). Studies of alcohol mentions in popular music have found them in at least one in five songs popular among youth, and specific brand mentions in a quarter of these (Primack, Nuzzo, Rice, & Sargent, 2012; Siegel, DeJong, et al., 2013; Siegel, Johnson, et al., 2013). Other studies have found that young people can easily access alcohol channels on YouTube (Barry et al., 2015) as well as alcohol-specific pages and feeds on Instagram and Twitter (Barry et al., 2016).

The constitutional context in the USA makes regulating alcohol advertising very challenging. Strong protections for "commercial speech" render total bans on alcohol advertising virtually impossible at the national level, although limited bans can be and have been implemented on publicly owned property (Center on Alcohol Marketing and Youth, 2012a). Thus the most active regulation of alcohol advertising comes from trade associations for the alcohol industry itself. The principal federal agency responsible for monitoring fairness and competition in the marketplace, the Federal Trade Commission, has consistently found that alcohol industry self-regulation is sufficiently protective of young people (Federal Trade Commission, 2003, 2008, 2014).

A number of peer-reviewed research studies, however, have found alcohol industry self-regulation less effective in the USA. A recent content analysis of a census of alcohol industry advertising in national magazines found very few violations of industry voluntary self-regulatory codes, but many examples of content that the authors found problematic, including degrading or sexualized images, promotion of risky behavior, and health claims associated with low calories (Smith, Cukier, & Jernigan, 2014). Another content analysis, of a sample of alcohol ads appearing in magazines popular among youth, found that the larger the youth audience, the more likely the alcohol ads were to contain risky content (Rhoades & Jernigan, 2013). Alcohol industry self-regulatory codes are highly subjective, and lay or public health bodies have found far more violations than industry code review boards (Babor, Xuan, Damon, & Noel, 2013; Donovan, Donovan, Howat, & Weller, 2007). The codes can also be loosened at any time at the industry's discretion, as the Beer Institute did in the USA in 2006 (Babor, Xuan, & Damon, 2010). A global review of peer-reviewed studies of the effectiveness of alcohol industry self-regulation of its marketing activities reviewed 100 studies, and found no evidence that this self-regulation was effective (Noel & Babor, 2016; Noel, Babor, & Robaina, 2016).

Youth exposure to this problematic content would make little difference in youth drinking if there were no evidence that alcohol advertising influenced young people's drinking. To date at least 25 longitudinal studies have found to a greater or lesser extent that the more young people are exposed to alcohol advertising of various kinds, the more likely they are to drink or, if already drinking, to drink more (Anderson, De Bruijn, Angus, Gordon, & Hastings, 2009; Smith & Foxcroft, 2009; Chang et al., 2014; Grenard, Dent, & Stacy, 2013; Jernigan, Noel, Landon, Thornton, & Lobstein, 2016). Results from these studies have been mixed, and they have been criticized by at least one alcohol and tobacco industry consultant for omitting key and relevant explanatory variables (such as price), measuring individual forms of marketing or promotion rather than a mix of potential exposures, using measures of exposure that are themselves endogenous to the models being tested (i.e., patronizing certain media or owning alcohol-promotional items, both of which represent behavioral choices on the part of youth and therefore are not independent of the behavioral choice of drinking), and selection bias (Nelson, 2010). However, the studies continue to proliferate, with longitudinal research published since the latest systematic review finding greater receptivity to Internet alcohol marketing associated with greater odds of initiating binge drinking (McClure et al., 2016), and hours of exposure to movie alcohol content associated with initiating alcohol use, progressing to consumption of a full drink, and engaging in heavy episodic or binge drinking (Jackson et al., 2018).

As a body of research, these longitudinal studies were an advance over previous cross-sectional or experimental research. The use of longitudinal designs increased the possibilities for testing causal hypotheses. One study was able to follow participants long enough to establish an association between early exposure and alcohol advertising, consumption, and youthful experience of negative consequences of alcohol use (Grenard et al., 2013). Another found that, in media markets with high levels of spending on alcohol marketing, young people's drinking continued to rise well into young adulthood, while in markets with less spending, drinking peaked at age 23 and then fell after that (Snyder, Milici, Slater, Sun, & Strizhakova, 2006). The studies have used varying populations—some national, some restricted to a single state or region—and have tested the effects of a wide range of exposures, including exposure to alcohol advertising on television and radio, in magazines, at sporting events, and in stores, as well as exposure to alcohol use in movies and ownership of alcohol-branded clothing or toys. More recent studies have found an even stronger relationship between exposure to alcohol marketing and youth progression from experimentation to binge or hazardous drinking, moving beyond the conclusion from earlier studies that exposure was related to initiation of drinking, and exploring various mechanisms of exposure such as receptivity—e.g., liking an ad, the ability to recall ads, participation in marketing by owning and wearing a branded alcohol promotional item, or liking or sharing alcohol-branded content in social media—or altered expectations of good things that will happen when one drinks (Jernigan et al., 2016).

The Importance of Branding and Brand Research

The gold standard in medical research is the randomized controlled trial. However, it is virtually impossible to employ such a design in a population where advertising exposure is pervasive, as is the case with young people in the USA. The next best design is looking at comparative exposure over time, which is what the longitudinal studies do.

However, the longitudinal studies to date share several shortcomings. Several of them rely on the young people's own reports of exposure to various media as opposed to more standard market research about youth exposure. They view advertising exposure as a linear variable, when evidence exists that, as with other forms of advertising, exposure to alcohol advertising becomes saturated over time, and its effects on behavior diminish with saturation, creating a nonlinear relationship between exposure and behavior (Ross, Maple, Siegel, et al., 2014; Ross, Ostroff, Siegel, et al., 2014). They ignore the content of the advertising, focusing solely on exposure. And finally, they aggregate exposure at the category level (i.e., beer, spirits, wine). From tobacco control's experience of the Joe Camel cigarette campaign in the USA, it is clear that particular branded advertising campaigns can have significant impact on young people (DiFranza et al., 1991). A relatively small number of brands—five percent of those advertising in magazines (Center on Alcohol Marketing and Youth, 2011a), eight percent on television (Center on Alcohol Marketing and Youth, 2010), and four percent on radio (Center on Alcohol Marketing and Youth, 2011b)—account for half or more of youth exposure to alcohol advertising in those media. By failing to differentiate these heavily youth-exposing brands from all the other brands, the longitudinal studies have most likely underestimated the impact of particular brands whose advertising may be more youth oriented.

The first ever survey of youth alcohol consumption by brand was fielded nationally in the USA in 2011 to address some of these limitations. Methods of this survey have been described in greater detail elsewhere (Siegel, DeJong, et al., 2013; Siegel, Johnson, et al., 2013). The survey generated 1031 responses from a national Internet panel of youth aged 13–20 about the quantity and frequency of consumption of 898 different brands of alcohol, as well as more general questions about their drinking behavior, risk-taking, media exposure, demographics, and parental drinking. To provide context for the findings of the main survey, the same research team also used online alcohol price data from 15 control states and 164 online stores to obtain estimates of the average price and strength (alcohol by volume) of 900 brands of alcohol available in the USA in 2011 (DiLoreto et al., 2012).

Topline results underscored the differences in underage consumption of alcohol by demographic subgroups. While for males six of the top ten brands were beer, in line with a long tradition of underage drinkers being most likely to consume beer in the USA, for girls six of the top ten were either "alcopops" (sweet fruity drinks such as Smirnoff Ice or Mike's Hard Lemonade) or distilled spirits products (Siegel, Ayers, DeJong, Naimi, & Jernigan, 2015; Siegel, Chen, et al., 2015). Among African-American youth, cognac and tequila brands, which are also more common in urban music (Siegel, DeJong, et al., 2013; Siegel, Johnson, et al., 2013), were more common than among non-Hispanic white youth, while among Hispanic youth Mexican beer (Corona) and tequila were more prominent (Siegel, Ayers, et al., 2015; Siegel, Chen, et al., 2015). Regarding the most commonly consumed brands by age group, beer and alcopops were most common among both 13–15-year-olds (four beers, one alcopop in the top five) and 16–18-year-olds (three beers, two alcopops), but 19–20-year-olds were more likely to drink spirits (two beers, one alcopop, two spirits brands in the top five; spirits brands comprising five of the top ten) (Siegel, Ayers, et al., 2015; Siegel, Chen, et al., 2015).

Beyond establishing the basic epidemiology of youth alcohol consumption by brand, the branded consumption survey sought to augment the findings of longitudinal surveys about the impact of exposure to alcohol marketing on youth with insights that only data regarding what brands youth consume could provide. Although the survey was cross-sectional and therefore could not be used to establish causal relationships, data from it were used to test various arguments against the finding that exposure to alcohol marketing influences youth alcohol consumption. Those arguments and survey findings related to them are described below.

Young people mimic adult consumption. Since adult consumption is a strong predictor of youth consumption, it stands to reason that young people would imitate the alcohol brand preferences of adults. This assumption is also supported by social modeling theory. Another aspect of this argument is that since alcohol advertising is aimed primarily at an adult audience, then youth exposure is an inevitable spillover from adult exposure, and youth and adult brand consumption could be expected to be very similar. Testing these propositions required calculating youth market shares based on the reported consumption in the youth survey, and then comparing that to adult market shares through the use of the commercially available Survey of the American Consumer conducted by GfK MRI, a large market research firm. This comparison revealed numerous brands—particularly alcopops—that were far more popular among youth than among adults. Corona Extra Light, Bacardi Malt Beverages, Smirnoff Malt Beverages, Mike's Hard Lemonade, Jack Daniel's Cocktails, Malibu Rums, and Natural Ice were all more than twice as likely to be consumed by youth than by adults (Siegel, Ayers, et al., 2015; Siegel, Chen, et al., 2015).

Young people drink the cheapest brands. The extensive price database built for this project (and available at http://www.youthalcoholbrands.org/price-database/) enabled comparison of youth consumption by brand and brand average price. Although youth are price sensitive, so that lower brand-specific prices were associated with greater likelihood of consumption in the past 30 days overall, within and across beverage types, the brands most commonly consumed by youth were not the cheapest. Only 1 of the 25 brands most popular among youth—Keystone Light, consumed by six percent of youth in the survey—was among the 88 cheapest brands. The most popular brands among youth—Bud Light, Smirnoff Malt Beverages, and Budweiser—ranked 253, 455, and 186 in cheapness of price, respectively. The clear conclusion from this finding is that price alone does not drive youth alcohol consumption (Albers, DeJong, Naimi, Siegel, & Jernigan, 2014).

Young people drink whatever is easiest for them to obtain. Alcohol industry sources routinely highlight studies finding that young people get alcohol for free, from social sources such as parties, their older friends, and their parents' liquor cabinets (Distilled Spirits Council of the United States, 2002). The youth brand survey included questions about where the young people obtained alcohol they drank most recently, and who made the choice about the brand of alcohol they consumed most recently. While 52 percent of youth reported getting the alcohol from someone else ("passive" sources—an adult aged 21 or above, another underage person, or a person they did not know), compared to 40% reporting a "transactional" source (primarily by giving someone else money to buy it or buying it at a store), roughly equal numbers of young people reported that they made the brand choice themselves whether they obtained it passively or from a transactional source (Roberts, Siegel, DeJong, Naimi, & Jernigan, 2014). Furthermore, the older the young people were, the more likely they were to have obtained the alcohol through a transaction. Regardless of source, youth brand choices were consistent: nine of the top ten brands obtained through transactions were the same as those that came from passive sources.

Comparing findings from the comparison of youth and adult consumption by brand with the two lists of brands consumed by youth when they obtained alcohol through a transaction and when they procured it passively, seven brands stood out whether or not they were making the brand choice as being more popular among youth than adults: Smirnoff Malt Beverages, Jack Daniel's Whiskey, Mike's, Absolut Vodkas, Heineken, Bacardi Malt Beverages, and Malibu Rums. It is worth noting that three of these seven are alcopops, a product category that has been hypothesized to be particularly attractive to youth (Mosher, 2012; Mosher & Johnsson, 2005).

Advertising exposure is not related to youth drinking behavior. Alcohol industry spokespeople and consultants consistently argue, as the tobacco industry did before them, that advertising only influences adult brand choices, and does not influence youth consumption (Nelson, 2010). This claim is disputed by published advertising research showing a nonlinear association between total alcohol purchases and advertising levels, including a study of advertising by Anheuser-Busch itself (Ackoff & Emshoff, 1975; Wind & Sharp, 2009). The brand survey asked young people which of 20 television programs popular with youth they had seen in the past 30 days, and also which magazines they routinely read. In magazines, for 18–20-year-old males and females, brands that delivered the most advertising to that age group were also often the most popular brands. For males, 11 of the top 25 brands exposed 18–20-year-olds more than any other group, while an additional six brands delivered exposure that was within 10% of that of the most heavily exposed group. For females, 16 of the top 25 brands exposed 18–20-year-olds to more advertising than any other age group, and two additional brands delivered exposure within 10% of that received by the most heavily exposed age group (Ross, Maple, Siegel, et al., 2014; Ross, Ostroff, Siegel, et al., 2014). On television, individuals who self-reported exposure to programming known to contain alcohol advertising for particular brands were three times more likely to consume a brand if they had been exposed to its advertising in the past year, even after controlling for demographic characteristics, magnitude of alcohol consumption, parental drinking, risk-taking behavior, media use patterns, autonomy of brand choice, brand-specific prices, and market share of the brand in the adult market (Ross, Maple, Siegel, et al., 2014; Ross, Ostroff, Siegel, et al., 2014). At the population level, brands that advertised on 20 television shows popular among youth were four times more likely to be consumed by youth than brands that did not advertise there (Ross et al., 2015).

Alcohol advertising does not target young people. These strong associations between youth exposure and alcohol advertising for a particular brand and youth consumption of that brand do not establish a causal relationship, nor do they address the advertisers' intent. It was not until internal documents surfaced from the tobacco industry that intent to target young people with tobacco advertising was established (Cummings, Morley, Horan, Steger, & Leavell, 2002). In the absence of such a smoking gun, another outcome of the tobacco control effort is instructive. The state of California sued R.J. Reynolds Tobacco Company in 2001 for violating the youth-targeting provisions of the Master Settlement Agreement negotiated between tobacco companies and attorneys general from 46 US states. Judicial decisions from that case, known as *Lockyer v. Reynolds*, created a judicial three-pronged test for establishing targeting: Is the exposure of the underage group equivalent (defined as within 10% points) to that of the closest of age group? Are there comparable products that do not target this age group? Can alternative advertising schedules be created that reduce youth exposure without affecting exposure of those of legal purchase age? Application of this definition to alcohol advertising on television in the USA from 2005 to 2011 demonstrated that alcopops, beer, and spirits advertising met the first test in four of seven years, while wine advertisers demonstrated that a comparable product existed that did not target youth. Finally, access to extensive television audience data from Nielsen permitted creation of alternative advertising schedules that reduced the exposure of 18–20-year-olds by nearly 32% (Ross, Ostroff, & Jernigan, 2014).

Furthermore, analysis of the magazine advertising behavior of brands most popular among young people found that these brands were more likely to advertise in magazines with larger underage readerships, compared to brands not as popular among youth, and that the likelihood of advertising grew with the percent of the magazine readership that was underage (King, Siegel, Ross, & Jernigan, 2017).

The content of alcohol advertising is oriented to adults and does not influence youth drinking. Alcohol industry self-regulatory codes ban content that has "primary appeal" or "special attractiveness" to youth, including specific bans against the use of Santa Claus, rites of passage, and symbols, language, music, and cartoons that meet the "primary appeal" criterion (Beer Institute, 2011; Distilled Spirits Council of the United States, 2011). However, the codes provide little insight into how to operationalize this criterion. A critical review of the media research literature identified six areas in which primary youth appeal could be defined: production value, character appeal, theme, product appeal, emotional appeal, and risky content. Based on these, Padon, Rimal, DeJong, Siegel, and Jernigan (2018) developed a "Content Appealing to Youth" (CAY) scoring methodology, and applied this to a sample of televised alcohol advertisements for brands popular and unpopular among youth that were played during the 20 television programs asked about in the youth alcohol brand consumption survey. Their finding, that brands popular among youth were more likely to have advertising with higher CAY scores (Padon et al., 2018), was replicated in a study asking a sample of 211 undergraduate and graduate students about magazine alcohol ads. Advertisements for brands popular among youth were significantly more likely to appeal to young people, according to the study respondents, than ads for unpopular brands (Siegel et al., 2016).

Preventing the Effects

In the face of substantial and growing evidence that alcohol marketing influences young people's drinking behavior, and that initiating drinking or binge drinking at a young age increases the likelihood of adverse outcomes from alcohol use, there are a number of potential courses of action. Existing research on youth alcohol consumption by brand and its relationship to alcohol marketing strengthens the case for greater restrictions on where and when alcohol advertising and promotion may occur. While the research itself does not establish that young people's drinking behavior is influenced by exposure to alcohol advertising, its findings only reinforce the substantial number of longitudinal studies that have shown correlations between exposure to alcohol advertising and youth alcohol consumption over time. To the extent that this relationship is nonlinear and has the greatest effect on the lower portions of the curve, the research points to the need for as comprehensive restrictions as are constitutionally feasible.

Globally, the World Health Organization has termed advertising restrictions one of the three most effective and cost-effective interventions for reducing harmful use of alcohol. The most recent WHO Global Status Report on Alcohol and Health used an advertising restrictiveness score (Esser & Jernigan, 2014) to show that, although countries appear to be moving in a slightly more restrictive direction, the largest number of countries continue to fall into the category of "least restrictive." A recent review of actions taken at country level to implement WHO's Global Strategy to Reduce the Harmful Use of Alcohol found no readily discernable trend from 2010 to 2015: some countries had increased and some had decreased their marketing restrictions, but the dominant trend was toward no action at all in this arena (Jernigan & Trangenstein, 2017).

The Pan American Health Organization (PAHO) recently released a technical note on recommended principles for regulatory control of alcohol marketing (Pan American Health Organization, 2017). These included seeking a comprehensive legally binding ban on all alcohol marketing as the only certain method of eliminating youth exposure, along with designation of a public agency or independent body free of conflict of interest to implement, monitor, and enforce such a ban. Short of this approach, the principles call for an approach similar to the French *Loi Évin*, which in 1991 began with a comprehensive ban and then wrote exceptions to that ban into French law, so that if advertisers wished to innovate, they would have to seek explicit change in the law to allow them to do so.

In the US context, the policy implications of the research on alcohol advertising's relationship with youth drinking point to the public health goal, already articulated in the Surgeon General's National Prevention Strategy, of reducing youth exposure to alcohol marketing (U.S. Surgeon General, 2011). Alcohol industry voluntary guidelines regarding the placement of alcohol advertising grew substantially stronger and more detailed from 1999, when the Federal Trade Commission first called attention to alcohol advertising placement practices, to 2011, the last time those codes were substantially revised (Federal Trade Commission, 1999, 2014). Researchers recently identified precisely where violations of the voluntary placement standards have been most likely to occur. They estimated that young people were exposed 15 billion times between 2005 and 2012 to advertising that was not compliant with the industry placement standards, and found that nearly all of this exposure could have been avoided had alcohol companies followed their codes in conducting systematic "look-backs" to ensure that advertising was not placed on programming, or on networks and at times of day, where underage audience exceeded the standard (Ross, Brewer, & Jernigan, 2016). At the national level, continued monitoring of and reporting on noncompliant advertising appear to be reducing the number of violations. Advertising placement decisions are often made as much as a year in advance; after a year of reporting quarterly on specific areas of noncompliance, noncompliant youth exposure fell by more than 60% (Ross, Henehan, Sims, & Jernigan, 2017).

However, the decline in noncompliant advertising is occurring in the larger context of increasing exposure to alcohol advertising on US television for persons of all ages, including youth. The origins of the industry's voluntary guidelines lie in a proportional 30% maximum for youth audience for its advertising, adopted in 2003 and based on how much of the US population at that time was below the legal purchase age of 21. This standard has been criticized for including the mostly nondrinking population of persons under age 12 in its proportional calculations; in contrast, the National Research Council, Institute of Medicine, and 24 state and territorial attorneys general have recommended that the industry move toward a 15% maximum based on the population between the ages of 12 and 20 (National Research Council and Institute of Medicine, 2004; Shurtleff et al., 2011). Modeling of the application of this stronger standard has shown that youth exposure can be reduced significantly, with virtually no impact on advertisers' ability to reach young adults aged 21–34, the group often cited as the target of much of alcohol advertising (Jernigan, Ostroff, & Ross, 2005).

Because of the devolution in the USA of substantial regulatory authority over alcohol to the states, there are numerous steps that states could be taking to reduce youth exposure. These include restricting outdoor advertising for alcohol in residential neighborhoods and near churches, schools, playgrounds, and other places frequented by young people; limiting signage visible from the exterior of retail outlets selling alcohol; and banning advertising and promotion on publicly owned property, including public postsecondary educational institutions. All of these are likely to withstand the particular challenges of contemporary judicial interpretations of the US constitution (Center on Alcohol Marketing and Youth, 2012a; Center for the Study of Law and Enforcement Policy of the Pacific Institute for Research and Evaluation, 2004). However, a comprehensive review of state actions as of 2012 found that most states had not exercised any of the powers, and no single state was taking full advantage of them (Center on Alcohol Marketing and Youth, 2012a).

At the individual as opposed to the population level, media literacy is one strategy for reducing youth susceptibility to promotional messaging for alcohol. A recent systematic review of research on alcohol media literacy programs found just ten interventions described in eight published evaluations that met inclusion criteria (Gordon, Jones, & Kervin, 2015). Theoretical principles and pedagogical and evaluation methods were sufficiently diverse among this group of studies to preclude statistical grouping of their results. The longest period of follow-up was three months (Austin & Johnson, 1997a, 1997b), and only one study measured the effects of the intervention on actual alcohol consumption. The review concluded that research in this area was emerging, and that more rigorous evaluations need to be conducted (Gordon et al., 2015).

Counter-advertising, which has been shown to be effective in reducing the risk of smoking initiation (Farrelly, Nonnemaker, Davis, & Hussin, 2009), has been much less explored as a method for preventing or delaying underage drinking. Two of the media literacy curricula described above incorporated creation of counter-advertising campaigns as culminating experiences in the process of teaching media deconstruction and counter-arguing skills (Goldberg, Niedermeier, Bechtel, & Gorn, 2006; Kupersmidt, Scull, & Benson, 2012). However, there have been no studies to date of the effectiveness of either youth-driven or youth-targeted counter-advertising at the population level in decreasing the likelihood of alcohol use or heavier drinking among youth.

Conclusion

Alcohol continues to take a substantial toll on young lives, both in the USA and throughout the world. There is substantial evidence at this point of an association between youth exposure to alcohol advertising and marketing and youth drinking behavior. There is a need for further longitudinal research that uses better measures of youth exposure and youth consumption by brand as opposed to in the aggregate. There is also a need for better evaluation of measures taken both at the population and at the individual level to reduce youth exposure and susceptibility to alcohol marketing.

However, given the well-established risks of youthful alcohol use, and the evidence of an association between exposure to alcohol marketing and progression among youth from experimentation to more hazardous forms of drinking, there is also a need for careful consideration by governments at all levels of the extent to which they are willing to restrict and reduce alcohol marketing in order to protect young people.

References

Ackoff, R. L., & Emshoff, J. R. (1975). Advertising research at Anheuser-Busch Inc. *Advertising Research, 16*(2), 1–15.

Albers, A. B., DeJong, W., Naimi, T. S., Siegel, M., & Jernigan, D. H. (2014). The relationship between alcohol price and brand choice among underage drinkers: Are the most popular alcoholic brands consumed by youth the cheapest? *Substance Use and Misuse, 49*(13), 1833–1843.

Anderson, P., De Bruijn, A., Angus, K., Gordon, R., & Hastings, G. (2009). Impact of alcohol advertising and media exposure on adolescent alcohol use: A systematic review of longitudinal studies. *Alcohol and Alcoholism, 44*(3), 229–243.

Austin, E. W., & Johnson, K. (1997a). Effects of general and alcohol-specific media literacy training on children's decision making about alcohol. *Journal of Health Communication, 2*(1), 17–42.

Austin, E. W., & Johnson, K. K. (1997b). Immediate and delayed effects of media literacy training on third grader's decision making for alcohol. *Health Communication, 9*(4), 323–349.

Babor, T. F., Xuan, Z., & Damon, D. (2010). Changes in the self-regulation guidelines of US Beer Code reduce the number of content violations reported in TV advertisements. *Journal of Public Affairs, 10*(1–2), 6–18.

Babor, T. F., Xuan, Z., Damon, D., & Noel, J. (2013). An empirical evaluation of the US Beer Institute's self-regulation code governing the content of beer advertising. *American Journal of Public Health, 103*(10), e45–e51.

Barry, A. E., Bates, A. M., Olusanya, O., Vinal, C. E., Martin, E., Peoples, J. E., … Montano, J. R. (2016). Alcohol marketing on twitter and instagram: Evidence of directly advertising to youth/adolescents. *Alcohol and Alcoholism, 51*(4), 487–492.

Barry, A. E., Johnson, E., Rabre, A., Darville, G., Donovan, K. M., & Efunbumi, O. (2015). Underage access to online alcohol marketing content: A youtube case study. *Alcohol and Alcoholism, 50*(1), 89–94.

Beer Institute. (2011). *Advertising and marketing code*. Washington, D.C.: Beer Institute.

Bergamini, E., Demidenko, E., & Sargent, J. D. (2013). Trends in tobacco and alcohol brand placements in the popular US movies, 1996 through 2009. *JAMA Pediatrics, 167*(7), 634–639.

Berey, B. L., Loparco, C., Leeman, R. F., & Grube, J. W. (2017). The myriad influences of alcohol advertising on adolescent drinking. *Current Addiction Reports, 4*(2), 172–183.

Center on Alcohol Marketing and Youth. (2010). *Youth exposure to alcohol advertising on television, 2001–2009*. Baltimore, MD: Center on Alcohol Marketing and Youth.

Center on Alcohol Marketing and Youth. (2011a). *Youth exposure to alcohol advertising in national magazines, 2001–2008*. Baltimore: Center on Alcohol Marketing and Youth.

Center on Alcohol Marketing and Youth. (2011b). *Youth exposure to alcohol product advertising on local radio in 75 U.S. markets, 2009*. Baltimore, MD: Center on Alcohol Marketing and Youth.

Center on Alcohol Marketing and Youth. (2012a). *State laws to reduce the impact of alcohol marketing on youth: Current status and model policies*. Baltimore, MD: Johns Hopkins Bloomberg School of Public Health.

Center on Alcohol Marketing and Youth. (2012b). *State laws to reduce the impact of alcohol marketing on youth: Current status and model policies*. Retrieved September 28, 2017, from http://www.camy.org/_docs/research-to-practice/promotion/legal-resources/state-ad-laws/CAMY_State_Alcohol_Ads_Report_2012.pdf.

Centers for Disease Control and Prevention. (2013). *Alcohol-related disease impact software*. Retrieved December 16, 2013, from http://apps.nccd.cdc.gov/DACH_ARDI/Default/Default.aspx.

Center for the Study of Law and Enforcement Policy of the Pacific Institute for Research and Evaluation. (2004). *Constitutionally defensible restrictions on alcohol advertising and alcohol sponsorship in state publications and on state-owned or state-leased lands 2004*. Retrieved January 12, 2012, from http://www.camy.org/bin/a/l/Commercial_Speech_Memo.pdf.

Chang, F. C., Lee, C. M., Chen, P. H., Chiu, C. H., Miao, N. F., Pan, Y. C., ... Lee, S. C. (2014). Using media exposure to predict the initiation and persistence of youth alcohol use in Taiwan. *International Journal of Drug Policy, 25*(3), 386–392.

Cummings, K. M., Morley, C. P., Horan, J. K., Steger, C., & Leavell, N.-R. (2002). Marketing to America's youth: Evidence from corporate documents. *Tobacco Control, 11*(suppl. 1), i5–i17.

DiFranza, J. R., Richards, J. W., Paulman, P. M., Wolf-Gillespie, N., Fletcher, C., Jaffe, R. D., & Murray, D. (1991). RJR Nabisco's cartoon camel promotes camel cigarettes to children. *Journal of the American Medical Association, 266*(22), 3149–3153.

DiLoreto, J. T., Siegel, M., Hinchey, D., Valerio, H., Kinzel, K., Lee, S., ... DeJong, W. (2012). Assessment of the average price and ethanol content of alcoholic beverages by brand—United States, 2011. *Alcoholism: Clinical and Experimental Research, 36*(7), 1288–1297.

Distilled Spirits Council of the United States. (2002). *Reducing underage drinking*. Retrieved August 20, 2014, from http://www.discus.org/responsibility/underage/.

Distilled Spirits Council of the United States. (2011). *Code of responsible practices for beverage alcohol advertising and marketing*. Retrieved December 16, 2013, from http://www.discus.org/assets/1/7/May_26_2011_DISCUS_Code_Word_Version1.pdf.

Donovan, K., Donovan, R., Howat, P., & Weller, N. (2007). Magazine alcohol advertising compliance with the Australian alcoholic beverages advertising code. *Drug and Alcohol Review, 26*(1), 73–81.

Elder, R. W., Lawrence, B., Ferguson, A., Naimi, T. S., Brewer, R. D., Chattopadhyay, S. K., ... Task Force on Community Preventive Services. (2010). The effectiveness of tax policy interventions for reducing excessive alcohol consumption and related harms. *American Journal of Preventive Medicine, 38*(2), 217–229.

Esser, M. B., & Jernigan, D. H. (2014). Assessing restrictiveness of national alcohol marketing policies. *Alcohol and Alcoholism, 49*(5), 557–562.

Farrelly, M. C., Nonnemaker, J., Davis, K. C., & Hussin, A. (2009). The influence of the National truth campaign on smoking initiation. *American Journal of Preventive Medicine, 36*(5), 379–384.

Federal Trade Commission. (1999). *Self-regulation in the alcohol industry: A federal trade commission report to congress*. Washington, D.C.: Federal Trade Commission.

Federal Trade Commission. (2003). *Alcohol marketing and advertising: A report to congress*. Washington, D.C.: Federal Trade Commission.

Federal Trade Commission. (2008). *Self-regulation in the alcohol industry: Report of the federal trade commission*. Washington, D.C.: Federal Trade Commission.

Federal Trade Commission. (2014). *Self-regulation in the alcohol industry*. Washington, D.C.: Federal Trade Commission.

Goldberg, M. E., Niedermeier, K. E., Bechtel, L. J., & Gorn, G. J. (2006). Heightening adolescent vigilance toward alcohol advertising to forestall alcohol use. *Journal of Public Policy & Marketing, 25*(2), 147–159.

Gordon, C. S., Jones, S. C., & Kervin, L. (2015). Effectiveness of alcohol media literacy programmes: A systematic literature review. *Health Education Research, 30*(3), 449–465.

Gore, F. M., Bloem, P. J., Patton, G. C., Ferguson, J., Joseph, V., Coffey, C., ... Mathers, C. D. (2011). Global burden of disease in young people aged 10–24 years: A systematic analysis. *Lancet, 377*(9783), 2093–2102.

Grant, B. F., & Dawson, D. (1997). Age of onset of alcohol use and its association with DSM-IV alcohol abuse and dependence: Results from the National longitudinal alcohol epidemiologic survey. *Journal of Substance Abuse, 9*, 103–110.

Grenard, J. L., Dent, C. W., & Stacy, A. W. (2013). Exposure to alcohol advertisements and teenage alcohol-related problems. *Pediatrics, 131*(2), e369–e379.

Grucza, R. A., Norberg, K. E., & Bierut, L. J. (2009). Binge drinking among youths and young adults in the United States: 1979–2006. *Journal of the American*

Academy of Children and Adolescent Psychiatry, 48(7), 692–702.

Hingson, R., Edwards, E. M., Heeren, T., & Rosenbloom, D. (2009). Age of drinking onset and injuries, motor vehicle crashes, and physical fights after drinking and when not drinking. *Alcoholism: Clinical and Experimental Research, 33*(5), 783–790.

Hollingworth, W., Ebel, B. E., McCarty, C. A., Garrison, M. M., Christakis, D. A., & Rivara, F. P. (2006). Prevention of deaths from harmful drinking in the United States: The potential effects of tax increases and advertising bans on young drinkers. *Journal of Studies on Alcohol, 67*(2), 300–308.

Jackson, K. M., Janssen, T., Barnett, N. P., Rogers, M. L., Hayes, K. L., & Sargent, J. (2018). Exposure to alcohol content in movies and initiation of early drinking milestones. *Alcoholism: Clinical and Experimental Research, 42*(1), 184–194.

Jernigan, D., Noel, J. K., Landon, J., Thornton, N., & Lobstein, T. (2016). Alcohol marketing and youth alcohol consumption: A systematic review of longitudinal studies published since 2008. *Addiction, 112*(Suppl 1), 7–20.

Jernigan, D., Ostroff, J., & Ross, C. (2005). Alcohol advertising and youth: A measured approach. *Journal of Public Health Policy, 26*(3), 312–325.

Jernigan, D., Padon, A., Ross, C. S., & Borzekowski, D. (2017). Self-reported youth and adult exposure to alcohol marketing in traditional and digital media: Results of a pilot survey. *Alcoholism: Clinical and Experimental Research, 41*(3), 618–625.

Jernigan, D. H., Ross, C. S., Ostroff, J., McKnight-Ely, L. R., & Brewer, R. D. (2013). Youth exposure to alcohol advertising on television—25 markets, United States, 2010. *Morbidity and Mortality Weekly Report, 62*(44), 877–880.

Jernigan, D. & Trangenstein, P. (2017). *Global developments in alcohol policies: Progress in implementation of the WHO global strategy to reduce the harmful use of alcohol since 2010*. Retrieved October 14, 2017, from http://www.who.int/substance_abuse/activities/fadab/msb_adab_gas_progress_report.pdf?ua=1.

King, C., Siegel, M., Ross, C. S., & Jernigan, D. H. (2017). Alcohol advertising in magazines and underage readership: Are underage youth disproportionately exposed? *Alcoholism: Clinical and Experimental Research, 41*(10), 1775–1782.

Kupersmidt, J. B., Scull, T. M., & Benson, J. W. (2012). Improving media message interpretation processing skills to promote healthy decision making about substance use: The effects of the middle school media ready curriculum. *Journal of Health Communication, 17*(5), 546–563.

McClure, A. C., Tanski, S. E., Li, Z., Jackson, K., Morgenstern, M., Li, Z., & Sargent, J. D. (2016). Internet alcohol marketing and underage alcohol use. *Pediatrics, 137*(2), e20152149.

Miech, R. A., Schulenberg, J. E., Johnston, L. D., Bachman, J. G., O'Malley, P. M. & Patrick, M. E. (2017). *National adolescent drug trends in 2017: Findings released.* Retrieved February 1, 2018, from http://www.monitoringthefuture.org/data/17data.html#2017data-drugs.

Miller, J. W., Naimi, T. S., Brewer, R. D., & Jones, S. E. (2007). Binge drinking and associated health risk behaviors among high school students. *Pediatrics, 119*(1), 76–85.

Mosher, J. F. (2012). Joe Camel in a bottle: Diageo, the Smirnoff brand, and the transformation of the youth alcohol market. *American Journal of Public Health, 102*(1), 56–63.

Mosher, J. F., & Johnsson, D. (2005). Flavored alcoholic beverages: An international marketing campaign that targets youth. *Journal of Public Health Policy, 26*(3), 326–342.

National Research Council and Institute of Medicine. (2004). *Reducing underage drinking: A collective responsibility*. Washington, D.C.: National Academies Press.

Nelson, J. P. (2010). What is learned from longitudinal studies of advertising and youth drinking and smoking? A critical assessment. *International Journal of Environmental Research and Public Health, 7*(3), 870–926.

Nelson, T. F., Naimi, T. S., Brewer, R. D., & Wechsler, H. (2005). The state sets the rate: The relationship among state-specific college binge drinking, state binge drinking rates, and selected state alcohol control policies. *American Journal of Public Health, 95*(3), 441–446.

Noel, J. K., & Babor, T. F. (2016). Does industry self-regulation protect young persons from exposure to alcohol marketing? A review of compliance and complaint studies. *Addiction, 112*(Suppl 1), 51–56.

Noel, J. K., Babor, T. F., & Robaina, K. (2016). Industry self-regulation of alcohol marketing: A systematic review of content and exposure research. *Addiction, 112*(Suppl. 1), 28–50.

Padon, A. A., Rimal, R. N., DeJong, W., Siegel, M., & Jernigan, D. (2018). Assessing youth-appealing content in alcohol advertisements: Application of a content appealing to youth (CAY) index. *Health Communication, 33*(2), 164–173.

Pan American Health Organization. (2017). *Technical note: Background on alcohol marketing regulation and monitoring for the protection of public health*. Retrieved October 14, 2017, from http://iris.paho.org/xmlui/handle/123456789/33972.

Primack, B. A., Nuzzo, E., Rice, K. R., & Sargent, J. D. (2012). Alcohol brand appearances in US popular music. *Addiction, 107*, 557–566.

Rhoades, E., & Jernigan, D. H. (2013). Risky messages in alcohol advertising, 2003–2007: Results from content analysis. *Journal of Adolescent Health, 52*(1), 116–121.

Roberts, S. P., Siegel, M. B., DeJong, W., Naimi, T. S., & Jernigan, D. H. (2014). The relationships between alcohol source, autonomy in brand selection, and brand preference among youth in the USA. *Alcohol and Alcoholism, 49*(5), 563–671.

Room, R., Jernigan, D., Carlini Cotrim, B., Gureje, O., Mäkelä, K., Marshall, M., ... Saxena, S. (2002). *Alcohol in developing societies: A public health approach.* Helsinki and Geneva: Finnish Foundation for Alcohol Studies and World Health Organization.

Ross, C. S., Brewer, R. D., & Jernigan, D. H. (2016). The potential impact of a "no-buy" list on youth exposure to alcohol advertising on cable television. *Journal of Studies on Alcohol and Drugs, 77*(1), 7–16.

Ross, C. S., Henehan, E. R., Sims, J. & Jernigan, D. H. (2017). *Alcohol advertising compliance on cable television, january–march (Q1), 2017.* Retrieved February 2, 2018, from http://www.camy.org/_docs/resources/reports/alcohol-advertising-monitoring/CAMY_CableTV_2016_Q1.pdf.

Ross, C. S., Maple, E., Siegel, M., DeJong, W., Naimi, T. S., Ostroff, J., ... Jernigan, D. H. (2014). The relationship between brand-specific alcohol advertising on television and brand-specific consumption among underage youth. *Alcoholism: Clinical and Experimental Research, 38*(8), 2234–2242.

Ross, C. S., Maple, E., Siegel, M., DeJong, W., Naimi, T. S., Padon, A. A., ... Jernigan, D. H. (2015). The relationship between population-level exposure to alcohol advertising on television and brand-specific consumption among underage youth in the U.S. *Alcohol and Alcoholism, 50*(3), 358–364.

Ross, C., Ostroff, J., & Jernigan, D. (2014). Evidence of underage targeting of alcohol advertising on television in the United States: Lessons from the Lockyer v. Reynolds decisions. *Journal of Public Health Policy, 35*(1), 105–118.

Ross, C. S., Ostroff, J., Siegel, M., DeJong, W., Naimi, T. S., & Jernigan, D. H. (2014). Exposure to magazine advertising for alcohol brands most commonly consumed by youth: Evidence of directed marketing. *Journal of Studies on Alcohol and Drugs, 75*(4), 615–622.

Schulenberg, J. E., Johnston, L. D., O'Malley, P. M., Bachman, J. G., Miech, R. A., & Patrick, M. E. (2017). *Monitoring the Future national survey results on drug use, 1975–2016: Volume II, College students and adults ages 19–55.* Ann Arbor, MI: Institute for Social Research, University of Michigan.

Shurtleff, M. L., Gansler, D. F., Horne, T., Jepsen, G., Biden, J. R., III, Rapadas, L., ... Phillips, G. (2011). *RE: Alcohol reports, paperwork comment; Project No. P114503. A communication from the chief legal officers of the following states: Arizona, Connecticut, Delaware, Guam, Hawaii, Idaho, Illinois, Iowa, Maryland, Massachusetts, Mississippi, Nevada, New Hampshire, New Mexico, New York, Oklahoma, Oregon, Rhode Island, South Carolina, Tennessee, Utah, Vermont, Washington, Wyoming.* Retrieved September 8, 2011, from https://www.ftc.gov/sites/default/files/documents/public_comments/alcohol-reports-project-no.p114503-00071%C2%A0/00071-58515.pdf.

Siegel, M., Ayers, A. J., DeJong, W., Naimi, T. S., & Jernigan, D. H. (2015). Differences in alcohol brand consumption among underage youth by age, gender, and race/ethnicity - United States, 2012. *Journal of Substance Use, 20*(6), 430–438.

Siegel, M., Chen, K., DeJong, W., Naimi, T. S., Ostroff, J., Ross, C. S., & Jernigan, D. H. (2015). Differences in alcohol brand consumption between underage youth and adults-United States, 2012. *Substance Use, 36*(1), 106–112.

Siegel, M., DeJong, W., Cioffi, D., Leon-Chi, L., Naimi, T. S., Padon, A. A., ... Xuan, Z. (2016). Do alcohol advertisements for brands popular among underage drinkers have greater appeal among youth and young adults? *Substance Abuse, 37*(1), 222–229.

Siegel, M., DeJong, W., Naimi, T. S., Fortunato, E. K., Albers, A. B., Heeren, T., ... Jernigan, D. H. (2013). Brand-specific consumption of alcohol among underage youth in the United States. *Alcoholism: Clinical and Experimental Research, 37*(7), 1195–1203.

Siegel, M., Johnson, R. M., Tyagi, K., Power, K., Lohsen, M. C., Ayers, A. J., & Jernigan, D. H. (2013). Alcohol brand references in U.S. popular music, 2009–2011. *Substance Use and Misuse, 48*(14), 1475–1484.

Smith, K. C., Cukier, S., & Jernigan, D. (2014). Regulating alcohol advertising: Content analysis of the adequacy of federal and self-regulation of magazine advertisements, 2008–2010. *American Journal of Public Health, 104*(11), 1901–1911.

Smith, L. A., & Foxcroft, D. R. (2009). The effect of alcohol advertising, marketing and portrayal on drinking behaviour in young people: Systematic review of prospective cohort studies. *BMC Public Health, 9*(51), 1–11.

Snyder, L., Milici, F., Slater, M., Sun, H., & Strizhakova, Y. (2006). Effects of alcohol exposure on youth drinking. *Archives of Pediatrics and Adolescent Medicine, 160*(1), 18–24.

Substance Abuse and Mental Health Services Administration (SAMHSA). (2017). *Results from the 2016 National survey on drug use and health: Detailed tables.* Retrieved February 1, 2018, from https://www.samhsa.gov/data/sites/default/files/NSDUH-DetTabs-2016/NSDUH-DetTabs-2016.htm.

U.S. Surgeon General. (2011). *National prevention strategy.* Retrieved June 29, 2014, from http://www.surgeongeneral.gov/initiatives/prevention/strategy/report.pdf.

Wind, Y., & Sharp, B. (2009). Advertising empirical generalizations: Implications for research and action. *Journal of Advertising Research, 49*(2), 246–252.

World Health Organization. (2014). *Global status report on alcohol and health—2014.* Retrieved May 21, 2014, from http://www.who.int/substance_abuse/publications/global_alcohol_report/msb_gsr_2014_1.pdf?ua=1.

Xuan, Z., Nelson, T. F., Heeren, T., Blanchette, J., Nelson, D. E., Gruenewald, P., & Naimi, T. S. (2013). Tax policy, adult binge drinking, and youth alcohol consumption in the United States. *Alcoholism: Clinical and Experimental Research, 37*(10), 1713–1719.

Part II

Effective Prevention Interventions and Strategies for Substance Use

Family Processes and Evidence-Based Prevention

J. Douglas Coatsworth and Melissa W. George

Background

Over the past three decades, prevention science has emerged as a key factor in reducing substance use and substance-use disorders worldwide. During this time, interventions targeting diverse developmental risk and protective processes have been developed and put to rigorous empirical evaluation. The science shows a mix of effective programs, practices, and policies from which organizations and communities can choose to address substance-use problems. Among these are a number of family-based programs that (1) are based on models of family risk, protection, and resilience processes (Masten, 2018); (2) indicate that families provide a nurturing environment critical for promoting human well-being (Biglan, Flay, Embry, & Sandler, 2012); (3) rely on a strong theoretical rationale for how these programs should reduce substance-use problems; and (4) draw from models of intervention practices from clinical and educational sciences. Family-based prevention science is both an applied and basic science. As an applied science, tests of family-based prevention programs have yielded strong findings that they can reduce social, emotional, and behavioral problems for children and youth (Durlak et al., 2007). As a basic science, randomized controlled trials of intervention models serve as strong tests of underlying theoretical propositions (Brown et al., 2008) and therefore inform theory development and developmental science. This iterative process is important in refining and strengthening programs over time.

Socialization within the Family: Family Structures, Family Processes, and Parenting

Families are one of the most important and proximal influences on the health and well-being of children and youth (Walsh, 2016). Family structure, family interactions, and parents' socialization practices all contribute substantially to whether children and adolescents engage in problem behaviors such as substance use (Ashby Wills & Yaeger, 2003).

Family Structures: Youth who live with a single parent or neither parent tend to have higher rates of substance use and abuse compared to youth who live with both biological parents (Ewing et al., 2015). However, studies do not always account for the diversity of family structures and the more nuanced way theory has developed to understand family functioning. Many families now include additional adults,

J. Douglas Coatsworth (✉)
Human Development and Family Studies, Colorado State University, Fort Collins, CO, USA
e-mail: Doug.Coatsworth@colostate.edu

M. W. George
Colorado State University, Fort Collins, CO, USA
e-mail: melissa.george@colostate.edu

such as grandparents, who take on family caregiving roles (DeLeire & Kalil, 2002). Moreover, most studies on family structure have been conducted in the United States and are limited in their ability to test theoretically relevant family processes as mediating mechanisms.

Family Functions: Families across the world function to provide their members some form of economic and material support, social placement, and emotional support (Georgas, 2006). Among the most important roles for the family is **socialization** of the child (Grusec, 2011). Socialization is a developmental process through which children learn and internalize the attitudes, values, and beliefs of their family and culture which generally results in learning to behave in socially approved and conventional ways. Some socialization experiences, however, can lead to problem behaviors such as substance use (Donovan, 2016).

Scholars (Grusec, 2011) have described five distinct socialization domains. **Protection** means families and parents take actions to protect children from physical and emotional threats in the environment. It also refers to environments in which adults respond sensitively when young children are physically or emotionally distressed, helping to build a secure parent-child attachment relationship. **Mutual reciprocity** of emotions and behaviors is created when parents respond appropriately to reasonable requests for attention by the child and, in turn, children respond positively and comply with requests or directives. **Control** is exerted by parents primarily through discipline and when used wisely children tend to develop and internalize standards of good conduct and become more likely to comply with societal rules and regulations. **Guided learning** involves helping children gain the requisite cognitive, social, and emotional skills to function well within their culture through formal education, or informally through exposure to social and emotional skills, and effective ways to solve social problems and challenging social situations. **Group participation** means children learn socially acceptable behaviors and societal values through the family and participation in other groups through positive modeling, ritual, and routine. This model emphasizes the role of the family as the key agent of communicating and facilitating the development of socially conventional attitudes, values, and behaviors in youth. Each domain is associated with distinct mechanisms of development and different child and youth developmental outcomes. Positive development occurs primarily through effective parenting and family processes within these domains and the development of positive parent-child relationships.

Key Family Processes

Studies have identified key family processes that help families and individuals build resilience, protect them from stressful life experiences, and promote health and well-being (Walsh, 2016). When these processes operate well, children and youth develop healthy behaviors, but when families lack skill for positive interaction youth are at risk of substance use.

Beliefs, Attitudes, and Values: Within families that use substances, children and adolescents may observe use, acquire favorable attitudes toward use, develop intentions to use, and begin using substances (Wills, Mariani, & Filer, 1996). Parents' promotion of prosocial values supporting nonuse or delayed use or disapproving values and attitudes about substance use predicts adolescent use (Bogenschneider, Wu, Raffaelli, & Tsay, 1998). Tolerant attitudes toward drug use have a direct effect on youth use and an indirect effect operating through association with peers (Bahr, Hoffmann, & Yang, 2005).

Organization Processes: The ways families organize themselves and respond to changes in the broader social environment influence the development of youth, including likelihood to use substances (Santisteban et al., 2003). Strong family organizational processes provide relational and structural supports for positive youth development, but when these are lacking problem behaviors may occur (Walsh, 2016). Flexible organization helps families adapt and draw on resources according to the changing developmental demands and stressors in their lives (Masten & Monn, 2015), but too much flexibility can manifest in chaotic functioning. Rigid family system is characterized by inequality in decision-making, and strictly defined rules. Both highly flexible and highly rigid family organizations are associated with greater substance use.

Cohesion reflects how family members are emotionally bonded. Families can range from being enmeshed or overly connected and dependent on each other to having healthy degrees of positive relationships and connection, and to disengaged and sharing little closeness, support, or loyalty (Olson, 2000). Youth from enmeshed or disengaged families are at elevated risk for substance use (Duncan, Tildesley, Duncan, & Hops, 1995).

Communication and Problem-Solving: Resilient families share emotional messages of warmth and love, and of sorrow and pain (Walsh, 2016). Families that provide clear, consistent messages about behavioral expectations and communicate openly with their children about uncertain or ambiguous circumstances promote healthy child and youth development (Masten, 2018). Parents also help reduce their children's risk for substance use when they communicate specifically about the risks of adolescent substance use (Miller-Day & Kam, 2010). Messages with less confrontation and criticism are more likely to be received (Turpyn & Chaplin, 2016).

Key Parenting Practices

Specific parenting behaviors are associated with socialization, key family resilience processes, and delaying or preventing adolescent substance use. Successful parenting requires an ability to respond and adjust practices sensitively according to the age and the developmental status of the child. Parenting knowledge, attitudes, and practices have been associated with healthy development of children and youth's physical health, cognitive, social, emotional, and behavioral competence (National Academies of Sciences, Engineering, and Medicine, 2016).

Parenting knowledge refers to caregivers' understanding of the milestones associated with healthy child development and parents' understanding of parent behaviors that promote healthy development.

Although basic studies are sparse (Sanders & Morawska, 2014), parenting and family-based interventions that change parenting knowledge can also show corresponding change in child behaviors (e.g., Dawson-McClure et al., 2015).

Parenting knowledge also refers to a specific aspect of parental monitoring (Dishion & McMahon, 1998) regarding whether parents know their children's whereabouts and activities. This kind of parental knowledge involves parents' solicitation and child's self-disclosure of information (Kerr & Stattin, 2000). Higher levels of parental knowledge are associated with lower levels of adolescent substance use, although the longitudinal relations are complex and bidirectional (Abar, Jackson, & Wood, 2014). For example, parental over-monitoring has negative effects on alcohol use and binge drinking (Donaldson, Handren, & Crano, 2016).

Parenting attitudes are the result of the knowledge, values, and expectations they have for their children's development. Parental tolerance or favorability toward adolescent use is associated with a higher likelihood of use (Lamb & Crano, 2014). Nonusing youth whose parents believed they were using were more likely to use one year later, while youth who were using but parents believed they were not were more likely to stop using one year later. These data indicate the importance of parental beliefs, attitudes, and expectations for influencing children and youth's initiation and use of substances.

Parenting practices and behaviors. Sensitive care and positive parenting are behaviors associated with healthy youth development and prevention of substance misuse. At early ages, infants and children require consistent sensitive and responsive parenting to help form secure attachments with a caregiver and create the foundations for long-term positive relations (Sroufe, Egeland, Carlson, & Collins, 2005). Interventions teach parents how to respond sensitively to infant and toddler's cries and requests for help (e.g., Olds, 2006). As children age, child and adolescent perceptions of their parents as loving, caring, and involved have better relationships with their parents which is the foundation for socialization and strongly linked to reduced likelihood of substance misuse (Donaldson et al., 2016). In contrast, harsh discipline and high conflict lead adolescents to disengage from the family and increase the likelihood of substance use (Ary, Duncan, Duncan, & Hops, 1999).

Family-Based Preventive Interventions: Rationale

Family-based prevention programs assume that teaching parenting practices, improving parent-child relationships, and promoting effective family functioning and management skills will lead to healthy youth development and prevent problem behaviors. Conceptually, most family-based preventive interventions draw from three main theoretical perspectives: family systems theory, attachment theory, and behavioral parent training models.

Family Systems Theory

A family systems perspective generally means interventions regard the entire family as a functional system and focus on the overall family rather than a single identified member. Problem behaviors are reflective of an imbalance in family processes and relationships (Bowen, 1985). There are several family systems concepts key to preventive interventions. **Interdependence** means family members are connected emotionally and behaviorally and influences on one member will have effect on other members. This idea has been instrumental in extending family-based preventive intervention strategies from training parents only to involving both parents and children. **Relationships** focus attention on the patterns and the quality of the interactions between individuals within the family. Interdependence and relationships also indicate that the relationship quality among two family members, such as mother and father, will influence the quality of relationship of others, such as mother and child. Distressed couples are more likely to use harsh discipline with their children (Kopystynska, Paschall, Barnett, & Curran, 2017), suggesting the need to consider the family unit when intervening (e.g., Feinberg,

2002). **Structure** describes how the relationships of the individuals in the family are aligned, and how this results in family organization. Each combination of members of the family creates a subsystem of the larger family system and each subsystem may have specific functions in keeping the family organized. For example, two parents can create a "parental subsystem" and function together to create family rules and socialize the children. Siblings are a different subsystem and their patterns of interactions with each other are different from how they act with parents. **Organization** of families reflects the ways subsystems interact and the ways rules define how they interact. **Wholism** suggests that the whole is greater than the sum of the parts and directs an intervention's focus to the broad organization and overall emotional climate of the family, rather than individual relationships.

Attachment Theory

Attachment theory guides many effective family-based preventive interventions to improve the well-being of mothers, mother-infant relationships, and parenting behaviors. Attachment theory emphasizes parental sensitivity, responsiveness, affection, and awareness of children's needs as central to building high-quality early child-parent relationships that predict positive development through childhood and adolescence (Sroufe et al., 2005). Family-based preventive interventions that incorporate attachment theory help parents respond sensitively to their children's attention-seeking behaviors, support prosocial behaviors, and reduce harsh, inconsistent, or hurtful interactions, (Miller-Heyl, MacPhee, & Fritz, 2002).

Behavioral Parent Training

Behavioral parent training models link parent management skills and beliefs to child development. The goal of behavioral parent training is to reduce parent coercive or negative interactions and increase parent positive behavior (Forgatch & Patterson, 2010), which over time changes the child's disruptive behaviors (McMahon, Wells,

& Kotler, 2006). Monitoring, communicating clear rules, and enforcing limits are also emphasized as key practices preventing the onset and escalation of adolescent substance use (Dishion, Nelson, & Bullock, 2004). When parents are able to use more effective discipline techniques, reinforce their children's prosocial behavior, engage in collaborative problem-solving, and maintain more involvement in the lives of their children, youth are less likely to use and abuse substances.

These three broad perspectives serve as the primary theoretical foundation for many family-based preventive interventions. Because of the diversity in family structures, cultures, and level of functioning, many approaches may draw from several theoretical perspectives.

Evidence

There is substantial evidence indicating that family-based preventive interventions are effective. Evidence derives from a number of elements. First, well-designed randomized controlled trials (RCT) demonstrate the utility of these interventions for altering family processes and influencing later substance use. Second, systematic reviews critically evaluate how well they meet various standards of evidence. Third, meta-analyses examine effects within and across interventions and investigate common program elements associated with better outcomes (Kaminski, Valle, Filene, & Boyle, 2008; Van Ryzin, Kumpfer, Fosco, & Greenberg, 2016; Van Ryzin, Roseth, Fosco, Lee, & Chen, 2016). These different forms of evidence demonstrate that family-based prevention programs work and illustrate differing strengths of these programs for changing family functioning and preventing youth behavior problems.

Standards of evidence: In 2005, the Society for Prevention Research (SPR) published a guide for scientists, community members, and policymakers to help provide consistency in how to classify the evidence for programs (Flay et al., 2005). Ten years later, SPR published a second edition clarifying additional elements, such as better standards for reporting results from trials, testing and reporting analyses examining mechanisms of program effects, and attention to cost analyses (Gottfredson et al., 2015). These reports define the criteria by which programs can be judged as "efficacious," or showing significant effects under tightly controlled conditions; as "effective" or showing effects when delivered by third parties under nonoptimal conditions; and as ready for "dissemination or scale-up," meaning programs with strong evidence can be implemented with fidelity. These rigorous standards help provide some common language and criteria by which prevention programs can be judged, but also have the goal of providing a means for helping to ensure that the best science is brought to practice.

Systematic Reviews: The purpose of a **systematic review** is to use specific and clear procedures to find, review, evaluate, and synthesize the results of relevant research. The International Standards on Drug Use Prevention from the United Nations Office on Drugs and Crime (UNODC), a systematic review of many different prevention approaches, concluded that family-focused programs work. Other systematic reviews have shown that universal family-based interventions are effective in preventing alcohol misuse in youth younger than 18 years old (Foxcroft & Tsertsvadze, 2012) and relatively short, parent-focused interventions can prevent and decrease adolescent tobacco, alcohol, and illicit substance use (Allen et al., 2016).

Some systematic reviews are organized in the form of a registry of interventions published in a document or on a website. These registries serve as relatively easily accessible resources for information about effective programs, with the drawback that some registries may be constructed with distinctly different criteria and may not be as rigorous as the published peer-reviewed literature or meta-analytic reviews. An example is The Blueprints for Healthy Youth Development registry (http://www.blueprintsprograms.com/) which uses very rigorous standards resulting in a list of very-high-quality programs organized into model programs (highest quality), or promising programs. A recently added category of model plus includes programs that have been independently replicated. Family-based interventions are well represented among the model programs on the Blueprints list. The European Monitoring Center for Drugs and Drug Addiction (http://www.emcdda.europa.eu/) includes a compendium of programs implemented in Europe. There are three levels of programs according to study design and analysis of process and outcome data. Another international resource is the UNODC-published compilation describing 24 family-based programs. These programs were chosen from a group of 150 programs and were selected by a panel of scholars as showing strong evidence (UNODC, 2009).

Systematic reviews also focus on characteristics of effective programs. For example, a group of scholars in conjunction with the UNODC (2009) identified principles guiding effective family-based interventions. These principles include such things as the intervention: is theory based; is matched to the needs and risk level of the potential participants; is age appropriate; provides adequate intensity and dosage; and is interactive, rather than exclusively didactic. The review also includes content and strategies common to effective programs delivered to parents, to youth, and to families together. Finally, the review identified strategies for high-quality implementation. An early systematic review conducted by the Center for Substance Abuse Prevention (1998) found that three family-based intervention types met the criteria for strong effects: (1) behavioral parent training, (2) family skill training, and (3) intensive family therapy. Subsequent review added home visitation and multicomponent interventions to the list of effective family-based interventions (Kumpfer & Alvarado, 2003).

Meta-analysis: Like systematic reviews, meta-analyses illustrate whether and how well specific programs or program types work. Early meta-analyses of family-based prevention programs (e.g., Tobler & Kumpfer, 2000) focused on parenting program effects on children's behavior problems and youth substance use compared to other types of programs. Results suggested that family programs were up to nine times as effective in reducing indicators of parenting and child behavior problems as child-only focused programs. Moreover, comparisons of different types of family-based interventions to other types of interventions showed that behavioral parent training programs had a medium effect whereas intensive in-home programs with families or parents showed very strong effects and family skill programs have stronger effects than parent training only (Tobler & Kumpfer, 2000). Although not specific to substance use, meta-analysis results also show that when positive parenting behaviors increase and negative parenting behaviors decrease, youth positive behaviors also increase and negative behaviors decrease (Durlak, Weissberg, Dymnicki, Taylor, & Schellinger, 2011). More recent meta-analyses have shown that interventions involving parents alone have a modest effect on preventing and decreasing adolescent tobacco, alcohol, and illicit substance use (Allen, et al., 2016). There is moderate evidence supporting positive effects of family-based interventions on preventing initiation of tobacco use among children and adolescents (Thomas, Baker, Thomas, & Lorenzetti, 2015) and marijuana use in the general population, but limited evidence for these programs influencing use among higher risk youth (Vermeulen-Smit, Verdurmen, & Engels, 2015). Van Ryzin, Kumpfer, et al. (2016), Van Ryzin, Roseth, et al. (2016) found that family-based interventions produced small to medium effects on average, with comparable effects for tobacco, alcohol, and a composite of other drugs including marijuana, hard drugs, and polydrug use.

Component meta-analysis: Some meta-analyses examine whether common content, strategies, or structures across programs relate to better outcomes. Among parent training programs for children aged 0–7, better outcomes were found when they focused on positive interactions, taught parents to communicate about emotions, taught effective and consistent discipline (e.g., timeout), and allowed parents to practice with their own children (Kaminski et al., 2008). More effective substance-use programs include components that include youth-focused activities designed to improve family relationships and foster youths' future orientation (Van Ryzin, Kumpfer, et al., 2016; Van Ryzin, Roseth, et al., 2016). Delivery mechanism, dosage, and whether programs were community or school based were not associated with better outcomes.

The evidence from independent reports of program evaluations, systematic reviews of the broader literature, and meta-analyses demonstrate the efficacy of family-based prevention programs for altering family and parenting practices and either delaying onset or reducing escalation of substance use. These findings are promising, yet point to room for improvement. For example, these analyses are beginning to illustrate for whom programs work, but more work is needed to fully understand for which populations our parenting and family-based prevention programs work (Garcia-Huidobro, Doty, Davis, Borowsky, & Allen, 2018). Additionally, many studies of substance-use prevention programs do not meet basic standards by which we can judge effectiveness because of weak designs, incomplete description of the theoretical and conceptual intervention models, or poor implementation. This suggests that there is more work to be done and often families who would benefit from receiving high-quality family programs are instead receiving less effective or ineffective programs.

Exemplary Family-Based Prevention Programs

Websites, such as Blueprints for Healthy Youth Development; compendia, such as the UNODC's "Compilation of evidence based family skills training programs"; and books (Van Ryzin, Kumpfer, et al., 2016; Van Ryzin, Roseth, et al., 2016) are excellent resources to learn more about specific programs. Here, we highlight a few programs with strong evidence and that illustrate the variety of family-based programs, across type, intensity, and age/developmental stage.

Early Interventions for New Parents

The Nurse Family Partnership program (Olds, 2006) is a home visitation program for poor, first-time mothers, delivered when mothers are pregnant and after the baby is born. It is guided by three theories. First, human ecology theory (Bronfenbrenner & Morris, 2006) helps to identify who should be in the program and poor, first-time mothers could benefit greatly by building connections to important sources of support like family, friends, and social agencies. Second, self-efficacy theory (Bandura, 1982) plays a role by helping mothers set small achievable goals they can manage, so they experience success, and can build their confidence in meeting the demands of parenthood and life. Third, attachment theory (Bowlby, 1969) plays an important role in guiding how to work with first-time mothers to develop sensitive, responsive, and engaged caregiving in the early years of parenthood.

Nurse Family Partnership activities are designed around three primary goals: (1) improving prenatal health to improve pregnancy outcomes; (2) improving sensitive and caring parenting to improve child health outcomes; and (3) improving parent life course by helping them plan for the future. Changing these factors is intended to lead to better intermediate outcomes in early childhood including fewer injuries and incidence of child abuse, and fewer problem behaviors. Improved early development should lead to fewer problems in adolescence, like delinquent behaviors and substance use (Olds, 2006).

Evidence for this program is based primarily on three randomized clinical trials in the United States. The first was in Elmira New York starting in 1978, the second in Memphis starting in 1990, and the third in Denver starting in 1994. All produced solid results regarding the efficacy of the program and those three studies launched the dissemination of the program nationally and internationally. The program is delivered in 43 states within the United States, the US Virgin Islands and 6 tribal nations. It is also implemented widely within the United Kingdom, Canada, Australia, and the Netherlands.

Behavior Parent Training in Childhood

The Positive Parenting Program "Triple P" (Sanders et al., 2008), one of the most widely used programs in the world, is a system of 20 different parenting programs for different ages, different levels of problems, and different contexts. It is based on social learning, cognitive behavioral and developmental theories of parenting, and child and youth behavior problems. The Triple P system operates on a tiered continuum of increasing strength and intensity (Sanders, 2012). Five levels of the programs range from very low intensity, such as media campaigns to reach a wide audience, to multi-session individual or group sessions with very-high-risk families experiencing high levels of stress. It is designed to maximize options and help parents make decisions about the kind of program they want based on their level of need and preference for access to the program. It can also be delivered in a targeted way to just a few families or to an entire population. In this way, Triple P is a system of interventions that has the potential to have a broad impact on the health of communities (Sanders et al., 2008).

Meta-analysis (Sanders, Kirby, Tellegen, & Day, 2014) of findings from all levels of the program across many different outcomes shows that effects of the program on parenting practices (e.g., parent-child relationships, and positive parenting methods) and for parenting satisfaction outcomes (e.g., parenting efficacy and parenting satisfaction) were in the medium to strong range and statistically significant. Long-term effects were similar, and the intervention was equally effective for families of different risk levels, in different modes, and in different countries. Effects were slightly stronger for targeted and treatment programming over universal interventions. For both short- and long-term outcomes on child social, emotional, and behavioral functioning, significant effects were found for all levels and for all variations of the program. As with parenting outcomes, results showed that there were no differences across risk levels, in different modes and in different countries. In general, the program of research with Triple P in diverse countries and cultures suggests that the strategy of using behavioral parenting principles can be adapted and used effectively across a wide range of cultural contexts (Sanders, 2012).

Family Skill Program for Early Adolescence/Adolescence

The Strengthening Families Program for Parents and Youth 10–14 (SFP 10–14; Molgaard, Spoth, & Redmond, 2000) is a universal family skill training program based on three main theoretical models: a biopsychosocial model, a resilience model, and a family process model. Together, these theoretical models suggest building family skills, during important developmental transition, such as: children moving from middle childhood into adolescence can buffer some of the stresses families may experience, and can also help youth build the skills they need to develop healthy habits and refrain from using substances.

SFP 10–14 has three primary program components: parent sessions, youth sessions, and family sessions. Skills unique to parents and youth and mutually beneficial to both are taught in these sessions. These components are designed to decrease risk factors and increase protective factors that will then improve parenting skills, youth skills, and family relationships. The long-term goals of this program are to reduce youth substance use, as well as antisocial behavior, and to improve academic performance.

Results from studies of SPF 10–14 show that it has powerful short-term effects in changing parenting strategies and youth attitudes, and long-term effects on youth substance use (Spoth & Redmond, 2002; Spoth, Redmond, Mason, Schainker, & Borduin, 2015). Short- and long-term (e.g., 4–6 years) effects have been found for alcohol use, lifetime drunkenness, and aggressive behavior and longer term effects on methamphetamine and prescription drug misuse. The program works by improving the quality of the relationships parents have with their youth and limiting youth exposures to substances, and therefore delaying the onset of substance use (Spoth et al., 2015).

Intensive Family Therapy for Adolescents

Multisystemic therapy, or MST (Henggeler, Schoenwald, Borduin, Rowland, & Cunningham, 2009), is an intensive family intervention implemented as an indicated intervention for youth who are showing early signs of aggressive and disruptive behavior or as a treatment for youth who have been in trouble with the authorities because of illegal behavior. MST is designed around a social ecological theory of problem development (Bronfenbrenner & Morris, 2006) and family systems theory that focuses on the relationships among family members and between family members and the social settings in which they live. The logic for MST is that by improving family functioning, other factors in the youth's social ecology that support problem behaviors (e.g., peers) will change, which will change behavior problems, criminal activity, and substance use.

The intervention serves youth aged 12–17 and their families. The treatment is intensive: therapists are available 24 h per day, 7 days per week. On average, contact ranges from 2 to 15 h per week and treatment lasts between 3 and 5 months. Therapists use proven intervention strategies such as structural and strategic family therapy, parent management training, behavioral therapy, and cognitive behavioral therapy (Henggeler et al., 2009).

MST shows strong effects on youth substance use and consequences including marijuana use, alcohol use, and substance-related arrests four years and 14 years following the intervention (Henggeler et al., 2009; Schaeffer & Borduin, 2005). These findings on substance use were so promising that MST has been adapted to focus more specifically on substance use and tested in early pilot trials (Randall, Cunningham, & Henggeler, 2018).

Challenges

Despite the promise evident in the strength of empirical findings of family-based programs, it remains a challenge to bring the full benefit of these programs to bear on larger populations. With relatively few exceptions, bringing family-based preventive interventions to scale has been difficult (Spoth et al., 2015). One of the biggest challenges to implementing family-based preventions on a large scale is *recruiting and retaining families*. Universal and selective family-based interventions typically have low rates of participation, meaning the program might not have the reach needed to influence the public's health. High-quality strategies can improve recruitment by several times (Dishion et al., 2008) and strategies for ensuring that families learn about the programs, managing logistics of delivering programs at convenient times and places, and reducing negative parental attitudes about the program availability (e.g., Shapiro, Prinz, & Sanders, 2015) can improve levels of involvement. Innovative strategies are now being used such as recruiting families via social media (Oesterle, Epstein, Haggerty, & Moreno, 2018) and testing different methods of recruitment in experimental trials (Winslow et al., 2016). Moreover, substantial work is being done to understand within-session process and between-session parent behaviors that affect the likelihood parents continue in the program (e.g., Coatsworth, Hemady, & George, 2018).

Adapting Interventions. A second challenge to broad dissemination of family-focused programs is that often when evidence-based programs are implemented under natural conditions by community organizations they are changed in some way. Sometimes as much as 80% of the program is changed (Durlak, 1998). Often program adaptations are reactive to logistical demands such as time and/or availability of staffing (Moore, Bumbarger, & Cooper, 2013). When adaptations are reactive rather than proactive to help the program better fit the context, changes tend to produce fewer positive effects. Proactive adaptations in consultation with a program developer can have positive results.

Programs may also be adapted for cultural reasons for example as attempts to increase the ecological validity of the program and to make aspects of an intervention more congruent with participants' life experiences (Castro & Yasui, 2017). Researchers are engaging community members in a process of adapting evidence-based programs to fit a new cultural context (e.g., Domenech Rodríguez, Baumann, & Schwartz, 2011) and use adaptation strategies that maintain theoretical congruence to the original program (Mejia, Leijten, Lachman, & Parra-Cardona, 2017). Cultural or local adaptations do not have to be detrimental to program efficacy and may even increase engagement, efficacy, and adoption or sustainability by the community (Barrera, Berkel, & Castro, 2017). Confronting challenges of adaptations of family-based interventions should be a priority if prevention science is to move toward a broader population approach (Gonzales, 2017).

The need to understand adaptations of evidence-based programs extends beyond the borders of the United States. There are an increasing number of "cross-national" programs created in one country, usually the United States, and implemented in another. Overall, the findings of replications of family-based programs have shown mixed results. Some positive results from replication studies have been shown for The Incredible Years (Axberg & Broberg, 2012), MST (Schoenwald, Heiblum, Saldana, & Henggeler, 2008), and Triple P (Chung, Leung, & Sanders, 2015), but negative or null results also have been found, sometimes for the same intervention. For example, Triple P results in Canada and Switzerland were less positive as were MST in Sweden and Canada (Sundell, Ferrer-Wreder, & Fraser, 2014). A trial of SFP 10–14 in Sweden failed to replicate the findings of the original program (Skärstrand, Sundell, & Andréasson, 2013), despite conferring with the developer, yet the adaptation appears to have changed the program's structure significantly (Segrott et al., 2014).

As the number of evaluations of these kinds of programs has grown, the ability to examine differences more carefully has also grown. A recent meta-analysis (Sundell, Beelmann, Hasson, & von Thiele Schwarz, 2016) of programs in Sweden and Germany compared effect sizes of novel programs, meaning they were developed within the country in which it was being evaluated; adopted programs or evidence-based programs were implemented with fidelity to their original form in the new country; and adapted programs or programs were changed to fit the current cultural context. Results indicated that novel programs, which were also the most frequent, showed the best effects. Programs that were adapted explicitly for cultural reasons were significantly more effective than international adopted programs without any adaptation. Although specifics about cultural adaptations have not been clearly articulated, international models exist (e.g., Ferrer-Wreder, Sundell, & Mansoory, 2012) and these at least pose some direction for careful adaptation while also shedding some light on potential methods for examining differences.

Several other challenges warrant brief description. First, like most areas of study, there is a need for replication. Currently the highest standard for achieving status of an evidence-based program is through the process of listing on the Blueprints for Healthy Youth Development. The top standard of Model Program Plus indicates that in addition to the replications that have been conducted by the program development team, a high-quality independent replication via RCT that has been conducted with strong data supporting the program effects is necessary. Second, measurement continues to be a challenge and greater attention to how best to measure complex constructs like parenting and family functioning is needed in prevention science (Lindhiem & Shaffer, 2017). Not only do these measures need to demonstrate strong psychometric properties (e.g., construct validity), but they also need to be sensitive to change and may need to possess these qualities for different subgroups (Eddy, 2017). Third, implementation of family-based prevention programming needs to be expanded to be integrated more completely into systems of care (Gonzales, 2017), such as within the primary care system (e.g., Smith & Polaha, 2017). Family-based preventive interventions do not have natural delivery systems so finding unique opportunities to "scale out" (Aarons, Sklar, Mustanski, Benbow, & Brown, 2017) these strong interventions is a necessary step to maximize their potential.

Conclusions

Evaluations from a growing number of family-focused programs support their efficacy in changing parenting practices, influencing family processes, and promoting healthy youth development while reducing the likelihood adolescents will use or misuse substances. Despite diversity of family structures and the many family processes that could be targeted in interventions, there appears to be some convergence on the kinds of program activities that produce change in critical family mechanisms that lead to healthier child and youth development. Although a growing number of Web-based and print resources point consumers to top-quality programs, additional work is required to move the science forward to find new outlets and models of family-based interventions that will extend their reach to other agencies serving families in need, thus broadening their public health impact.

References

Aarons, G. A., Sklar, M., Mustanski, B., Benbow, N., & Brown, C. H. (2017). "Scaling-out" evidence-based interventions to new populations or new health care delivery systems. *Implementation Science, 12*(1), 111.

Abar, C. C., Jackson, K. M., & Wood, M. (2014). Reciprocal relations between perceived parental knowledge and adolescent substance use and delinquency: The moderating role of parent–teen relationship quality. *Developmental Psychology, 50*(9), 2176.

Allen, M., Garcia-Huidobro, D., Porta, C., Curran, D., Patel, R., Miller, J., & Borowski, I. (2016). Effective parenting interventions to reduce youth substance use: A systemic review. *Pediatrics, 138*, e20154425. https://doi.org/10.1542/peds.2015-4425

Ary, D. V., Duncan, T. E., Duncan, S. C., & Hops, H. (1999). Adolescent problem behavior: The influence of parents and peers. *Behaviour Research and Therapy, 37*(3), 217–230.

Ashby Wills, T., & Yaeger, A. M. (2003). Family factors and adolescent substance use: Models and mechanisms. *Current Directions in Psychological Science, 12*(6), 222–226.

Axberg, U., & Broberg, A. G. (2012). Evaluation of "the incredible years" in Sweden: The transferability of an American parent-training program to Sweden. *Scandinavian Journal of Psychology, 53*(3), 224–232.

Bahr, S. J., Hoffmann, J. P., & Yang, X. (2005). Parental and peer influences on the risk of adolescent drug use. *Journal of Primary Prevention, 26*(6), 529–551.

Bandura, A. (1982). Self-efficacy mechanism in human agency. *American Psychologist, 37*(2), 122–147. https://doi.org/10.1037/0003-066X.37.2.122

Barrera, M., Berkel, C., & Castro, F. G. (2017). Directions for the advancement of culturally adapted preventive interventions: Local adaptations, engagement, and sustainability. *Prevention Science, 18*(6), 640–648.

Biglan, A., Flay, B. R., Embry, D. D., & Sandler, I. N. (2012). The critical role of nurturing environments for promoting human well-being. *American Psychologist, 67*(4), 257.

Bogenschneider, K., Wu, M. Y., Raffaelli, M., & Tsay, J. C. (1998). Parent influences on adolescent peer orientation and substance use: The interface of parenting practices and values. *Child Development, 69*(6), 1672–1688.

Bowen, M. (1985). *Family therapy in clinical practice*. Northvale, NJ: Aaronson.

Bowlby, J. (1969). *Attachment. Attachment and loss (vol. 1)*. New York: Basic Books.

Bronfenbrenner, U., & Morris, P. A. (2006). The bioecological model of human development. In W. Damon & R. M. Lerner (Eds.), *Handbook of child psychology. Vol. 1: Theoretical models of human development* (6th ed., pp. 793–828). New York, NY: John Wiley.

Brown, C. H., Wang, W., Kellam, S. G., Muthén, B. O., Petras, H., Toyinbo, P., … Sloboda, Z. (2008). Methods for testing theory and evaluating impact in randomized field trials: Intent-to-treat analyses for integrating the perspectives of person, place, and time. *Drug & Alcohol Dependence, 95*, S74–S104.

Castro, F. G., & Yasui, M. (2017). Advances in EBI development for diverse populations: Towards a science of intervention adaptation. *Prevention Science, 18*(6), 623–629.

Center for Substance Abuse Prevention. (1998). *Preventing substance abuse among children and adolescents: Family-centered approaches Prevention Enhancement Protocols System (PEPS) (DHHS Publication No. SMA 3223-FY'98)*. Washington, DC: U.S. Government Printing Office.

Chung, S., Leung, C., & Sanders, M. (2015). The Triple P–Positive Parenting Programme: The effectiveness of group Triple P and brief parent discussion group in school settings in Hong Kong. *Journal of Children's Services, 10*(4), 339–352.

Coatsworth, J. D., Hemady, K., & George, M. W. (2018). Predictors of Group Leaders' Perceptions of Parents' Initial and Dynamic Engagement in a Family Preventive Intervention. *Prevention Science, 28*, 609–619.

Dawson-McClure, S., Calzada, E., Huang, K.-Y., Kamboukos, D., Rhule, D., Kolawole, B., … Brotman, L. M. (2015). A population-level approach to promoting healthy child development and school success in low-income, urban neighborhoods: Impact on parenting and child conduct problems. *Prevention Science, 16*(2), 279–290.

DeLeire, T., & Kalil, A. (2002). Good things come in threes: Single-parent multigenerational family structure and adolescent adjustment. *Demography, 39*(2), 393–413.

Donovan, J. E. (2016). Child and adolescent socialization into substance use. In *The oxford handbook of adolescent substance abuse*. Oxford: Oxford University Press.

Dishion, T. J., & McMahon, R. J. (1998). Parental monitoring and the prevention of child and adolescent problem behavior: A conceptual and empirical formulation. *Clinical Child and Family Psychology Review, 1*(1), 61–75.

Dishion, T. J., Nelson, S. E., & Bullock, B. M. (2004). Premature adolescent autonomy: Parent disengagement and deviant peer process in the amplification of problem behaviour. *Journal of Adolescence, 27*(5), 515–530.

Dishion, T. J., Shaw, D., Connell, A., Gardner, F., Weaver, C., & Wilson, M. (2008). The family check-up With high-risk indigent families: Preventing problem behavior by increasing parents' positive behavior support in early childhood. *Child Development, 79*, 1395–1414.

Domenech Rodríguez, M. M., Baumann, A. A., & Schwartz, A. L. (2011). Cultural adaptation of an evidence based intervention: From theory to practice in a Latino/a community context. *American Journal of Community Psychology, 47*(1–2), 170–186.

Donaldson, C. D., Handren, L. M., & Crano, W. D. (2016). The enduring impact of parents' monitoring, warmth, expectancies, and alcohol use on their children's future binge drinking and arrests: A longitudinal analysis. *Prevention Science, 17*(5), 606–614.

Duncan, T. E., Tildesley, E., Duncan, S. C., & Hops, H. (1995). The consistency of family and peer influences on the development of substance use in adolescence. *Addiction, 90*(12), 1647–1660.

Durlak, J. A. (1998). Why program implementation is important. *Journal of Prevention & Intervention in the Community, 17*, 5–18.

Durlak, J. A., Taylor, R. D., Kawashima, K., Pachan, M. P., DuPre, E. P., Celio, C. I., … Weissberg, R. P. (2007). Effects of positive youth development programs on school, family, and community systems. *American Journal of Community Psychology, 40*, 269–286.

Durlak, J. A., Weissberg, R. P., Dymnicki, A. B., Taylor, R. D., & Schellinger, K. B. (2011). The impact of enhancing students' social and emotional learning: A meta-analysis of school-based universal interventions. *Child Development, 82*(1), 405–432.

Eddy, J. M. (2017). Facing a Fundamental Problem in Prevention Science: the Measurement of a Key Construct. *Prevention Science, 18*(3), 322–325.

Ewing, B. A., Osilla, K. C., Pedersen, E. R., Hunter, S. B., Miles, J. N., & D'Amico, E. J. (2015). Longitudinal family effects on substance use among an at-risk adolescent sample. *Addictive Behaviors, 41*, 185–191.

Feinberg, M. E. (2002). Coparenting and the transition to parenthood: A framework for prevention. *Clinical Child and Family Psychology Review, 5*, 173–195.

Ferrer-Wreder, L., Sundell, K., & Mansoory, S. (2012). Tinkering with perfection: Theory development in the intervention cultural adaptation field. *Child and Youth Care Forum, 41*, 149–171. https://doi.org/10.1007/s10566-011-9162-6

Flay BR, Biglan A, Boruch RF, Castro FG, Gottfredson D, Kellam S, … &, Ji P. (2005) Standards of evidence: Criteria for efficacy, effectiveness and dissemination. *Prevention Science, 6*, 151–175. doi: https://doi.org/10.1007/s11121-005-5553-y

Forgatch, M. S., & Patterson, G. R. (2010). Parent management training—Oregon model: An intervention for antisocial behaviors in children and adolescents. In J. R. Weisz & A. E. Kazdin (Eds.), *Evidenced-based psychotherapies for children and adolescents* (Vol. 2, pp. 159–178). New York: Guilford.

Foxcroft, D. R., & Tsertsvadze, A. (2012). Universal alcohol misuse prevention programmes for children and adolescents: Cochrane systematic reviews. *Perspectives in Public Health, 132*, 128–134.

Garcia-Huidobro, D., Doty, J. L., Davis, L., Borowsky, I. W., & Allen, M. L. (2018). For whom do parenting interventions to prevent adolescent substance use work? *Prevention Science, 19*, 570–578.

Gonzales, N. A. (2017). Expanding the cultural adaptation framework for population-level impact. *Prevention Science, 18*(6), 689–693. http:\\doi.org\10.1007/s11121-017-0808-y

Georgas, J. (2006). Families and family change. In J. E. Georgas, J. W. Berry, F. J. Van de Vijver, Ç. E. Kağitçibaşi, & Y. H. Poortinga (Eds.), *Families across cultures: A 30-nation psychological study (3–50)*. Cambridge: Cambridge University Press.

Gottfredson, D. C., Cook, T. D., Gardner, F. E. M., Gorman-Smith, D., Howe, G. W., Sandler, I. N., & Zafft, K. M. (2015). Standards of evidence for efficacy, effectiveness, and scale-up research in prevention science: Next generation. *Prevention Science, 7*, 893–926. https://doi.org/10.1007/s11121-015-0555-x

Grusec, J. E. (2011). Socialization processes in the family: Social and emotional development. *Annual Review of Psychology, 62*, 243–269.

Henggeler, S. W., Schoenwald, S. K., Borduin, C. M., Rowland, M. D., & Cunningham, P. B. (2009). *Multisystemic therapy for antisocial behavior in children and adolescents* (2nd ed.). New York: Guilford Press.

Kaminski, J. W., Valle, L. A., Filene, J. H., & Boyle, C. L. (2008). A meta-analytic review of components associated with parent training program effectiveness. *Journal of Abnormal Child Psychology, 36*(4), 567–589.

Kerr, M., & Stattin, H. (2000). What parents know, how they know it, and several forms of adolescent adjustment: further support for a reinterpretation of monitoring. *Developmental Psychology, 36*(3), 366.

Kopystynska, O., Paschall, K. W., Barnett, M. A., & Curran, M. A. (2017). Patterns of interparental conflict, parenting, and children's emotional insecurity: A person-centered approach. *Journal of Family*

Psychology, 31(7), 922–932. https://doi.org/10.1037/fam0000343

Kumpfer, K. L., & Alvarado, R. (2003). Family-strengthening approaches for the prevention of youth problem behaviors. *American Psychologist, 58*(6–7), 457–465.

Lamb, C. S., & Crano, W. D. (2014). Parents' beliefs and children's marijuana use: Evidence for a self-fulfilling prophecy effect. *Addictive Behaviors, 39*(1), 127–132.

Lindhiem, O., & Shaffer, A. (2017). Introduction to the special series: Current directions for measuring parenting constructs to inform prevention science. *Prevention Science, 18*(3), 253–256.

Masten, A. S. (2018). Resilience theory and research on children and families: Past, present, and promise. *Journal of Family Theory & Review, 10*(1), 12–31.

Masten, A. S., & Monn, A. R. (2015). Child and family resilience: A call for integrated science, practice, and professional training. *Family Relations, 64*(1), 5–21.

McMahon, R. J., Wells, K. C., & Kotler, J. S. (2006). Conduct problems. In E. J. Mash & R. A. Barkley (Eds.), *Treatment of childhood disorders* (Vol. 3, pp. 137–268). New York: Guilford Press.

Mejia, A., Leijten, P., Lachman, J. M., & Parra-Cardona, J. R. (2017). Different strokes for different folks? Contrasting approaches to cultural adaptation of parenting interventions. *Prevention Science, 18*(6), 630–639.

Miller-Day, M., & Kam, J. A. (2010). More than just openness: Developing and validating a measure of targeted parent–child communication about alcohol. *Health Communication, 25*(4), 293–302.

Miller-Heyl, J., MacPhee, D., & Fritz, J. (2002). *DARE to be You: A systems approach to the early prevention of problem behaviors*. New York: Kluwer/Plenum.

Molgaard, V., Spoth, R., & Redmond, C. (2000). Competency training: The strengthening families program for parents and youth 10–14. In *OJJDP family strengthening series, juvenile justice bulletin* (p. 11). Washington, DC: U.S. Dept. of Justice, Office of Justice Programs, Office of Juvenile Justice and Delinquency Prevention Retrieved from https://www.ncjrs.gov/pdffiles1/ojjdp/182208.pdf

Moore, J. E., Bumbarger, B. K., & Cooper, B. R. (2013). Examining adaptations of evidence-based programs in natural contexts. *The Journal of Primary Prevention, 34*(3), 147–161.

National Academies of Sciences, Engineering, and Medicine. (2016). *Parenting matters: Supporting parents of children ages 0–8*. Washington, DC: National Academies Press.

Oesterle, S., Epstein, M., Haggerty, K. P., & Moreno, M. A. (2018). Using Facebook to recruit parents to participate in a family program to prevent teen drug use. *Prevention Science, 19*(4), 559–569.

Olds, D. L. (2006). The nurse–family partnership: An evidence-based preventive intervention. *Infant Mental Health Journal, 27*(1), 5–25.

Olson, D. H. (2000). Circumplex model of marital and family sytems. *Journal of Family Therapy, 22*, 144–167.

Randall, J., Cunningham, P. B., & Henggeler, S. W. (2018). The development and transportability of multisystemic therapy-substance abuse: A treatment for adolescents with substance use disorders. *Journal of Child & Adolescent Substance Abuse, 27*(2), 59–66. https://doi.org/10.1080/1067828X.2017.1411301

Sanders, M. R. (2012). Development, evaluation, and multinational dissemination of the Triple P-Positive Parenting Program. *Annual Review of Clinical Psychology, 8*, 1–35. https://doi.org/10.1146/annurev-clinpsy-032511-143104

Sanders, M. R., Morawska, A. (2014). Can changing parental knowledge, dysfunctional expectations and attributions, and emotion regulation improve outcomes for children? In: Tremblay, R. E., Boivin, M., Peters, RDeV, Tremblay RE (Eds.), (topic ed.). *Encyclopedia on early childhood development*. Retrieved April 22, 2017, from http://www.child-encyclopedia.com/parenting-skills/according-experts/can-changing-parental-knowledge-dysfunctional-expectations-and

Sanders, M. R., Ralph, A., Sofronoff, K., Gardiner, P., Thompson, R., Dwyer, S., & Bidwell, K. (2008). Every family: A population approach to reducing behavioral and emotional problems in children making the transition to school. *The Journal of Primary Prevention, 29*, 197–222.

Sanders, M. R., Kirby, J. N., Tellegen, C. L., & Day, J. J. (2014). The Triple P-Positive Parenting Program: A systematic review and meta-analysis of a multi-level system of parenting support. *Clinical Psychology Review, 34*(4), 337–357.

Santisteban, D. A., Coatsworth, J. D., Perez-Vidal, A., Kurtines, W. M., Schwartz, S. J., LaPerriere, A., & Szapocznik, J. (2003). Efficacy of brief strategic family therapy in modifying Hispanic adolescent behavior problems and substance use. *Journal of Family Psychology, 17*(1), 121.

Schaeffer, C. M., & Borduin, C. M. (2005). Long-term follow-up to a randomized clinical trial of multisystemic therapy with serious and violent juvenile offenders. *Journal of Consulting and Clinical Psychology, 73*(3), 445–453. https://doi.org/10.1037/0022-006X.73.3.445

Shapiro, C. J., Prinz, R. J., & Sanders, M. R. (2015). Sustaining use of an evidence-based parenting intervention: Practitioner perspectives. *Journal of Child and Family Studies, 24*, 1615–1624.

Schoenwald, S. K., Heiblum, N., Saldana, L., & Henggeler, S. W. (2008). The international implementation of multisystemic therapy. *Evaluation & the Health Professions, 31*(2), 211–225.

Segrott, J., Holliday, J., Rothwell, H., Foxcroft, D., Murphy, S., Scourfield, J., … Moore, L. (2014). Cultural adaptation and intervention integrity: a response to Skärstrand, Sundell and Andréasson. *The European Journal of Public Health, 24*(3), 354–355.

Skärstrand, E., Sundell, K., & Andréasson, S. (2013). Evaluation of a Swedish version of the strengthening families programme. *The European Journal of Public Health, 24*(4), 578–584.

Smith, J. D., & Polaha, J. (2017). Using implementation science to guide the integration of evidence-based family interventions into primary care. *Families, Systems, & Health, 35*(2), 125.

Spoth, R., & Redmond, C. (2002). Project Family prevention trials based in community-university partnerships: Toward scaled-up preventive interventions. *Prevention Science, 3*(3), 203–221.

Spoth, R., Redmond, C., Mason, W. A., Schainker, L., & Borduin, L. (2015). Research on the Strengthening Families Program for Parents and Youth 10-14: Long-term effects, mechanisms, translation to public health, PROSPER partnership scale up. In L. M. Scheier (Ed.), *Handbook of drug prevention* (pp. 267–292). Washington, DC: American Psychological Association.

Sroufe, L. A., Egeland, B., Carlson, E., & Collins, W. A. (2005). *The development of the person: The Minnesota study of risk and adaptation from birth to adulthood.* New York: Guilford Publications.

Sundell, K., Ferrer-Wreder, L., & Fraser, M. W. (2014). Going global: A model for evaluating empirically supported family-based interventions in new contexts. *Evaluation & the Health Professions, 37*(2), 203–230.

Sundell, K., Beelmann, A., Hasson, H., & von Thiele Schwarz, U. (2016). Novel programs, international adoptions, or contextual adaptations? Meta-analytical results from German and Swedish intervention research. *Journal of Clinical Child & Adolescent Psychology, 45*(6), 784–796.

Thomas, R. E., Baker, P. R. A., Thomas, B. C., & Lorenzetti, D. L. (2015). Family-based programmes for preventing smoking by children and adolescents. *Cochrane Database of Systematic Reviews*, (2), CD004493. https://doi.org/10.1002/14651858.CD004493.pub3

Tobler, N. S., & Kumpfer, K. L. (2000). *Meta-analyses of family approaches to substance abuse prevention.* Rockville, MD: Tech. Rep., CSAP.

Turpyn, C. C., & Chaplin, T. M. (2016). Mindful parenting and parents' emotion expression: effects on adolescent risk behaviors. *Mindfulness, 7*(1), 246–254.

United Nations Office of Drugs and Crime. (2009). *Compilation of evidence based family skills training programs.* Vienna, Austria: United Nations Publications.

Van Ryzin, M. J., Kumpfer, K. L., Fosco, G. M., & Greenberg, M. T. (Eds.). (2016). *Family-based prevention programs for children and adolescents: Theory, research, and large-scale dissemination.* Washington, DC: Psychology Press.

Van Ryzin, M. J., Roseth, C. J., Fosco, G. M., Lee, Y.-K., & Chen, I. C. (2016). A component-centered meta-analysis of family-based prevention programs for adolescent substance use. *Clinical Psychology Review, 45*, 72–80. https://doi.org/10.1016/j.cpr.2016.03.007

Vermeulen-Smit, E., Verdurmen, J. E. E., & Engels, R. C. M. E. (2015). The effectiveness of family interventions in preventing adolescent illicit drug use: A systematic review and meta-analysis of randomized controlled trials. *Clinical Child and Family Psychology Review, 18*(3), 218–239.

Walsh, F. (2016). *Strengthening family resilience.* New York: Guilford Publications.

Wills, T. A., Mariani, J., & Filer, M. (1996). The role of family and peer relationships in adolescent substance use. In *Handbook of social support and the family* (pp. 521–549). Boston, MA: Springer.

Winslow, E. B., Poloskov, E., Begay, R., Tein, J. Y., Sandler, I., & Wolchik, S. (2016). A randomized trial of methods to engage Mexican American parents into a school-based parenting intervention. *Journal of Consulting and Clinical Psychology, 84*, 1094.

The School: A Setting for Evidence-Based Prevention Interventions and Policies

Zili Sloboda and Christopher L. Ringwalt

Why Schools Are an Important Setting for Psychoactive Substance-Use Prevention

With the exception of their own homes, most children spend more time at school than anywhere else. Schools and other educational institutions have, therefore, a particular responsibility for the children enrolled in them. This includes teaching students what they need to know to become fully functional and independent citizens as adults and fulfilling their responsibilities at home and, eventually, in the workplace. In so doing schools reinforce the positive behaviors that children learn at home and in the community. Schools are thus society's most important agent of socialization, outside of the family. Indeed, when families experience problems, or because work limits the amount of time parents can spend with their children, schools may become the *prime* agent of socialization. Schools are also in an excellent position to help students develop negative beliefs about and attitudes towards all behaviors that put them at risk—including

Z. Sloboda (✉)
Applied Prevention Science International, Inc., Ontario, OH, USA
e-mail: zili.sloboda@apsintl.org

C. L. Ringwalt
Injury Prevention Research Center, University of North Carolina, Chapel Hill, NC, USA
e-mail: cringwal@email.unc.edu

substance use—and to strengthen their positive attitudes towards prosocial behaviors. Students in preschool settings, as well as those in lower and middle schools, are under almost constant adult supervision, which provides school staff with an exceptional opportunity to shape their behaviors by rewarding their appropriate behavior and intervening when they see antisocial behavior.

Psychoactive Substance Use

As children move from the preschool into the school years they become more autonomous, are exposed to a wider variety of people and experiences, and develop greater cognitive skills. Preventive interventions have been developed that address the challenges and opportunities associated with spending a large portion of the day in school. One challenge that may present itself to children during the elementary, middle, junior high, and high school years is the possibility of exposure to psychoactive substances.

What do we mean by "psychoactive substance use" and why should this issue be of concern, particularly to schools? All psychoactive substances exert their effects by altering the functioning of the central nervous system (CNS), which consists of the brain and spinal cord. The blood-brain barrier (BBB) allows only certain substances to pass from the blood to the brain through a series of tightly compressed cells that permit the passage of only certain chemicals. This barrier protects the brain not only from foreign substances in the blood that may injure the brain but also from naturally occurring hormones and neurotransmitters that flow through the body and maintain a constant environment in which the brain can function. The BBB keeps out substances with large molecular water-soluble structures such as aspirins or antibiotics. However, substances with small molecular structures and that are fat soluble, such as most psychoactive substances, can easily pass through the BBB. Because of this, psychoactive substances can have a direct effect on brain functioning.

The primary characteristic of psychoactive substances is that when they cross the BBB they alter mood, thoughts, judgments, sensory perceptions, and behavior. Psychoactive substances include alcohol and tobacco, and certain prescription medications as well as marijuana, heroin, and methamphetamines. The effects of psychoactive substances may be both positive and negative. By understanding their positive effects, we begin to understand the attraction that individuals have for these substances. However, we also need to understand the substances' negative effects, particularly on the developing brain. The effects themselves depend on the type of substance that is consumed.

Psychoactive substance use can disrupt brain function in areas critical to motivation, memory, learning, judgment, and behavior control. One of the brain areas still maturing during adolescence is the prefrontal cortex—the part of the brain that enables us to assess situations, make sound decisions, and keep emotions and desires under control (Dwyer, McQuown, and Leslie (2009); Hiller-Sturmhofel & Swartzwelder, 2004/2005; Huang, Kandel, Kandel, & Levine, 2013). The introduction of psychoactive substance during adolescence can interfere with the ongoing development of the brain as well as contemporaneous brain function, thus contributing to increased risk for making poor decisions. Moreover, such use can result in profound and long-lasting adverse consequences (Fishbein, Rose, Darcey, Belcher, & VanMeter, 2016) including vulnerability to physical and social and emotional problems. Therefore, school-based prevention programming for older children is concerned with early protection against all the pharmacological, psychological, social, and health effects of substance use.

Schools and Cognitive Skills

Schools come in all shapes and sizes and configurations, but their typical purpose is to prepare children and youth in basic academic skills and to become fully contributing members of their families, workplaces, communities, and their society. In general, schools represent the first major transition into the greater society for children after the family, and for many children schools are the source of major influences on their lives well into adolescence and early adulthood.

However, schools and education may accomplish much more than this. A 2007 World Bank Policy Report (Hanushek & Woessmann, 2007) found by means of analyses of educational data and national economies that "there is strong evidence that the *cognitive skills* of the population—rather than mere *school attainment*—are powerfully related to individual earnings, to the distribution of income, and to economic growth" (Hanuskek & Woessman, p. 1). Cognitive skills address students' ability to:

- Think for themselves and to address problems in a reasoned and carefully considered fashion, both alone and in collaboration with others.
- Reason, conceptualize, and solve problems using unfamiliar information or new procedures.
- Draw conclusions and come up with solutions by analyzing the relationships among given problems, issues, or conditions.

The World Bank report continues: "International comparisons incorporating expanded data on cognitive skills reveal much larger skill deficits in developing countries than are generally derived from just school enrollment and [academic achievement or] attainment. The magnitude of change needed makes clear that closing the economic gap with developed countries will require major structural changes in schooling institutions" (Hanuskek & Woessman, p. 1). The changes suggested may require such measures as:

- Increasing budgets for public schools.
- Ensuring that all students, regardless of economic status or gender, have access to at least a high school education.
- Reducing class sizes.
- Developing students' skills related to the analysis of the information they are taught, as opposed to learning it by rote.
- Increasing teachers' pay and educational expectations.
- Offering meals—both breakfast and lunch—in communities whose students may be likely to come to school hungry.

Schools should do considerably more than just teach students information and improve their cognitive skills. There are many complex interactions among a person's biological, personal, social, and environmental characteristics that affect human behavior. These interactions shape children's and youth's values, beliefs, attitudes, intentions, and behaviors, all of which are important to the physical, emotional, and social development from childhood to adolescence, and then from adolescence to adulthood. Like the family, the school can influence how children and youth perceive the acceptability and unacceptability of various positive and negative behaviors. So, school interventions can affect an individual's vulnerability to and risk for problem behaviors in general, and substance use in particular.

School Culture and Climate

Every school, of course, is much greater than the sum of its physical parts, or even the teachers and staff who work in it. Each school has many important characteristics that shape its students' behaviors. The school's setting, for example, can affect whether the students feel—and are—safe and healthy there. Students' perceptions of physical and emotional safety at school, connections to caring, respectful and dedicated teachers and staff, and engagement in meaningful and rewarding activities all serve to enhance school bonding. Schools with a positive culture and climate are much more likely to have students who are psychologically attached to them, and this school bonding is necessary if the school's socialization function is to be successfully realized.

Schools with a positive climate and culture have a shared vision to which everyone contributes. Considerable research has been conducted on these very intangible notions (e.g., Battistich, Schaps, Watson, Solomon, & Lewis, 2000). One set of researchers has concluded that the key aspects of school climate that are most linked to students' academic achievement are their perceptions of safety and support, the degree to which they are challenged, and the extent to which they consider themselves socially competent and capable (Schaps & Solomon, 2003). Students must also believe that their school has rigorous academic standards and high expectations of them. They should feel challenged, invested, and motivated to succeed, and appreciate the relationship between their academic achievement at school and their life goals. Students should be taught emotional intelligence, which means having the ability to identify, assess, and control one's own emotions, and to understand, assess, and respond appropriately to the emotions of others, both singly and in groups. Finally, an effective school is one in which students are given meaningful opportunities to contribute to the welfare of the school.

Students cannot learn if they feel unsafe in their school environment. Their physical safety is just the beginning—although too many schools are indeed not safe, either for students or faculty. That is, many students and faculty live with the threat of violence and aggressive or delinquent behavior (Gottfredson & Gottfredson, 2001). Included in the threat of violence is, of course, both sexual coercion and harassment, as it relates to both girls and boys. Thus, students need to know that they are safe from the threat of any kind of psychological or emotional harm or sexual violation or harassment, from either peers or staff. In addition, they must feel socially safe—which means that they are in an environment that does not allow, and takes active steps to prevent or stop, bullying and teasing. Teasing and bullying are now taking a wide variety of forms, including the use of electronic media like Facebook and Twitter to send harassing text and pictures. Schools should assume responsibility for the prevention of a wide array of behaviors that may compromise their students' physical and mental health—not just substance use.

Students must also believe that they are fairly and equitably treated by those in authority over them. That is, they should be able to feel that school administrators and teachers treat all students in the same manner, and that no students are treated favorably because of their special status—for example, because they are outstanding athletes or students, or belong to a particular racial or ethnic group. Further, the school must be orderly; that is, there should be clear rules of and expectations related to behaviors that are known to all. For example, students should not be concerned that they may be punished for breaking a rule—such as coming late to class, or threatening another student—that is inconsistently enforced. Thus, all rules should apply equally to all students.

Finally, students must feel that they are supported (Hyde, Gorka, Manuck, & Hariri, 2011). Their feelings of safety and security at school come in part from being well connected to a social network that includes both peers and school staff. Students should also feel a strong attachment to their school, insofar as they know their place and role in the school and enjoy positive relationships with teachers and peers. In addition, they should know where and to whom to turn for help when they need it, and how to access it. They should expect that the help they receive will be given them in a thoughtful, sensitive, and respectful fashion that ensures their rights of confidentiality, and that it will help them respond effectively to the problems and adversities they face.

Schools and Prevention

It is thus clear that schools have a vital role to play in the prevention of substance use (Bosworth & Sloboda, 2015; Rohrbach & Dyal, 2015). The primary responsibility that schools can assume to prevent substance use is to create and maintain a positive school climate with the characteristics discussed above. But schools have a major role to play in substance-use prevention in at least three additional key areas. The first is demand reduction: that is, preventing or at least delaying youths' substance use by attempting to instill anti-substance-use values, norms, beliefs, and attitudes, and by giving them the skills to say "no" effectively to peers who may invite them to use substances. Most school-based substance-use prevention programs have demanded reduction as their primary, and often exclusive, goal. Schools also have some responsibility for supply reduction—that is, developing reasonable, clear, and consistently enforced policies targeting the use and sale of all substances, including alcohol and tobacco, on and near school grounds and at all school-sponsored events. Third, schools have a responsibility to their students to reduce the adverse consequences associated with use. Schools can treat students who are problem users with sensitivity and compassion, by referring them to appropriate counseling and treatment, and by helping them stop using and remain substance free. Schools can begin teaching students, from a very young age, the dangers of exposure to second-hand smoke and of riding with an adult or peer who is under the influence of psychoactive substances. Older children can also be taught a repertoire of behaviors to successfully avoid situations where they may be invited to ride with a driver who has been drinking. In countries with a relatively low drinking age or where the drinking age is not adequately or consistently enforced, students can be taught to drink in moderation and to take conscious steps, including periodic snacking and hydration, to mitigate the effects of alcohol on their body; these are sometimes called "harm reduction" or "protective behavioral" strategies. But schools that elect to teach these strategies should take great care to send the message that underage drinking is neither legal, safe, nor normative.

Theories of Individual Behavior Change

Changing behavior, particularly behaviors that are associated with health outcomes, has received a great deal of attention since the 1940s. These theories have been effectively incorporated into substance-use prevention programs since the late 1970s. The particular utility of behavior change theories in regard to school-based substance-use prevention interventions is that they address, in a systematic fashion, the question of how students make decisions about behaviors that affect their health, and provide a guide, or roadmap, as to how to support positive decisions and how to change bad ones.

Theories of behavior change seek to predict human behavior from a certain set of potentially measurable factors related to individuals or groups and their social and physical environments. They provide a guide as to how best to reinforce decisions that lead to positive behaviors. They also suggest points at which efforts to change behavior may be successful.

The most often cited theory of behavior change noted in prevention is the theory of planned behavior, developed in the 1970s by Ajzen and Fishbein (1972, 2008). In general this theory states that behavioral beliefs about the consequences of a behavior are influenced by both individuals' values and normative beliefs about what others think about the behavior, and what the individuals' motivations are regarding the behavior. These factors affect the individual's intent to engage in a behavior. The degree to which individuals will follow through with their intention is driven by whether they feel they can perform the behavior and whether there are environmental or other constraints or enhancers that affect their performance of the behavior. The model specifies the factors that affect a person's intentions to perform a behavior, including attitudes, subjective norms, and perceived behavioral control. The interplay of these three preliminary causal components is theorized to affect an individual's intention to perform the behavior and then, if the individual has the skills and resources to engage in the behavior, the intention is realized, and the behavior occurs. The theory suggests that attitudes alone are not sufficient to impel an action. Subjective norms and perceived behavioral control also play a key role in one's intention to behavior.

Reconceptualization of Risk and Protection

In 1992 two significant works were published on the determinants of substance use that had a major impact on planning for and developing prevention programming. The first was a publication by Hawkins, Catalano, and Miller (1992) that summarized the findings to date of longitudinal studies that had followed adolescents over time to determine the correlates of initiating substance use. The second was a monograph published by the National Institute on Drug Abuse that was edited by Glantz & Pickens (1992) and that highlighted factors that were associated with the progression from substance use to abuse and dependence.

The emergence of the "eco-biodevelopmental" framework for explaining human behavior in the early years of the twenty-first century (Fishbein et al., 2016; Shonkoff, 2010) has prompted a reconceptualization of prevention that builds on and more fully transforms the concepts of risk and protection to those of vulnerability and resilience (Sloboda, Glantz, & Tarter, 2012). These new frameworks focus more on the underlying mechanisms of behaviors such as substance use and serve to elucidate their etiology showing that we develop attitudes, beliefs, and behaviors in response to our interface with micro- and macro-level environments. Key micro-level environments include individuals' family and school, and macro-level environments include their physical, social, and economic settings. Merging this framework with the theoretical behavioral models and what we know about learning processes suggests an approach to prevention that increases the abilities of primary socialization agents including parents, teachers, peers, and employers, and the contexts or settings in which they function, to have positive influences on those for whom they are responsible—children, students, workers, and communities (Hyde et al., 2011; Hyde et al., 2013; Sloboda, 2015; Trentacosta, Hyde, Shaw, & Cheong, 2009).

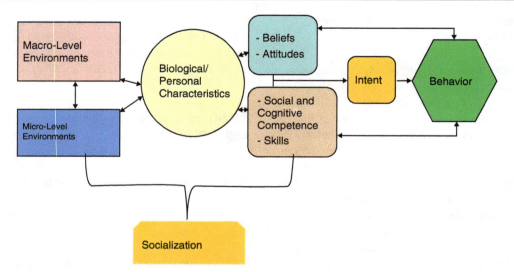

The model suggests that genetic and other biological factors play a significant role in the achievement of developmental benchmarks, that is, the goal of each stage of development, from infancy to early adulthood. Development in children includes intellectual ability; language development; cognitive, emotional, and psychological functioning; and attainment of social competency skills. The extent to which developmental benchmarks are met determines our level of vulnerability to influences from our environment. Such vulnerability can vary within an individual and across developmental periods. Children who don't reach early developmental benchmarks are most likely the most vulnerable, as failure to achieve these early benchmarks will increase their difficulty in reaching later ones. Influences from the micro- and/or macro-level environmental can both decrease and enhance this vulnerability. It is the combination of these environmental influences and personal characteristics of individuals that shapes beliefs, attitudes, and behavior. As these environmental experiences heightened stress or adversity, the risk for substance use is increased. It is important to emphasize that the two levels of influence—the macro- and micro-level—do not operate independently to influence behavior, but they also affect one another. For instance, the stability of a family that experiences financial stress will be threatened, thus challenging parenting behaviors. These processes of multidirectional influences suggest that prevention interventions should serve as socialization agents in two ways. First, prevention interventions should operate to help family and school staff to improve their interactions with each other and with the children and adolescents for whom they are responsible. Second, they should intervene directly with children, adolescents, and adults with prevention messages through the media, substance-use prevention school curricula, and enforcement of appropriate policies, regulations, and laws.

School Prevention Objectives

As supported by cognitive theories, effective substance-use prevention strategies are designed to address children's different development stages. For example, for children in middle childhood, substance-use prevention strategies should focus on the delivery of simple, straightforward instructions—e.g., doctors give you medicine when you are sick to make you well; medicine can be bad for you if you take it without a doctor telling you to; and giving medicine to others is dangerous, even if they ask for it. In the early middle child years, teachers can implement strategies designed to reward prosocial behavior and sanction impulsive or otherwise inappropriate behaviors. In so doing, teachers can help children succeed as students.

Early adolescents are sufficiently sophisticated to understand the importance of developing positive values and attitudes that are contrary to substance use, and on which they can base their decisions as to whether to use. Students also can learn their school's policies concerning both legal and illegal substances, and the consequences of infractions.

For later adolescence, students should be able to use their values, decision-making skills, and various life skills—particularly their assertiveness or "resistance" skills—in situations where substances are being used or where they may be invited to use these substances. They should also learn society's penalties for the use of substances that are unlawful for adolescents and adults. Finally, they can be taught a variety of strategies to reduce the adverse consequences of, or harms associated with, substance use.

Clearly evidence-based prevention interventions must be carefully matched to the developmental stage of the participating children to be effective. Prevention science is thus built on child development theory and practice, and incorporates our understanding of how best to reach children at each stage of their development.

Research on Effective School-Based Prevention

There are over two decades of research and evaluation in schools that demonstrate which interventions are supported by evidence that they work. The results of these studies have helped to identify the key components of effective substance-use prevention programs, and how these programs should be delivered if they are to be effective. The studies have also shown for what specific populations of children and youth, and at what ages, these interventions are most effective.

Evidence-Based Substance-Use Prevention Curricula: Standards for Selection

Until 2013, when the United Nations Office on Drugs and Crime (UNODC) developed the International Standards on Drug Use Prevention, no one body had reviewed and summarized research findings from the prevention science literature. The Standards established rigorous criteria for assessing research evidence of effectiveness and summarized the scientific evidence, describing effective interventions and policies and their characteristics by various targeted age groups and settings (discussed later). The Standards used a rating system based on the rigor of the research methods applied in the evaluation process from "excellent," "very good," and "good" ratings for effectiveness that are supported by meta-analyses and systematic reviews, multiple randomized controlled trials, and quasi-experimental methods, primarily comprising time series analyses. Ratings of "good" and "adequate" were used for single randomized control trials or evaluations conducted by means of acceptable methodologies.

The International Standards document does not advocate for a particular program but rather presents the content, structure, and delivery strategy used in the evaluated interventions. The findings are presented within development age groups (infancy and early childhood, middle childhood, early adolescence, and late adolescence and adulthood) and developmental age groups within settings in which the interventions are delivered (family, school, workplace, community, and the health sector). What is presented below is an enhanced summary of the findings from the Standards document.

Evidence-Based Prevention Interventions for Schools

There are three aspects of the school environment that lend themselves specifically to substance-use prevention intervention: (1) *school culture*, that is, norms, beliefs, and expectancies, and *school bonding*, that is, connecting the individual to the school experience and community; (2) *school policy* or *social control*, the most common approach establishing disciplinary policies and procedures; and (3) classroom *curricula* or manualized programs. These are discussed below.

School Culture and School Bonding

Earlier we discussed the etiology model that describes the processes associated with the initiation of substance use as an individual–environmental interaction (Fishbein et al., 2016; Sloboda, 2015; Tarter et al., 1999). Effective programs that impact the macro-school environment to make it more attractive to students help them develop more prosocial attitudes and affiliations and to engage in more prosocial behaviors. These programs focus on increasing self-efficacy and school bonding while at the same time they decrease the likelihood that students will use alcohol, tobacco, or other psychoactive substances (Campello, Sloboda, Heikkil, & Brotherhood, 2014). The targets for effective strategies to create a positive normative environment for children include the following (Fletcher, 2015; Greenberg et al. 2003):

- Ensuring that the school environment is inclusive and emotionally and physically safe.
- Promoting positive relationships between students, teachers, and other school staff in which there is mutual respect, caring, and a shared sense of belonging and commitment to the school experience.
- Setting and supporting health norms, behaviors, and relationships including creating nonsubstance-using settings.

In general, the content of these approaches includes strategies to respond to and correct inappropriate behavior and those that acknowledge and reward appropriate behavior. Training of school staff to implement these programs is required to assure fidelity, consistency, and sustainability.

School Bonding

Although programs to impact school culture also increase school bonding, there are a number of programs that focus primarily on school bonding *per se* such as skills, opportunities and recognition (SOAR) program (Hawkins, Catalano, Kosterman, Abbott, & Hill, 1999), the Incredible Years (Webster-Stratton, Reid, & Hammond, 2001), and Early Risers Skills for Success (August, Lee, Bloomquist, Realmuto, & Hektner, 2003). Common elements or principles of school bonding programs include the following:

- Focusing on the early years, that is, preschool to middle school.
- Enhancing competency in reading and math.
- Providing interpersonal skills to enable students to relate positively with peers and adults.
- Involving parents in communication and parenting skills and in school activities.

As an example, the SOAR program developed at the University of Washington by the Social Development Research Group emphasizes positive personal development and academic success. SOAR provides opportunities for the active involvement of elementary school-aged children in their families and in school with consistent positive recognition for their positive attitudes and behavior. The program includes components for students, teachers, and parents. The student component is designed to develop acceptable social skills both in school and at home. The teacher component focuses on improving classroom management and instruction methods to increase academic skills and behavior. The parent component emphasizes developmentally appropriate parenting skills. The investigators found that students in the full implementation program improved their attachment to school and their academic performance, and had lower rates of heavy drinking and violent behavior (Hawkins et al., 1999).

Classroom Climate

While these interventions address school climate and culture, other interventions address classroom climate. The most widely recognized intervention of this type is the Good Behavior Game (GBG). The purpose of this classroom management program, which targets children in elementary and early middle school, is to socialize them into their roles as students. In particular, the program seeks to reduce aggressive or otherwise disruptive classroom behavior by establishing a set of rules of appropriate conduct, teaching students how to behave and work together effectively as members of a team, and how to monitor their own as well as their team's behavior. The teacher also specifies incentives for positive behavior for both the individual student and the team as a whole. Evaluations have demonstrated that the program reduces substance use and violence and enhances students' mental health (Kellam et al., 2014).

GBG is a classroom environment improvement program. Typically classroom environment improvement programs are delivered in early years of school when children are around 6–9 years old. They include strategies to respond to and correct inappropriate behavior in the classroom setting, and to acknowledge and reward appropriate behavior.

Like all evidence-based programs that are delivered in classroom settings, GBG actively engages students. Teachers are required to receive training in the delivery of GBG to ensure that it is administered correctly. In particular, the program seeks to reduce aggressive or otherwise disruptive classroom behavior by establishing a set of rules of appropriate conduct, teaching students how to behave and work together effectively as members of a team, and showing students how to monitor their own as well as their team's behavior. The teacher also specifies incentives for positive behavior for both the individual student and the team as a whole. Evaluations have demonstrated that the program reduces substance use and violence, and enhances students' mental health.

School Policies

Another approach to addressing the school and classroom environment is through the enforcement of reasonable and appropriate school policies. School policies related to substance use are an integral and vital part of the school's comprehensive substance-use prevention programming (Adams, Jason, Pokorny, & Hunt, 2009; Evans-Whipp et al., 2004; Evans-Whipp, Plenty, Catalano, Herrenkohl, & Toumbourou, 2013; Galanti, Coppo, Jonsson, Bremberg, & Faggiano, 2013). Unfortunately, they are all too often developed in a casual and unsystematic manner, buried in the school's manual of policies, and then inconsistently or arbitrarily enforced. Policies are particularly important for at last three reasons. First, those that restrict the use of substances help establish social norms that substance use will not be tolerated. If students see no smoking or drinking whatsoever on school grounds or at school-sponsored events, their exposure to potential role models who are exhibiting the behavior will decrease. As such, their normative beliefs that substance use is inappropriate should strengthen. Second, to reference the model of the determinants of behavior yet again, policies can also be conceptualized as acting like environmental constraints, insofar as they reduce access to substances. Third, policies can also act as a deterrent to substance use and possession.

The structure of substance use school policies often includes a statement of purpose, which might include language referencing the need to establish and maintain a safe, healthy, and substance use-free environment to support the healthy development of all students and to ensure that they achieve their academic potential. Many policies also commit the school to implementing programs and policies that represent known principles of effectiveness, and, where possible, are supported by evidence. One of the most important objectives in school policy is to ensure that the policy is communicated to everyone in the school community who would be affected, including students, staff, and visitors. Policies should specify the range and types of substances they include and cover substance use and possession not only at school but also at school-sponsored events. Policies should also make clear what types of substance-related incidents will be sanctioned—for example, the possession or sale of various types of substances, or a reasonable suspicion that a student has come to school impaired. Policies should also be clear about whom, and at what point in the process, families and law enforcement authorities will be notified concerning an event related to substance use, possession, and sales. These policies should also specify clear consequences for violations by students that will be consistently enforced. Policies should be readily available to, and understood by, all members of the school community. These policies should not be punitive in nature but instead have the goal of keeping students who use substances in school.

In that regard, students using substances should be given the opportunity to stop doing so in a supportive environment in which their behaviors—including timely attendance, completion of homework assignments, and academic performance—are closely monitored. Many schools have established teams of faculty and staff that meet regularly with these students to review their progress. Students with substance-use problems should also be referred for counseling or substance-use treatment, as appropriate. It is also critical that all members of the school community, including students and their families, be aware of the school's substance-use policies, including how the school will respond to violations. A school's call or note to a student's parents, informing them that their son or daughter is involved with substances, can be particularly challenging if there is any possibility that the parents' response may be punitive.

Prevention Curricula

Probably the most frequently occurring prevention approach is the use of a classroom curriculum that focuses on the prevention of substance use. As such, many types of classroom curricula have been developed and evaluated over the past 25 years. Several researchers have conducted meta-analyses of the data from these evaluations (Durlak, Weissberg, Dymnicki, Taylor, & Schellinger, 2011; Faggiano, Minozzi, Versino, & Buscemi, 2014; Gottfredson & Wilson, 2003; Lemstra et al., 2010; Porath-Waller, Beasley, & Beimess, 2010; Tobler, 1986, 1992; Tobler, Lessard, Marshall, Ochshorn, & Roona, 1999) while others have conducted program content analyses (Dusenbury & Falco, 1995; Sloboda & David, 1997; United Nations Office on Drugs and Crime, 2013/2015) to determine common elements of effective interventions. There have been consistent findings across all of these approaches.

Common elements of effective school-based curriculum include the following:

- Dispelling exaggerated misconceptions regarding the normative nature and expectancies of substance use (i.e., the prevalence and positive/negative effects of use).
- Affecting perceptions of risks associated with substance use for children and adolescents (i.e., emphasizing the effects students will experience now not when they are adults).
- Providing and practicing what are called life skills that include making good decisions, especially in regard to initiating or continuing substance use; communicating these decisions in an effective, non-alienating manner; and resistance skills to refuse the use of tobacco, alcohol, and illicit drugs.
- Providing interventions and boosters over multiple years into middle and high school, when students are most at risk.

Most available evidence-based school substance-use prevention curricula are considered universal as they target general populations that include students at different levels of risk for initiating the use of alcohol, tobacco, or other psychoactive substances. There are a number of indicated programs that target students who are considered at higher risk to initiate the use of these substances because they are not doing well in school and are experiencing high numbers of absences, suspensions, or expulsions. There are few that could be considered selective programs, that is, that address students who may have initiated low levels of substance use or are expressing other problem behaviors.

There are several examples of effective universal curricula available. These include Life Skills Training (LST) (Botvin, Baker, Dusenbury, Tortu, & Botvin, 1995) and Project Toward No Drug Abuse (Project TND) (Sussman, Dent, Stacy, & Craig, 1998). LST, which was developed at Cornell University by Botvin and his group, has been one of the most cited effective universal curricula in the United States. LST is a program that enhances key competencies of the participants. It consists of a 24-session elementary school program delivered over 3 years (third or fourth to sixth grades) and/or a 30-session middle school also to be delivered over 3 years (sixth or seventh to eighth grades). LST has been evaluated with a number of diverse populations with consistently good results.

Another curriculum that we will describe is Project TND. The purpose of this curriculum is to teach a number of skills, including self-control, decision-making, and substance-use resistance, and to strengthen motivations not to use substances, which is another way of saying to increase anti-substance-use attitudes. Project TND, which uses interactive methods, is taught in 12 weekly sessions of about 40 minutes each, and is thus designed to fit comfortably within a traditional 45–50-minute class period. While it has been tested on students from early adolescence through young adulthood, it is designed primarily for universal and selective populations of adolescents in school settings. We are paying particular attention to this curriculum because it is one of relatively few that are available for adolescent populations. Like all evidence-based substance-use prevention curricula, LST and TND are manualized and require training by those implementing them.

Despite the availability of evidence-based and effective substance-use interventions and policies that can be integrated into schools, their implementation and delivery have been disappointing (Hallfors, Sporer, Pankratz, & Godette, 2000; Hanley et al., 2010; Ringwalt et al., 2008; Ringwalt, Ennett, Vincus, Rohrbach, & Simons-Rudolph, 2004). Some of these barriers relate to the characteristics of the schools and potential implementers but also to the characteristics of the interventions (Payne, Gottfredson, & Gottfredson, 2006; Powers, Bowen, & Bowen, 2010; Sloboda, Dusenbury, & Petras, 2014).

What Doesn't Work in Prevention

Three decades of evaluations of school-based substance-use prevention curricula have also taught us a great deal about what does not work. This is almost as helpful as finding out what works, because many schools have wasted a lot of time and resources on prevention programs and strategies that have gathered no or very scant evidence of effectiveness, and some program evaluations have found results that are exactly the opposite of those that were expected.

Lecturing and "Knowledge Only"

Lecturing does not work and teaching knowledge about substance use alone will not directly change behavior. Teachers need to be a "guide on the side, not a sage on the stage." Also ineffective are unstructured class discussions, in which it is easy for the teacher to lose control of the class (as well as the amount of time allotted for a particular discussion). Also generally considered ineffective are efforts to increase students' knowledge by providing facts concerning specific substances, such as amphetamines (speed) or crack cocaine. For example, a well-meaning school staff might hold up a poster that displays pills that represent various types of controlled substances, and then describe their effects. Such efforts may merely serve to make students more intelligent consumers of prescription drugs. For that reason, some prevention curricula barely mention specific substances at all, although that may be difficult in a school with an epidemic of a particularly popular substance, where the school's administration may be eager to include one or more lessons that pertain specifically to it.

Peer-led Groups, Posters/Pamphlets

Several other strategies have shown little evidence of effectiveness. For a time schools were excited about the notion of using students instead of staff to teach substance-use prevention curricula. The notion for this approach was that younger students would relate and listen more attentively to their older peers than to adults. But studies as to which teaching method is better have proven to be inconclusive. Also found to be ineffective are posters and pamphlets that were developed without using evidence-based media strategies. These typically seek to increase knowledge, but may or may not be read or properly understood.

Ex-Substance Users, Self-Esteem

Also ineffective as a substance-use prevention strategy is the use of ex-substance users, or indeed any motivational speakers, to provide testimonials or other types of speeches about substance use. While one-time events of this nature may be particularly popular with schools, insofar as they are cheap, easy, and popular and do not require much class time, these individuals simply lack credibility with increasingly sophisticated student audience. If they talk about the horrible consequences of substance use, students will discount what they say, because most students know peers who take substances without any apparent bad effects. Besides, young people generally believe that they can "handle" any substances they take. At worst, the testimonials of former or recovering substance users can inadvertently promote substance use by glamorizing the dangers that the speaker faced when still a user (or, perhaps, a dealer). Or the students may think "you used drugs, went through treated, and you are okay now. So what's the problem?"

Also lacking evidence of effectiveness are two approaches that were very popular in the United States for a time: to build students' self-esteem and drug testing. Self-esteem strategies have generally failed for at least two reasons: it is very difficult to change self-esteem within the context of a curriculum, and the relationship between self-esteem and substance use is weak—substance-using students, indeed, may have a very positive sense of themselves. While there is no harm in seeking to increase students' self-esteem, it should be part of a much more comprehensive set of objectives (Schroeder, Laflin, & Weis, 1993).

Random Drug Testing

Another ineffective popular strategy is random drug testing (Goldberg et al., 2007; James-Burdumy, Goesling, Deke, & Einspruch, 2010; Terry-McElrath, O'Malley, & Johnston, 2013). Despite its considerable cost, many people supported the widespread dissemination of drug testing because of its potential as a deterrent. The reason for the support of this approach was that if students knew they were likely to be tested for the presence of a variety of substances, they would be less likely to use and, indeed, would have a credible excuse not to use if invited to do so by peers. But controlled evaluations of the effects of drug testing have generally failed to yield anticipated—perhaps because students knew that the likelihood that they might be tested in any given week was relatively low. This is not to say that drug testing is never useful—it certainly can be quite effective as an intervention but not a prevention tool. This is particularly relevant within the context of students who are being subjected to testing for cause—that is, when they have been suspected of using (or have previously been identified as users) and are being monitored to ensure that they are remaining drug free. But from the perspective of primary prevention, drug testing has not been found to be effective particularly in relationship to its costs and the burdens associated with administration. These include not only the cost of the test itself but also monitoring students while they provide samples, and then establishing what is called a "chain of custody" to ensure that samples are not mislabeled or lost (Yamaguchi et al., 2003).

Media-Based "Scare Tactics," and One-Time Events

Our final set of ineffective strategies are scare tactics and one-time school events that address substance use and its consequences. Scare tactics to deter high-risk behaviors have been found to be ineffective through numerous studies. However, this approach had been used for the prevention of substance use and still are. We found that years ago media ads targeting youth presented exaggerated consequences of using various types of drugs, which contradicted young peoples' own experiences and that of their peers. As a result, these overblown messages lost all credibility.

Our final strategy to avoid constitutes any stand-alone, single-event activity that takes the place of activities that are ongoing, comprehensive, and developmentally appropriate. These include motivational speeches, fairs, and speech contests, and the use of drug-detecting dogs.

Selecting and Adapting the Right Substance-Use Prevention Curriculum for Your School

Administrators should first recognize that substance use is not the sole problem of the school. There are two types of substance-use challenges for schools: substance use in the schools and substance use by students and staff. School administrators sometimes think that if substances are not used in the schools they are really a community and not a school problem. However, as noted in the first section of the chapter, the effects of psychoactive substance use on the developing brain, regardless of whether the substances are used outside or inside the school, are detrimental to making good decisions and to learning. Students who use these substances are at higher risk of poor academic performance and dropping out (Gasper, 2011; Townsend, Flisher, & King, 2007). But schools don't have to address its substance-use problems alone. Findings from prevention research studies show that school-based programming is more effective when supported by community and/or family components such as PROSPER (Crowley, Greenberg, Feinberg, Spoth, & Redmond, 2012; Spoth et al., 2013) or Communities That Care (Hawkins, Oesterle, Brown, Abbott, & Catalano, 2014), which have demonstrated the sustained effectiveness of prevention programming by building community prevention implementation systems that support multiple community-based interventions, including those in schools.

School Readiness

One place to begin with school-based prevention interventions and policies is by assessing school readiness to adopt and implement substance-use prevention programs and strategies. Here are some key questions to consider. Is there administrative support for making room for substance-use prevention programming during the school day? Is there human capital with the requisite skills available to implement the programs? What about resources to pay for materials related to programming, teacher training, substitute teachers to cover classrooms during the training, and follow-up technical assistance? Is there high-quality training and technical assistance available to guide school personnel in implementing prevention programs successfully, and in responding to challenges as they arise? All of these factors should be assessed prior to selecting a prevention approach.

It is important that the administration of the school, and also the school district or regional authority, provides the support and leadership necessary for adopting, implementing, and sustaining a prevention program. But many other factors should also be in place. The school should have an articulated vision as to what kind of environment it seeks to have in order to support the educational and social development of the students entrusted to its care. This vision should be accompanied by related goals, one of which should ensure that the school environment is free of alcohol, tobacco, and other substances. Plans need to be in place as to who will lead and be responsible for the effort to adopt and implement prevention policies and programs. The plan should include an assessment of the ability of the school to implement the program. What teachers or staff are required to do it? Do they have sufficient education and training? Are they available? How much time will the program require, and of whom? Finally, an assessment should be made of the organizational support available for the program.

Before initiating a program of evidence-based prevention interventions and policies, there are a number of other issues that need to be considered. These include the timing of the interventions, delivery by peers and/or adults, use of interactive teaching approaches, targeting multiple substances, focusing on minority groups, durability and sustainability of interventions, and implementation fidelity (Botvin & Griffin, 2003).

This last item is of particular importance and a challenge to the effective implementation of evidence-based prevention in schools and in other settings (Durlak & Dupre, 2008; Fagan & Mihalic, 2003; Mihalic, Fagan, & Argamaso, 2008; Ringwalt, Vincus, Hanley, Ennett, Bowling, & Haws 2010; Ringwalt, Pankratz, Jackson-Newsom, Gottfredson, Hansen, Giles, & Dusenbury 2010; Rohrbach, Ringwalt, Ennett, & Vincus, 2005). What is meant by the term "implementation fidelity" is the extent to which the curriculum content, structure, and delivery style are consistent with those of the original tested prevention intervention, as specified in the teachers' curriculum guide or manual. This has particular relevance to school-based prevention curricula. Often, when an evidence-based curriculum is taken from a research setting to the "real world," changes are made to meet the needs of the school, the targeted participants, or the instructor. It is therefore very important to have a thorough understanding of the curriculum design and key elements of the program. Having training in the curriculum by experts helps instructors understand the theoretical foundation of the curriculum and program design. The establishment of a monitoring system to assess program implementation and provide ongoing technical assistance when fidelity falters will enhance the likelihood of an effective implementation. However, the reality of integrating these interventions in a variety of cultural and language settings may require tailoring or adapting an intervention to increase the likelihood that the participants will view the program as relevant and that the desired outcomes will be achieved. Tailoring that includes addressing cultural beliefs, values, language, and visual images does not mean altering the basic content or delivery strategies of the intervention (Barrera & Catro, 2006; Castro, Barrera, & Martinez, 2004). The Substance Abuse and Mental Health Services Administration (2017) has some pointers about adapting a program for a new community:

- Change capacity before changing the program. It may be easier to change the program, but improving local capacity to deliver it as it is designed is a safer choice.
- Consult with the program developer to determine what experience and/or advice he or she has about adapting the program to a particular setting or circumstance.
- There is a greater likelihood of effectiveness when a program retains all the core component(s) of the original intervention.
- There is a greater likelihood of success if an adaptation does not violate an established evidence-based prevention principle.

Finally, school administrators should be mindful of the fact that the field of psychoactive substance-use prevention is relatively new. The knowledge that is accumulating from prevention researchers changes as intervention strategies and statistical methodologies become more sophisticated. In addition, the research that serves to guide prevention intervention development, that is, epidemiology and behavioral science, is also evolving. Finally, our children's cultural worlds and influences are ever changing. Programs that may be effective for adolescents today may not be so for their younger siblings when they enter their teen years. Such changes suggest constant attention to updating prevention messages and strategies.

References

Adams, M. L., Jason, L. A., Pokorny, S., & Hunt, Y. (2009). The relationship between school policies and youth tobacco use. *Journal of School Health, 79*, 17–23.

Ajzen, I., & Fishbein, M. (1972). Attitudes and normative beliefs as factors influencing behavioral intentions. *Journal of Personality and Social Psychology, 21*, 1–9.

Ajzen, I., & Fishbein, M. (2008). Attitudinal and normative variables as predictors of specific behaviors. In R. H. Fazio & R. E. Petty (Eds.), *Attitudes: Their structure, function, and consequences* (pp. 425–443). New York, NY: Psychology Press.

August, G. J., Lee, S. S., Bloomquist, M. L., Realmuto, G. M., & Hektner, J. M. (2003). Dissemination of an evidence-based prevention innovation for aggressive children living in culturally diverse, urban neighborhoods: The early risers effectiveness study. *Prevention Science, 4*, 271–286.

Barrera, M., & Catro, F. (2006). A heuristic framework for the cultural adaptation of interventions. *Clinical Psychology Scientific Practice, 13*, 311–316.

Battistich, V., Schaps, E., Watson, M., Solomon, D., & Lewis, C. (2000). Effects of the child development project on students' drug use and other problem behaviors. *The Journal of Primary Prevention, 21*, 75–99.

Bosworth, K., & Sloboda, Z. (2015). Prevention science 1970-present. In K. Bosworth (Ed.), *Prevention science in school settings: Complex relationships and processes* (pp. 125–149). New York, NY: Springer.

Botvin, G. J., Baker, E., Dusenbury, L., Tortu, S., & Botvin, E. M. (1995). Long-term follow-up results of a randomized drug abuse prevention trial in a white middle-class population. *Journal of the American Medical Association, 273*, 1106–1112.

Botvin, G. J. & Griffin, K. W. (2003). Drug abuse prevention curricula in schools. In Sloboda, Z. & Bukoski, W.J. (Eds.). Handbook of Drug Abuse Prevention: Theory, Science, and Practice. New York: Kluwer Academic/Plenum Publishers; pp. 45–74.

Campello, G., Sloboda, Z., Heikkil, H., & Brotherhood, A. (2014). International standards on drug use prevention: The future of drug use prevention worldwide. *International Journal of Prevention and Treatment of Substance Use Disorders, 1*, 6–27.

Castro, F. G., Barrera, M., Jr., & Martinez, C. R., Jr. (2004). The cultural adaptation of prevention interventions: Resolving tensions between fidelity and fit. *Prevention Science, 5*, 41–45.

Crowley, D. M., Greenberg, M. T., Feinberg, M. E., Spoth, R. L., & Redmond, C. R. (2012). The effect of the PROSPER partnership model on cultivating local stakeholders' knowledge of evidence-based programs: A five-year longitudinal study of 28 communities. *Prevention Science, 13*, 96–105.

Durlak, J. A., & Dupre, E. P. (2008). Implementation matters: A review of research on the influence of implementation on program outcomes and the factors affecting implementation. *American Journal of Community Psychology, 41*, 327–350.

Durlak, J. A., Weissberg, R. P., Dymnicki, A. B., Taylor, R. D., & Schellinger, K. B. (2011). The impact of enhancing students' social and emotional learning: A meta-analysis of school-based universal interventions. *Child Development, 82*, 405–432.

Dusenbury, L., & Falco, M. (1995). Eleven components of effective drug abuse prevention curricula. *Journal of School Health, 65*, 420–425.

Dwyer, J. B., McQuown, S. C., & Leslie, F. M. (2009). The dynamic effects of nicotine on the developing brain. *Pharmacology & Therapeutics, 122*(2), 125–139.

Evans-Whipp, T., Beyers, J. M., Lloyd, S., Lafazia, A. N., Toumbourou, J. W., Arthur, M. W., & Catalano, R. F. (2004). A review of school drug policies and their impact on youth substance use. *Health Promotion International, 19*, 227–234.

Evans-Whipp, T. J., Plenty, S. M., Catalano, R. F., Herrenkohl, T. I., & Toumbourou, J. W. (2013). The impact of school alcohol policy on student drinking. *Health Education Research, 28*, 651–662.

Fagan, A. A., & Mihalic, S. (2003). Strategies for enhancing the adoption of school-based prevention programs: Lessons learned from the blueprints for violence prevention replications of the life skills training program. *Journal of Community Psychology, 31*, 235–253.

Faggiano, F., Minozzi, S., Versino, E., & Buscemi, D. (2014). Universal school-based prevention for illicit drug use. *Cochrane Database of Systematic Reviews, 12*, CD003020. https://doi.org/10.1002/14651858.CD003020.pub3

Fishbein, D. H., Rose, E. J., Darcey, V., Belcher, A., & VanMeter, J. (2016). Neurodevelopmental precursors and consequences of substance use during adolescence: Promises and pitfalls of longitudinal neuroimaging strategies. *Frontiers in Human Neuroscience, 10*, 296. https://doi.org/10.3389/fnhum.2016.00296

Fletcher, A. (2015). School culture and classroom climate. In K. Bosworth (Ed.), *Prevention science in school settings: Complex relationships and processes* (pp. 273–286). New York, NY: Springer.

Galanti, M. R., Coppo, A., Jonsson, E., Bremberg, S., & Faggiano, F. (2013). Anti-tobacco policy in schools: Upcoming preventive strategy or prevention myth? A review of 31 studies. *Tobacco Control, 23*, 295–301.

Gasper, J. (2011). Revisiting the relationship between adolescent substance use and high school dropout. *Journal of substance Use Issues, 41*, 587.

Glantz, M. D. & Pickens, R. W. (1992). Vulnerability to drug abuse: Introduction and Overview. In Glantz, M. D. & Pickens, R. W. (Eds.). Vulnerability to Drug Abuse. Washington, D.C.: American Psychological Association Books; pp. 1–14.

Goldberg, L., Elliot, D. L., MacKinnon, D. P., Moe, E. L., Kuehl, K. S., Yoon, M., ... Williams, J. (2007). Outcomes of a prospective trial of student-athlete drug testing: The Student Athlete Testing Using Random Notification (SATURN) study. *Journal of Adolescent Health, 41*, 421–429.

Gottfredson, D. C., & Wilson, D. B. (2003). Characteristics of effective school-based substance abuse prevention. *Prevention Science, 4*, 27–38.

Gottfredson, G. D., & Gottfredson, D. C. (2001). What schools do to prevent problem behavior and promote safe environments. *Journal of Educational and Psychological Consultation, 12*, 313–344.

Greenberg, M. T., Weissberg, R. P., O'Brien, M. U., Zins, J. E., Fredericks, L., Resnik, H., & Elias, M. J. (2003). Enhancing school-based prevention and youth development through coordinated social, emotional, and academic learning. *American Psychologist, 58*, 466.

Hallfors, D., Sporer, A., Pankratz, M., & Godette, D. (2000). *Drug free schools survey: Report of results*. Chapel Hill, NC: School of Public Health, Department of Maternal and Child Health, University of North Carolina.

Hanley, S. M., Ringwalt, C., Ennett, S. T., Vincus, A. A., Bowling, J. M., Haws, S. W., & Rohrback, L. A. (2010). The prevalence of evidence-based substance use prevention curriculum in the national elementary schools. *Journal of Drug Education, 40*, 51–60.

Hanushek, E. A. & Woessmann, L. (2007). The role of education quality for economic growth. *World Bank Policy Research Working Paper No. 4122*. Retrieved SSRN, from https://ssrn.com/abstract=960379

Hawkins, J. D., Catalano, R. F., & Miller, J. Y. (1992). Risk and protective factors for alcohol and other drug problems in adolescence and early adulthood: Implications for substance abuse prevention. *Psychological Bulletin, 112,* 64–105.

Hawkins, J. D., Catalano, R. F., Kosterman, R., Abbott, R., & Hill, K. G. (1999). Preventing adolescent health-risk behaviors by strengthening protection during childhood. *Archives of Pediatric and Adolescent Medicine, 153,* 226–234.

Hawkins, J. D., Oesterle, S., Brown, E., Abbott, R., & Catalano, R. F. (2014). Youth problem behaviors 8 years after implementing the communities that care prevention system. A community randomized trial. *Journal of the American Medical Association Pediatrics, 168,* 122–129.

Hiller-Sturmhofel, S., & Swartzwelder, S. (2004/2005). Alcohol's effects on the adolescent brain. In *What can be learned from animal models.* Bethesda, MD, National Institute on Alcohol Abuse and Alcoholism. Retrieved from https://pubs.niaaa.nih.gov/publications/arh284/213-221.htm

Huang, Y. Y., Kandel, D. B., Kandel, E. R., & Levine, A. (2013). Nicotine primes the effect of cocaine on the induction of LTP in the amygdala. *Neuropharmacology, 74,* 126–134.

Hyde, L. W., Gorka, A., Manuck, S. B., & Hariri, A. R. (2011). Perceived social support moderates the link between threat-related amygdala reactivity and trait anxiety. *Neuropsychologia, 49,* 651–656.

Hyde, L. W., Shaw, D. S., Gardner, F., Cheong, J., Dishion, T. J., & Wilson, M. N. (2013). Dimensions of callousness in early childhood: Links to problem behavior and family intervention effectiveness. *Development and Psychopathology, 25,* 347–363.

James-Burdumy, S., Goesling, B., Deke, J., & Einspruch, E. (2010). *The effectiveness of mandatory-random student drug testing (NCEE 2010–4025).* Washington, DC: National Center for Education Evaluation and Regional Assistance, Institute of Education Sciences, U.S. Department of Education.

Kellam, S. G., Wang, W., Mackenzie, A. C. L., Brown, C. H., Ompad, D. C., Or, F., … Windham, A. (2014). The impact of the good behavior game, a universal classroom based preventive intervention in first and second grades, on high risk sexual behaviors and drug abuse and dependence disorders in young adulthood. *Prevention Science, 15*(Suppl 1), S6–S18.

Lemstra, M., Bennett, N., Nannapaneni, U., Neudorf, C., Warren, L., Kershaw, T., & Scott, C. (2010). A systematic review of school-based marijuana and alcohol prevention programs targeting adolescents aged 10-15. *Addiction Research & Theory, 18,* 84–96.

Mihalic, S. F., Fagan, A. A., & Argamaso, S. (2008). Implementing the lifeskills training drug prevention program: Factors related to implementation fidelity. *Implementation Science, 3,* 1–16.

Payne, A. A., Gottfredson, D. C., & Gottfredson, G. D. (2006). School predictors of the intensity of implementation of school-based prevention programs: Results from a national study. *Prevention Science, 7,* 225–237.

Porath-Waller, A., Beasley, E., & Beimess, D. J. (2010). A meta-analytic review of school-based prevention for cannabis use. *Health Education Behavior, 37,* 709–723.

Powers, J. D., Bowen, N. K., & Bowen, G. L. (2010). Evidence-based programs in school settings: Barriers and recent advances. *Journal of Evidence-Based Social Work, 7,* 313–331.

Ringwalt, C. L., Ennett, S. T., Vincus, A. A., Rohrbach, L. A., & Simons-Rudolph, A. (2004). Who's calling the shots? Decision-makers and the adoption of effective school-based substance use prevention curricula. *Journal of Drug Education, 34,* 19–31.

Ringwalt, C., Hanley, S. M., Vincus, A. A., Ennett, S. T., Rohrbach, L. A., & Bowling, J. M. (2008). The prevalence of effective substance use prevention curricula in the Nation's high schools. *Journal of Primary Prevention, 29,* 479–488.

Ringwalt, C., Vincus, A. A., Hanley, S. M., Ennett, S. T., Bowling, J. M., & Haws, S. W. (2010). The prevalence of evidence-based prevention curricula in U.S. middle schools in 2008. *Prevention Science, 12,* 63–69.

Ringwalt, C. L., Pankratz, M. M., Jackson-Newsom, J., Gottfredson, N. C., Hansen, W. B., Giles, S. M., & Dusenbury, L. (2010). Three-year trajectory of teachers' fidelity to a drug prevention curriculum. *Prevention Science, 11,* 67–76.

Rohrbach, L. A., & Dyal, S. R. (2015). Scaling up evidence-based prevention interventions. In K. Bosworth (Ed.), *Prevention science in school settings: Complex relationships and processes* (pp. 175–197). New York, NY: Springer.

Rohrbach, L. A., Ringwalt, C. L., Ennett, S. T., & Vincus, A. A. (2005). Factors associated with adoption of evidence-based substance use prevention curricula in U.S. school districts. *Health Education Research, 20,* 514–526.

Schaps, E., & Solomon, D. (2003). The role of the school's social environment in preventing student drug use. *The Journal of Primary Prevention, 23,* 299–328.

Schroeder, D. S., Laflin, M. T., & Weis, D. L. (1993). Is there a relationship between self-esteem and drug use? Methodological and statistical limitations of the research. *Journal of Drug Issues, 23,* 645–665.

Shonkoff, J. (2010). Building a new biodevelopmental framework to guide the future of early childhood policy. *Child Development, 81,* 357–367.

Sloboda, Z. (2015). Vulnerability and risks: Implications for understanding etiology and drug use prevention. In L. M. Scheier (Ed.), *Handbook of adolescent drug use prevention: research, intervention strategies, and practice* (pp. 85–100). Washington, DC: American Psychological Association.

Sloboda, Z., & David, S. L. (1997). *Preventing drug abuse among children and adolescents: A research-based guide* (NIH Publication No. 97–4212). Washington, DC: National Institute of Health.

Sloboda, Z., Dusenbury, L., & Petras, H. (2014). Implementation science and the effective delivery of evidence-based prevention. In Z. Sloboda & H. Petras (Eds.), *Advances in prevention science: Defining prevention science* (Vol. 1). New York: Springer.

Sloboda, Z., Glantz, M. D., & Tarter, R. E. (2012). Revisiting the concepts of risk and protective factors for understanding the etiology and development of substance use and substance use disorders: Implications for prevention. *Substance Use & Misuse, 47*, 944–962.

Spoth, R., Redmond, C., Shin, C., Greenberg, M., Feinberg, M., & Schainker, L. (2013). PROSPER community-university partnerships delivery system effects on substance misuse through 6½ years past baseline from a cluster randomized controlled intervention trial. *Preventive Medicine, 56*, 190–196.

Sussman, S., Dent, C. W., Stacy, A. W., & Craig, S. (1998). One-year outcomes of project towards no drug abuse. *Preventive Medicine, 27*, 632–642.

Tarter, R., Vanyukov, M., Giancola, P., Dawes, M., Blackson, T., Mezzich, A., & Clark, D. B. (1999). Etiology of early age onset substance use disorder: A maturational perspective. *Development and Psychopathology, 11*, 657–683.

Terry-McElrath, Y. M., O'Malley, P. M., & Johnston, L. D. (2013). Middle and high school drug testing and student illicit drug use: a national study 1998-2011. *The Journal of Adolescent Health, 52*, 707–715.

Tobler, N. S. (1986). Meta-analysis of 143 adolescent drug prevention programs: Quantitative outcome results of program participants compared to a control or comparison group. *Journal of Drug Issues, 16*, 537–567.

Tobler, N. S. (1992). Drug prevention programs can work: Research findings. *Journal of Addictive Diseases, 11*, 1–28.

Tobler, N. S., Lessard, T., Marshall, D., Ochshorn, P., & Roona, M. (1999). Effectiveness of school-based drug prevention programs for marijuana use. *School Psychology International, 20*, 105–137.

Townsend, L., Flisher, A. J., & King, G. (2007). A systematic review of the relationship between high school dropout and substance use. *Clinical Child and Family Psychology Review, 10*, 295–317.

Trentacosta, C. J., Hyde, L. W., Shaw, D. S., & Cheong, J. (2009). Adolescent dispositions for antisocial behavior in context: the roles of neighborhood dangerousness and parental knowledge. *Journal of Abnormal Psychology, 118*, 564–575.

United Nations Office on Drugs and Crime. (2013/2015). *International standards for drug use prevention.* Retrieved from https://www.unodc.org/unodc/en/prevention/prevention-standards.html

Webster-Stratton, C., Reid, J., & Hammond, M. (2001). Preventing conduct problems, promoting social competence: A parent and teacher training partnership in Head Start. *Journal of Clinical Child Psychology, 30*, 282–302.

Yamaguchi, R., Johnston, L. D., & O'Malley, P. M. (2003). Relationship between student illicit drug use and school drug-testing policies. *Journal of School Health, 73*, 159–164.

Substance Use Policy Interventions: Intended and Unintended Consequences

Mallie J. Paschall, Rebecca Yau, and Christopher L. Ringwalt

Policy approaches to preventing and reducing substance use focus on limiting the availability of substances and/or on direct deterrence of substance use. The purpose of such policies is to increase the resources necessary to obtain substances or the potential costs for possessing or consuming substances. Regulatory policies, practices, and enforcement may also affect community norms regarding the acceptability of substance use. The purpose of availability policies is to restrict or reduce the ease with which people can obtain substances or increase the economic costs of obtaining substances. The purpose of deterrence policies is to increase the personal consequences or anticipated consequences for purchasing, possessing, or consuming substances, and for supplying youth with substances. According to deterrence theory, the effectiveness of such penalties is affected by their severity, the probability of their imposition, and the swiftness with which they are imposed (e.g., Akers, 2012). Many policies have both availability and deterrence properties, which can affect individual decisions based on perceived costs of substance use, and normative beliefs regarding the acceptability of substance use (Paschall, Grube, & Kypri, 2009; Paschall, Lipperman-Kreda, & Grube, 2014; Paschall, Lipperman-Kreda, Grube, & Thomas, 2014; Paschall, Grube, & Biglan, 2017).

Introduction

The chapter considers the effects of policy interventions on overall levels of consumption and excessive substance use, but does not focus on consequences of substance use (e.g., injuries, chronic diseases, deaths) as these are considered more extensively in other chapters. Additionally, policy interventions related to prescription drug use are discussed separately at the end of this chapter, as policies related to prescription drugs differ from those of other substances we discuss in this chapter.

We examine six types of substance use policies in this chapter, including bans, age restrictions, price increases and taxes, days and hours of sale restrictions, government monopolies, and advertising restrictions. Bans prohibit the production, sale, and possession of a substance and may be specific to geographic areas (e.g., a country, region, city) and specific places such as public buildings and parks. Age restrictions make it illegal for people under a certain age to purchase, possess, or use a substance. Price increases and taxes can prevent or reduce substance use by increasing the total cost of a substance for the end user. Days and hours of sale restrictions limit the

M. J. Paschall (✉) · R. Yau
Prevention Research Center, Pacific Institute for Research and Evaluation, Berkeley, CA, USA
e-mail: paschall@prev.org; ryau@prev.org

C. L. Ringwalt
Injury Prevention Research Center, University of North Carolina, Chapel Hill, NC, USA
e-mail: cringwal@email.unc.edu

commercial availability of a substance during certain time periods. Government monopolies can limit the availability of a substance by constraining the number of outlets and hours of operation where a substance is sold and by regulating its price. Advertising restrictions limit the extent to which a substance is marketed through advertisements in various types of media, and may focus on advertising content that targets youth. The following sections provide a review of evidence related to the intended and intended consequences of these policies for each type of substance.

Alcohol

Bans. Alcohol use bans encompass the prohibition of all production and sale of alcohol, the proscription of alcohol use for religious reasons, and restrictions on alcohol use in certain places. Alcohol prohibition and proscription currently exist in Islamic countries such as Iran, Kuwait, Libya, Pakistan, Saudi Arabia, and Yemen, which have the lowest annual levels of alcohol use in the world per capita (≤0.2 L) (World Health Organization, 2016). Even without a national prohibition policy, proscription of alcohol use for religious reasons is associated with substantially lower levels of alcohol consumption in countries like Turkey and states like Utah (Centers for Disease Control and Prevention, 2017; World Health Organization, 2016). Prohibition of alcohol occurred in the United States (U.S.), Canada, Iceland, Finland, Norway, and Russia and USSR during the first quarter of the twentieth century in response to high levels of consumption and mortality due to liver cirrhosis and chronic alcoholism. In the U.S., prohibition through the Volstead Act significantly reduced both per capita consumption and liver cirrhosis mortality, effects that persisted years after the Act was repealed in 1933 (Blocker Jr, 2006).

Unintended consequences of prohibition included the illegal production, sale, and consumption of alcohol, and an increase in organized crime and violence related to these illegal activities. These consequences were due in part to inadequate enforcement of prohibition laws (Blocker Jr, 2006). Prohibition also changed drinking contexts from saloons, where men typically drank beer or liquor, to private homes, where a greater number of women began to consume alcohol (Blocker Jr, 2006). Thus the effects of total alcohol bans yielded mixed results.

Place-based alcohol use bans (e.g., no alcohol allowed at community or sporting events, substance-free residence halls on college campuses) may also constitute an effective strategy for reducing hazardous drinking, though research on this type of policy is very limited. Some studies have found lower rates of alcohol sales and service to underage youth and pseudo-intoxicated patrons at community and sporting events where more restrictive alcohol control policies were in place (Lenk et al., 2010; Toomey, Erickson, Patrek, Fletcher, & Wagenaar, 2005), suggesting that alcohol bans at such events could substantially reduce underage and excessive drinking. Epidemiological youth surveys (e.g., California Healthy Kids Survey, Oregon Healthy Teens Survey) consistently show lower levels of alcohol use on school campuses compared to overall drinking levels, suggesting that alcohol use bans at public and private schools may be effective.

A possible unintended consequence of place-based bans is the "displacement" of alcohol use to other locations, such as private settings or parties where hazardous drinking among youth is prevalent and may be more challenging to monitor (LaBrie, Hummer, Pedersen, Lac, & Chithambo, 2012; Paschall, Grube, Black, & Ringwalt, 2007; Paschall & Saltz, 2007; Pemberton, Colliver, Robbins, & Gfroerer, 2008).

Age Restrictions. Setting a minimum legal drinking age for alcohol purchase and consumption reduces alcohol use among young people by decreasing the overall prevalence of alcohol use and binge drinking, as well as the frequency of alcohol consumption (Babor, 2010; Carpenter & Dobkin, 2011; DeJong & Blanchette, 2014; Hingson & White, 2014; Wagenaar & Toomey, 2002). However, the effectiveness of setting a minimum legal drinking age depends on the level of enforcement of this policy (Babor, 2010).

One study found that an unintended consequence of increasing the minimum legal drinking age was an increase in prevalence of marijuana use among high school seniors (DiNardo &

Lemieux, 2001). Additionally, claims have been made that raising the minimum legal drinking age in the U.S. to 21 years old has increased risky drinking behaviors (e.g., binge drinking) especially for off-campus college gatherings (Amethyst Initiative, 2010). However, we found no empirical evidence supporting these claims.

Price Increases and Taxes. Increasing the price of alcoholic beverages has been found to be associated with reductions in overall alcohol consumption (Babor, 2010; Giesbrecht et al., 2016; Martineau, Tyner, Lorenc, Petticrew, & Lock, 2013; Xu & Chaloupka, 2011) and heavy drinking (Wagenaar, Salois, & Komro, 2009; Xu & Chaloupka, 2011). However, very limited research has been conducted to determine whether minimum pricing requirements (i.e., setting a minimum price that must be charged for alcoholic beverages) are associated with reductions in drinking behavior (Babor, 2010). One study conducted in Saskatchewan, Canada, indicates that increases in minimum price were associated with reduced alcoholic beverage consumption (Stockwell et al., 2012). However, two studies of bans on happy-hour promotions suggest that they had no effect on alcohol consumption, but these studies were methodologically weak (Babor, 2010).

One potential unintended consequence of bans on happy-hour promotions is that people may consume higher quantities of alcohol before going out to a bar or some other venue where alcohol is sold (sometimes called "pre-loading," "pre-gaming," or "pre-partying") in order to reduce the total cost of drinking (Wells, Graham, & Purcell, 2009). Although research indicates that pre-partying is common among young adults and college students (e.g., Paschall & Saltz, 2007; Reed et al., 2011), and difficulties related to obtaining alcohol at a bar or other venue are a motive for pre-partying (LaBrie et al., 2012), no studies have explicitly examined the effects of alcohol price increases on this behavior.

Days and Hours of Sale Restrictions. Regulations addressing the day of the week and the time of day of sales of a substance constitute a type of policy intended to reduce the use of the substance by limiting its commercial availability to certain time periods. Prior research shows that the success of using regulations to limit the days and times that alcohol is available for sale may depend on the community's location. Specifically, these regulations tend to be more successful in reducing consumption when implemented in communities surrounded by others with similar times of alcohol availability (Martineau et al., 2013). One review study investigated the effect of increasing the hours of sales on various alcohol-related harms, and found a corresponding increase in alcohol consumption (Hahn et al., 2010). Another review investigated the effects of changing days of sales on consumption and alcohol-related harms, and found that an increase in days of alcohol sales was associated with an increase in excessive alcohol use and negative consequences (Middleton et al., 2010). Conversely, a study in Brazil found that prohibiting the sale of alcohol at bars after 11 pm was significantly associated with reductions in both the local homicide rate and violent assaults against women (Duailibi et al., 2007).

Government Monopolies. Government control of alcohol sales affects both the commercial availability and price of alcohol. The overall evidence indicates that creating or maintaining government monopolies related to alcohol sales is an effective strategy for reducing alcohol use. The privatization (i.e., ending government monopolies) of alcohol sales has been associated with increased total or excessive alcohol consumption (Babor, 2010; Martineau et al., 2013), while the presence of government monopolies is associated with decreased total consumption (Martineau et al., 2013; Pacula, Kilmer, Wagenaar, Chaloupka, & Caulkins, 2014) and binge drinking (Babor, 2010).

As with other policies limiting commercial alcohol availability, restricting days and times of alcohol sales and government monopolies may have the unintended consequence of increasing consumption in private settings, where potentially hazardous drinking may occur. However, no research has been conducted to assess possible unintended consequences of these policies.

Advertising Restrictions. A review of 26 studies suggests that people who live in communities with a high density of alcohol outlets and alcohol advertising consume more alcohol, though these findings were not conclusive (Bryden, Roberts, McKee, & Petticrew, 2012). A review of 14 studies indicates that reducing alcohol advertising near schools can help to reduce alcohol use among youth (Knai, Petticrew, Durand, Eastmure, & Mays, 2015). The review also indicates that alcohol warning labels have little or no effect on alcohol use. The authors concluded that limiting alcohol availability, increasing alcohol prices, and enforcing alcohol policies have a much greater impact on alcohol consumption than advertising and marketing restrictions. A more recent review of 12 longitudinal studies shows that greater youth exposure to alcohol marketing is associated with initiation of alcohol use, binge drinking, and any drinking in the previous 30 days (Jernigan, Noel, Landon, Thornton, & Lobstein, 2017). There has been no research on the unintended consequences of alcohol advertising restrictions.

Tobacco

Bans. Smoke-free policies are a strategy frequently employed to prevent or reduce tobacco use. These policies exist in a variety of settings including public spaces, residences, and workplaces (Hoffman & Tan, 2015). The preponderance of evidence from studies in the U.S. and other countries indicates that smoking bans reduce both smoking prevalence and cigarette consumption (Hoffman & Tan, 2015).

While bans on sales of specific types of tobacco products are not frequently employed, they may be effective. Beginning November 2010, New York City banned the sales of all flavored tobacco products (excluding those that were menthol flavored). New York City Youth Risk Behavior Survey results indicated that among youth aged 13–17, following the ban, there were significantly lower odds of ever trying a flavored tobacco product and ever using any tobacco products compared with before the ban. However, the odds of current smoking before the ban and after the ban did not differ significantly (Farley & Johns, 2016).

We are unaware of any research on the unintended consequences of bans on tobacco use, although black markets for cigarettes and other tobacco products could be at least partly attributable to tobacco use bans.

Age Restrictions. Studies investigating the restriction of tobacco sales to youth have yielded mixed results (Brownson, Haire-Joshu, & Luke, 2006); any positive effect of sales restrictions on tobacco use may depend on the enforcement of (Hoffman & Tan, 2015) or compliance with these restrictions (Levy, Chaloupka, & Gitchell, 2004). However, one systematic review found that compliance with youth access laws was not associated with prevalence of teenage smoking (Fichtenberg & Glantz, 2002). There is no known research on the unintended consequences of age restriction policies on tobacco use.

Price Increases and Taxes. Increasing the price of tobacco has been found to be associated with reductions in the number of cigarettes smoked (Brownson et al., 2006) and smoking prevalence (Brownson et al., 2006; Hoffman & Tan, 2015), while increasing the number of people who quit smoking (Boyle, 2010; Hoffman & Tan, 2015).

An unintended consequence of taxation on tobacco use is that smokers may also change their habits to use cheaper products (e.g., generic brands, loose tobacco) to avoid the costs caused by increased taxes (Hawken, Kulick, & Prieger, 2013). When one specific type of tobacco product (e.g., cigarettes) is more heavily taxed than other products (e.g., cigars), increases in prevalence of use of the less heavily taxed products have been observed (Hawken et al., 2013). Increasing cigarette taxes can also contribute to tax avoidance by smuggling cigarettes from other countries, which creates black markets (Birkett, 2014; Stehr, 2005).

Days and Hours of Sale Restrictions. To the best of our knowledge, there has not been any research conducted on days or hours of tobacco sales regulations and tobacco use, even with research using tobacco sales as a proxy for tobacco use.

Government Monopolies. Though a relatively small number of jurisdictions have ever exercised a monopoly on certain types of tobacco products (e.g., cigarettes), prior studies investigating the former Soviet Union have found that privatization of tobacco manufacturing was associated with increases in smoking prevalence (Gilmore, Fooks, & McKee, 2011).

Advertising Restrictions. A large body of research indicates that tobacco marketing affects the initiation of tobacco use among youth and their progression to regular use (National Cancer Institute, 2008). Econometric studies also show an association between tobacco advertising and consumption (National Cancer Institute, 2008). Research also indicates that comprehensive tobacco advertising bans may reduce tobacco consumption, while partial bans have limited or no effect on consumption (National Cancer Institute, 2008; Saffer & Chaloupka, 2000; Stewart, 1993). Government mandated tobacco warning labels, especially pictorial labels, appear to increase smokers' awareness of smoking health risks and motivation to quit smoking (Fong, Hammond, & Hitchman, 2009; Hammond, 2011). We are not aware of any research on unintended consequences of tobacco advertising restrictions.

Marijuana

Bans. There is mixed evidence regarding whether or not lifting medical marijuana bans increases marijuana use. One study found that lifting bans on medical marijuana was not associated with increase in the use of marijuana use generally (Harper, Strumpf, & Kaufman, 2012). However, two other studies, which stratified results by age, found differences between states with and without medical marijuana laws. Among those aged 21 or older, there was an increase in past-month use of marijuana (Choi, 2014; Wen, Hockenberry, & Cummings, 2015) and marijuana abuse or dependence (Wen et al., 2015). Among those under 21, there were no increases in past-month marijuana use (Choi, 2014; Wen et al., 2015), abuse, or dependence (Wen et al., 2015). However, a study based on data from the National Survey on Drug Use and Health (NSDUH) found that medical marijuana legalization was associated with an increase in past-year marijuana use initiation among 12 to 20-year-olds, but not among respondents aged 21 or older (Wen et al., 2015). One explanation for these seemingly incongruent findings is that among youth, states that pass medical marijuana laws may already have a higher prevalence of marijuana use than those that do not have medical marijuana laws; the prevalence of youth marijuana use in states that had passed medical marijuana laws were not significantly different before and after the laws passed (Hasin et al., 2015).

Very limited evidence exists related to lifting bans on recreational marijuana use. One study based in Washington state attempted to determine whether the legalization of recreational marijuana use increased marijuana use prevalence, but data collection concluded before the laws were fully implemented (Mason et al., 2016). Another study using data from the U.S. Monitoring the Future surveys examined the association between legalization of recreational marijuana use and prevalence of marijuana use in the past 30 days in the states of Colorado and Washington among students in eight, tenth, and twelfth grades. There was no association found in Colorado. In Washington, legalization of recreational marijuana use was associated with increased prevalence of marijuana use among eighth and tenth graders (Cerdá et al., 2017).

A negative and presumably unintended consequence of marijuana use bans is the association with over-incarceration of individuals, especially African-American males, for possession, use, and illegal sale of marijuana (Gilmore & Betts, 2012). This negative consequence has been very costly to society in terms of over-crowded prisons and its associated detrimental effects on thousands of African-American males.

The study based on NSDUH data mentioned above suggests that legalizing medical marijuana is associated with an increase in the frequency of binge drinking, though it was not associated with the total number of drinks (Wen et al., 2015). Additionally, there were no observed effects of medical marijuana legalization on alcohol abuse and dependence, nonmedical use of prescription pain medication, heroin use or cocaine use (Wen et al., 2015). Another study found that among adults 21 or older, states legalizing medical marijuana had increased prevalence of alcohol abuse or dependence (Choi, 2014). This relationship did not exist among those aged 20 or younger, nor was there any association with smoking or binge drinking for different age groups. A third study also found that there was no effect of legalizing medical marijuana on drinking or binge drinking, even after stratifying by age (Anderson, Hansen, & Rees, 2013). One unintended positive consequence of lifting bans on medical marijuana is that the misuse of prescription opiates has apparently decreased in states that allow medical marijuana use (Powell, Pacula, & Jacobson, 2015). A recent review of research on the potential effects of marijuana policies on alcohol use in the U.S. suggests that an unintended consequence of legalization of marijuana for either medical or recreational use is that the legalization may lead to marijuana being both substituted for alcohol and used complementarily with alcohol (Guttmannova et al., 2016).

Age Restrictions. Regulations concerning the use of medical marijuana typically have not included any age restrictions. Despite the lack of age restrictions, it appears that medical marijuana laws are not associated with increased marijuana use among adolescents (Hasin et al., 2015; Lynne-Landsman, Livingston, & Wagenaar, 2013). As of 2016, in the U.S., *recreational* marijuana use is legal only for those aged 21 and older in Alaska (Division of Public Health, 2016), California (Hecht, 2016), Colorado (Colorado, 2016), Oregon (Oregon Liquor Control Commission, 2016a, 2016b, 2016c), Maine (Graham & Writers, 2016), Massachusetts (Gilbert, 2016), Nevada (Gilbert, 2016), Washington (Visit Spokane, 2016), and the District of Columbia (Metropolitan Police Department, 2016). However, no research has been conducted either in the U.S. or elsewhere on whether or not changing the minimum legal using age may affect the prevalence of marijuana use, nor is there any research on the unintended consequences of age restrictions on marijuana use.

Price Increases and Taxes. The effect of marijuana price increases or taxation on marijuana use is unknown. The tax rate of recreational marijuana in the U.S. in 2016 ranges from 0% in the District of Columbia to 37% in Washington State (Henchman & Scarboro, 2016). Medical marijuana can also be taxed, though the tax rate is generally lower than recreational marijuana (Henchman & Scarboro, 2016). There is no known research on the unintended consequences of pricing regulations on marijuana use.

Days and Hours of Sale Restrictions. Research on the effectiveness of limiting the times that marijuana is available for retail sale is limited. One state in the U.S. limits recreational marijuana sales from 8 a.m. to midnight (Ghosh et al., 2016), but it appears that no work has been done to determine if variations in sales hours have any effect on marijuana use patterns.

Government Monopolies. The effectiveness of government monopolies on reducing marijuana use is unknown. In the U.S., state-run monopolies of marijuana are not permitted because of the Controlled Substances Act (Pacula et al., 2014); therefore no research on government monopolies of marijuana exists from the U.S. To the best of our knowledge, no government monopolies for marijuana exist outside of the U.S.

Advertising Restrictions. Although restrictions or prohibitions on marijuana advertising and marketing exist in states and communities across the U.S. and in other countries, no research has investigated possible effects of these policies on marijuana use.

Other Illegal Drugs

Bans. Illegal drug bans appear to have varying degrees of effectiveness. For example, the reported lifetime prevalence of cocaine and opiate use in various countries ranged from 0% to 14.5% (Bucello et al., 2010) and 0% to 17.9% (Nelson et al., 2010), respectively. In 2014, the worldwide annual prevalence of cocaine use, amphetamine and prescription stimulant use, and 3,4-methylenedioxy-methamphetamine (also known as "Ecstasy") was estimated to be 0.38%, 0.8%, and 0.4%, respectively (United Nations Office on Drugs and Crime, 2016). Unintended consequences of bans on illegal drugs include black markets, crime related to illegal drug trafficking, and related drug abuse and addiction.

Because the sale and use of drugs such as cocaine, heroin, and Ecstasy is illegal for all age groups in the U.S. and other countries, there is no basis for policies such as age restrictions, price increases and taxes, days and hours of sale restrictions, government monopolies, and advertising restrictions.

Directions for Future Research

Overall. In general, there has been relatively little research on the unintended consequences of substance use policy interventions. For example, one review of studies investigating alcohol taxes found that very few studies have investigated differential impacts by ethnicity and socioeconomic status (Giesbrecht et al., 2016) or other subgroups, such as those based on age.

Bans on substances create black markets, but the consequences of black markets are not a well-researched topic. Some research does suggest that black markets can lead to increases in crime, violence, and decreased product quality, which may result in unintentional poisoning (Hall, 2010; Hawken et al., 2013; Miron & Zwiebel, 1995). However, the effects of the establishment of a black market on both substance use and other consequences need to be more thoroughly examined.

Additionally, research concerning the enforcement of bans affecting the supply-side equation of substance use is limited. Strategies in the U.S. used to enforce bans include aerial spraying and interdiction to reduce the production and trafficking of illegal drugs (Office of National Drug Control Policy, 1999). While these supply-side actions may decrease the supply and availability of a given substance, no research has been conducted to determine whether substance use actually decreases as a result of such actions.

Many substance use policies have been investigated singularly, leaving questions about the effectiveness of combined substance use policies and enforcement efforts. Some research does suggest that more comprehensive alcohol and tobacco policy interventions and related enforcement activities at the community and national levels can have a beneficial effect on alcohol and tobacco consumption and related harms (e.g., Flewelling et al., 2013; Holder et al., 2000; Levy, Chaloupka, & Gitchell, 2004; Naimi et al., 2014; Paschall, Grube, & Kypri, 2009). Additional studies are needed, however, to assess optimal combinations of substance use policies and the possible unintended consequences of multicomponent policy interventions.

There will continue to be opportunities to conduct such research in the U.S. through both natural and controlled experiments because of the substantial variability in substance use policies within and among the 50 states and the District of Columbia. For example, the potential effect of variations in the taxes levied on substances at the county and city levels should be further investigated (e.g., certain states allow for cigarette taxes to be levied at the county or city level, (Boonn, 2016; The Tax Burden on Tobacco, 2014), as well as regulations addressing days and hours of operation. This heterogeneity can be utilized to gain a more comprehensive understanding of the role of policy interventions in decreasing substance use.

Variations in substance use policies within and between countries will also provide a basis for future research into the intended and unintended effects of substance use policy interventions. Ongoing investigations such as the International Alcohol Control Policy Evaluation Study will provide useful information on the effects of alcohol policies within and among participating countries, and can be utilized to investigate unintended policy effects as well (Casswell et al., 2012).

Alcohol

A number of policies targeting reductions in the availability of alcohol were not addressed in the initial section due to limited research related to their effectiveness. Such policies include social host and keg registration laws, which may help to reduce the social availability of alcohol and underage drinking in potentially hazardous private settings (Paschall, Lipperman-Kreda, & Grube, 2014; Paschall, Lipperman-Kreda, Grube, & Thomas, 2014; Ringwalt & Paschall, 2011). Responsible beverage service (RBS) training programs may also help to reduce sales and service of alcohol to underage youth and intoxicated patrons, though research to date suggests that RBS training alone only has short-term effects, and may be more effective if coupled with enforcement operations, including minor decoy operations and undercover operations in bars (Toomey et al., 2001; Toomey et al., 2008).

Additionally, research indicates that more comprehensive alcohol policies may reduce binge drinking among adults and college students (Naimi et al., 2014; Nelson, Naimi, Brewer, & Wechsler, 2004), and both alcohol use and binge drinking among youth (Paschall, Lipperman-Kreda, & Grube, 2014; Paschall, Lipperman-Kreda, Grube, & Thomas, 2014; Xuan et al., 2015). Research is needed to investigate whether these reductions are related to presence of specific policies or simply through the number of policies that are present.

Research related to the effectiveness of alcohol policy enforcement is also needed. For example, undercover operations in bars may help to reduce the service of alcohol to clearly intoxicated patrons and excessive drinking, but very few studies have addressed this question (Fell, Fisher, Yao, & McKnight, 2017; McKnight & Streff, 1994). The effects of social host and keg registration law enforcement on underage and hazardous drinking also have not been investigated.

Finally, Campbell et al. (2009) reviewed five studies that investigated association between alcohol outlet density and alcohol consumption or sales (a proxy for consumption). All five studies concluded that increasing outlet density was associated with an increase in alcohol consumption. However, all of these studies were conducted in 2000 or earlier, and results were mixed depending on the type of alcohol. The U.S.-based studies found associations only between outlet density and spirit and wine consumption or sales. The United Kingdom-based study found associations only for beer and hard cider consumption, while the Canada-based study found an association between outlet density and overall alcohol consumption (Campbell et al., 2009). Further research is needed to determine if policies intending to reduce alcohol availability from commercial sources by restricting outlet density help to reduce overall alcohol consumption or consumption of specific types of alcohol.

Tobacco

E-cigarettes were first patented in 2004, and usage of these devices has increased since then (Franck, Budlovsky, Windle, Filion, & Eisenberg, 2014; Yamin, Bitton, & Bates, 2010). Worldwide, different countries have placed different levels of regulations on e-cigarettes. For example, as of 2015, 25 countries have banned all e-cigarette sales (World Health Organization, 2015), but sales are still allowed in various countries (Davidson, 2015). However, the research on e-cigarette regulatory policies and use is limited, and more is needed to determine if policy strategies aimed at reducing e-cigarette use should be similar to those addressing traditional cigarettes.

Furthermore, research is needed to determine if different policies have different effects depending on type of tobacco product (e.g., cigarettes, cigars, smokeless tobacco, flavored products), or if policies targeting specific types of tobacco products can reduce both the use of the specific product and tobacco use overall.

Bans on using smokeless tobacco exist in various athletic venues in the U.S. Minor league baseball has banned its use in stadiums since 1993 (Sanders, 2015). As of 2016, the cities of Boston (Freyer, 2015), Chicago (Chapman, 2016), Los Angeles (Becerra, 2016), New York (Berkman, 2016), and San Francisco (Baggarly & Almond, 2016) have banned smokeless tobacco use in athletic venues. Starting in January 2017, California banned chewing tobacco use in all athletic venues (Baggarly & Almond, 2016; Sanders, 2015). Studies are needed to determine whether these bans reduce smokeless tobacco use both overall and specifically among people entering the stadiums. Research should also be conducted to see if place-based bans are effective strategies for reducing tobacco use in general.

Marijuana

The landscape of marijuana use policies is currently changing rapidly in the U.S. In 1996, California became the first state in the U.S. to legalize medical marijuana. Less than twenty years later, Colorado and Washington were the first states to legalize recreational use of marijuana (Schuermeyer et al., 2014), and as of 2016, eight states and the District of Columbia have legalized recreational marijuana use by adults 21 or older (Gilbert, 2016; McGinty et al., 2016). Very limited research exists on the effects of the legalization of marijuana for recreational use (e.g., Cerdá et al., 2017). However, medical use of marijuana has been legal in some states for a much longer time period than recreational use, and some lessons can be gleaned from the legalization of medical marijuana.

States with laws legalizing medical marijuana have higher marijuana use prevalence than those without these laws (Cerdá, Wall, Keyes, Galea, & Hasin, 2012; Schuermeyer et al., 2014). While studies have found that the legalization of marijuana for medical and recreational use may lead to the perception that marijuana use is harmless (Schauer, King, Bunnell, Promoff, & McAfee, 2016) and acceptable (Paschall, Grube, & Biglan, 2017), research still needs to be conducted to determine whether these shifts in attitudes lead to increased marijuana use. Furthermore, research should be conducted to determine if different policies have different effects depending on type of marijuana product (e.g., edible vs. smoked product).

Within the U.S., there is considerable variability in implementation and enforcement of marijuana legislation, even within individual states. For example, in Oregon, recreational possession and use of marijuana is permitted for adults aged 21 or older (Oregon Liquor Control Commission, 2016a, 2016b, 2016c). However, individual cities and counties within Oregon can choose to prohibit the production, processing, or sales of marijuana within their jurisdictions (Oregon Liquor Control Commission, 2016a, 2016b, 2016c). Research should be conducted within states with heterogeneous marijuana policies to determine whether and how different policies and related enforcement activities have an effect on marijuana use. Furthermore, future work can be done to determine whether changes in the tax rates of recreational marijuana change the prevalence of both marijuana use overall and recreational marijuana use. Additionally, future research is needed to determine whether variations in day of week and time of day availability of recreational marijuana affect prevalence and patterns of recreational marijuana use.

Prescription Drugs

The Centers for Disease and Prevention (CDC) have recommended several promising state-level policies that are designed to reduce the misuse and abuse of prescription drugs, while also maintaining patients' right to safe and effective pain treatment (National Center for Injury Prevention and Control, 2011). These include prescription monitoring programs (PMPs), patient review and restriction programs (PRRPs), policies to prevent the abuse and diversion of prescription drugs, and health care provider accountability. As this review will reveal, the evidence base for these practices varies considerably.

Prescription Monitoring Programs (PMP). Of these, policies related to PMPs have been the most closely studied. PMPs are state-maintained databases that serve as depositories for information designed to prevent the misuse, abuse, and diversion of these substances. They typically contain information entered by the state's pharmacies concerning the nature, dose, and duration of each controlled substance (Schedule II through V) dispensed, as well as contact information for the patient, provider, and dispenser. They are designed to be used by medical providers and dispensers who wish to know their patients' history of filled controlled substances, from whom their patients received prescriptions for these substances, and what pharmacies dispensed them. This information may be used both to determine whether to write or fill a prescription for a controlled substance for a given patient, and to identify patients at high risk for abuse who might benefit from an early intervention. Policies addressing PMPs typically concern how expeditiously these data are entered into a database; who should register with and consult the database, under what circumstances, and how frequently; and measures to increase ease of access to the PMP, including the development of mechanisms to integrate and automate PMP information into providers' daily practice (Compton, Volkow, Throckmorton, & Lurie, 2013) and the interoperability of PMPs across state lines.

A comprehensive review of PMPs has yielded evidence that the programs are successful in reducing the supply and thus availability and potential abuse of prescriptions stimulants and pain relievers. Further, greater reductions were observed in states with proactive than reactive regulations in regard to PMPs. Proactive regulations, for this study, included identifying patients at risk of abuse and generating unsolicited reports to their medical providers (Simeone & Holland, 2006). In another study, which compared 14 states with PMPs to 36 states without them, patients in states with PMPs were less likely (odds ratio = 0.78) to be admitted to an inpatient drug abuse rehabilitation program than those in non-PMP states (Reisman, Shenoy, Atherly, & Flowers, 2009). In a third study that compared states with and without PMPs, reports to the state's Poison Center of intentional exposure to opioids increased by 1.9% per quarter in states without a PMP, whereas they decreased by 0.2% in states with a PMP (Reifler et al., 2012).

Patient Review and Restriction Programs (PRRP). PRRPs target patients typically who are nested within Medicaid or other state benefits programs like workmen's compensation. Eligible patients manifest signs of the inappropriate use of controlled substances, secure prescriptions from multiple providers ("doctor shoppers") or fill them at multiple dispensers ("pharmacy hoppers"). Such programs often "lock in" these patients to a single provider, dispenser, and even an emergency department "home" for at least a 12-month period, and will decline to reimburse any services that the locked in patient may seek elsewhere. The purpose of the program is to enhance care coordination for high-risk patients and reduce the potential for abuse and diversion.

One evaluation of the PRRP in North Carolina's Medicaid program found an 84% reduction during the locked in period, relative to baseline, in the likelihood that patients would file an opioid claim in any given month. The monthly number of opioid prescriptions decreased by 1.1, and the number of pharmacies visited decreased by 0.6 (Skinner et al., 2016). However, concerns have been raised by another small study that a substantial proportion of locked in Medicaid patients may choose to exit the program due to these restrictions (Dreyer, Michalski, & Williams, 2015).

Similar to PRRPs are programs that are now being implemented in some hospital emergency departments (EDs), which are designed to identify frequent visitors with chronic noncancer pain who may be seeking prescriptions for opioid analgesics. An evaluation was conducted in a set of EDs with linked medical records of an intervention in which a flag was placed in the charts of patients randomized to an intervention warning their providers of their status. During the study's follow-up year, patients in the intervention relative to the control group received opioids on 16–26% of their return visits, and they averaged 11.9–16.6 return visits, respectively (Ringwalt et al., 2015).

Policies. Laws and regulations to prevent the abuse and diversion of controlled substances include those that target the operation of so-called "pill mills," which give patients prescriptions for controlled substances, often after only cursory examinations. In one study that was designed to test Florida's law designed to suppress these medical practices, the investigators reported modest but significant reductions in both the volume and strength (in morphine milligram equivalents) of opioids prescribed, most notably among providers and patients whose use at baseline was highest (Rutkow et al., 2015).

Many other policies are being implemented by the states that have yet to be subjected to even uncontrolled evaluations, particularly in Medicaid programs. For example, some states are limiting the quantity of controlled substances that can be dispensed in any given prescription, and others require prior authorization of single prescriptions for opioid analgesics. Prior authorization procedures require a third party review of the justification for prescriptions for a given controlled substance before claims are accepted by insurers. One policy that has received attention is the use of "step therapy" programs, which introduce opioid-naïve patients to the analgesics in a tiered, stepwise fashion. Thus patients with no experience of opioids will be prescribed immediate-release opioid medications—which are most appropriate for acute, sporadic, or breakthrough pain—before graduating to extended-release, long-acting medications (Keast, Nesser, & Farmer, 2015). Other states are implementing drug utilization reviews to identify patients manifesting potentially problematic use and then notifying their providers; they may also identify potentially problematic providers whose prescribing behaviors may warrant examination by their state medical boards. To prevent the diversion of prescription drugs to young children, the Poison Prevention Packaging Act (Title 16 CFR parts 1700 through 1702) was enacted in 1970. The Act requires that containers for prescription drugs—as well as for a variety of other potentially harmful household products—be designed in such a way that a child under five years of age would find difficult to open.

Generally speaking, the quality of the methodology of many of the evaluations of policies and regulations related to opioid overdose prevention is poor. A recent review of the research has lamented the lack of experimental or interrupted time series designs, small sample sizes, inadequate statistical tests, short-term follow-ups, and the presence of potential confounders from secular trends and the contemporaneous implementation of other opioid overdose prevention policies and practices. Also of concern are the nonbehavioral outcomes often used, and the lack of attention to prevention policies' effects on provider and patient behaviors and, of ultimate interest, mortality and morbidity attributable to opioid overdoses. The authors conclude that methodologically rigorous studies are greatly needed to improve the quality of recommended strategies from promising to evidence-based (Haegerich, Paulozzi, Manns, & Jones, 2014).

Also of concern is the potential for the iatrogenic effects of these policies. As patients' behaviors in regard to securing and filling controlled substances comes under increased scrutiny, the potential for patients suffering from chronic pain to be denied the palliative care they require to function effectively commensurately increases. Some patients may legitimately need long-term opioid therapy, particularly if the kinds of alternatives to pain relief that are currently being explored are inadequate. They may also have legitimate reasons to secure pain medications from multiple providers, especially if they are suffering from multiple complaints that require attention from multiple specialized clinicians. While these clinicians should be particularly careful to consult their state's PMP, their patients should not be expected to suffer because they fail to coordinate their medications. We know very little about the effects on patients of various policies designed to constrain their inappropriate drug-seeking behavior, and the extent to which these policies may have the inadvertent effect of inducing them to turn to heroin and other illicit substances.

Health Care Provider Accountability. Providers are also finding their prescribing practices under closer scrutiny. While the evidence for what is called the "chilling effect" (Goodin, Blumenschein, Freeman, & Talbert, 2012) of prevention policies is lacking, there is anecdotal evidence that providers may be failing to accept pain patients in their practice, may push them out prematurely, or may fail to reduce their pain medication in appropriately small increments—a practice known as "tapering." Again, these patients may be at high risk for overdose-related morbidity and mortality. Policies that effectively reduce morbidity and mortality at the population level may ill-serve particular patients.

In summary, there are a variety of promising strategies designed to combat the epidemic of opioid overdose that are supported by evidence of varying strength and methodological rigor. Relatively few of these strategies can practically be subjected to the randomized trials that constitute the gold standard of evaluation research. Many others, like enhancements to PMPs and their use to proactively notify prescribers that their patients may exhibit drug-seeking behavior, and regulatory authorities that prescribers' behaviors may be unusual or excessive, can be tested using interrupted time series designs. But these studies can only be conducted within the context of an environment that is constantly changing and evolving, as multiple efforts are simultaneously being brought to bear on the epidemic. Thus the causal attribution of positive effects noted for any given strategy will almost inevitably be an ambiguous process. Clearly, practitioners interested in preventing opioid overdose are not in a position to await the arrival of unimpeachable evidence of the effectiveness of any given strategy. Instead, they are fully justified in selecting and implementing an array of promising strategies, as long as they remain vigilant to the possibility that some of these strategies may have iatrogenic as well as positive effects.

Acknowledgments The writing of this chapter was supported by grants from the National Institute on Alcohol Abuse and Alcoholism (NIAAA Grant Nos. P60-AA006282, R01AA021726, and T32-AA014125). The content is solely the responsibility of the authors and does not necessarily represent the official views of the NIAAA or the National Institutes of Health.

References

Akers, R. L. (2012). *Criminological theories: Introduction and evaluation*. New York, NY: Routledge, Taylor, and Francis.

Amethyst Initiative. (2010). *Amethyst initiative: Rethink the drinking age*.

Anderson, D. M., Hansen, B., & Rees, D. I. (2013). Medical marijuana laws, traffic fatalities, and alcohol consumption. *Journal of Law and Economics, 56*(2), 333–369.

Babor, T. (2010). *Alcohol: No ordinary commodity: Research and public policy*. Oxford: Oxford University Press.

Baggarly, A. & Almond, E. (2016). No dipping in giants baseball? Tobacco ban set to hit AT&T Park. The Mercury News. Retrieved March 30, from http://www.mercurynews.com/2016/03/30/no-dipping-in-giants-baseball-tobacco-ban-set-to-hit-att-park/.

Becerra, H. (2016). *Smokeless Tobacco at Dodger Stadium? You're out of here!* Los Angeles Times. Retrieved January 26, 2016, from http://www.latimes.com/local/lanow/la-me-ln-city-to-consider-ban-on-chewing-tobacco-20160126-story.html.

Berkman, S. (2016). It's official: Smokeless tobacco is out. *The New York Times*. Retrieved April 6, 2016, from http://www.nytimes.com/2016/04/07/sports/baseball/smokeless-tobacco-ban-new-york-yankees-mets.html.

Birkett, N. J. (2014). The impact of taxation reduction on smoking in youth between 1990 and 1999: Results from a Reconstructed Cohort Analysis of the Canadian Community Health Surveys. *PLoS One, 9*(4), e93412.

Blocker, J. S., Jr. (2006). Did prohibition really work? Alcohol prohibition as a public health innovation. *American Journal of Public Health, 96*(2), 233–243.

Boonn, A. (2016). *Local government cigarette tax rates & fees. Campaign for tobacco-free kids*. Retrieved from http://www.tobaccofreekids.org/research/factsheets/pdf/0304.pdf.

Boyle, P. (2010). *Tobacco: Science, policy and public health*. Oxford: Oxford university press.

Brownson, R. C., Haire-Joshu, D., & Luke, D. A. (2006). Shaping the context of health: A review of environmental and policy approaches in the prevention of chronic diseases. *Annual Reviews of Public Health, 27*, 341–370.

Bryden, A., Roberts, B., McKee, M., & Petticrew, M. (2012). A systematic review of the influence on alcohol use of community level availability and marketing of alcohol. *Health & Place, 18*(2), 349–357.

Bucello, C., Degenhardt, L., Calabria, B., Nelson, P., Roberts, A., Medina-Mora, M. E., & Compton, W. M. (2010). *What do we know about the extent of cocaine use and dependence? Results of a global systematic review. Technical report 308*. Sydney: National Drug and Alcohol Research Centre, University of New South Wales https://ndarc.med.unsw.edu.au/sites/default/files/ndarc/resources/TR.308.pdf

Campbell, C. A., Hahn, R. A., Elder, R., Brewer, R., Chattopadhyay, S., Fielding, J., ... The Task Force on Community Preventive Services. (2009). The effectiveness of limiting alcohol outlet density as a means of reducing excessive consumption and alcohol-related harms. *American Journal of Preventive Medicine, 37*(6), 556–569.

Carpenter, C., & Dobkin, C. (2011). The minimum legal drinking age and public health. *Journal of Economic Perspectives, 25*(2), 133–156.

Casswell, S., Meier, P., MacKintosh, A. M., Brown, A., Hastings, G., Thamarangsi, T., ... Wall, M. (2012). The International Alcohol Control (IAC) study—evaluating the impact of alcohol policies. *Alcoholism: Clinical and Experimental Research, 36*(8), 1462–1467.

Centers for Disease Control and Prevention. (2017). *BRFSS prevalence & trends data*. Retrieved January 3, 2017, from https://www.cdc.gov/brfss/brfssprevalence/index.html.

Cerdá, M., Wall, M., Feng, T., Keyes, K. M., Sarvet, A., Schulenberg, J., ... Hasin, D. (2017). Association of state recreational marijuana laws with adolescent marijuana use. *Journal of the American Medical Association Pediatrics, 171*(2), 142–149.

Cerdá, M., Wall, M., Keyes, K. M., Galea, S., & Hasin, D. (2012). Medical marijuana laws in 50 states: Investigating the relationship between state legalization of medical marijuana and marijuana use, abuse and dependence. *Drug and Alcohol Dependence, 120*(1), 22–27.

Chapman, S. (2016). Knocking smokeless tobacco out of the Ballpark. *Chicago Tribune*. Retrieved March 25, 2016. http://www.chicagotribune.com/news/opinion/chapman/ct-smokeless-tobacco-ban-ballpark-baseball-mlb-perspec-0327-jm-20160325-column.html.

Choi, A. (2014). The impact of medical marijuana laws on marijuana use and other risky health behaviors. *Health & Healthcare in America: From Economics to Policy. Ashecon*

Colorado. (2016). *Laws and youth|Colorado Marijuana*. Accessed December 12, 2016, from https://www.colorado.gov/pacific/marijuana/laws-and-youth.

Compton, W. M., Volkow, N. D., Throckmorton, D. C., & Lurie, P. (2013). Expanded access to opioid overdose intervention: Research, practice, and policy needs. *Annals of Internal Medicine, 158*(1), 65–66.

Davidson, L. (2015). Vaping takes off as E-cigarette sales break through £6bn. *The Telegraph*. Retrieved June 23, 2015, from http://cloud.highcharts.com/show/odiwuz/2.

DeJong, W., & Blanchette, J. (2014). Case closed: Research evidence on the positive public impact of the age 21 minimum legal drinking age in the United States. *Journal of Studies on Alcohol and Drugs, 75*(s17), 108–115.

DiNardo, J., & Lemieux, T. (2001). Alcohol, marijuana, and American youth: The unintended consequences of government regulation. *Journal of Health Economics, 20*(6), 991–1010.

Division of Public Health. (2016). *Know the laws about marijuana*. Retrieved December 12, 2016, from http://dhss.alaska.gov/dph/Director/Pages/marijuana/law.aspx.

Dreyer, T. R. F., Michalski, T., & Williams, B. C. (2015). Patient outcomes in a medicaid managed care lock-in program. *Journal of Managed Care & Specialty Pharmacy, 21*(11), 1006–1012.

Duailibi, S., Ponicki, W., Grube, J., Pinsky, I., Laranjeira, R., & Raw, M. (2007). The effect of restricting opening hours on alcohol-related violence. *American Journal of Public Health, 97*(12), 2276–2280.

Farley, S. M. & Johns, M. (2016). New York City flavoured tobacco product sales ban evaluation. *Tobacco Control*, tobaccocontrol-2015-052418.

Fell, J. C., Fisher, D. A., Yao, J., & McKnight, A. S. (2017). Evaluation of responsible beverage service and enforcement program: Effects on bar patron intoxication and potential impaired driving by young adults. *Traffic Injury Prevention, 18*(6), 557–565. https://doi.org/10.1080/15389588.2017.1285401

Fichtenberg, C. M., & Glantz, S. A. (2002). Youth access interventions do not affect youth smoking. *Pediatrics, 109*(6), 1088–1092.

Flewelling, R. L., Grube, J. W., Paschall, M. J., Biglan, A., Kraft, A., Black, C., ... Ruscoe, J. (2013). Reducing youth access to alcohol: Findings from a community-based randomized trial. *American Journal of Community Psychology, 51*(1–2), 264–277.

Fong, G. T., Hammond, D., & Hitchman, S. C. (2009). The impact of pictures on the effectiveness of tobacco warnings. *Bulletin of the World Health Organization, 87*, 640–643. https://doi.org/10.2471/BLT.09.069575

Franck, C., Budlovsky, T., Windle, S. B., Filion, K. B., & Eisenberg, M. J. (2014). Electronic cigarettes in North America history, use, and implications for smoking cessation. *Circulation, 129*(19), 1945–1952.

Freyer, F. J. (2015). Boston bans chewing tobacco in Ballparks, including Fenway. *The Boston Globe*. Retrieved September 2, 2015, from https://www.bostonglobe.com/metro/2015/09/02/boston-bans-chewing-tobacco-ballparks-including-fenway/KEgAULnyWsVt5Pji2w5JdI/story.html.

Ghosh, T., Van Dyke, M., Maffey, A., Whitley, E., Gillim-Ross, L., & Wolk, L. (2016). The public health framework of legalized marijuana in Colorado. *American Journal of Public Health, 106*(1), 21–27.

Giesbrecht, N., Wettlaufer, A., Cukier, S., Geddie, G., Gonçalves, A.-H., & Reisdorfer, E. (2016). Do alcohol pricing and availability policies have differential effects on sub-populations? A commentary. *The International Journal of Alcohol and Drug Research, 5*(3), 89–99.

Gilbert, B. 2016. 4 States just voted to make marijuana completely legal—Here's what we know. *Business Insider*. Retrieved November 9, 2016, from http://www.businessinsider.com/marijuana-states-legalized-weed-2016-11.

Gilmore, A. B., Fooks, G., & McKee, M. (2011). A review of the impacts of tobacco industry privatisation: Implications for policy. *Global Public Health, 6*(6), 621–642.

Gilmore, B. G., & Betts, R. D. (2012). Deconstructing carmona: The US war on drugs and black men as non-citizens. *Val. UL Rev., 47*, 777.

Goodin, A., Blumenschein, K., Freeman, P. R., & Talbert, J. (2012). Consumer/patient encounters with prescription drug monitoring programs: Evidence from a medicaid population. *Pain Physician, 15*(3 Suppl), ES169.

Graham, G. & Writers, M. D. S. 2016. Maine voters legalize recreational use of marijuana by razor-thin margin. *The Portland Press Herald/Maine Sunday Telegram*. Retrieved November 10, 2016, from http://www.pressherald.com/2016/11/10/absentee-ballots-from-overseas-may-be-key-to-maine-marijuana-vote/.

Guttmannova, K., Lee, C. M., Kilmer, J. R., Fleming, C. B., Rhew, I. C., Kosterman, R., & Larmier, M. E. (2016). Impacts of changing marijuana policies on alcohol use in the United States. *Alcoholism: Clinical and Experimental Research, 40*(1), 33–46.

Haegerich, T. M., Paulozzi, L. J., Manns, B. J., & Jones, C. M. (2014). What we know, and don't know, about the impact of state policy and systems-level interventions on prescription drug overdose. *Drug and Alcohol Dependence, 145*, 34–47.

Hahn, R. A., Kuzara, J. L., Elder, R., Brewer, R., Chattopadhyay, S., Fielding, J., ... Lawrence, B. (2010). Effectiveness of policies restricting hours of alcohol sales in preventing excessive alcohol consumption and related harms. *American Journal of Preventive Medicine, 39*(6), 590–604.

Hall, W. (2010). What are the policy lessons of national alcohol prohibition in the United States, 1920–1933? *Addiction, 105*(7), 1164–1173.

Hammond, D. 2011. Health warning messages on tobacco products: A review. *Tobacco Control*, tc. 2010.037630

Harper, S., Strumpf, E. C., & Kaufman, J. S. (2012). Do medical marijuana laws increase marijuana use? Replication study and extension. *Annals of Epidemiology, 22*(3), 207–212.

Hasin, D. S., Wall, M., Keyes, K. M., Cerdá, M., Schulenberg, J., O'Malley, P. M., ... Feng, T. (2015). Medical marijuana laws and adolescent marijuana use in the USA from 1991 to 2014: Results from annual, repeated cross-sectional surveys. *The Lancet Psychiatry, 2*(7), 601–608.

Hawken, A., Kulick, J., & Prieger, J. E. 2013. Unintended consequences of cigarette taxation and regulation. *Available at SSRN 2354772*

Hecht, P. 2016. California legalized recreational marijuana. What does that mean for you? *The Sacramento Bee*. Retrieved November 9, 2016, from http://www.sacbee.com/news/state/california/california-weed/article113420578.html.

Henchman, J., & Scarboro, M. 2016. Marijuana legalization and taxes: Lessons for other states from Colorado and Washington. *Tax Foundation*. Retrieved May 12, 2016, from http://taxfoundation.org/article/marijuana-legalization-and-taxes-lessons-other-states-colorado-and-washington.

Hingson, R., & White, A. (2014). New research findings since the 2007 surgeon general's call to action to prevent and reduce underage drinking: A review. *Journal of Studies on Alcohol and Drugs, 75*(1), 158–169.

Hoffman, S. J., & Tan, C. (2015). Overview of systematic reviews on the health-related effects of government tobacco control policies. *BMC Public Health, 15*(1), 1.

Holder, H. D., Gruenewald, P. J., Ponicki, W. R., Treno, A. J., Grube, J. W., Saltz, R. F., ... Sanchez, L. (2000). Effect of community-based interventions on high-risk drinking and alcohol-related injuries. *Journal of the American Medical Association, 284*(18), 2341–2347.

Jernigan, D., Noel, J., Landon, J., Thornton, N., & Lobstein, T. (2017). Alcohol marketing and youth alcohol consumption: A systematic review on longitudinal studies published since 2008. *Addiction, 112*(Supplement 1), 7–20.

Keast, S. L., Nesser, N., & Farmer, K. (2015). Strategies aimed at controlling misuse and abuse of opioid prescription medications in a state medicaid program: A policymaker's perspective. *The American Journal of Drug and Alcohol Abuse, 41*(1), 1–6.

Knai, C., Petticrew, M., Durand, M. A., Eastmure, E., & Mays, N. (2015). Are the public health responsibility deal alcohol pledges likely to improve public health? An evidence synthesis. *Addiction, 110*(8), 1232–1246.

LaBrie, J. W., Hummer, J. F., Pedersen, E. R., Lac, A., & Chithambo, T. (2012). Measuring college students' motives behind prepartying drinking: Development and validation of the prepartying motivations inventory. *Addictive Behaviors, 37*(8), 962–969.

Lenk, K. M., Toomey, T. L., Erickson, D. J., Kilian, G. R., Nelson, T. F., & Fabian, L. E. A. (2010). Alcohol control policies and practices at professional sports stadiums. *Public Health Reports, 125*(5), 665.

Levy, D. T., Chaloupka, F., & Gitchell, J. (2004). The effects of tobacco control policies on smoking rates: A tobacco control scorecard. *Journal of Public Health Management and Practice, 10*(4), 338–353.

Lynne-Landsman, S. D., Livingston, M. D., & Wagenaar, A. C. (2013). Effects of state medical marijuana laws on adolescent marijuana use. *American Journal of Public Health, 103*(8), 1500–1506.

Martineau, F., Tyner, E., Lorenc, T., Petticrew, M., & Lock, K. (2013). Population-level interventions to reduce alcohol-related harm: An overview of systematic reviews. *Preventive Medicine, 57*(4), 278–296.

Mason, W. A., Fleming, C. B., Ringle, J. L., Hanson, K., Gross, T. J., & Haggerty, K. P. (2016). Prevalence of marijuana and other substance use before and after Washington state's change from legal medical marijuana to legal medical and nonmedical marijuana: Cohort comparisons in a sample of adolescents. *Substance Abuse, 37*(2), 330–335.

McGinty, E. E., Samples, H., Bandara, S. N., Saloner, B., Bachhuber, M. A., & Barry, C. L. (2016). The emerging public discourse on state legalization of marijuana for recreational use in the US: Analysis of news media coverage, 2010–2014. *Preventive Medicine, 90*, 114–120.

McKnight, A. J., & Streff, F. M. (1994). The effect of enforcement upon service of alcohol to intoxicated patrons of bars and restaurants. *Accident Analysis & Prevention, 26*(1), 79–88.

Metropolitan Police Department. (2016). *The facts on DC marijuana laws*. Retrieved December 12, 2016. / marijuana

Middleton, J. C., Hahn, R. A., Kuzara, J. L., Elder, R., Brewer, R., Chattopadhyay, S., ... Lawrence, B. (2010). Effectiveness of policies maintaining or restricting days of alcohol sales on excessive alcohol consumption and related harms. *American Journal of Preventive Medicine, 39*(6), 575–589.

Miron, J. A., & Zwiebel, J. (1995). The economic case against drug prohibition. *The Journal of Economic Perspectives, 9*(4), 175–192.

Naimi, T. S., Blanchette, J., Nelson, T. F., Nguyen, T., Oussayef, N., Heeren, T. C., ... Xuan, Z. (2014). A new scale of the US alcohol policy environment and its relationship to binge drinking. *American Journal of Preventive Medicine, 46*(1), 10–16.

National Cancer Institute. (2008). *Monograph 19: The role of the media in promoting and reducing tobacco use*. 07-6242

National Center for Injury Prevention and Control. (2011). *Policy impact: Prescription painkiller overdoses*. Atlanta, GA: Centers for Disease Control and Prevention Retrieved from https://www.cdc.gov/drugoverdose/pdf/policyimpact-prescriptionpainkillerod-a.pdf

Nelson, P., McLaren, J., Degenhardt, L., Bucello, C., Calabria, B., Roberts, A., ... Wiessing, L. (2010). *What do we know about the extent of opioid use and dependence? Results of a global systematic review. Technical report 309*. Sydney: National Drug and Alcohol Research Centre, University of New South Wales Retrieved from https://ndarc.med.unsw.edu.au/sites/default/files/ndarc/resources/TR.309.pdf

Nelson, T. F., Naimi, T. S., Brewer, R. D., & Wechsler, H. (2004). The state sets the rate. *American Journal of Public Health, 95*(3), 441–446.

Office of National Drug Control Policy. (1999). *1999 National drug control strategy*. Retrieved from https://www.ncjrs.gov/ondcppubs/publications/policy/99ndcs/contents.html.

Oregon Liquor Control Commission. (2016a). *Record of cities/counties prohibiting licensed recreational marijuana facilities*. Retrieved from https://www.oregon.gov/olcc/marijuana/Documents/Cities_Counties_RMJOptOut.pdf.

Oregon Liquor Control Commission. (2016b). *Recreational marijuana FAQs: Local government opt-out*. Retrieved December 13, 2016, from http://www.oregon.gov/olcc/marijuana/Pages/FAQs-Local-Government-Opt-Out.aspx.

Oregon Liquor Control Commission. (2016c). *Recreational marijuana FAQs: Personal use*. Retrieved December 12, 2016, from https://www.oregon.gov/olcc/marijuana/Pages/FAQs-Personal-Use.aspx.

Pacula, R. L., Kilmer, B., Wagenaar, A. C., Chaloupka, F. J., & Caulkins, J. P. (2014). Developing public health regulations for marijuana: Lessons from alcohol and tobacco. *American Journal of Public Health, 104*(6), 1021–1028.

Paschall, M. J., Grube, J. W., & Biglan, A. (2017). Medical marijuana legalization and use among Oregon youth. *Journal of Primary Prevention, 38*(3), 329–341.

Paschall, M. J., Grube, J. W., Black, C., & Ringwalt, C. L. (2007). Is commercial alcohol availability related to adolescent alcohol sources and alcohol use? Findings from a multi-level study. *Journal of Adolescent Health, 41*(2), 168–174.

Paschall, M. J., Grube, J. W., & Kypri, K. (2009). Alcohol control policies and alcohol consumption by youth: A multi-national study. *Addiction, 104*(11), 1849–1855.

Paschall, M. J., Lipperman-Kreda, S., & Grube, J. W. (2014). Effects of the local alcohol environment on adolescents' drinking behaviors and beliefs. *Addiction, 109*(3), 407–416.

Paschall, M. J., Lipperman-Kreda, S., Grube, J. W., & Thomas, S. (2014). Relationships between social host laws and underage drinking: Findings from a study of 50 California cities. *Journal of Studies on Alcohol and Drugs, 75*(6), 901–907.

Paschall, M. J., & Saltz, R. F. (2007). Relationships between college settings and student alcohol use before, during and after events: A multi-level study. *Drug and Alcohol Review, 26*(6), 635–644.

Pemberton, M. R., Colliver, J. D., Robbins, T. M., & Gfroerer, J. C. (2008). *Underage alcohol use: Findings from the 2002–2006 national surveys on drug use and health*. Rockville, MD: Substance Abuse and Mental Health Services Administration, Office of Applied Studies.

Powell, D., Pacula, R. L., & Jacobson, M. 2015. *Do medical marijuana laws reduce addiction and deaths related to pain killers? Product page*. http://www.rand.org/pubs/working_papers/WR1130.html.

Reed, M. B., Clapp, J. D., Weber, M., Trim, R., Lange, J., & Shillington, A. M. (2011). Predictors of partying prior to bar attendance and subsequent BrAC. *Addictive Behaviors, 36*(12), 1341–1343.

Reifler, L. M., Droz, D., Bailey, J. E., Schnoll, S. H., Fant, R., Dart, R. C., & Bucher Bartelson, B. (2012). Do prescription monitoring programs impact state trends in opioid abuse/misuse? *Pain Medicine, 13*(3), 434–442.

Reisman, R. M., Shenoy, P. J., Atherly, A. J., & Flowers, C. R. (2009). Prescription opioid usage and abuse relationships: An evaluation of state prescription drug monitoring program efficacy. *Substance Abuse: Research and Treatment, 3*, 41.

Ringwalt, C., Shanahan, M., Wodarski, S., Jones, J., Schaffer, D., Fusaro, A., ... Ford, M. (2015). A randomized controlled trial of an emergency department intervention for patients with chronic noncancer pain. *The Journal of Emergency Medicine, 49*(6), 974–983.

Ringwalt, C. L., & Paschall, M. J. (2011). The utility of keg registration laws: A cross-sectional study. *Journal of Adolescent Health, 48*(1), 106–108.

Rutkow, L., Chang, H.-Y., Daubresse, M., Webster, D. W., Stuart, E. A., & Caleb Alexander, G. (2015). Effect of Florida's prescription drug monitoring program and pill mill laws on opioid prescribing and use. *Journal of the American Medical Association Internal Medicine, 175*(10), 1642–1649.

Saffer, H., & Chaloupka, F. (2000). The effect of tobacco advertising bans on tobacco consumption. *Journal of Health Economics, 19*(6), 1117–1137.

Sanders, J. 2015. California to MLB: Ditch the dip. San Diego Union-Tribune, October 14. http://www.sandiegouniontribune.com/sports/padres/sdut-california-bans-chewing-tobacco-baseball-2015oct14-story.html.

Schauer, G. L., King, B. A., Bunnell, R. E., Promoff, G., & McAfee, T. A. (2016). Toking, vaping, and eating for health or fun: Marijuana use patterns in adults, US, 2014. *American Journal of Preventive Medicine, 50*(1), 1–8.

Schuermeyer, J., Salomonsen-Sautel, S., Price, R. K., Balan, S., Thurstone, C., Min, S.-J., & Sakai, J. T. (2014). Temporal trends in marijuana attitudes, availability and use in colorado compared to non-medical marijuana states: 2003–11. *Drug and Alcohol Dependence, 140*, 145–155.

Simeone, R., & Holland, L. (2006). *An evaluation of prescription drug monitoring programs*. Albany, NY: Simeone Associates. Retrieved on September 11, 2012.

Skinner, A. C., Ringwalt, C., Naumann, R. B., Roberts, A. W., Moss, L. A., Sachdeva, N., ... Farley, J. (2016). Reducing opioid misuse: Evaluation of a medicaid controlled substance lock-in program. *The Journal of Pain, 17*(11), 1150–1155.

Stehr, M. (2005). Cigarette tax avoidance and evasion. *Journal of Health Economics, 24*(2), 277–297.

Stewart, M. J. (1993). The effect on tobacco consumption of advertising bans in OECD countries. *International Journal of Advertising, 12*(2), 155–180.

Stockwell, T., Zhao, J., Giesbrecht, N., Macdonald, S., Thomas, G., & Wettlaufer, A. (2012). The raising of minimum alcohol prices in Saskatchewan, Canada: Impacts on consumption and implications for public health. *American Journal of Public Health, 102*(12), e103–e110.

The Tax Burden on Tobacco. (2014). Arlington, VA: Orzechowski and Walker. Retrieved from http://www.taxadmin.org/assets/docs/Tobacco/papers/tax_burden_2014.pdf.

Toomey, T. L., Erickson, D. J., Patrek, W., Fletcher, L. A., & Wagenaar, A. C. (2005). Illegal alcohol sales and use of alcohol control policies at community festivals. *Public Health Reports, 120*(2), 165.

Toomey, T. L., Wagenaar, A. C., Gehan, J. P., Kilian, G., Murray, D. M., & Perry, C. L. (2001). Project ARM: Alcohol risk management to prevent sales to underage and intoxicated patrons. *Health Education & Behavior, 28*(2), 186–199.

Toomey, T. L., Erickson, D. J., Lenk, K. M., Kilian, G. R., Perry, C. L., & Wagenaar, A. C. (2008). A randomized trial to evaluate a management training program to prevent illegal alcohol sales. *Addiction, 103*(3), 405–413.

United Nations Office on Drugs and Crime. (2016). World drug report 2016. United Nations. Retrieved from https://www.unodc.org/doc/wdr2016/WORLD_DRUG_REPORT_2016_web.pdf.

Visit Spokane. (2016). Marijuana FAQ | Legal Cannabis in Washington | Smoke Pot | Weed. Retrieved December 12, 2016, from http://www.visitspokane.com/learn-about-the-spokane-region/marijuana-in-washington/.

Wagenaar, A. C., Salois, M. J., & Komro, K. A. (2009). Effects of beverage alcohol price and tax levels on drinking: A meta-analysis of 1003 estimates from 112 studies. *Addiction, 104*(2), 179–190.

Wagenaar, A. C., & Toomey, T. L. (2002). Effects of minimum drinking age laws: Review and analyses of the literature from 1960 to 2000. *Journal of Studies on Alcohol, Supplement*, (14), 206–225.

Wells, S., Graham, K., & Purcell, J. (2009). Policy implications of the widespread practice of 'pre-drinking' or 'pre-gaming' before going to public drinking establishments—are current prevention strategies backfiring? *Addiction, 104*(1), 4–9.

Wen, H., Hockenberry, J. M., & Cummings, J. R. (2015). The effect of medical marijuana laws on adolescent and adult use of marijuana, alcohol, and other substances. *Journal of Health Economics, 42*, 64–80.

World Health Organization. (2015). *WHO report on the global tobacco epidemic, 2015: Raising taxes on tobacco*. Geneva: WHO.

World Health Organization. (2016). *World health statistics 2016: Monitoring health for the SDGs*. Geneva: WHO.

Xu, X., & Chaloupka, F. J. (2011). The effects of prices on alcohol use and its consequences. *Alcohol Research & Health, 34*(2), 236–245.

Xuan, Z., Blanchette, J. G., Nelson, T. F., Nguyen, T. H., Hadland, S. E., Oussayef, N. L., ... Naimi, T. S. (2015). Youth drinking in the United States: Relationships with alcohol policies and adult drinking. *Pediatrics, 136*(1), 18–27.

Yamin, C. K., Bitton, A., & Bates, D. W. (2010). E-cigarettes: A rapidly growing internet phenomenon. *Annals of Internal Medicine, 153*(9), 607–609.

Brief Interventions as Evidence-Based Prevention Strategies

Emily E. Tanner-Smith and Sean P. Grant

The consumption of alcohol and other illicit drugs is a critical public health issue. In 2009, an estimated 4% of all global deaths were attributable to alcohol or illicit drug consumption (WHO, 2009). In the United States, an estimated 27 million people aged 12 or older (10.2% of the population) used an illicit drug in the past month, and 60.9 million (23% of the population) were heavy episodic drinkers in the past month (or "binge drinkers," defined as drinking five or more drinks on the same occasion) (SAMHSA, 2015). Illicit drug use and heavy episodic drinking are associated with numerous detrimental sequelae, including the development of subsequent substance use disorders (SUDs), psychiatric conditions, injuries, unemployment, loss of work productivity, and criminal justice system involvement (Boden & Fergusson, 2011; Bouchery, Harwood, Sacks, Simon, & Brewer, 2011; Cherpitel, Martin, Macdonald, Brubacher, & Stenstrom, 2013; Degenhardt & Hall, 2012; Rehm et al., 2010; UNODC, 2012). Given their prevalence and societal impact, discovering effective interventions for substance use is currently a policy priority.

E. E. Tanner-Smith (✉)
Department of Counseling Psychology and Human Services, College of Education, University of Oregon, Eugene, OR, USA
e-mail: etanners@uoregon.edu

S. P. Grant
Indiana University, Indianapolis, IN, Indiana
e-mail: spgrant@iu.edu

Strategies to prevent the development of problems with alcohol and other psychoactive substances are equally important as interventions to treat and manage the symptoms of those with established disorders. A wide range of prevention approaches can be used for addressing alcohol and illicit drug use (hereafter referred to as substance use) (Stockings et al., 2016). An Institute of Medicine framework provides a useful classification scheme for these various prevention approaches based on the targeted population (Mrazek & Haggerty, 1994): universal prevention programs are delivered to participants regardless of their current substance use, selected prevention programs are provided to participants identified as being members of subgroups of the population at high risk of unhealthy substance use, and indicated prevention programs are geared toward individuals already exhibiting high-risk substance use behaviors.

Brief interventions (BIs) represent one promising and prominent family of substance use prevention approaches that can be delivered at the universal, selected, and indicated prevention levels, although most BIs are delivered as selected or indicated based on screening for risk. We define BIs for substance use broadly as interventions delivered in a circumscribed time frame that aim to promote changes in substance use behaviors or their determinants. Although researchers and practitioners vary in their definitions of what counts as "brief" (e.g., Kazemi, Levine,

Dmochowski, Shou, & Angbing, 2013; Moyer, 2013), most BIs typically involve only a single session or contact with recipients, although multiple sessions may be required with higher-risk clients. As described in more detail below, BIs tend to vary on other key characteristics of interventions, such as procedures, materials, delivery personnel, format of delivery, location, dosage, underlying theory of change, and general intervention philosophy (Hoffmann et al., 2014). BIs are often appealing to substance use researchers and practitioners given their flexibility, transportability across settings and contexts, and brevity in delivery and implementation (Aalto, Pekuri, & Seppä, 2001; Neighbors, Barnett, Rohsenow, Colby, & Monti, 2010).

This chapter aims to summarize existing research on BIs for preventing substance use. Although BIs have also been used to prevent tobacco use and other health behaviors (e.g., Colby et al., 2005; Marcus et al., 2001; Petry, Weinstock, Ledgerwood, & Morasco, 2008; Stanley & Brown, 2012), this chapter focuses specifically on the evidence of BIs for preventing alcohol and other illicit substance use. We will describe the types of services that BIs for substance use typically provide, followed by a review of the current evidence base on the effectiveness of BIs in promoting substance use-related behavior change. We then discuss the current gaps in the evidence base regarding BIs for substance use prevention, highlighting important areas for future research.

Brief Intervention Strategies for Substance Use Prevention

The intervention philosophies and theories of change underlying BIs vary across different approaches. BIs are most often based on the Transtheoretical Model of Change (Prochaska, DiClemente, & Norcross, 1992), which posits that individuals move through a series of nonlinear stages when undergoing behavior change, namely precontemplation, contemplation, preparation, action, and maintenance. Individuals in the precontemplation stage have no intention to make behavior changes in the foreseeable future; those in the contemplation stage are considering making changes in the near future (typically within 6 months); those in the preparation stage intend to make behavior changes in the immediate future; those in the action stage are making or have recently made specific behavior modifications; and those in the maintenance stage have made behavior changes recently and are actively working to maintain those behavior changes. BIs based on this model are matched to an individual's specific stage of change. For instance, individuals in the contemplation stage are aware that they have unhealthy levels of substance use, but are not currently committed to taking action to change their substance use behaviors. Strategies such as decisional balance exercises (identifying the pros/cons of substance use) or goal-setting exercises (developing goals for behavior change) may therefore be appropriate for helping individuals in the contemplation stage move to the action stage. However, these types of activities may be inappropriate for participants in the precontemplation stage who have no intention to change their behavior and/or do not perceive a problem with their current substance use. Motivational interviewing and motivational enhancement techniques are commonly used in BIs that draw on the Transtheoretical Model of Change. Motivational enhancement approaches involve supportive and nonconfrontational therapeutic techniques that encourage motivation to change based on clients' readiness to change and self-efficacy for behavior change (Miller & Rollnick, 1991). BIs using these motivational enhancement approaches therefore aim to guide individuals through all stages of change until they ultimately are successful in maintaining changes in substance use behaviors.

In addition to the Transtheoretical Model, theories from other fields of psychology have influenced the design of BIs for substance use. For instance, many BIs are also based on cognitive and behavioral theories—most notably classical conditioning. BIs that draw on these theories typically involve cognitive behavioral therapy procedures focusing on teaching skills and cognitive restructuring techniques for dealing with stimuli that might trigger substance use relapse or substance cravings (Marlatt & Witkiewitz, 2005). BIs influenced by theories from social psychology often rely on social norms approaches, which attempt to correct mismatches between descriptive norms (clients' perceptions of peers' substance use behaviors) and injunctive norms (clients' perceptions of peers' attitudes toward substance use) (Cialdini, Kallgren, & Reno, 1991). Despite such diversity in these theories of change underlying most BIs, they share a foundation in psychological science's emphasis on mental abilities, capacities, and motivations as determinants of self-evaluating and self-regulating substance use behaviors.

BIs are often not delivered as isolated services, but are instead combined with approaches to identify those at risk of substance use problems and referring those with diagnosable disorders to appropriate treatment. Indeed, most selected and indicated BI prevention approaches are combined with screening assessments. In 2003, the Substance Abuse and Mental Health Services Administration launched the Screening, Brief Intervention, and Referral to Treatment (SBIRT) initiative to promote a comprehensive early intervention strategy for addressing substance use. In the SBIRT model, screening involves assessing the severity of an individual's substance use, information that can then be used to identify the appropriate level of intervention or treatment. Those identified via screening tools to exhibit unhealthy use receive a BI, with the possibility of tailoring the content of that BI to a particular individual or population based on the screening tool used and risk factors identified. Screening and BIs may be supplemented with referral to additional treatment or specialty care, based on the severity of substance use identified in screening and/or lack of behavior change following the BI. Because BIs are not always (but often) accompanied by screening and/or referral to treatment, this chapter focuses specifically on BIs (see SAMHSA, 2013, for additional resources related specifically to SBIRT). However, as described in greater detail below, it is worth noting the current lack of evidence that SBIRT is successful in increasing the use of substance use services (Glass et al., 2015) or improving clinical outcomes (Saitz, 2010) for adults exhibiting severe substance use in general healthcare settings.

Common Therapeutic Activities in Brief Interventions

Because BIs are a broad family of interventions that may be based on diverse underlying theories of change, the active ingredients or core components in BIs can also vary widely (McCambridge, 2013). Indeed, as noted previously, BIs based on the Transtheoretical Model often include specific tailoring of intervention content to individuals based on their readiness to change. Table 11.1 provides a list of some of the most common types of therapeutic components used in BIs for substance use, which we briefly describe here.

Decisional balance exercises involve working with a client to list the pros and cons of substance use, and to subjectively weigh the importance or salience of each positive and negative aspect of substance use (Migneault, Pallonen, & Velicer, 1997; Miller, 1999). These exercises are intended to promote behavior change by highlighting individuals' potential ambivalence about their current substance use, clarifying various motivational factors related to substance use, and encouraging potential behavior change.

Table 11.1 Commonly used therapeutic components in brief interventions for substance use

Decisional balance
Goal-setting or contracting
Personalized feedback
Feedback on substance use
Personalized normative feedback
Provision of information
Blood alcohol concentration/tolerance
Calories associated with alcohol
Consequences of substance use
Financial costs
Risk factors for substance use disorders
Skills training
Peer refusal skills
Moderation skills

Goal-setting or contracting exercises involve working with a client to agree upon goals for reducing substance use; typically these exercises focus on moderation or harm reduction (not abstinence). These exercises are designed to promote behavior change by explicitly specifying target goals and intentions to change behavior (Locke & Latham, 2002).

Personalized feedback involves providing individuals with tailored reports based on their responses to initial screening and assessment instruments (Walters & Neighbors, 2005). This feedback often involves a summary of clients' actual substance use, but may also provide normative feedback (i.e., information about perceived and actual substance use by peers). Personalized normative feedback can then provide information about perceived peer group norms of substance use, and compare individuals' own substance use to those norms. The peer reference group can vary in proximity—including proximal peer groups such as college campus norms or state-level age-matched groups, or more distal peer groups such as national, age-matched groups. Researchers and providers typically utilize the most proximal referent group for which data are available. These feedback components aim to promote behavior change by highlighting potential discrepancies between individuals' descriptive and injunctive norms around substance use.

Another common type of therapeutic activity includes the provision of information intended to motivate behavior change. These therapeutic components are often based on psychoeducational approaches to substance use intervention, which aim to promote behavior change by providing education and information intended to promote healthy behavior decision-making. The type of information provided can vary substantially, but might include, for instance, providing information regarding the risk factors for developing a clinical substance use disorder; economic, physical, psychological, and/or social consequences associated with substance use; financial costs associated with substance use (which can be personalized, based on individuals' responses to screening instruments that can be translated into annual costs); information about the calories in alcoholic drinks; and information about how to calculate blood alcohol concentration levels, or other information about substance use tolerance levels.

Skills training components are also commonly used in BIs, which are based on cognitive behavioral principles of teaching and rehearsal of various skills. This might include a focus on peer refusal skills, whereby individuals identify social settings and situations in which substance use may be likely, and practice skills for refusing substance use offers from peers. Other skills developed might focus on moderation strategies, such as identifying triggers for substance use or strategies for reducing the amount of substances consumed. These skills training components aim to promote behavior change by providing the cognitive and behavioral skills needed to navigate social environments that may cue unhealthy behaviors, and may be tailored based on the age, gender, race, or culture of participants.

Review of the Evidence Base for Brief Interventions

It is no surprise that there is a large and growing body of empirical research examining the effects of BIs in reducing substance use, given the brevity with which BIs can be delivered, and their transportability to diverse settings such as high schools, universities, primary health care, emergency departments, and other general healthcare settings. There has been fairly consistent evidence that alcohol BIs can lead to reductions in unhealthy alcohol use, although the magnitude of effects can vary across age of population (adolescent, young adult, adult), baseline alcohol severity (low, risky, dependent), and setting (school, community, primary care). To date, however, the evidence base for (non-alcohol) substance use-focused BIs has been less consistent. Here we review findings from recent systematic reviews and meta-analyses that have synthesized literature on BIs for substance use, supplemented with a discussion of relevant primary studies where appropriate.

One recent systematic review and meta-analysis of 185 randomized and controlled quasi-experimental evaluations of alcohol BIs among adolescents and young adults (primarily college samples of young adults) reported that alcohol BIs led to an average improvement in the magnitude of 0.27 standard deviations among adolescent samples and 0.17 standard deviations for young adult/college student samples (Tanner-Smith & Lipsey, 2015). These beneficial intervention effects were remarkably consistent across delivery provider, length of the BI, and type of youth participants. Overall, the modest beneficial effects of alcohol BIs for youth persisted for up to one year after the end of the intervention. This meta-analysis also reported that multiple behavior-focused BIs targeting both alcohol and illicit drugs (typically marijuana or mixed illicit substances) were efficacious in reducing both of these behaviors among adolescents and young adults (Tanner-Smith, Steinka-Fry, Hennessy, Lipsey, & Winters, 2015).

However, findings from this meta-analysis of alcohol BIs for adolescents and young adults indicated that effects varied across different types of BIs and for BIs delivered in different settings. Namely, alcohol BIs that used motivational interviewing, personalized normative feedback, and cognitive behavioral therapy approaches were consistently effective in reducing alcohol use; however, alcohol BIs targeting twenty-first birthday celebrations among college students had no (beneficial or harmful) effects in terms of reducing drinking during students' twenty-first birthday celebrations (Steinka-Fry, Tanner-Smith, & Grant, 2015). This meta-analysis further highlighted the small and inconclusive evidence base regarding the efficacy of alcohol BIs for adolescents when delivered in emergency departments (Tanner-Smith & Lipsey, 2015; see also Newton et al., 2013).

Other systematic reviews and meta-analyses have reported similar findings, indicating that alcohol BIs can lead to modest reductions in self-reported drinking among youth (e.g., Barnett, Sussman, Smith, Rohrbach, & Spruijt-Metz, 2012; Patton et al., 2014). Although the US Preventive Services Task Force (Moyer, 2013) concluded that there was insufficient evidence on the effects of alcohol BIs delivered in primary care for adolescents, the results from the more recent Tanner-Smith and Lipsey (2015) meta-analysis that synthesized the most current evidence base suggest that BIs may indeed be efficacious for adolescents in primary care.

Alcohol BIs have also been found to be generally efficacious in reducing self-reported drinking in adults exhibiting unhealthy alcohol use, typically defined as heavy episodic drinking and/or beginning to exhibit abuse, tolerance, or withdrawal symptoms of alcohol use disorder. For instance, in a systematic review and meta-analysis of 22 alcohol BIs trials in primary care for adults, Kaner et al. (2007) reported average reductions of 38 grams—or 2.7 standard drinks—per week, which persisted for up to one year of follow-up after the BI. This is similar in magnitude to effects reported in other meta-analyses of the alcohol BI literature among adults (e.g., Bertholet, Daeppen, Wietlisbach, Fleming, & Burnand, 2005; D'Onofrio & Degutis, 2002; Donoghue, Patton, Phillips, Deluca, & Drummond, 2014; Moyer, 2013). A recent review of systematic reviews and meta-analyses examining the effects of alcohol BIs in primary care also similarly concluded that they are efficacious in reducing drinking, particularly among middle-aged males (O'Donnell et al., 2014). Several reviews also conclude with recommendations to use BIs for alcohol-related problems in emergency departments with adult clients (D'Onofrio & Degutis, 2002; Nilsen et al., 2008).

Despite fairly consistent evidence regarding the beneficial effects of alcohol BIs in reducing self-reported drinking among adolescents, young adults, and adults, to date there is a much smaller evidence base regarding the effectiveness of BIs targeting substances other than alcohol (as noted by Saitz et al., 2010; Saitz, 2014a). For instance, a recent systematic review of the drug BI literature located only five randomized trials examining drug BI efficacy (Young et al., 2014). This systematic review concluded that although individual studies often reported reductions in cannabis and other drug use among participants, inconsistent measurement and reporting across studies precluded any meaningful synthesis that would permit strong conclusions regarding the current evidence base. Several high-quality trials have been published since the completion of that review, however. For instance, one recent trial examined the effects of a preventive BI for cannabis among adolescents in primary care, which reported small but significant beneficial effects on cannabis use equivalent to a 0.12 standard deviation improvement (Walton et al., 2014). In recent drug BI trials with adults in primary care settings, however, some studies have failed to find beneficial effects on unhealthy drug use, healthcare utilization, or self-help group attendance (Bogenschutz et al., 2014; Roy-Byrne et al., 2014; Saitz et al., 2014), whereas other studies have reported significant reductions in drug use equivalent to 3.5 fewer days of drug use per month (Gelberg et al., 2015). The inconsistency in the evidence base for drug BIs for adults in primary care settings has led some scholars to call for a return to the drawing board on how to reduce drug use in primary care settings (Hingson & Compton, 2014). It is important to note, however, that to date there have been few studies examining the effects of drug BIs, or multiple substance BIs, in other (nonprimary care) settings, or for adolescent and young adult samples. Thus, in returning to the drawing board, it is important to bring a renewed attention to the active ingredients and mechanisms of change in the BIs employed in trials and in real-world practice (Gaume, McCambridge, Bertholet, & Daeppen, 2014), while acknowledging that those active ingredients will likely need tailoring for different clients, contexts, and behavior change targets. We discuss some of these theoretically important mediators and moderators in the section below.

Moderators and Mediators of Effects

It is unrealistic to expect that BIs can or should produce consistent reductions in substance use for all types of clients in all contexts. Indeed, recent initiatives to promote precision medicine reflect the growing need for more nuanced understandings of individual characteristics associated with behavioral intervention effects, with the goal of promoting targeted and personalized intervention approaches (The White House, 2015). For the BI literature, this suggests a need for more refined research examining the moderators of intervention effects (for whom and under what contexts are BIs more or less effective), as well as mechanisms of action (what active ingredients and mediators drive the effects of BIs on behavior change).

Several individual or client characteristics are likely important moderators of the effects of BIs. Perhaps the most important client characteristic is risk level or severity of substance use. As noted in a recent systematic review, alcohol BIs in primary care settings are efficacious for adults with unhealthy alcohol use levels, but may not be appropriate for adults who exhibit heavy drinking or more severe alcohol use disorders (Saitz, 2010). Even among less heavy users, however, BI effects may vary for occasional users, risky users, or those meeting SUD diagnostic criteria (e.g., Doumas, Haustveit, & Coll, 2010). Other important client characteristics include gender (Kaner et al., 2007), race/ethnicity (Murphy, Dennhardt, Skidmore, Martens, & McDevitt-Murphy, 2010), and age or developmental stage (Tanner-Smith & Lipsey, 2015). Any future BI trials with variability in participant samples on these characteristics should thus consistently test whether these client level characteristics moderate intervention effects. Furthermore, future BI trials should always report intervention effects separately for these subgroups (regardless of the statistical significance of tests for moderation), to aid future meta-analyses that will synthesize these subgroup effects.

In addition to these more nuanced understandings of the types of clients for whom BIs may be more or less effective, there is a need for more refined analyses to identify the underlying mechanisms in BIs that elicit behavior change (Gaume et al., 2014). Although clients' readiness to change is sometimes posited as a potential mediator of BI effects, to date there has been minimal evidence to support this claim, and thus readiness to change may be more appropriately explored as a moderator of BI effects (Barnett et al., 2010; Borsari, Murphy, & Carey, 2009). Drawing on the Transtheoretical Model, social norms theory, and principles of motivational enhancement, other potential mediators to be explored include participants' descriptive and injunctive norms, beliefs and attitudes toward substance use, change talk during the intervention, and experiences of discrepancy during the intervention (Apodaca & Longabaugh, 2009; Barnett et al., 2010; Neighbors, Lee, Lewis, Fossos, & Walter, 2009; Turrisi et al., 2009). Future BI trials should specify logic models or theories of change, and test for potential mediators of intervention effects based on those logic models.

Directions for Advancing the BI Evidence Base

Despite the burgeoning literature of rigorous experimental and quasi-experimental evaluations examining the effects of BIs, there are several notable gaps in the current evidence base. First and foremost, more high-quality trials are needed to examine the overall effects of drug BIs on adolescents, young adults, and adult samples—and trials are needed to examine the feasibility and outcomes of drug BIs implemented in diverse settings (e.g., primary care, schools, community centers). Most prior trials and meta-analyses have focused exclusively on alcohol BIs; thus the evidence base for drug BIs is still nascent. Future trials on drug BIs should attend carefully to the measurement and reporting of participants' risk level, readiness to change, and the active ingredients or therapeutic components included in the BI—which may be important mediators or moderators of BI effects. In addition to this need for more research on the overall effects of drug BIs, however, future studies on BIs for substance use (whether alcohol, drug, or multiple behavior-targeted BIs) also need to attend to issues related to mediators and moderators of effects, outcome measurement, and implementation feasibility. We describe each of these areas below, highlighting research needs and opportunities.

Outcomes and Expected Effects

Two primary limitations in the current BI literature are the reliance on self-reported measures of substance use, and the inconsistent measurement and operationalization of substance use outcomes. The vast majority of BI trials to date have relied solely on self-reported measures of alcohol or illicit drug use (Tanner-Smith & Risser, 2016). Given the potential for reporting and social desirability bias in self-reported measures of substance use, future trials need to include biomarker outcomes (e.g., ethyl glucuronide, phosphatidylethanolamine) to at least verify and validate any self-reported assessments (Bradley & Lapham, 2016; Magura, Achtyes, Batts, Platt, & Moore, 2015).

Furthermore, there is a need for a core outcome set of validated and reliable measures of alcohol and other substance use. Prevention intervention trials—including those that evaluate BIs—do not consistently assess the same outcomes, and researchers often use measures of varying quality. For example, several Cochrane Collaboration reviews examining the effectiveness of interventions targeting adolescent alcohol use identified extensive heterogeneity of outcomes measured and found that key, relevant outcomes were typically not measured or reported (Foxcroft & Tsertsvadze, 2011a, 2011b, 2011c; Siegfried et al., 2014). In addition, researchers use different measures and even different definitions of outcomes. One review found at least 10 different definitions of an "alcohol-use outcome variable" across 20 trials—introducing a new definition of "alcohol use" on average every two trials—while another review found that less than 50% of the instruments or questionnaires used for measurement of alcohol misuse were validated (Foxcroft & Tsertsvadze, 2011a, 2011b). Such heterogeneous choice of outcome domains and outcome measures of varying quality hinders the ability of intervention trials to detect effects that may exist, synthesize or compare results across trials, and produce meaningful information for evidence-based policy and practice (Williamson et al., 2012; Williamson, Altman, Blazeby, Clarke, & Gargon, 2012).

Outcome measurement in effectiveness evaluations must be improved so the field can better understand the overall effects of substance use interventions (Foxcroft, Ireland, Lister-Sharp, Lowe, & Breen, 2003). Failing to consistently measure certain domains (e.g., age of substance use initiation, rates of substance-related risk behaviors, and substance-related injuries or accidents; Siegfried et al., 2014) that are important to stakeholders in substance use prevention—as well as the inconsistent use of valid, responsive, and practical measures for these outcome domains—hinders the ability of trials to detect effects that may exist and produce meaningful results for evidence-based policy and practice (Williamson, Altman, Blazeby, Clarke, Devane, et al., 2012; Williamson, Altman, Blazeby, Clarke, & Gargon, 2012). Groups developing core outcome sets could engage stakeholders (e.g., researchers, practitioners, and clients) to determine which outcomes each stakeholder group finds most important and the minimal clinically important difference (MCID) for these outcomes (Grant et al., 2016). These consensus-based core outcome sets and MCIDs could then be used to inform interpretations of effect sizes in systematic reviews that are sensitive to the views of important stakeholder groups, as well as to select outcomes for clinical audit and performance measurement (Grant, Mayo-Wilson, & Montgomery, 2016). Such a core outcome set must of course be sensitive to measures that need to vary across clients and contexts and by purpose. Expected sustainability of effects postintervention is also another important consideration, given the populations, targeted at-risk periods, and brevity of BIs (Grant, Pedersen, Osilla, Kulesza, & D'Amico, 2016a, 2016b).

Another important direction for future research is to examine the effects of substance use BIs on healthcare utilization and uptake rates, particularly when those BIs are combined with referrals to treatment (consistent with the SBIRT model). Indeed, despite evidence that alcohol BIs can be effective in reducing alcohol use, to date there is limited evidence regarding their effects on subsequent treatment utilization. In a meta-analysis of 13 trials, Glass et al. (2015) found no evidence that alcohol BIs were associated with increased or decreased utilization of alcohol-related care. Findings like this reflect a potential failure of BIs to adequately refer clients to other treatment services, which is a key link in the SBIRT process. Thus, in addition to behavioral measures of substance use, BI trials should also consider conducting longer term follow-up to measure other treatment utilization outcomes.

Implementation

Given prominent national efforts to integrate substance use interventions into medical and other settings (Hunter, Schwartz, & Friedmann, 2016), it is imperative to go beyond clinical effects and to actually consider implementation of BIs in real-world settings. Even in primary care settings, the best evidence supports efficacy rather than effectiveness in contexts that better resemble real-world practice (Saitz, 2014b). Process evaluations should be embedded within outcomes evaluations of BIs in order to provide critical information on how effective BIs might be reproduced in specific contexts (Moore et al., 2015). In addition, systematic reviews that involve qualitative meta-syntheses of primary literature offer an explicit, transparent method for developing robust descriptive and analytic themes about intervention implementation across a body of literature (Grant, Mayo-Wilson, & Montgomery, 2016). For instance, they can identify barriers and facilitators to implementation of BIs in specific contexts, such as adequate resources, training providers, and tools to screen and identify those at risk without stereotyping (Johnson, Jackson, Guillaume, Meier, & Goyder, 2011). A future focus on implementation can therefore inform the development of tools that help providers on the ground in delivering BIs. For example, clinical decision support tools can incorporate insights from qualitative meta-syntheses on implementation of the BI literature tailored to the specific barriers and facilitators individual clinicians might face.

Summary and Conclusion

Brief interventions (BIs) are promising approaches for preventing and reducing substance use. Most BIs rely on the Transtheoretical Model of Change and align therapeutic content with individuals' underlying stage of behavior change. Common therapeutic activities in BIs are decisional balance, goal-setting, personalized feedback, provision of information, and skills training activities. Despite fairly robust evidence that alcohol BIs can effectively reduce drinking among adolescents and adults, to date it is unclear whether and how BIs may affect other types of substance use among individuals. Indeed, given that BIs may not be universally effective, this chapter sought to identify important directions for future research. Most notably, the field is in need of high-quality research that explores mediators and moderators of BI effects on substance use, which will ultimately be useful in identifying mechanisms of change in these interventions and clarifying which subpopulations are most appropriate for targeting with BIs. Given their brevity in delivery and implementation, and transportability across settings and contexts, BIs are a promising family of interventions for substance use prevention efforts.

References

Aalto, M., Pekuri, P., & Seppä, K. (2001). Primary health care nurses' and physicians' attitudes, knowledge and beliefs regarding brief intervention for heavy drinkers. *Addiction, 96*(2), 305–311. https://doi.org/10.1046/j.1360-0443.2001.96230514.x

Apodaca, T. R., & Longabaugh, R. (2009). Mechanisms of change in motivational interviewing: A review and preliminary evaluation of the evidence. *Addiction, 104*(5), 705–715. https://doi.org/10.1111/j.1360-0443.2009.02527.x

Barnett, N. P., Apodaca, T. R., Magill, M., Colby, S. M., Gwaltney, C., Rohsenow, D. J., & Monti, P. M. (2010). Moderators and mediators of two brief interventions for alcohol in the emergency department. *Addiction, 105*(3), 452–465. https://doi.org/10.1111/j.1360-0443.2009.02814.x

Barnett, E., Sussman, S., Smith, C., Rohrbach, L. A., & Spruijt-Metz, D. (2012). Motivational interviewing for adolescent substance use: A review of the literature. *Addictive Behaviors, 37*(12), 1325–1334. https://doi.org/10.1016/j.addbeh.2012.07.001

Bertholet, N., Daeppen, J.-B., Wietlisbach, V., Fleming, M., & Burnand, B. (2005). Reduction of alcohol consumption by brief alcohol intervention in primary care: Systematic review and meta-analysis. *Archives of Internal Medicine, 165*, 986–995.

Boden, J. M., & Fergusson, D. M. (2011). Alcohol and depression. *Addiction, 106*(5), 906–914.

Bogenschutz, M. P., Donovan, D. M., Mandler, R. N., Perl, H. I., Forcehimes, A. A., Crandall, C., … Douaihy, A. (2014). Brief intervention for patients with problematic drug use presenting in emergency departments: A randomized clinical trial. *JAMA Internal Medicine, 174*(11), 1736. https://doi.org/10.1001/jamainternmed.2014.4052

Borsari, B., Murphy, J. G., & Carey, K. B. (2009). Readiness to change in brief motivational interventions: A requisite condition for drinking reductions? *Addictive Behaviors, 34*(2), 232–235. https://doi.org/10.1016/j.addbeh.2008.10.010

Bouchery, E. E., Harwood, H. J., Sacks, J. J., Simon, C. J., & Brewer, R. D. (2011). Economic costs of excessive alcohol consumption in the U.S., 2006. *American Journal of Preventive Medicine, 41*(5), 516–524. https://doi.org/10.1016/j.amepre.2011.06.045

Bradley, K. A., & Lapham, G. T. (2016). Is it time for a more ambitious research agenda for decreasing alcohol-related harm among young adults? *Addiction, 111*(9), 1531–1532. https://doi.org/10.1111/add.13235

Cherpitel, C. J., Martin, G., Macdonald, S., Brubacher, J. R., & Stenstrom, R. (2013). Alcohol and drug use as predictors of intentional injuries in two emergency departments in British Columbia: Alcohol and drug use as predictors. *The American Journal on Addictions, 22*(2), 87–92. https://doi.org/10.1111/j.1521-0391.2013.00316.x

Cialdini, R. B., Kallgren, C. A., & Reno, R. R. (1991). A focus theory of normative conduct: A theoretical refinement and reevaluation of the role of norms in human behavior. *Advances in Experimental Social Psychology, 24*, 201–234.

Colby, S. M., Monti, P. M., O'Leary Tevyaw, T., Barnett, N. P., Spirito, A., Rohsenow, D. J., … Lewander, W. (2005). Brief motivational intervention for adolescent smokers in medical settings. *Addictive Behaviors, 30*(5), 865–874. https://doi.org/10.1016/j.addbeh.2004.10.001

Degenhardt, L., & Hall, W. (2012). Extent of illicit drug use and dependence, and their contribution to the global burden of disease. *The Lancet, 379*(9810), 55–70. https://doi.org/10.1016/S0140-6736(11)61138-0

D'Onofrio, G., & Degutis, L. C. (2002). Preventive care in the emergency department: Screening and brief intervention for alcohol problems in the emergency department: A systematic review. *Academic Emergency Medicine, 9*(6), 627–638. https://doi.org/10.1197/aemj.9.6.627

Donoghue, K., Patton, R., Phillips, T., Deluca, P., & Drummond, C. (2014). The effectiveness of electronic screening and brief intervention for reducing levels of alcohol consumption: A systematic review and meta-analysis. *Journal of Medical Internet Research, 16*(6), e142. https://doi.org/10.2196/jmir.3193

Doumas, D. M., Haustveit, T., & Coll, K. M. (2010). Reducing heavy drinking among first year intercollegiate athletes: A randomized controlled trial of web-based normative feedback. *Journal of Applied Sport Psychology, 22*(3), 247–261. https://doi.org/10.1080/10413201003666454

Foxcroft, D. R., Ireland, D., Lister-Sharp, D. J., Lowe, G., & Breen, R. (2003). Longer-term primary prevention for alcohol misuse in young people: A systematic review. *Addiction, 98*(4), 397–411. https://doi.org/10.1046/j.1360-0443.2003.00355.x

Foxcroft, D. R., & Tsertsvadze, A. (2011a). Universal family-based prevention programs for alcohol misuse in young people. *Cochrane Database of Systematic Reviews, 9*, CD009308. https://doi.org/10.1002/14651858.CD009308

Foxcroft, D. R., & Tsertsvadze, A. (2011b). Universal multi-component prevention programs for alcohol misuse in young people. *Cochrane Database of Systematic Reviews, 9*, CD009307. https://doi.org/10.1002/14651858.CD009307

Foxcroft, D. R., & Tsertsvadze, A. (2011c). Universal school-based prevention programs for alcohol misuse in young people. *Cochrane Database of Systematic Reviews, 9*, CD009113. https://doi.org/10.1002/14651858.CD009113

Gaume, J., McCambridge, J., Bertholet, N., & Daeppen, J. B. (2014). Mechanisms of action of brief alcohol interventions remain largely unknown-a narrative review. *Frontiers in Psychiatry, 5*, 108. https://doi.org/10.3389/fpsyt.2014.00108

Gelberg, L., Andersen, R. M., Afifi, A. A., Leake, B. D., Arangua, L., Vahidi, M., ... Baumeister, S. E. (2015). Project QUIT (Quit Using Drugs Intervention Trial): A randomized controlled trial of a primary care-based multi-component brief intervention to reduce risky drug use. *Addiction, 110*(11), 1777–1790. https://doi.org/10.1111/add.12993

Glass, J. E., Hamilton, A. M., Powell, B. J., Perron, B. E., Brown, R. T., & Ilgen, M. A. (2015). Specialty substance use disorder services following brief alcohol intervention: A meta-analysis of randomized controlled trials: SBI and referral to treatment. *Addiction, 110*(9), 1404–1415. https://doi.org/10.1111/add.12950

Grant, S., Mayo-Wilson, E., & Montgomery, P. (2016). Implementing quality improvement for psychosocial interventions. *JAMA, 315*(9), 943–943. https://doi.org/10.1001/jama.2015.17855

Grant, S., Pedersen, E. R., Osilla, K. C., Kulesza, M., & D'Amico, E. J. (2016a). Reviewing and interpreting the effects of brief alcohol interventions: Comment on a Cochrane review about motivational interviewing for young adults. *Addiction, 111*(9), 1521–1527. https://doi.org/10.1111/add.13136

Grant, S., Pedersen, E. R., Osilla, K. C., Kulesza, M., & D'Amico, E. J. (2016b). It is time to develop appropriate tools for assessing minimal clinically important differences, performance bias and quality of evidence in reviews of behavioral interventions. *Addiction, 111*(9), 1533–1535. https://doi.org/10.1111/add.13380

Hingson, R., & Compton, W. M. (2014). Screening and brief intervention and referral to treatment for drug use in primary care: Back to the drawing board. *JAMA, 312*(5), 488–489. https://doi.org/10.1001/jama.2014.7863

Hoffmann, T. C., Glasziou, P. P., Boutron, I., Milne, R., Perera, R., Moher, D., ... Lamb, S. E. (2014). Better reporting of interventions: Template for intervention description and replication (TIDieR) checklist and guide. *BMJ, 348*, g1687. https://doi.org/10.1136/bmj.g1687

Hunter, S. B., Schwartz, R. P., & Friedmann, P. D. (2016). Introduction to the special issue on the studies on the implementation of integrated models of alcohol, tobacco, and/or drug use interventions and medical care. *Journal of Substance Abuse Treatment, 60*, 1–5. https://doi.org/10.1016/j.jsat.2015.10.001

Johnson, M., Jackson, R., Guillaume, L., Meier, P., & Goyder, E. (2011). Barriers and facilitators to implementing screening and brief intervention for alcohol misuse: A systematic review of qualitative evidence. *Journal of Public Health, 33*(3), 412–421. https://doi.org/10.1093/pubmed/fdq095

Kaner, E. F., Beyer, F., Dickinson, H. O., Pienaar, E., Campbell, F., Schlesinger, C., ... Burnand, B. (2007). Effectiveness of brief alcohol interventions in primary care populations. *Cochrane Database of Systematic Reviews, 2*, CD004148. https://doi.org/10.1002/14651858.CD004148.pub3

Kazemi, D. M., Levine, M. J., Dmochowski, J., Shou, Q., & Angbing, I. (2013). Brief motivational intervention for high-risk drinking and illicit drug use in mandated and voluntary freshman. *Journal of Substance Use, 18*(5), 392–404.

Locke, E. A., & Latham, G. P. (2002). Building a practically useful theory of goal setting and task motivation: A 35-year odyssey. *American Psychologist, 57*(9), 705–717. https://doi.org/10.1037//0003-066X.57.9.705

Magura, S., Achtyes, E. D., Batts, K., Platt, T., & Moore, T. L. (2015). Adding urine and saliva toxicology to SBIRT for drug screening of new patients. *The American Journal on Addictions, 24*(5), 396–399. https://doi.org/10.1111/ajad.12252

Marcus, A. C., Heimendinger, J., Wolfe, P., Fairclough, D., Rimer, B. K., Morra, M., ... Julesberg, K. (2001). A randomized trial of a brief intervention to increase fruit and vegetable intake: A replication study among callers to the CIS. *Preventive Medicine, 33*(3), 204–216. https://doi.org/10.1006/pmed.2001.0873

Marlatt, G. A., & Witkiewitz, K. (2005). Relapse prevention for alcohol and drug problems. In G. A. Marlatt & D. M. Donovan (Eds.), *Relapse prevention: Maintenance strategies in the treatment of addictive behaviors* (2nd ed., pp. 1–44). New York, NY: The Guilford Press.

McCambridge, J. (2013). Brief intervention content matters. *Drug and Alcohol Review, 32*(4), 339–341. https://doi.org/10.1111/dar.12044

Migneault, J. P., Pallonen, U. E., & Velicer, W. F. (1997). Decisional balance and stage of change for adolescent drinking. *Addictive Behaviors, 22*(3), 339–351.

Miller, W. R. (1999). *Enhancing motivation for change in substance abuse treatment* (Treatment Improvement Protocol (TIP) Series 35, DHHS Publication No. (SMA) 99–3354). Rockville, MD: U.S. Department of Health and Human Services, Substance Abuse and Mental Health Services Administration.

Miller, W. R., & Rollnick, S. (1991). *Motivational interviewing: Preparing people to change addictive behavior.* New York, NY: Guilford Press.

Moore, G. F., Audrey, S., Barker, M., Bond, L., Bonell, C., Hardeman, W., ... Baird, J. (2015). Process evaluation of complex interventions: Medical research council guidance. *BMJ, 350*, h1258. https://doi.org/10.1136/bmj.h1258

Moyer, V. A. (2013). Screening and behavioral counseling interventions in primary care to reduce alcohol misuse: U.S. preventive services task force recommendation statement. *Annals of Internal Medicine, 159*, 210–218. https://doi.org/10.7326/0003-4819-159-3-201308060-00652

Mrazek, P. J., & Haggerty, R. J. (Eds.). (1994). *Reducing risks for mental disorders: Frontiers for preventive intervention research.* Washington, DC: National Academies Press, Institute of Medicine.

Murphy, J. G., Dennhardt, A. A., Skidmore, J. R., Martens, M. P., & McDevitt-Murphy, M. E. (2010). Computerized versus motivational interviewing alcohol interventions: Impact on discrepancy, motivation, and drinking. *Psychology of Addictive Behaviors, 24*(4), 628–639. https://doi.org/10.1037/a0021347

Neighbors, C. J., Barnett, N. P., Rohsenow, D. J., Colby, S. M., & Monti, P. M. (2010). Cost-effectiveness of a motivational intervention for alcohol-involved youth in a hospital emergency department. *Journal of Studies on Alcohol and Drugs, 71*(3), 384–394.

Neighbors, C., Lee, C. M., Lewis, M. A., Fossos, N., & Walter, T. (2009). Internet-based personalized feedback to reduce 21st-birthday drinking: A randomized controlled trial of an event-specific prevention intervention. *Journal of Consulting and Clinical Psychology, 77*(1), 51–63. https://doi.org/10.1037/a0014386

Newton, A. S., Dong, K., Mabood, N., Ata, N., Ali, S., Gokiert, R., ... Wild, T. C. (2013). Brief emergency department interventions for youth who use alcohol and other drugs: A systematic review. *Pediatric Emergency Care, 29*(5), 673–684. https://doi.org/10.1097/PEC.0b013d31828ed325

Nilsen, P., Baird, J., Mello, M. J., Nirenberg, T., Woolard, R., Bendtsen, P., & Longabaugh, R. (2008). A systematic review of emergency care brief alcohol interventions for injury patients. *Journal of Substance Abuse Treatment, 35*(2), 184–201. https://doi.org/10.1016/j.jsat.2007.09.008

O'Donnell, A., Anderson, P., Newbury-Birch, D., Schulte, B., Schmidt, C., Reimer, J., & Kaner, E. (2014). The impact of brief alcohol interventions in primary healthcare: A systematic review of reviews. *Alcohol and Alcoholism, 49*(1), 66–78. https://doi.org/10.1093/alcalc/agt170

Patton, R., Deluca, P., Kaner, E., Newbury-Birch, D., Phillips, T., & Drummond, C. (2014). Alcohol screening and brief intervention for adolescents: The how, what and where of reducing alcohol consumption and related harm among young people. *Alcohol and Alcoholism, 49*(2), 207–212. https://doi.org/10.1093/alcalc/agt165

Petry, N. M., Weinstock, J., Ledgerwood, D. M., & Morasco, B. (2008). A randomized trial of brief interventions for problem and pathological gamblers. *Journal of Consulting and Clinical Psychology, 76*(2), 318–328. https://doi.org/10.1037/0022-006X.76.2.318

Prochaska, J. O., DiClemente, C. C., & Norcross, J. C. (1992). In search of how people change: Applications to addictive behaviors. *American Psychologist, 47*(9), 1102–1114.

Rehm, J., Baliunas, D., Borges, G. L. G., Graham, K., Irving, H., Kehoe, T., ... Taylor, B. (2010). The relation between different dimensions of alcohol consumption and burden of disease: An overview. *Addiction, 105*(5), 817–843. https://doi.org/10.1111/j.1360-0443.2010.02899.x

Roy-Byrne, P., Bumgardner, K., Krupski, A., Dunn, C., Ries, R., Donovan, D., ... Zarkin, G. A. (2014). Brief intervention for problem drug use in safety-net primary care settings: A randomized clinical trial. *JAMA, 312*(5), 492. https://doi.org/10.1001/jama.2014.7860

Saitz, R. (2010). Alcohol screening and brief intervention in primary care: Absence of evidence for efficacy in people with dependence or very heavy drinking. *Drug and Alcohol Review, 29*(6), 631–640. https://doi.org/10.1111/j.1465-3362.2010.00217.x

Saitz, R. (2014a). Screening and brief intervention for unhealthy drug use: Little or no efficacy. *Frontiers in Psychiatry, 5*, 121. https://doi.org/10.3389/fpsyt.2014.00121

Saitz, R. (2014b). The best evidence for alcohol screening and brief intervention in primary care supports efficacy, at best, not effectiveness: You say tomāto, I say tomăto? That's not all it's about. *Addiction Science & Clinical Practice, 9*, 14. https://doi.org/10.1186/1940-0640-9-14

Saitz, R., Alford, D. P., Bernstein, J., Cheng, D. M., Samet, J., & Palfai, T. (2010). Screening and brief intervention for unhealthy drug use in primary care settings: Randomized clinical trials are needed. *Journal of Addiction Medicine, 4*(3), 123–130. https://doi.org/10.1097/ADM.0b013e3181db6b67

Saitz, R., Palfai, T. P. A., Cheng, D. M., Alford, D. P., Bernstein, J. A., Lloyd-Travaglini, C. A., ... Samet, J. H. (2014). Screening and brief intervention for drug use in primary care: The ASPIRE randomized clinical trial. *JAMA, 312*(5), 502. https://doi.org/10.1001/jama.2014.7862

Siegfried, N., Pienaar, D. C., Ataguba, J. E., Volmink, J., Kredo, T., Jere, M., & Parry, C. D. H. (2014). Restricting or banning alcohol advertising to reduce alcohol consumption in adults and adolescents. *Cochrane Database of Systematic Reviews, 11*, CD010704. https://doi.org/10.1002/14651858.cd010704.pub2

Stanley, B., & Brown, G. K. (2012). Safety planning intervention: A brief intervention to mitigate suicide risk. *Cognitive and Behavioral Practice, 19*(2), 256–264. https://doi.org/10.1016/j.cbpra.2011.01.001

Steinka-Fry, K. T., Tanner-Smith, E. E., & Grant, S. (2015). Effects of 21st birthday brief interventions on college student celebratory drinking: A systematic review and meta-analysis. *Addictive Behaviors, 50*, 13–21. https://doi.org/10.1016/j.addbeh.2015.06.001

Stockings, E., Hall, W. D., Lynskey, M., Morley, K. I., Reavley, N., Strang, J., ... Degenhardt, L. (2016). Prevention, early intervention, harm reduction, and treatment of substance use in young people. *Lancet Psychiatry, 3*, 280–296.

Substance Abuse and Mental Health Services Administration (SAMHSA). (2013). *Systems-level implementation of screening, brief intervention, and referral to treatment* (Technical Assistance Publication (TAP) Series 33. HHS Publication No. (SMA) 13–4741). Rockville, MD: Substance Abuse and Mental Health Services Administration.

Substance Abuse and Mental Health Services Administration (SAMHSA). (2015). *Behavioral health trends in the United States: Results from the 2014 National Survey on Drug Use and Health*. Rockville, MD: Center for Behavioral Health Statistics and Quality, Substance Abuse and Mental Health Services Administration Retrieved from http://www.samhsa.gov/data/

Tanner-Smith, E. E., & Lipsey, M. W. (2015). Brief alcohol interventions for adolescents and young adults: A systematic review and meta-analysis. *Journal of Substance Abuse Treatment, 51*, 1–18. https://doi.org/10.1016/j.jsat.2014.09.001

Tanner-Smith, E. E., & Risser, M. D. (2016). A meta-analysis of brief alcohol interventions for adolescents and young adults: Variability in effects across alcohol measures. *The American Journal of Drug and Alcohol Abuse, 42*(2), 140–151. https://doi.org/10.3109/00952990.2015.1136638

Tanner-Smith, E. E., Steinka-Fry, K. T., Hennessy, E. A., Lipsey, M. W., & Winters, K. C. (2015). Can brief alcohol interventions for youth also address concurrent illicit drug use? Results from a meta-analysis. *Journal of Youth and Adolescence, 44*(5), 1011–1023. https://doi.org/10.1007/s10964-015-0252-x

Turrisi, R., Larimer, M. E., Mallett, K. A., Kilmer, J. R., Ray, A. E., Mastroleo, N. R., ... Montoya, H. (2009). A randomized clinical trial evaluating a combined alcohol intervention for high-risk college students. *Journal of Studies on Alcohol and Drugs, 70*(4), 555–567.

The White House. (2015). *The precision medicine initiative*. Retrieved from https://www.whitehouse.gov/precision-medicine

United Nations Office on Drugs and Crime (UNODC). (2012). *World drug report 2012. United Nations Publication, Sales No. E.12.XI.1*. Vienna, Austria: UNODC.

Walters, S. T., & Neighbors, C. (2005). Feedback interventions for college alcohol misuse: What, why and for whom? *Addictive Behaviors, 30*(6), 1168–1182. https://doi.org/10.1016/j.addbeh.2004.12.005

Walton, M. A., Resko, S., Barry, K. L., Chermack, S. T., Zucker, R. A., Zimmerman, M. A., ... Blow, F. C. (2014). A randomized controlled trial testing the efficacy of a brief cannabis universal prevention program among adolescents in primary care: Efficacy of a brief cannabis universal prevention program. *Addiction, 109*(5), 786–797. https://doi.org/10.1111/add.12469

Williamson, P., Altman, D., Blazeby, J., Clarke, M., & Gargon, E. (2012). Driving up the quality and relevance of research through the use of agreed core outcomes. *Journal of Health Services Research & Policy, 17*(1), 1–2. https://doi.org/10.1258/jhsrp.2011.011131

Williamson, P. R., Altman, D. G., Blazeby, J. M., Clarke, M., Devane, D., Gargon, E., & Tugwell, P. (2012). Developing core outcome sets for clinical trials: Issues to consider. *Trials, 13*(1), 132.

World Health Organization. (2009). *Global health risks mortality and burden of disease attributable to selected major risks*. Geneva: World Health Organization Retrieved from http://site.ebrary.com/id/10363978

Young, M. M., Stevens, A., Galipeau, J., Pirie, T., Garritty, C., Singh, K., ... Moher, D. (2014). Effectiveness of brief interventions as part of the Screening, Brief Intervention and Referral to Treatment (SBIRT) model for reducing the nonmedical use of psychoactive substances: A systematic review. *Systematic Reviews, 3*(1), 22. https://doi.org/10.1186/2046-4053-1-22

ATOD Prevention in Diverse Communities: Research and Receptivity

12

Anna Pagano, Raul Caetano, and Juliet P. Lee

Introduction-Ethnic Diversity in the USA

With the majority of its current population descended from non-indigenous people who arrived within only the last few hundred years, the USA has been considered an example of the settler colonial type of nation (Dunbar-Ortiz, 2014). Since the establishment of British colonies in the early seventeenth century, different groups have come to the USA under different circumstances. An estimated 300,000 enslaved Africans were brought to the USA by force and kept as slaves between 1626 and 1862, when they were emancipated by federal law (Emory University, 2013). For many immigrants, circumstances in their country of origin were the determining factors, such as lack of economic opportunities, sometimes famine (e.g., Ireland), sometimes, war. Many have come in search of better educational and economic opportunities, while others have come as refugees fleeing religious or political persecution. Beginning in the early 1800s the US population received Irish, German, Scandinavian, Italian, Polish, Asian, and Latin American immigrants. Migration from China was spurred by the Gold Rush of the late 1800s; a century later, many thousands of people fled warfare in Indochina to arrive to the USA as refugees.

Little by little, the earlier European immigrant groups such as Italians and the Irish were assimilated into US society. Non-white and/or multiracial groups such as African-Americans, Asian-Americans, and Hispanics, however, have been diacritically marked as "others" and marginalized from this process of European-dominant identity consolidation (Barth, 1998). These groups are identified today as racial/ethnic minorities that, together with American-Indians and Alaska Natives, are affected by considerable health disparities in relation to whites.

The socioeconomic and health disadvantages affecting racial/ethnic minority groups and indigenous people are rooted in past and present social adversity. African-Americans have a history marked by slavery and enduring racism. The history of American-Indians and Alaska Natives has also been distinctly affected by continuing racism and cultural domination. Discrimination has affected Asians and Hispanics as well, but these two groups have distinct histories of immigration to the USA, as do more recent immigrants of African descent. Recent immigrants, especially the foreign born, have unique challenges associated with acculturation to the US complex processes of adaptation and adoption of US cultural norms can be stressful, adding an important factor of risk that compounds existing health disparities and

A. Pagano (✉) · R. Caetano · J. P. Lee
Prevention Research Center, Pacific Institute for Research and Evaluation, Berkeley, CA, USA
e-mail: apagano@prev.org; Raul.Caetano@utsouthwestern.edu; jlee@prev.org

alcohol-related problems (Berry, 1997; Schwartz, Unger, Zamboanga, & Szapocznik, 2010).

While racial and ethnic minority groups and indigenous people are often described and studied within ATOD research as if homogeneous, they are quite diverse. American-Indians and Alaska Natives belong to many different tribes and nations with a variety of cultures and languages. Asians and Hispanics come from many countries with different cultural traditions. African-Americans are also diverse, with a sizeable subgroup of immigrants from the Caribbean and African nations. Although the US Census forces people into limited racial and ethnic categories, and health policies incorporate these categories, social reality is more complex.

The US population continues to be quite diverse. Data from the Census Bureau's March 2015 Current Population Survey show that whites are still a majority, and constituted 62% of the population in 2014. The same data show that blacks/African-Americans accounted for 12%, Hispanics for 18%, Asians for 6%, and American-Indians/Alaska Natives for 1%. About 2% of the population is identified as having two or more races (Kaiser Family Foundation, 2015).

This means that in 2014 roughly 36% of the US population belonged to a racial/ethnic minority group or tribal nation. Further, the Census Bureau estimates that by 2044 more than half of the US population will belong to a racial/ethnic minority group or tribal nation (Colby & Ortman, 2014). The proportion of the US population who is foreign born, many of whom belong to a racial/ethnic minority group, is also substantial, comprising 13% of the total population in 2010 (Grieco et al., 2012). Most of these individuals came from Latin America and the Caribbean (53%) and Asia (28%). Half of the foreign born are 18–44 years of age, a group that is at higher risk for substance use, although when compared to the US born the foreign born are usually at lower risk for problems related to substance use (Breslau & Chang, 2006; Ojeda, Patterson, & Strathdee, 2008). The foreign-born population is not evenly distributed across the country; more than half live in just four states: 25% in California, 11% in New York, 10% in Texas, and 9% in Florida. Prevention programs with racial/ethnic minorities or indigenous people should take nativity into consideration, especially so in these states. However, even states with a smaller proportion of foreign-born residents may have geographical regions such as large metropolitan areas that may be at variance with this population pattern.

Why Conduct ATOD Prevention Research in Ethnically Diverse Communities?

Conducting prevention research in ethnically diverse communities provides unique knowledge about the effectiveness of prevention programs in these communities, helping to ensure equitable access to evidence-based interventions. Prevention interventions may require adaptation to adequately address variations in socioeconomic, cultural, geographic, and policy contexts that can affect communities' access to and use of alcohol, tobacco, and other drugs. Such community-level variation in ATOD use can produce an unequal health burden over the life course. Just as ATOD-related problems vary, few if any preventive interventions are universally effective since implementation and success or failure of interventions are context dependent.

Many sociodemographic and cultural characteristics of racial/ethnic groups have been identified as protective or risk factors associated with substance use and the level and types of substance use-related problems these groups develop. For instance, religious affiliations that support abstention from drinking have been often linked to the higher rate of abstention among African-Americans (Herd, 1996; Herd & Grube, 1996). Family cohesion has been identified as a protective factor against substance use and problems among Hispanic-Americans (Caetano, Clark, & Tam, 1998; Marsiglia, Kulis, Parsai, & Garcia, 2009; Sale et al., 2005). Other factors may exacerbate risky ATOD (alcohol and other drug) use among racial/ethnic minorities, such as racial/ethnic discrimination (Chae et al., 2008; Mulia & Zemore, 2012; Okamoto, Ritt-Olson, Soto, Baezconde-Garbanati, & Unger, 2009), acculturation stress (Buchanan & Smokowski, 2009; Lee et al., 2013), and lower socioeconomic status (Jones-Webb, Hsiao, & Hannan, 1995).

Neighborhood factors may also play a role in ethnic minorities' ATOD problems, which occur at rates disproportionate to their ATOD use (Mulia, Ye, Greenfield, & Zemore, 2009) (Goldstick et al., 2015). First, there is often greater alcohol availability in low-income and ethnic minority neighborhoods due to a higher density of alcohol outlets such as bars and liquor stores (Berke et al., 2010; LaVeist & Wallace Jr., 2000). Higher concentration of alcohol outlets is related to greater incidence of intimate partner violence (Cunradi, Mair, Ponicki, & Remer, 2012), child maltreatment (Freisthler, Needell, & Gruenewald, 2005), and drunk driving (Gruenewald, Johnson, & Treno, 2002) which may occur far from the premises, as well as death and injuries from assaults that occur in closer proximity to alcohol outlets (Mair, Gruenewald, Ponicki, & Remer, 2013; Morrison, Mair, Lee, & Gruenewald, 2015). Researchers have also demonstrated the presence of targeted marketing by alcohol and tobacco companies to racial/ethnic minorities, which is observable at the neighborhood level (Alaniz, 1998; Moore, Williams, & Qualls, 1996).

Furthermore, racial/ethnic minorities in need of treatment for substance-use disorders (SUD) face greater barriers to accessing SUD services (Schmidt, Greenfield, & Mulia, 2006; Wells, Klap, Koike, & Sherbourne, 2001). These barriers include few affordable public services, long waiting lists, linguistic barriers in the case of individuals with LEP (limited English proficiency) (Guerrero, Pan, Curtis, & Lizano, 2011), and often transportation barriers (Guerrero, Kao, & Perron, 2013). Reduced access to prevention and treatment services for substance-use disorders can lead to more complicated and costly SUD-related mental and physical health problems down the line (Ettner et al., 2006).

Figure 12.1, adapted from Alegría et al. (1998), shows a schematic representation of the various factors that influence drinking and problems among ethnically diverse populations. The associations shown in the figure are not meant to be exhaustive. Also, most of the represented factors affect substance use by all individuals, although some ethnically defined communities face greater exposure to specific factors, such as poverty, crime, residential segregation, and discrimination. Also, the effect of potential or known risk factors can vary across communities and can be exacerbated by socioeconomic disadvantage and lack of access to health care. The implication of this factor for the development and implementation of prevention efforts in ethnically diverse communities is that there is no "one size fits all." Prevention interventions in ethnically diverse communities must take into account the social and cultural characteristics as well as the receptivity of these communities where such actions are being implemented. Receptivity by the community is often linked to the degree of congruence between the prevention actions being implemented and the community's social, cultural, and political contexts.

From a public health prevention perspective, the most important circles in Fig. 12.1 are the three at the top, that is, those that identify (from left to right) general environmental factors, substance-use contexts, and individual. While the latter group is not intervened upon directly by public health substance-use prevention polices, individual characteristics interact in dynamic ways with the factors in the other two circles. For instance, a previous study indicated that for Hispanics with DUI involvement, the home was a frequent place of drinking before the "last DUI event" (Caetano & Raspberry, 2001). For whites with DUI involvement, the most frequent place of drinking before the last DUI event was a bar. Further, those who are underage seldom drink alcohol in public venues such as bars. Being underage increases the likelihood that drinking will take place mostly in unsupervised locales such as parking lots, parks, or parties (Coleman & Cater, 2005; Mayer, Forster,

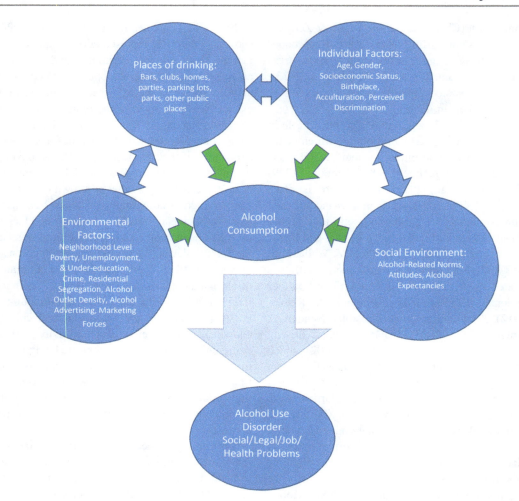

Fig. 12.1 Conceptual framework of alcohol consumption, alcohol-related problems, and treatment (adapted from Alegría and McGuire 2003)

Murray, & Wagenaar, 1998). Ethnicity may also be associated with drinking locations. For instance, one study found that European-American adolescents were more likely to engage in outdoor drinking, while their African-American peers were more likely to consume alcohol either alone or in school or work settings (Stewart & Power, 2003). Finally, the three circles of interest are shown with arrows representing reciprocal associations. For example, an environmental level factor such as residential segregation can have an impact on alcohol availability (LaVeist & Wallace Jr, 2000) and illicit drug use (Cooper, Friedman, Tempalski, & Friedman, 2007).

Cultural Competence

Given the cultural diversity of the US population, cultural competence is an important attribute of a well-trained health professional workforce, including prevention researchers. The Substance Abuse and Mental Health Services Administration (SAMHSA) has paid considerable attention to the development of knowledge related to cultural competence, including definitions and criteria for assessment of training in this area. SAMHSA defines cultural competence as "the ability to interact effectively with people of different cultures." It means to be respectful and responsive to the health beliefs and practices—and cultural and linguistic needs—of diverse population groups. Further, according to SAMHSA, recognition of the unique cultures of population groups does not apply to race/ethnicity only but should also include other factors such as gender, age, sexual orientation, and religion (Substance Abuse and Mental Health Services Administration, 2016).

To work effectively with racial/ethnically diverse communities, prevention researchers must understand and respect the cultural contexts of their community partners. Knowledge about culture need not exist a priori, but the prevention researcher must be willing to learn from community members and be skilled enough to adapt prevention actions to the cultural characteristics of the community. Attention to how community members communicate with one another, refer to substance use in the community, and identify cultural processes that they believe are protective for preventing substance use are all steps in this learning process. Epidemiological and ethnographic studies of the community can also provide important guidance for developing prevention actions. These studies can provide crucial understanding about risk and protective factors affecting substance use in the community.

Cultural competence is an attribute not only of individual researchers and service providers, but also of organizations. It is difficult, if not impossible, for a prevention practitioner to be culturally competent and work successfully in an organization that does not value such an approach. If the organization is not culturally competent, chances are that the prevention framework adopted and implemented by the organization will also fail to exhibit such competence. The National Center for Cultural Competence (NCCC) at Georgetown University Center for Child and Human Development has identified characteristics of culturally competent organizations (National Center for Cultural Competence, 2007). According to the NCCC, these organizations possess the characteristics listed in Box 1, below. Essentially, they have a mission, policies, and practices that incorporate cultural competence and active community participation and engagement. They also have a culturally competent workforce, provide fiscal support and professional development to strengthen cultural competence, and have capacity to collect and analyze data in a culturally meaningful way. Unfortunately, few of the organizations working with prevention intervention in minority communities have all of these characteristics.

> **Box 1. Characteristics of Culturally Competent Organizations**
>
> Have a mission statement for the organization that articulates principles, rationale, and values for cultural and linguistic competence in all aspects of the organization.
>
> Implement specific policies and procedures that integrate cultural and linguistic competence into each core function of the organization.
>
> Identify, use, and/or adapt evidence-based and promising practices that are culturally and linguistically competent.
>
> Develop structures and strategies to ensure consumer and community participation in the planning, delivery, and evaluation of the organization's core function.
>
> Implement policies and procedures to recruit, hire, and maintain a diverse and culturally and linguistically competent workforce.
>
> Provide fiscal support, professional development, and incentives for the improvement of cultural and linguistic competence at the board, program, and faculty and/or staff levels.
>
> Dedicate resources for both individual and organizational self-assessment of cultural and linguistic competence.
>
> Develop the capacity to collect and analyze data using variables that have meaningful impact on culturally and linguistically diverse groups.
>
> Practice principles of community engagement that result in the reciprocal transfer of knowledge and skills between all collaborators, partners, and key stakeholders.

ATOD Prevention Research Within Ethnically Diverse Communities

Personal choices and behaviors influence only part of what determines an individual's health status, while social determinants of health—economic and social conditions—influence the health of people and communities as a whole (Cerdá, Tracy, Ahern, & Galea, 2014; Marmot, 2005; Phelan, Link, & Tehranifar, 2010). Many unfavorable health outcomes that affect communities—particularly low-income and communities of color—are due to the circumstances in which people live, work, age, socialize, and form relationships. Negative health outcomes are exacerbated by gaps in healthcare and social welfare systems serving minority communities.

To maximize effectiveness, ATOD prevention efforts in ethnically diverse communities should be responsive not only to community-specific cultural factors, but also to aspects of the socioeconomic and physical environments in which the communities are embedded and which shape their ATOD availability and use patterns (Blume, 2016; Galvan & Caetano, 2003). Interactions between individuals and environmental factors constitute an "ecology" of ATOD use (Gruenewald, Millar, & Treno, 1993) that both constitutes health disparities and holds important clues to their amelioration.

Prevention interventions based on public health research can affect ATOD use in diverse communities in several ways. For instance, these interventions can reduce alcohol and tobacco retailers' market power by limiting advertising in ethnic minority and indigenous communities. In Chicago, a community-university coalition used research data to address excessive alcohol and tobacco advertising concentrated in African-American and Latino-predominant neighborhoods (Hackbarth et al., 2001). The coalition mapped billboards with alcohol or tobacco content located near schools, parks, or playgrounds throughout the city, and presented this data to the Chicago City Council. Although the coalition faced pushback from the advertising companies who had placed the ads, they succeeded in convincing the Council to pass a stringent zoning ordinance limiting the billboards.

Another example of intervening in the alcohol marketing environment is responsible beverage service (RBS) interventions, in which retailers are trained to avoid selling alcohol to minors or intoxicated patrons. The Sacramento Neighborhood Alcohol Prevention Project implemented RBS interventions in two predominantly Hispanic neighborhoods (Treno, Gruenewald, Lee, & Remer, 2007). The intervention reduced sales to minors in the target area over time, thus restricting supply and reducing alcohol availability to priority populations for alcohol intervention.

Moore et al. (2012) observed that underage American-Indian youth were easily able to buy alcohol at stores located on- and off-reservations in California. To reduce alcohol availability, the researchers implemented a "reminder and reward" program through which underage-appearing American-Indian individuals attempted to purchase alcohol. If they were not asked for identification, the research team sent the store a reminder that their staff was violating underage drinking laws. If identification was requested, the store received a gift card reward. The intervention eventually resulted in 100% store compliance. As with the RBS intervention described in the previous section, Moore and colleagues' apparent minor intervention affected both the legal and economic environments simultaneously.

ATOD prevention research can also address aspects of the natural and built environment that constitute barriers or supports to ATOD use and problem use, such as urban versus rural locations. Alcohol availability may be reduced in rural locations (Dixon & Chartier, 2016), while living in poorly maintained urban buildings may contribute to heavier drinking (Bernstein, Galea, Ahern, Tracy, & Vlahov, 2007). Although the physical environment may be inalterable, interventions can address the way people interact with their physical environments. For instance, community gardening interventions in inner-city neighborhoods aim to strengthen interpersonal bonds, improve residents' mental health, and repurpose areas of disuse that invite ATOD consumption and illicit drug dealing (Garvin, Branas, Keddem, Sellman, & Cannuscio, 2013; Rose & Thompson, 2012).

Prevention interventions may reduce ATOD use by tapping into culturally based ATOD norms. ATOD norms often differ among ethnic communities, and among gender and age groups within these communities. For instance, within many Latino cultures, it has traditionally been more socially acceptable for men than for women to engage in public heavy drinking (Canino, 1994). Among certain ethnic groups in Nigeria, male elders have traditionally been expected to drink more at public gatherings than younger men (Oshodin, 1995). In regard to ethnic minority communities in the USA, ATOD consumption norms may vary further according to whether community members were born in the USA or elsewhere, how long they have resided in the host country, and their immigration status (which affects access to employment, and therefore shapes living conditions and access to alcohol and other drugs).

In a recent review of advances in substance-abuse prevention and treatment among racial/ethnic and sexual minority populations, Blume (2016) discussed the importance of culturally meaningful programs that focus on the family rather than individuals. Lee and colleagues used a family focus in their MI (motivational interviewing) intervention for Latino immigrant men who were regularly engaging in heavy drinking (Lee et al., 2011). Rather than focusing on individual motivations for heavy drinking, the culturally adapted intervention focused on immigration-related stressors such as separation from family and friends. Rather than discussing personal benefits of reducing alcohol intake, the tool encouraged men to think about their responsibility to spouses and children back home, their ability to support their families through remittances, and their culturally salient role as family provider.

Implementation Considerations

Implementing effective, culturally appropriate ATOD interventions across diverse communities generally requires adaptation and careful attention to context-specific aspects of implementation that may influence outcomes. These include (but are not limited to) *fidelity*, or the extent to which the implemented program retains its original principles and characteristics; *adaptability*, or the extent to which a program can be altered to reflect community context; *compatibility*, or the degree to which the program is congruent with community characteristics; and *participant responsiveness*, or community receptivity to the program (Durlak & DuPre, 2008).

Evaluation to determine community receptivity is a key component of implementation analysis. An example of this is a community-specific adaptation of the Community Readiness Model or CRM, first developed at Colorado State University's Tri-Ethnic Center for Prevention Research (Oetting et al., 1995). The adapted CRM was deployed as part of a community mobilization intervention to prevent youth inhalant use in rural Alaska (Ogilvie et al., 2008). Community mobilization was the first of a three-step intervention that also included environmental prevention strategies in home, school, and retail settings, and a school-based life skill curriculum for preadolescents. At this stage, the CRM was used to assess community members' readiness to engage in concrete action to prevent youth inhalant use. Prior to initiating the mobilization intervention in four communities with significant proportions of Alaska Natives, researchers conducted community readiness assessments with key informants representing community systems identified as locally influential. These included 7–9 community experts in each of the following areas: behavioral health, court system, elders, faith organizations, families, health care, law enforcement, media, policymakers, retailers, schools, social services, and tribal leaders. Researchers then used CRM assessment scores to initiate a dialogue with community members, including specially appointed community prevention officers, about how they envisioned a successful mobilization strategy. They repeated the assessment post-intervention with the same community experts (or, if they were unavailable, experts from the same community subsystems), and again shared with the community the change in readiness pre- and post-mobilization. Significant positive changes in community readiness were found for each of the four communities. In other words, community receptivity to the planned preventive interventions had increased through mobilization efforts.

Fidelity and adaptability are other important considerations when implementing evidence-based interventions across different communities; there is a tension between consistency of format and flexibility of content (Castro, Barrera Jr., & Martinez Jr., 2004). In the previous example, the CRM assessment tool was adjusted substantively to reflect characteristics of the community where interventions were being deployed as well as the health problem being addressed. Researchers worked with colleagues at Colorado State University's Tri-Ethnic Prevention Research Center to ensure that the tool maintained its validity. Part of how they did this was to retain the original nine stages and six dimensions of community readiness from the CRM. The final steps in adjusting the tool consisted of pretesting it among local community members, soliciting their feedback on how to improve it (e.g., simplifying language and clarifying details of inhalant use), consulting Colorado state experts once again, and then creating a final version of the tool. These final steps, which exemplify an iterative cycle of negotiation between fidelity and adaptability, also helped to ensure local compatibility of the intervention. Further examples of iterative consultation with community members to adapt ATOD interventions in a culturally appropriate way abound in the literature (Gilder et al., 2011; Jumper-Reeves, Dustman, Harthun, Kulis, & Brown, 2014; Netto, Bhopal, Lederle, Khatoon, & Jackson, 2010; Okamoto, Kulis, Marsiglia, Holleran Steiker, & Dustman, 2014; Ringwalt & Bliss, 2006).

Community-Based Participatory Research

Thus far, we have focused on ATOD prevention research and program implementation in ethnically diverse communities. In so doing, we have highlighted community-responsive approaches used by prevention researchers. Based on these examples and on our own work, we believe that community participation should be an integral part of program design and implementation. Grassroots engagement has great potential to deepen the investigation of the social determinants of health and move intervention strategies into innovative modalities and structures, perhaps with high risks but also with potential for high rewards, to address seemingly intractable health issues. Grassroots engagement may support community ownership and institutionalization of intervention strategies, and develop new leadership capacities to improve community well-being.

Community-based participatory research, or CBPR, is a community-driven process in which researchers and community members work as a team. CBPR is an approach to research, rather than a method or methodology. Together, the team of community members and researchers (1) determines the subject of the research, (2) chooses and sometimes creates the research methods, (3) collects and analyzes the data, and (4) takes action to change fundamental social structures and relationships (Cornwall & Jewkes, 1995).

The CBPR movement in research and prevention was developed in recognition of a need for more participation by community members in the research process (Israel, Schulz, Parker, & Becker, 2001). CBPR promotes researchers building relationships with communities and developing interventions that derive from the communities' assessments of their needs, rather than from external experts' assumptions about what is needed (O'Fallon & Dearry, 2002). Through participation in research, community members can bring their life experiences to the research process and therefore more accurately identify health issues unique to that community and the root causes of these conditions, increasing the likelihood that research findings will effect structural changes for the benefit of the community's health. The participation of community members in public health research is critical to understanding the concrete ways that inequality and disparity are related to health in any community.

Biggs (1989) delineated four levels of community participation in CBPR projects: *contractual*—community members are contracted into projects of researchers to take part in their inquiries or experiments; *consultative*—community members are asked for their opinions and not consulted by researchers before interventions are designed; *collaborative*—researchers and community members work together on projects designed, initiated, and managed by researchers; and *collegiate*—researchers and community members work together as colleagues with different skills to offer, in a process of mutual learning where local people have control over the process.

In the collegiate form of CBPR, which is the most inclusive and egalitarian, popular education is typically used to develop a collective analysis based on the life experiences of those involved in the project. Popular education is rooted in the principles and philosophy of Paulo Freire (1970) and liberation struggles of marginalized and excluded peoples. It is a form of political education that uses a framework of action and reflection to generate collective social changes meant to empower the community. Popular education is based on principles of democracy and promotes participation, interaction, social action, and critical thinking skills of analysis. Through the use of popular education, participants can share their individual experiences and analyze the roots of existing social problems collectively (Travers, 1997). Popular education provides the methods, tools, and theory needed to help groups of people understand their experiences within a specific social and political context and move from blaming themselves to having a perspective on the environmental and structural causes of the problems they face. Using a popular education approach, communities can develop strategies to address these root causes while enhancing their confidence and ability to effect positive change on their own behalf.

Within US-based prevention research, there has been increasing interest in community-engaged approaches (Myser, 2004); however, it is often unclear how "the community" should be represented in research products such as publications and presentations (Mair et al., 2010). Typically, when community members are engaged in community-based research, their involvement is limited to focus groups and key informant interviews conducted by a research expert who extracts information from participants on preselected topics. The results of this research may be analyzed and interpreted by the professional researchers, possibly with consultation from other professionals within the community, and utilized to improve outreach for health education, prevention programs, and other interventions. Dutta (2007) refers to this type of approach as a *cultural sensitivity approach*, while Peterson (2010) refers to it as *cultural tailoring* and contrasts it with a *culturally centered approach* in which "alternative theories of health are generated by engaging in meaning-making with cultural participants."

A culturally centered, collegiate approach to ATOD preventive interventions ideally should entail an initial phase in which researchers and community partners engage in dialogue regarding the latter's perceptions of ATOD use in their community. To what extent do community partners see ATOD use as a source of health problems? What changes, if any, would they like to see in ATOD use and its consequences within the community? What are their ideas about acceptable and feasible ways to address ATOD-related problems?

To initiate this dialogue with the community, researchers typically approach key community leaders and co-establish a conduit for maintaining productive collaboration. CBPR projects often begin by inviting community leaders, perhaps from community-serving health and/or social service organizations, to participate in a community advisory board (CAB). The first meetings with the CAB might concern characteristics of ATOD use in the community and perceived problems, followed by preliminary plans to engage the wider community. This may take the form of a needs assessment, such as conducting a survey at a community event. It may also involve information gathering about ATOD availability, for example via systematic observations and assessment of alcohol or tobacco outlets and their proximity to schools, parks, or residential areas (Lee, Lipperman-Kreda, Saephan, & Kirkpatrick, 2013). The needs assessment might also involve conducting community focus groups to gather baseline data on perceived impacts of ATOD use and misuse, and soliciting data from local criminal justice agencies and hospitals on baseline prevalence and incidence rates of ATOD-related health problems. Community members can then be enlisted to co-create an intervention plan that they believe will be effective and elicit high community receptivity. At the implementation stage, community-based researchers can help to recruit program participants, collect data, conduct formative and summative assessments, analyze data, and disseminate the data to community and scientific forums.

Conclusions

There is a need for increased support of ATOD prevention research within racial/ethnic minority and indigenous communities. In this chapter, we have discussed reasons why this research is important; presented "best practices" of cultural competence in ATOD prevention research and services; reviewed examples of successful ATOD preventive interventions conducted in racial/ethnic minority and indigenous communities; provided reflections on implementation; and reviewed CBPR principles and practices.

There are several ways to improve ATOD preventive intervention studies in diverse communities. First, we as prevention researchers should devote increased effort, when possible given resource constraints, to pre-intervention studies of community contexts. To construct an effective intervention, researchers must understand the everyday contexts of ATOD use, misuse, and related problems for communities. Ethnographic research, in which researchers spend time in communities making relevant observations and speaking with community members, is one of the most effective ways to gather information on context. If feasible, community members should be included in the design and implementation of the intervention. Their insider insights are invaluable for creating interventions that will be acceptable to community members, effective and sustainable after the research project has ended.

Of course, none of this is simple. CBPR approaches are resource intensive, especially in the initial stages, and usually involve negotiating a series of local social and political challenges. Nevertheless, it is our position that studies with more community involvement lead to increased participant buy-in and a greater chance of success.

Additionally, the most effective interventions address community-level contextual factors, which we reviewed above, in addition to individual behaviors, knowledge, and attitudes regarding ATOD use. ATOD use and resulting community health problems should be engaged from a public health perspective—that is, using a host-agent-environment model—and addressed through environmental interventions (Aguirre-Molina & Gorman, 1996; Holder, 1994). This approach not only is more effective than behavioral interventions alone, but also avoids stigmatizing low-income minority communities the way a primary focus on individual behaviors might. If the field of ATOD prevention in diverse communities is to move forward, interventions should address social determinants of ATOD-related health problems with the goal of empowering communities to achieve greater health equity.

References

Aguirre-Molina, M., & Gorman, D. M. (1996). Community-based approaches for the prevention of alcohol, tobacco, and other drug use. *Annual Review of Public Health, 17*(1), 337–358.

Alaniz, M. L. (1998). Alcohol availability and targeted advertising in racial/ethnic minority communities. *Alcohol Research and Health, 22*(4), 286.

Alegría, M., Vera, M., Negrón, G., Burgos, M., Albizu, C., Canino, G., … Roman, A. (1998). Methodological and conceptual issues in understanding female Hispanic drug users. In C. Wetherington & A. Roman (Eds.), *Drug addiction research and the health of women* (pp. 529–551). Bethesda, MD: National Institute on Drug Abuse.

Alegría, M., & McGuire, T. (2003). Rethinking a Universal Framework in the Psychiatric Symptom-Disorder Relationship. Journal of Health and Social Behavior, 44(3), 257–274.

Barth, F. (1998). *Ethnic groups and boundaries: The social organization of culture difference*. Long Grove, IL: Waveland Press.

Berke, E. M., Tanski, S. E., Demidenko, E., Alford-Teaster, J., Shi, X., & Sargent, J. D. (2010). Alcohol retail density and demographic predictors of health disparities: A geographic analysis. *American Journal of Public Health, 100*(10), 1967–1971.

Bernstein, K. T., Galea, S., Ahern, J., Tracy, M., & Vlahov, D. (2007). The built environment and alcohol consumption in urban neighborhoods. *Drug and Alcohol Dependence, 91*(2), 244–252.

Berry, J. W. (1997). Immigration, acculturation, and adaptation. *Applied Psychology, 46*(1), 5–34.

Biggs, S. D. (1989). *Resource-poor farmer participation in research: A synthesis of experiences from nine national agricultural research systems* (Vol. 3). Hague: OFCOR: International Service for National Agricultural Research.

Blume, A. W. (2016). Advances in substance abuse prevention and treatment interventions among racial, ethnic, and sexual minority populations. *Alcohol Research: Current Reviews, 38*(1), 47–54.

Breslau, J., & Chang, D. F. (2006). Psychiatric disorders among foreign-born and US-born Asian-Americans in a US national survey. *Social Psychiatry and Psychiatric Epidemiology, 41*(12), 943–950.

Buchanan, R. L., & Smokowski, P. R. (2009). Pathways from acculturation stress to substance use among latino adolescents. *Substance Use & Misuse, 44*(5), 740–762.

Caetano, R., Clark, C. L., & Tam, T. (1998). Alcohol consumption among racial/ethnic minorities: Theory and research. *Alcohol Research and Health, 22*(4), 233.

Caetano, R., & Raspberry, K. (2001). DUI-arrest characteristics among white and Mexican-American DUI offenders mandated for treatment. *Journal of Studies on Alcohol, 62*(6), 750–753.

Canino, G. (1994). Alcohol use and misuse among Hispanic women: Selected factors, processes, and studies. *International Journal of the Addictions, 29*(9), 1083–1100.

Castro, F., Barrera, M., Jr., & Martinez, C., Jr. (2004). The cultural adaptation of prevention interventions: Resolving tensions between fidelity and fit. *Prevention Science, 5*(1), 41–45.

Cerdá, M., Tracy, M., Ahern, J., & Galea, S. (2014). Addressing population health and health inequalities: the role of fundamental causes. *American Journal of Public Health, 104*(S4), S609–S619.

Chae, D. H., Takeuchi, D. T., Barbeau, E. M., Bennett, G. G., Lindsey, J. C., Stoddard, A. M., & Krieger, N. (2008). Alcohol disorders among Asian Americans: associations with unfair treatment, racial/ethnic discrimination, and ethnic identification (the national Latino and Asian Americans study, 2002–2003). *Journal of Epidemiology and Community Health, 62*(11), 973–979.

Colby, S. L., & Ortman, J. M. (2014). *Projections of the size and composition of the U.S. population: 2014–2060 current population reports* (pp. 25–1143). Washington, DC.

Coleman, L., & Cater, S. (2005). Underage 'binge' drinking: A qualitative study into motivations and outcomes. *Drugs: Education, Prevention and Policy, 12*(2), 125–136.

Cooper, H. L. F., Friedman, S. R., Tempalski, B., & Friedman, R. (2007). Residential segregation and injection drug use prevalence among black adults in US metropolitan areas. *American Journal of Public Health, 97*(2), 344–352.

Cornwall, A., & Jewkes, R. (1995). What is participatory research? *Social Science & Medicine, 41*(12), 1667–1676.

Cunradi, C. B., Mair, C., Ponicki, W., & Remer, L. (2012). Alcohol outlet density and intimate partner violence-related emergency department visits. *Alcoholism: Clinical and Experimental Research, 36*(5), 847–853.

Dixon, M. A., & Chartier, K. G. (2016). Alcohol use patterns among urban and rural residents: demographic and social influences. *Alcohol Research: Current Reviews, 38*(1), 69.

Dunbar-Ortiz, R. (2014). *An indigenous peoples' history of the United States*. Boston, MA: Beacon Press.

Durlak, J., & DuPre, E. (2008). Implementation matters: A review of research on the influence of implementation on program outcomes and the factors affecting implementation. *American Journal of Community Psychology, 41*(3–4), 327–350.

Dutta, M. J. (2007). Communicating about culture and health: Theorizing culture-centered and cultural sensitivity approaches. *Communication Theory, 17*(3), 304–328.

Emory University. (2013). *Table, 1501 to 1866*. Voyages: The Transatlantic Slave Trade Retrieved from http://www.slavevoyages.org/assessment/estimates

Ettner, S. L., Huang, D., Evans, E., Rose Ash, D., Hardy, M., Jourabchi, M., & Hser, Y.-I. (2006). Benefit–cost in the California treatment outcome project: Does substance abuse treatment "pay for itself"? *Health Services Research, 41*(1), 192–213.

Freire, P. (1970). *Pedagogy of the oppressed*. New York: Continuum.

Freisthler, B., Needell, B., & Gruenewald, P. J. (2005). Is the physical availability of alcohol and illicit drugs related to neighborhood rates of child maltreatment? *Child Abuse & Neglect, 29*(9), 1049–1060.

Galvan, F. H., & Caetano, R. (2003). Alcohol use and related problems among ethnic minorities in the United States. *Alcohol Research & Health, 27*(1), 87–94.

Garvin, E., Branas, C., Keddem, S., Sellman, J., & Cannuscio, C. (2013). More than just an eyesore: Local insights and solutions on vacant land and urban health. *Journal of Urban Health, 90*(3), 412–426.

Gilder, D. A., Luna, J. A., Calac, D., Moore, R. S., Monti, P. M., & Ehlers, C. L. (2011). Acceptability of the use of motivational interviewing to reduce underage drinking in a Native American community. *Substance Use & Misuse, 46*(6), 836–842.

Goldstick, J. E., Brenner, A. B., Lipton, R. I., Mistry, R., Aiyer, S. M., Reischl, T. M., & Zimmerman, M. A. (2015). A spatial analysis of heterogeneity in the link between alcohol outlets and assault victimization: Differences across victim subpopulations. *Violence and Victims, 30*(4), 649–662.

Grieco, E. M., Acosta, Y. D., de la Cruz, G. P., Gambino, G., Gryn, T., Larsen, J. L., Trevelyan, E. N., & Walters, N. P. (2012). *The Foreign-Born Population in the United States: 2010 American Community Survey Reports*. Washington, DC.

Gruenewald, P. J., Johnson, F. W., & Treno, A. J. (2002). Outlets, drinking and driving: a multilevel analysis of availability. *Journal of Studies on Alcohol, 63*(4), 460–468.

Gruenewald, P. J., Millar, A. B., & Treno, A. J. (1993). Alcohol availability and the ecology of drinking behavior. *Alcohol Research and Health, 17*(1), 39.

Guerrero, E. G., Kao, D., & Perron, B. E. (2013). Travel distance to outpatient substance use disorder treatment facilities for Spanish-speaking clients. *International Journal of Drug Policy, 24*(1), 38–45.

Guerrero, E. G., Pan, K. B., Curtis, A., & Lizano, E. L. (2011). Availability of substance abuse treatment services in Spanish: A GIS analysis of Latino communities in Los Angeles County, California. *Substance Abuse Treatment, Prevention, and Policy, 6*(1), 1–8.

Hackbarth, D. P., Schnopp-Wyatt, D., Katz, D., Williams, J., Silvestri, B., & Pfleger, M. (2001). Collaborative research and action to control the geographic placement of outdoor advertising of alcohol and tobacco products in Chicago. *Public Health Reports, 116*(6), 558–567.

Herd, D. (1996). The influence of religious affiliation on sociocultural predictors of drinking among Black and White Americans. *Substance Use & Misuse, 31*(1), 35–63.

Herd, D., & Grube, J. (1996). Black identity and drinking in the US: A national study. *Addiction, 91*(6), 845–857.

Holder, H. (1994). Public health approaches to the reduction of alcohol problems. *Substance Abuse, 15*(2), 123–138.

Israel, B. A., Schulz, A. J., Parker, E. A., & Becker, A. B. (2001). Community-based participatory research: Policy recommendations for promoting a partnership approach in health research. *Education for health, 14*(2), 182–197.

Jones-Webb, R. J., Hsiao, C.-Y., & Hannan, P. (1995). Relationships between socioeconomic status and drinking problems among black and white men. *Alcoholism: Clinical and Experimental Research, 19*(3), 623–627.

Jumper-Reeves, L., Dustman, P., Harthun, M., Kulis, S., & Brown, E. (2014). American Indian cultures: How CBPR illuminated intertribal cultural elements fundamental to an adaptation effort. *Prevention Science, 15*(4), 547–556.

Kaiser Family Foundation. (2015). *Population distribution by race/ethnicity*. Retrieved from http://kff.org/other/state-indicator/distribution-by-raceethnicity

LaVeist, T. A., & Wallace, J. M., Jr. (2000). Health risk and inequitable distribution of liquor stores in African American neighborhood. *Social Science & Medicine, 51*(4), 613–617.

Lee, C. S., Colby, S. M., Rohsenow, D. J., López, S. R., Hernández, L., & Caetano, R. (2013). Acculturation stress and drinking problems among urban heavy drinking Latinos in the northeast. *Journal of Ethnicity in Substance Abuse, 12*(4), 308–320.

Lee, C. S., Lopez, S. R., Hernandez, L., Colby, S. M., Caetano, R., Borrelli, B., & Rohsenow, D. (2011). A cultural adaptation of motivational interviewing to address heavy drinking among Hispanics. *Cultural Diversity & Ethnic Minority Psychology, 17*(3), 317–324.

Lee, J. P., Lipperman-Kreda, S., Saephan, S., & Kirkpatrick, S. (2013). Tobacco environment for southeast Asian American youth: Results from a participatory research project. *Journal of Ethnicity in Substance Abuse, 12*(1), 30–50.

Mair, C., Gruenewald, P. J., Ponicki, W. R., & Remer, L. (2013). Varying impacts of alcohol outlet densities on violent assaults: Explaining differences across neighborhoods. *Journal of Studies on Alcohol and Drugs, 74*(1), 50–58.

Mair, C., Roux, A. V. D., Osypuk, T. L., Rapp, S. R., Seeman, T., & Watson, K. E. (2010). Is neighborhood racial/ethnic composition associated with depressive symptoms? The multi-ethnic study of atherosclerosis. *Social Science & Medicine, 71*(3), 541–550.

Marmot, M. (2005). Social determinants of health inequalities. *The Lancet, 365*(9464), 1099–1104.

Marsiglia, F. F., Kulis, S., Parsai, M. V. P., & Garcia, C. K. (2009). Cohesion and conflict: Family influences on adolescent alcohol use in immigrant Latino families. *Journal of Ethnicity in Substance Use, 8*, 400–412.

Mayer, R. R., Forster, J. L., Murray, D. M., & Wagenaar, A. C. (1998). Social settings and situations of underage drinking. *Journal of Studies on Alcohol, 59*(2), 207–215.

Moore, D. J., Williams, J. D., & Qualls, W. J. (1996). Target marketing of tobacco and alcohol-related products to ethnic minority groups in the United States. *Ethnicity and Disease, 6*, 83–98.

Moore, R. S., Roberts, J., McGaffigan, R., Calac, D., Grube, J. W., Gilder, D. A., & Ehlers, C. L. (2012). Implementing a reward and reminder underage drinking prevention program in convenience stores near Southern California American Indian reservations. *American Journal of Drug and Alcohol Abuse, 38*(5), 456–460.

Morrison, C., Mair, C. F., Lee, J. P., & Gruenewald, P. J. (2015). Are barroom and neighborhood characteristics independently related to local-area assaults? *Alcoholism: Clinical and Experimental Research, 39*(12), 2463–2470.

Mulia, N., Ye, Y., Greenfield, T. K., & Zemore, S. E. (2009). Disparities in alcohol-related problems among white, black, and Hispanic Americans. *Alcoholism: Clinical and Experimental Research, 33*(4), 654–662.

Mulia, N., & Zemore, S. E. (2012). Social adversity, stress, and alcohol problems: are racial/ethnic minorities and the poor more vulnerable? *Journal of Studies on Alcohol and Drugs, 73*(4), 570–580.

Myser, C. (2004). Community-based participatory research in United States bioethics: Steps toward more democratic theory and policy. *American Journal of Bioethics, 4*(2), 67–68.

National Center for Cultural Competence. (2007). *A guide to infusing cultural & linguistic competence in health promotion training*. Washington, DC: Georgetown University Center for Child & Human Development.

Netto, G., Bhopal, R., Lederle, N., Khatoon, J., & Jackson, A. (2010). How can health promotion interventions be adapted for minority ethnic communities? Five principles for guiding the development of behavioural interventions. *Health Promotion International, 25*(2), 248–257.

O'Fallon, L. R., & Dearry, A. (2002). Community-based participatory research as a tool to advance environmental health sciences. *Environmental Health Perspectives, 110*(Suppl 2), 155.

Oetting, E. R., Donnermeyer, J. F., Plested, B. A., Edwards, R. W., Kelly, K., & Beauvais, F. (1995). Assessing community readiness for prevention. *International Journal of the Addictions, 30*(6), 659–683.

Ogilvie, K. A., Moore, R. S., Ogilvie, D. C., Johnson, K. W., Collins, D. A., & Shamblen, S. R. (2008). Changing community readiness to prevent the abuse of inhalants and other harmful legal products in Alaska. *Journal of Community Health, 33*(4), 248–258.

Ojeda, V. D., Patterson, T. L., & Strathdee, S. A. (2008). The influence of perceived risk to health and immigration-related characteristics on substance use among Latino and other immigrants. *American Journal of Public Health, 98*(5), 862–868.

Okamoto, J., Ritt-Olson, A., Soto, D., Baezconde-Garbanati, L., & Unger, J. B. (2009). Perceived discrimination and substance use among Latino adolescents. *American Journal of Health Behavior, 33*(6), 718–727.

Okamoto, S. K., Kulis, S., Marsiglia, F. F., Holleran Steiker, L., & Dustman, P. (2014). A continuum of approaches toward developing culturally focused prevention interventions: From adaptation to grounding. *The Journal of Primary Prevention, 35*(2), 103–112.

Oshodin, O. G. (1995). Nigeria. In D. B. Heath (Ed.), *International handbook on alcohol and culture* (pp. 213–233). Westport, CT: Greenwood Press.

Peterson, J. C. (2010). CBPR in Indian country: Tensions and implications for health communication. *Health Communication, 25*(1), 50–60.

Phelan, J. C., Link, B. G., & Tehranifar, P. (2010). Social conditions as fundamental causes of health inequalities theory, evidence, and policy implications. *Journal of Health and Social Behavior, 51*(1 suppl), S28–S40.

Ringwalt, C., & Bliss, K. (2006). The cultural tailoring of a substance use prevention curriculum for American Indian Youth. *Journal of Drug Education, 36*(2), 159–177.

Rose, V. K., & Thompson, L. M. (2012). Space, place and people: A community development approach to mental health promotion in a disadvantaged community. *Community Development Journal, 47*(4), 604–611.

Sale, E., Sambrano, S., Springer, J. F., Peña, C., Pan, W., & Kasim, R. (2005). Family protection and prevention of alcohol use among Hispanic youth at high risk. *American Journal of Community Psychology, 36*(3), 195–205.

Schmidt, L., Greenfield, T., & Mulia, N. (2006). Unequal treatment: Racial and ethnic disparities in alcoholism treatment services. *Alcohol Research & Health, 29*(1), 49–54.

Schwartz, S. J., Unger, J. B., Zamboanga, B. L., & Szapocznik, J. (2010). Rethinking the concept of acculturation: Implications for theory and research. *American Psychologist, 65*(4), 237–251.

Stewart, C., & Power, T. G. (2003). Ethnic, social class, and gender differences in adolescent drinking: Examining multiple aspects of consumption. *Journal of Adolescent Research, 18*(6), 575–598.

Substance Abuse and Mental Health Services Administration. (2016). *Cultural competence*. Retrieved March 18, 2017, from https://www.samhsa.gov/capt/applying-strategic-prevention/cultural-competence

Travers, K. D. (1997). Reducing inequities through participatory research and community empowerment. *Health Education & Behavior, 24*(3), 344–356.

Treno, A. J., Gruenewald, P. J., Lee, J. P., & Remer, L. G. (2007). The sacramento neighborhood alcohol prevention project: Outcomes from a community prevention trial. *Journal of Studies on Alcohol and Drugs, 68*(2), 197–207.

Wells, K., Klap, R., Koike, A., & Sherbourne, C. (2001). Ethnic disparities in unmet need for alcoholism, drug abuse, and mental health care. *American Journal of Psychiatry, 158*(12), 2027–2032.

Part III
Methodological Challenges

Qualitative Methods in the Study of Psychoactive Substance Use: Origins and Contributions—Implications for Substance-Use Prevention

13

J. Bryan Page and Zili Sloboda

Introduction-Early Documentation of Drug and Alcohol Use

Human beings have been using fermented juice, plant extracts, smoke, and vegetal material for mind- and body-altering purposes for at least 20,000 years. The origins of these behaviors are so cloaked in humankind's deep past that the stories of how we came to use drugs are products of eons of oral tradition retelling, complete with full mythological and legendary embellishment. We can imagine how humankind first accidentally discovered fermentation, resulting eventually in wine and beer, but we have no narrative descriptions of how it happened (Singer & Page, 2014). In the case of the narrative describing the origins of ayahuasca, the vine used to make a hallucinogenic drink used in the Amazon region, however, the description is specific and mythological. Its central action involves the death and burial of a defeated king who caused the hallucinogenic plant to grow out of his hair (Luna & Amaringo, 1999). Myriad cultural traditions repeat myriad narratives like this to explain how their people came to possess drugs that comprise their own pharmacopoeias.

Curiosity about how and why other peoples have various preferences for drugs emerged at about the time that writers began to chronicle contact between people of very different cultural backgrounds (Page & Singer, 2010). Herodotus' apparent description of cannabis use among the Scythians exemplifies this kind of writing about unfamiliar drug-use patterns. Hesiod chronicled use of the opium poppy even earlier, about the eighth century BCE (Kritikos & Papadaki, 1967). Friar Ramon Pané, who accompanied Christopher Columbus on his second expedition to the New World, recorded a direct observation of a shaman using a snuff that caused strong intoxication (Ott, 1993), providing the first eyewitness account of drug use by people in the Americas. Later he described tobacco consumption on the same journey. Bernardino de Sahagún (1956), 20 centuries after Herodotus, took an interest in the drugs used among Aztec and other Mexican natives, deciding to chronicle the extensive psychotropic pharmacopoeia of New Spain.

The Emergence of the Social Sciences: Anthropology and Sociology

Accounts written by explorers, travelers, and priests dominated the descriptions of drug use until the twentieth century (Page & Singer, 2010),

J. Bryan Page (✉)
Department of Anthropology, University of Miami, Coral Gables, FL, USA
e-mail: bryan.page@miami.edu

Z. Sloboda
Applied Prevention Science International, Ontario, OH, USA
e-mail: zili.sloboda@apsintl.org

and they continued to vary greatly in content and quality. Late in the nineteenth century, social and behavioral science disciplines began to emerge in the context of what had previously been called history. Anthropology and sociology both developed in the 1800s, at first relying on large data sources, such as museums, in the case of anthropology, and national statistics, in the case of sociology. Grand theorists were prominent in these processes. Auguste Comte and Max Weber exemplified sociological writers, while Edward Burnett Tylor and James George Frazer interpreted museum artifacts to try to define anthropology's key paradigm—culture.

The growth of emphasis on empirically verifiable facts in the later nineteenth and early twentieth centuries led these relatively young disciplines to focus on the procurement of new knowledge and perspectives, rather than relying on information already collected. With these emphases came a demand for rigor in the collection of data and observations, corresponding to the growing realization in the laboratory sciences that, for findings to be generalizable, they had to be replicable. Anthropology and sociology appeared to converge in this regard, with Franz Boas, the founder of the North American tradition of cultural anthropology, and Bronislaw Malinowski, the founder of British social anthropology, setting high standards for rigorous and industrious collection of cultural data, and Emile Durkheim setting similar standards for data collection among sociologists. Durkheim is sometimes called the "the mother's brother of anthropology" because of his interest in non-Western cultural patterns.

These individuals set standards for collecting highly detailed information on patterns of culture, establishing anthropology as a field observational discipline. Disciples of Boas and Malinowski produced many of the classic ethnographic monographs of the early to middle twentieth century (e.g., Evans-Pritchard, 1940; Mead, 1928). Durkheim's influence on sociology eventually led to the development of qualitative research in large-scale societies (Bulmer, 1984), as exemplified in Park (1915) and Park, Burgess, and McKenzie (1925) as proponents of the Chicago School of urban sociology. A distinguished anthropologist, Robert Redfield, also developed his career under the influence of Park and others.

Ethnography as pursued by the anthropologists and sociologists of the early twentieth century consisted primarily of placing oneself in positions to watch what the people under study do, and to ask them what they think about what they are doing. The ethnographer records narrative notes about his/her observations, including the conversations informally elicited during observations. These narrative notes constitute one kind of database that, when fully collected and coded for retrievability, helps the ethnographer to identify and document patterns of behavior. In addition to this staple of ethnographic field work, the ethnographer may engage in an assessment of the physical environment, mapping of key landmarks and features that are relevant to the topics being studied, house-to-house surveys, photographs (only with permission), individual, extensive conversations with key informants, open-ended interviews with individuals in the community of interest, and group interviews. In all cases, the process of ethnography is true to its etymology, as it comes from the Greek "ethnos" which means "people" and "grafia" which means "write down." Ethnographers in the field are constantly writing, drawing, or otherwise recording what they see and hear the best they can.

Application of Anthropology and Qualitative Research Methods to the Study of the Epidemiology of Use of Psychoactive Substances

With the establishment of ethnographic inquiry as a useful and rigorously applied technique in social and behavioral research, its power to gather and process sources of new knowledge gained increasingly wide and varied applications. The first anthropologists who applied the power of ethnography to the study of drug use included Robert Harry Lowie (1919), Weston La Barre (1938; 1975), and Richard Evans Schultes (1938, 1976). Lowie's primary interest was to collect as complete an ethnography of the Crow tribe as possible. In the course of accomplishing that goal, however, he encountered a highly elaborate and culturally salient tradition of tobacco use, cultivation, and ritual, which resulted in a separate volume entitled *The Tobacco Society of the Crow Indians* (Lowie, 1919). LaBarre and Schultes, on the other hand, had chosen to focus on patterns of drug use as they fit into Native American cultural contexts. Their approach set a precedent for subsequent studies of drug use, in which anthropologists attempted to write about the patterns they studied in terms of how they fit into cultural context. Later (in the 1960s) testimony and depositions by LaBarre and Schultes proved crucial in convincing the Federal Government to allow the Native American Church to conduct rituals in which the participants used peyote, or *Lophophora williamsii*. These anthropologists were the first to suggest that even very strong mind-altering drugs could be safely used if that use occurred in a well-defined cultural context with clear culturally defined purposes for that use (Page & Singer, 2010). Later anthropologists (e.g., Dobkin de Rios, 1972; Furst, 1972, 1976) reinforced those interpretations of "exotic" drug use.

Ethnography of drug use was not exclusively the province of anthropologists. One of its sociological proponents, Howard Becker (1953) wrote about his experience as a jazz drummer observing the process of becoming a marihuana user. Twenty-three years later, this paper strongly influenced Page as he struggled with his dissertation (Page, 1976). Becker's article clarified that the psychotropic effects of smoking marihuana needed some interpretation on the part of more experienced older peers, so that the novices would learn what to appreciate about the first experience of smoking marihuana. Based on this seminal work and further observations, Becker (1963) suggested provocative theories about the origins of deviance.

Another sociologist, Alfred Lindesmith (1968), in the context of a large study of injecting drug users in Chicago, used open-ended interviewing to derive a qualitative perspective on the nature of addiction. He developed a theory of addiction that held that much of the reported symptoms of withdrawal constituted a cultural complex of shared experience among heroin users (Lindesmith, 1968). His use of open-ended interviewing suggested new and useful strategies for gaining insight into the behavior of street-based drug users. Open-ended interviews, in which the interviewer initiates the conversation, but then stands back to give the respondent as full an opportunity as possible to structure his/her response according to his/her own interpretation of the topic, have formed large parts of the ethnographic data collected since the 1940s on drug use. By the 1970s, ethnographers of drug users were recording and transcribing these interviews verbatim for thorough qualitative analysis.

William Spradley (1970) introduced an analysis of life experience among what he called "Urban Nomads," the drunks regularly found along Skid Road in Seattle in the late 1960s. He used a form of componential analysis, a strategy for understanding cultural processes that involved identifying components of a set of experiences, and learned ways to reassemble them into authentic "nomad" experiences. This technique was derived from the techniques used by linguists to discover within-system meaning, and it inspired other anthropologists (e.g., Agar, 1973; James, 1972, 1976) to use techniques called ethnoscience (cf. James, 1977) to analyze how addicts and other street-based people structured their lives.

Agar (1973) engaged patients at the Lexington Center for Treatment of Opiate Dependency in a qualitative process that investigated the logic and sequence of events in the procurement and consumption of heroin. The insights gained by using these methods enabled Agar to present an understandable structure of activities to his audience that succeeded in helping them understand the lifestyle and behavior of street heroin addicts.

The technique he used for accomplishing this success began with a procedure called free listing, in which a gathered panel of individuals who have experience in the cultural complex of interest contribute a list of significant words and concepts from that complex. The group reviews the list and points out synonyms and areas of overlap, and this process results in a list of key terms that the group consensually agrees are significant in the cultural complex (in this case, the cultural complex was the procurement of heroin). Participants in the group then individually are asked to sort through a stack of cards that each has one of the identified words or concepts. Participants sort the cards into piles that reflect a separate, identifiable part of the cultural complex of interest. The results of this sorting process yield a set of card clusters, forming a cognitive map of the cultural complex being studied. The map produced by Agar's participants called the entire procurement process "getting off." Within that concept, the Lexington patients identified several component parts, including "the hustle," which denoted the behaviors and concepts involved in getting money for drugs. "Copping" (actually procuring the drugs) came next, followed by "finding a place," the process of identifying a safe haven for administering the drugs. "Getting high" involved the administration of drugs, which completed the process of "getting off." Page, Chitwood, Smith, Kane, and McBride (1990) found this cognitive map useful in characterizing new sources of HIV risk among IDUs in Miami.

Formalization of Anthropologic Methods in Understanding Psychoactive Substance Use

Standard practice in the conduct of anthropological research involves employing qualitative methods, especially as an ethnographic study begins. Qualitative methods have the objective of identifying and characterizing key aspects of the cultural complex under study. The process whereby investigations accomplish this objective is in essence inductive. As the investigator becomes increasingly familiar with the complex of knowledge and practice under study, an understanding or comprehension of those phenomena takes shape. The most efficient strategy for pursuing this objective employs techniques of direct observation of the behaviors of interest and conversations with the people engaged in those behaviors about intentions, meaning, and underlying beliefs with regard to the behaviors being studied. Once fully identified and characterized in terms of meaning and beliefs, it is possible to devise quantitative instruments to determine how widespread the behaviors are, and to what degree practitioners of these behaviors agree on their meaning and importance. Other techniques that contribute to a thorough characterization of behavior include participant observation, which involves ongoing presence in the cultural context where the behaviors of interest take place, and in-depth interviews, which give the investigator the opportunity to probe questions of meaning and belief in extended conversations, either with individuals or small groups of participants in the cultural complex of interest.

All of the varieties of data mentioned above primarily entail the accumulation of large bodies of text. Field notes written about participant observational experiences include descriptions of settings in terms of terrain, built structures, odors and aromas, weather, sounds and music, clothing, human interactions, and many other observable aspects of a place and time where behaviors under study take place. These notes accumulate as the field researcher repeatedly goes into those settings and describes what is going on there. The notes form large bodies of textual descriptions that provide the investigator with the wherewithal to review times and places of interest. Efficient retrieval of the content in field notes is crucial to the qualitative analytical process Therefore, field notes must be systematized for retrievability. Codes embedded in the text constitute a highly efficient way to build retrievability into large volumes of text. These codes can take the form of numeric strings, alphanumeric strings, or alphabetic strings. Likewise, the notes taken on informal conversations with people in the settings of interest will require codes for retrievability, as will open-ended formal interviews with individuals or small groups. In the author's experience, the *Human Relations Area Files* (Murdock et al., 2016) offers a coding system in its Outline of Cultural Materials (hereafter, OCM) that provides numeric codes for a wide variety of aspects of the human condition. The OCM's coding system includes more than 750 topical codes that cover the full range of the human condition.

Because 750 codes would be far more than the number necessary for most individual research projects, it is especially useful to select between 100 and 200 content codes that are likely to be relevant to a specific project and use those as the embedded markers for content items. Word processing software can retrieve these codes without confusing content areas with within-word alphabetic strings. More elaborate software, such as Atlas TI and Nvivo, can also be helpful in the retrieving and arraying of qualitative concepts as they appear in textual data.

Narrative texts also become voluminous rapidly as a qualitative study progresses. Anthropological investigators often have open-ended interviews with individuals or groups transcribed verbatim, resulting in extensive bodies of text. OCM-derived codes embedded in these textual materials also help with retrieval and analysis of laboriously collected in-depth interviews.

Field notes, informal interviews, and individual and group in-depth interviews are the staples of qualitative research, especially research on the consumption of drugs and alcohol. They are the principal tools for determining the etiology of drug-using patterns and the meaning of those patterns to the users themselves. They also provide the investigator with a sense of the cultural contexts in which people take up drug use. Set (the expectations that drug users have for their drug-using experience) and setting (the place and social context in which drug consumers ingest their drugs of choice) have been recognized for almost a half century (see Zinberg & Weil, 1969) as key factors in how people respond to the drugs that they consume. The combination of observational field notes, individual, open-ended interviews, and small group interviews helps the investigator to link personal and group expectations to the choice of circumstances for drug use and ultimately the kinds of effects experienced by the users. This combination also helps to explain some important details of the process of ingesting drugs, as in Page's characterization of injecting behavior (Page, Smith, & Kane, 1990) and Koester's (1994) explanation for heroin users' reluctance to carry personal needle/syringe sets while out in the streets.

By the early 1970s, the National Institute on Drug Abuse had identified ethnographic research on emergent patterns of drug use as essential to its array of research strategies for understanding and attempting to prevent drug use. One of the first initiatives funded by that agency involved investigations of the effects of long-term, heavy use of cannabis (Carter, Coggins, & Doughty, 1980; Rubin & Comitas, 1975; Stephanis, Dornbush, & Fink, 1977). To varying degrees, all three studies relied on ethnographic methods to conduct their studies focusing on the negative effects of long-term cannabis consumption (Page & Singer, 2010). Observation of study participants in natural habitat gave the investigators a sense of how cannabis smoking fit into the rest of their lives. Elicitation of life histories helped the researchers determine the life stage at which the study participants began smoking cannabis and hypothesize why they began to use the drug.

Illegal and otherwise rarely used drugs attracted the attention of some anthropologists, while others, notably Heath (1991), Marshall (1979, 1983), and Wilbert (1990), focused on drugs that are both commonly used and in most cases legal. Because they brought their holistic, observational, and context-focused attention to bear on patterns of drug use in culturally distinct contexts, their analyses of the drug-use patterns they studied led to provocative perspectives on drugs that seem familiar. In Heath's case, his mere observation and recording of how the Camba of the early 1950s used alcohol led to controversy about the impact of heavy drinking. Marshall's studies of drinking in Micronesia (1979) and Melanesia (1983) documented the negative impact of recently introduced distilled spirits in these cultural contexts. Wilbert's (1990) descriptions of tobacco use in a Venezuelan indigenous group called the Warao bear almost no resemblance to the patterns of tobacco use familiar to the people of Western civilization. Rather than using tobacco as a day-in, day-out constant drug, the Warao use it in heavy doses to induce visions.

Anthropologists' perspectives on how peoples around the world use drugs, both familiar and unfamiliar, help to point out where the problems lie in the society-wide patterns of drug use. In the absence of generally accepted guidance for users within a ritual context of drug use, use patterns become damaging and uncontrolled. The Camba of 1952 only drank in ritual contexts, and Heath (1991) found no evidence of alcoholism or health sequelae of alcohol use. Wilbert (1990) saw no evidence among the Warao of the disease complexes that affect Western tobacco smokers. In non-Western culture after non-Western culture, people use strong drugs without discernible public health impact (see also Weil, 1972). These peoples' protection against negative consequences of drug use comes from the fact that the patterns of drug use that they practice are fully endorsed by most or all members of the group. This endorsement involves universally agreed-upon, well-defined structures of behavior surrounding drug use, typically of ritual nature. They suggest an approach to gaining control of how people use drugs in cultural contexts where no ritual restrictions are in place. Obviously, traditions that have hundreds of years' experience with a drug will have established wisdom about a drug's effects that contemporary Western societies cannot match. Nevertheless, carefully defined rules of consumption, including acceptable ages, social circumstances, and purposes for use, could benefit the overall shape of drug use in environments where no such rules have been established or enforced. This perspective on how people consume the human pharmacopoeia in cultural context represents an important contribution by anthropologists such as LaBarre, Schultes, and Heath.

The HIV pandemic, as it emerged in the early 1980s, required the services of people trained in ethnographic methods, especially because the behaviors eventually linked to HIV contagion tended to happen out of sight, in spaces of intimacy, and involving behaviors that were objects of social disapproval. Ethnographers are adept at gaining access to an "up close and personal" view of human behavior, and this skill seemed necessary in order to learn about the cultural circumstances of HIV contagion. Direct observation of risk became the principal method used by Page and his colleagues (Page, Chitwood, et al., 1990; Page, Smith, & Kane, 1990) to determine that the circumstances of risk occurred in cultural contexts that presented a number of risks of exposure beyond the use of a previously used needle/syringe. Other anthropologists, including Koester (1994), Bourgois (1998), and Carlson, Siegal, and Falck (1995), engaged in similar studies, adding in their own work to the understanding of HIV risk among injecting drug users (IDUs). As a spin-off of their work, the danger of hepatitis C infection among IDUs received additional attention (Bourgois, Prince, & Moss, 2004; Koester, Glanz, & Baron, 2005).

By following IDUs through their daily activities, Page and Salazar (1999) used ethnographic methods to answer the question of high seroprevalence rates in a population that had always had legal access to needle/syringes. The Valencian IDUs studied by Page and Salazar had life circumstances that tended to track them into situations of great risk. Young men who still lived in their households of orientation were not permitted to inject heroin at home, and therefore they sought locales (called "chutaderos") in the city that afforded some privacy and had available used needle/syringes. These young men often were only able to cobble together just enough money to buy their desired drugs, but not enough to buy new needles. In the chutaderos they could find used needle/syringes, which they employed to inject their recently acquired drugs. To learn about the shape of risk in Valencia, the ethnographic team had to follow Valencian IDUs through their day to determine how circumstances tracked them into risk.

Other patterns of drug use, ranging from the consumption of black tar heroin (Ciccarone & Bourgois, 2003) to marijuana joints soaked in formaldehyde (Singer et al., 2005; Singer, Juvalis, & Weeks, 2000) to small cigars (Page & Evans, 2003; Singer et al., 2007), have been discovered and characterized using ethnographic methods. Each has significance for public health, and each discovery has given the efforts to prevent drug-related health problems and reduce harm.

Application of Qualitative Research Methods to Prevention

The contributions of qualitative research to our understanding of the epidemiology of substance use and its progression to abuse and dependence as well as to the transmissions of infections such as HIV and hepatitis B and C have led to progress in the treatment of substance-use disorders and to these life-threatening diseases. However, the importance of qualitative methods to substance-use prevention has not received the attention it so deserves. The field of prevention science is an evolving field that has had its origins in the late 1980s and early 1990s (references) and has become fully recognized through the establishment of the US and European Union Societies for Prevention Research (SPR, 2011). Prevention science draws on several related fields such as epidemiology, psychology, sociology, and neurobiology, and encompasses methodological and statistical approaches that are both taken from these other fields and are unique to the field of prevention.

The qualitative foundations from substance-use epidemiology have not been easily transferred to substance-use prevention. The most likely reason may be related to the many challenges that have plagued substance-use prevention researchers over the past 40 years attempting to demonstrate effectiveness of prevention interventions that demanded not only costly longitudinal designs but also biological evidence supporting no-use outcomes. Nevertheless, more and more prevention researchers are looking to mixed method approaches, combining qualitative and quantitative, to understand not only the outcomes of the prevention interventions but also what factors may have played a role in the receptivity to the intervention itself (Castro, Morera, Kellisong, & Aguirre, 2014). Ethnographic research has informed not only the prevention field about the influences of micro- and macro-level environments (family, school, peers, and neighborhood, and culture and laws and regulations, respectively) on individuals and their susceptibility to substance use but also about how to plan and implement prevention interventions effectively and interpreting the outcomes from evaluations of the prevention interventions. The most often used qualitative data collection methods used in prevention include key informant interviews, focus group discussions, and ethnographic studies.

Over the last several years more and more attention has been placed on qualitative studies in the planning process for prevention programming from the assessment of needs and the availability of prevention-related resources through to implementation and, of course, monitoring and evaluation and interpretation of findings from these data collection efforts.

Identifying the Target Populations for Prevention

A prevention professional needs to know the prevalence of the problem—how extensive is the problem and what substances are being used—and the incidence of use—who is initiating the use of different substances and what types of substances are they using. Understanding the problem and who is involved will then serve to inform the prevention professional's assessment about existing prevention services and whether they are reaching the target population, if they are evidence-based prevention interventions and/or policies, and whether existing social or health programs are available in which evidence-based prevention interventions can be integrated.

Use of archival data such as admissions to treatment programs, arrest information, emergency department admissions, medical examiner or coroner reports, reports to poison control or toxicology centers, reports on infectious diseases, and school reports of absenteeism due to the use of alcohol, tobacco, or drugs all serve to help define the problem. This information along with any available survey information on the general and/or student population serves further to define the needs of the defined population being targeted for prevention interventions. These quantitative data along with qualitative information gathered through key informant interviews with those knowledgeable about the target population and substance use such as treatment providers, law enforcement officers, health service providers, school administrators, and local leaders enrich the interpretation of quantitative data and the additional information from focus group discussions can provide a "rich" picture on the substances being used in the population and the consequences of such use.

The field of substance-use prevention has identified population groups that require different forms of prevention interventions based on the level of risk. The Society for Prevention Research has defined these as universal prevention—an intervention delivered without regard to the level of risk of individuals in the population; selective prevention—an intervention designed for a subgroup of the population with elevated levels on one or more risk factors; and indicated prevention—an intervention designed for a particular subgroup in the population that upon examination is found to be exhibiting prodromal signs or symptoms of problems due to their exposure to particular risks (SPR, 2011).

Each form of prevention focuses on different segments of the human population. With universal prevention interventions, the focus is on individuals who have not yet tried drugs for the first time. Obviously, the audience for these efforts are young, mostly children. In most societies, drug use is reserved for adults, primarily because children's brains are more vulnerable to the effects of psychoactive substances. Therefore, people all over the world discourage children from drinking, smoking, or otherwise administering drugs to themselves through both formal and informal means such as reducing the availability and access to these substances. Success then begins with reinforcing the naturally occurring influences that keep children from using drugs as a routine part of their inculcation process, including parenting programs, school policies and curricula, and community policies limiting access and availability of these substances.

An anthropological perspective on the process of children learning about substance use can be very useful in identifying aspects of the process that are amenable to change through education, modification of family and neighborhood environment, and attention to children's interaction with peers. Perspectives on family- and peer-dominated environments have provided useful insights into how children learn to use drugs such as tobacco and marihuana (cf. Page & Evans, 2003; True, Krauskopf, Carter, & Doughty, 1980). In their investigation of how middle schoolers begin using tobacco, Page and Evans came to perceive peer influence as implicit rather than directive. Young informants described as aspirational their entry into social contexts where tobacco use was happening. Upon entry, no one urged them to take up tobacco smoking. Rather, they were already primed to accept a cigarette or small cigar if offered, because that was what the group they considered "cool" was doing. In the streets of San José, we saw younger boys hang around the periphery of the group of older peers, waiting for an opening to be accepted in the group of marihuana smokers. In both cases, in very disparate parts of the world, the motivation to use these drugs—tobacco and marihuana—emanated not so much from curiosity about the drugs, but rather the desire for affiliation with the group that was using them. These findings suggest that prevention efforts should focus on how children who are moving into middle-school age categories identify and become attracted to groups who use drugs.

Selective prevention's focus is on keeping those at risk from progressing to substance use. Since the 1970s, adolescents who get into trouble in school, or whose parents suspect they have been using drugs have been referred to interventions that have predominantly taken the form of one-on-one counseling, peer group therapy, or family therapy, usually with the focal adolescent as an outpatient. Other behavioral interventions have been developed around findings from anthropological work addressing an understanding of important cultural influences on families and youth. In part, because of etiologic research on drug use among Cuban adolescents (cf. Page, 1980; Page, 1990), Szapocznik and his colleagues began to formulate selective preventive strategies based on two primary concepts: families' internal structure and the relationship between the adolescent and his/her cultural surroundings (Coatsworth, Duncan, Pantin, & Szapocznik, 2006; Robbins et al., 2009). This development extended both to local communities in Miami (Pantin et al., 2009) and to an application in Ecuador. Elsewhere, Marsiglia, Ayers, Baldwin-White, and Booth (2016) have incorporated cultural components in their approach to prevention of substance use among Mexican-American adolescents.

Indicated prevention has historically received the most attention, primarily because the people who are evidencing substance use are the easiest to identify. They are the ones who exhibit behaviors that bring them to the attention of family members, teachers, law enforcement, and workplace colleagues These behaviors may include truancy from school, absenteeism from work, public intoxication, loss of control, and compulsion to use their substances of choice. They also present the most difficult problems for those attempting to help them. Those in need of indicated prevention, whether they are sober or still using their drugs, have a high likelihood of continuing to use unless they receive a preventive intervention. Ethnographic insights into the lives of substance users and abusers have made important contributions of potential use to these prevention efforts.

Understanding the Processes Involved in the Prevention Intervention Process

Although the use of qualitative methods has been used more extensively in gaining an understanding of the prevention process in that area of HIV transmission (Carlson, Wang, Siegal, Falck, & Guo, 1994; Power, 1998), it has received the least attention in the area of substance-use prevention. What is meant by the "process of prevention" is the impact of the intervention on the changes that take place during the intervention period on those factors or elements of the intervention that are targeted by the intervention itself. These factors include constructs that include attitudes about substance use, beliefs about the normative nature of substance use among peers, beliefs in one's ability to "resist" offers of substances, or use of appropriate parenting skills under pressure. Mediation analysis has received increasing attention in the field of prevention to examine the relationship between these factors or short-term outcomes of an intervention and the long-term outcome of actual substance use (Fairchild & MacKinnon, 2014; Stephens et al., 2009). However, the question of the target group's receptivity to the prevention messages has been much less explored. Stephens et al. (2009) examined the impact of the perceptions of the instructor or source of the prevention messages on students' receptivity to a new substance-use prevention curriculum. They found using survey questions that measured perceptions of credibility—items asked about whether the instructor understood what the world was like for "kids my age"; whether it was easy to talk to the instructor; whether the student thought the instructor gave real/true information; and whether he/she was enthusiastic. It was found that the perceptions of the instructor significantly affected refusal, communication and decision-making skills, normative beliefs, perceived consequences of use, and actual substance use. The authors conclude, "Our study is also based solely on quantitative data, leading us to make assumptions about how the students are processing information about the instructor and the information presented by the instructor based on a limited number of measured variables. Further research should look at the extent to which students are using the central processing route when presented with program content. This type of research calls for designs that allow the researcher to 'get into the heads' of students participating in the program to elicit the types of thought processes they use during various program activities. Questions to be addressed by this type of research include whether students continue thinking about the program outside of the classroom setting and how they come to conclusions about their own use and the use of substances by adolescents in general given their experience with program content and activities." Such research would benefit greatly from the application of qualitative methods.

Another avenue for qualitative research in the area of receptivity is the differential response to the elements of the prevention intervention examined by the characteristics of the environments in which the target population lives. For instance, to what extent does the experience of living in neighborhoods in which substance use is widespread or if the participants' family members or friends are substance users or are involved in the sales or distribution of drugs or even the legal sales of tobacco and alcohol have an impact on preventive messages? In the case of a workplace intervention, where alcohol is a part of the workplace norm either during or after work or as a reward for services, what impact do those circumstances have on prevention messages (e.g., Emory et al., 2015; Zhao et al., 2016)? We know that having substance-using peers impacts not only substance use among youth but also the outcomes of treatment for substance abusers (e.g., Dishion, Capaldi, Spracklen, & Li, 1995; Ennett et al., 2006; Kandel, 1978).

Interpreting the Findings from Evaluation Studies

Another opportunity for qualitative methods to be integrated into prevention is through the interpretation of findings from evaluation studies. Not only would such studies provide a better and richer understanding of the outcomes, they would also serve a key role in the early development of the evaluation itself. However the history of using "mixed methods" in prevention is relatively new and evolving. Castro et al. (2014) provide both a concise history of using mixed methods and a guide for effective use of these methods. The authors indicate that qualitative methods have generally not been employed effectively in substance-use prevention. In fact in their review of 57 studies found during the period 2007–2012 to employ mixed methods, only 14 had these key words in their abstracts—"mixed methods," "prevention," and "intervention" were available as full-text documents, and focused on an empirical intervention study. Of these only two were studies of substance-use interventions. A review of the qualitative methods used in these studies indicated weaknesses in their use and integrating qualitative with quantitative approaches. Mixed method research in the health area in general has not been supported until recently (Creswell, Klassen, Plano Clark, and Smith (2011). Castro et al. (2014) make five recommendations for those in prevention research when using mixed methods:

1. Specify the intended mixed method design. Investigators should not only be specific about the mixed methods that are to be used but also provide the rationale for the choice of the methods and how they relate to the purposes of the study.
2. Specify the sampling plan and methodological procedures for the qualitative component. Many of the weaknesses of the mixed method studies that were reviewed were related to the sampling plans for the qualitative parts of the studies. They were found not to be selected to appropriately represent the study population and/or were not large enough to achieve their objectives.
3. Use a study design that has greater internal validity. Most of the studies that were reviewed failed to meet the criteria for internal validity. For this reason, it is recommended that mixed method research should be developed in line with controlled randomized trials or well-operationalized multivariate model study and that the data analysis plan be explicit as to how qualitative and quantitative data will be integrated to achieve the objectives of the study (Castro & Coe, 2007).
4. Maximize integration in accord with the study purpose. This recommendation strongly underscores what was said above by having an a priori purposeful design that integrates the two methodologies across all major study components from its conceptualization through data collection, implementation, data analysis, and data interpretation. This planning aims to maximize the usefulness of the mixed method approach.
5. Training and mentorship in mixed method research: Clearly utilization of a mixed method approach requires training.

Conclusions

In response to the growing realization that qualitative perspectives are especially important in understanding human patterns of substance use, new initiatives to address substance use and substance use-related problems often include ethnographic components, because, to quote Mike Agar, "Ethnography is how we learn to ask the hip questions." Ethnography's armamentarium of methods has proven especially effective in finding out what is going on in difficult-to-reach cultural contexts and defining what actions need implementation to prevent psychoactive substance use and its related harms. The marriage between qualitative methods and quantitative approaches remains tricky and difficult. In an attempt to provide guidance for combining qual and quant, however, an initiative headed by Kagawa Singer, Dressler, George, and Elwood (2015) has made an effort to establish rigorous approaches to include culture in health research. The document (The Cultural Framework for Health: An integrative approach for research and program design and evaluation available at the NIH website) that resulted from that effort presents a wide range of ways to operationalize culture, providing for fidelity to the complexity and ubiquity of that concept, and facilitate the combining of qualitative and quantitative modes of inquiry. Contributors to this *Framework* include highly active researchers who have contributed their experience and innovations to a potentially very helpful handbook for health research involving culture. The Framework along with Creswell and colleagues' Best Practices for Mixed Methods Research in the Health Sciences Future (2011) provides directions for substance-use prevention researchers that would not only move them toward an increasingly seamless combination of qualitative and quantitative methods but, more importantly, also improve the development and delivery of prevention interventions and our understanding of the receptivity of the participants to their messages.

References

Agar, M. (1973). *Ripping and running: A formal ethnography of urban heroin addicts*. New York: Academic Press.

Becker, H. (1953). Becoming a marihuana user. *American Journal of Sociology, 59*, 235–242.

Becker, H. (1963). *Outsiders: Studies of the Sociology of Deviance*. New York: Macmillan, The Free Press.

Bourgois, P. (1998). Just another night in a shooting gallery. *Theory, Culture and Society, 15*, 37–66.

Bourgois, P., Prince, B., & Moss, A. (2004). The everyday violence of hepatitis C among young women who inject drugs in San Francisco. *Human Organization, 63*, 253–264.

Bulmer, M. (1984). *The Chicago School of Sociology: Institutionalization, diversity, and the rise of sociological research*. Chicago: University of Chicago Press.

Carlson, R. G., Siegal, H. A., & Falck, R. S. (1995). Qualitative research methods in drug and AIDS prevention research: An overview. In E. Lambert, R. S. Ashery, & R. H. Needle (Eds.), *Qualitative methods in drug abuse and HIV research, NIDA research monograph #157; NIH Pub. No. 95–4025*. Washington, DC: Supt. of Docs., U.S. Govt. Printing Office.

Carlson, R., Wang, J., Siegal, H., Falck, R., & Guo, J. (1994). An ethnographic approach to targeted sampling: problems and solutions in aids prevention research among injection drug and crack-cocaine users. *Human Organization, 53*(3), 279–286.

Carter, W. E., Coggins, W. J., & Doughty, P. L. (1980). *Cannabis in Costa Rica*. Philadelphia, PA: ISHI Press.

Castro, F. G., & Coe, K. (2007). Traditions and alcohol use: A mixed methods analysis. *Cultural Diversity and Ethnic Minority Psychology, 13*, 269–284.

Castro, F. G., Morera, O. F., Kellisong, J. G., & Aguirre, K. M. (2014). Mixed methods research design for prevention science: Methods, critiques, and recommendations. In Z. Sloboda & H. Petras (Eds.), *Defining prevention science, advances in prevention science* (pp. 452–490). New York: Springer.

Ciccarone, D., & Bourgois, P. (2003). Explaining the geographical variation of HIV among injection drug users in the United States. *Substance Use and Misuse, 38*, 2049–2063.

Coatsworth, J. D., Duncan, L. G., Pantin, J., & Szapocznik, J. (2006). Patterns of retention in a preventive intervention with ethnic minority families. *Journal of Primary Prevention, 27*, 171–193.

Creswell, J. W., Klassen, A. C., Plano Clark, V. L., & Smith, K. C. (2011). *Best practices for mixed methods research in the health sciences*. Bethesda, MD: National Institutes of Health.

Dishion, T. J., Capaldi, D., Spracklen, K. M., & Li, F. (1995). Peer ecology of male adolescent drug use. *Development and Psychopathology, 7*, 803–824.

Dobkin de Rios, M. (1972). *Visionary vine: Psychedelic Healing in the Peruvian Amazon*. San Francisco: Chandler Publishing Company.

Emory, K. T., Messer, K., Vera, L., Ojeda, N., Elder, J. P., Usita, P., & Pierce, J. P. (2015). Receptivity to cigarette and tobacco control messages and adolescent smoking initiation. *Tobacco Control, 24*(3), 281–284.

Ennett, S. T., Bauman, K. E., Hussong, A., Faris, R., Foshee, V. A., DuRant, R. H., & Cai, L. (2006). The peer context of adolescent substance use: Findings from social network analysis. *Journal of Research on Adolescence, 28*, 159–186.

Evans-Pritchard, E. E. (1940). *The Nuer: A description of the modes of livelihood and political institutions of a Nilotic People*. Oxford: Clarendon Press.

Fairchild, A. J., & MacKinnon, D. P. (2014). Using mediation and moderation analyses to enhance prevention research. In Z. Sloboda & H. Petras (Eds.), *Defining prevention science* (pp. 537–556). New York: Springer.

Furst, P. T. (1972). *Flesh of the Gods: The ritual use of Hallucinogens*. New York: Praeger Publishers.

Furst, P. T. (1976). *Hallucinogens and culture*. San Francisco, CA: Chandler and Sharp.

Heath, D. (1991). Continuity and change in drinking patterns of the bolivian camba. In D. Pittman & H. White (Eds.), *Society, culture and drinking patterns reexamined: Alcohol, culture and social control monograph series* (pp. 78–86). New Brunswick: Rutgers Center for Alcohol Studies.

James, J. (1972). Two domains of streetwalker argot. *Anthropological Linguistics, 14*, 174–175.

James, J. (1976). Prostitution and addiction: An interdisciplinary approach. *Addictive Diseases: An International Journal, 2*, 601–618.

James, J. (1977). Ethnography and social problems. In R. S. Weppner (Ed.), *Street ethnography: Selected studies of crime and drug use in natural settings* (pp. 179–200). Beverly Hills, CA: Sage.

Kagawa Singer, M., Dressler, W. W., George, S., & Elwood, W. N. (2015). *The cultural framework for health: An integrative approach for research and program design and evaluation*. Bethesda, MD: Office of Behavioral and Social Science Research.

Kandel, D. B. (1978). Homophily, selection and socialization in adolescent friendships. *American Journal of Sociology, 84*, 427–436.

Koester, S. (1994). Copping, running, and paraphernalia laws: Contextual variables and needle risk behavior among injection drug users. *Human Organization, 53*, 287–295.

Koester, S., Glanz, J., & Baron, A. (2005). Drug sharing among heroin networks: Implications for HIV and hepatitis B and C prevention. *AIDS and Behavior, 9*, 27–39.

Kritikos, P. G., & Papadaki, S. P. (1967). History of poppy and of opium and their expansion in antiquity in eastern Mediterranean area 2. *Bulletin on Narcotics, 19*, 17–38.

La Barre, W. (1975). *The Peyote cult*. Hamden, CT: Archon Books.

Lindesmith, A. R. (1968). *Addiction and opiates*. Chicago, IL: Aldine.

Lowie, R. H. (1919). *The tobacco society of the crow Indians*. New York: The Trustees.

Luna, L. E., & Amaringo, P. (1999). *Ayahuasca visions: The religious Iconography of a Peruvian Shaman*. Berkeley, CA: North Atlantic Press.

Marshall, M. (1979). *Weekend warriors: Alcohol in a Micronesian Culture*. Palo Alto, CA: Mayfield Publishing.

Marshall, M. (1983). *Through a glass darkly: Beer and modernization in Papua New Guinea*. Boroko: Institute of Applied Social and Economic Research.

Marsiglia, F. F., Ayers, S. L., Baldwin-White, A., & Booth, J. (2016). Changing Latino adolescents' substance use norms and behaviors: the effects of synchronized youth and parent drug use prevention interventions. *Prevention Science, 17*, 1–12.

Mead, M. (1928). *Coming of age in Samoa*. New York: Morrow.

Murdock, G. P., Ford, C. S., Hudson, A. E., Kennedy, R., Simmons, L. W., & Whiting, J. W. M. (2016). *Outline of cultural materials*. New Haven, CT: Human Relations Area Files. Retrieved from http://hraf.yale.edu/resources/reference/outline-of-cultural-materials/#outline-of-cultural-materials8211-origin-prin

Ott, J. (1993). *Pharmacotheon: Ethnogenic drugs, their plant sources, and history*. Kennewick, WA: Natural Products Company.

Page, J. B. (1976). *Costa Rican marijuana users and the amotivational syndrome hypothesis*. Ann Arbor: University Microfilms.

Page, J. B. (1980). The children of exile: Relationships between the acculturation process and drug use among Cuban youth. *Youth and Society, 11*, 431–447.

Page, J. B. (1990). Streetside drug use among Cuban drug users in Miami, Florida. In R. Glick & J. Moore (Eds.), *Drug use in Hispanic Communities* (pp. 169–191). New Brunswick: Rutgers Press.

Page, J. B., Chitwood, D. D., Smith, P. C., Kane, N., & McBride, D. C. (1990). Intravenous drug abuse and HIV infection in Miami. *Medical Anthropology Quarterly, 4*(1), 56–71.

Page, J. B., & Evans, S. (2003). Cigars, cigarillos, and youth: Emergent patterns of subcultural complexes. *Journal of Ethnicity in Substance Abuse, 2*, 63–76.

Page, J. B., &. Salazar, J. (1999). Use of needles and syringes in Miami and Valencia: Observations of high and low availability. *Medical Anthropology Quarterly, 4*, 413–435.

Page, J. B., & Singer, M. (2010). *Comprehending drug use: Ethnographic research at the social margins*. New Brunswick, NJ: Rutgers University Press.

Page, J. B., Smith, P. C., & Kane, N. (1990). Shooting galleries, their proprietors, and implications for prevention of AIDS. *Drugs and Society, 5*, 69–86.

Pantin, H., Prado, G., Lopez, B., Huang, S., Tapia, M. I., Schwartz, S. J., … Branchini, J. (2009). A randomized controlled trial of Familias Unidas for Hispanic adolescents with behavior problems. *Psychosomatic Medicine, 71*, 987–995.

Park, R. E. (1915). The City: Suggestions for the investigation of behavior in the city environment. *American Journal of Sociology, 20*, 579–583.

Park, R. E., Burgess, E., & McKenzie, R. (1925). *The City*. Chicago, IL: University of Chicago Press.

Power, R. (1998). The role of qualitative research in HIV/AIDS. *AIDS, 12*(7), 687–695.

Robbins, M. S., Szapocznik, J., Horigian, V. E., Feaster, D. J., Puccinelli, M., Jacobs, P., … Brigham, G. (2009). Brief strategic family therapy for adolescent drug abusers: A multi-site effectiveness study. *Contemporary Clinical Trials, 30*, 269–278.

Rubin, V., & Comitas, L. (1975). *Ganja in Jamaica*. The Hague: Mouton.

de Sahagún, B. (1956). *Historia general de las Cosas De Nueva España* (Vol. 3, p. 292). Mexico City: Editorial Porrua.

Schultes, R. E. (1938). The appeal of peyote (Lophophora williamsii) as a medicine. *American Anthropologist, 40*, 698–715.

Schultes, R. E. (1976). *Hallucinogenic plants*. New York: Golden Press.

Singer, M., Clair, S., Schensul, J., Huebner, C., Eiserman, J., Pino, R., & Garcia, J. (2005). Dust in the wind: The growing use of embalming fluid among youth in Hartford, CT. *Substance Use and Misuse, 40*, 1035–1050.

Singer, M., Juvalis, J. A., & Weeks, M. (2000). High on Illy: Studying an emergent drug problem in Hartford, CT. *Medical Anthropology, 18*, 365–388.

Singer, M., Mirhej, G., Page, J. B., Hastings, E., Salaheen, H., & Prado, G. (2007). Black 'N Mild and carcinogenic: Cigar smoking among inner city young adults in Harford, CT. *Journal of Ethnicity and Substance Abuse, 6*, 81–94.

Singer, M., & Page, J. B. (2014). *The social value of drug addicts: Uses of the useless*. Walnut Creek, CA: Left Coast Press.

Society for Prevention Research. (2011). *Standards of knowledge for the science of prevention*. Retrieved from http://www.preventionresearch.org.

Spradley, J. (1970). *You Owe yourself a drunk: An ethnography of Urban Nomads*. Prospect Heights, IL: Waveland Press.

Stephanis, C., Dornbush, R. L., & Fink, M. (1977). *Hashish: A study of long-term use*. New York: Raven Press.

Stephens, P. C., Sloboda, Z., Stephens, R. C., Teasdale, B., Grey, S. F., Hawthorne, R. D., & William, J. (2009). Universal school-based substance abuse prevention programs: Modeling targeted mediators and outcomes for adolescent cigarette, alcohol and marijuana use. *Drug and Alcohol Dependence, 102*, 19–29.

Stephens, P. C., Sloboda, Z., Grey, S., Stephens, R., Hammond, A., Hawthorne, R., … Williams, J. (2009). Is the receptivity of substance abuse prevention programming affected by students' perceptions of the instructor? *Health Education & Behavior, 36*(4), 724–745.

True, W. R., Krauskopf, D., Carter, W. E., & Doughty, P. L. (1980). Marijuana and user lifestyles. In W. E. Carter (Ed.), *Cannabis in Costa Rica* (pp. 98–115). Philadelphia: ISHI Press.

Weil, A. (1972). *The natural mind: A new way of looking at drugs and the higher consciousness*. Boston: Houghton Mifflin Company.

Wilbert, J. (1990). Tobacco and shamanistic ecstasy among the Warao Indians of Venezuela. In P. T. Furst (Ed.), *Flesh of the Gods: The ritual use of Hallucinogens* (pp. 55–83). Prospect Heights, IL: Waveland Press.

Zhao, X., Alexander, T. N., Hoffman, L., Jones, C., Delahanty, J., Walker, M., … Talbert, E. (2016). Youth receptivity to FDAs the real cost tobacco prevention campaign: evidence from message pretesting. *Journal of Health Communications, 21*(11), 1153–1160.

Zinberg, N., & Weil, A. (1969). Cannabis – 1st Controlled Experiment. New Society 13(329):84–86.

Monitoring Trends: Use of Local Data

14

Jane Mounteney and Paul Griffiths

Introduction

Considerable efforts are made both internationally and at national levels to monitor the nature, scale, and dynamics of substance-use behaviours and associated problems (EMCDDA, 2017a; UNODC, 2016). A set of special methods have been developed to meet the considerable practical and methodological challenges of monitoring these complex set of behaviours together with their associated health and social outcomes in populations that are often stigmatised, hidden, and/or socially excluded. These approaches can be grouped under the heading 'drug or substance-use epidemiology' and collectively represent adaptions of standard approaches or new methods designed to overcome the difficulties inherent to this area (for a comprehensive review of this topic see Sloboda, 2005). Importantly from a technical point of view, as substance use is usually a behaviour subject to social, criminal, or legal sanctions, the potential data sets available,

J. Mounteney (✉)
Head of Public Health Unit, European Monitoring Centre for Drugs and Drug Addiction, Lisbon, Portugal
e-mail: Jane.Mounteney@emcdda.europa.eu

P. Griffiths
Scientific Director, European Monitoring Centre for Drugs and Drug Addiction (EMCDDA), Lisbon, Portugal
e-mail: Paul.Griffiths@emcdda.europa.eu

outcomes of interest, and information needs with implications for policy and interventions are broader than those found in many health-related areas of inquiry. Thus, as well as behavioural data on substance use and data on substance use-associated morbidity and mortality, information on the illicit drug market and from the criminal justice system is usually included in information systems in this area.

In this chapter we provide an overview of the established and some innovative approaches to collecting information in this area. For the purposes of clarity we consider substance-use epidemiology within a general paradigm of drug monitoring, although the reader should be aware that this includes some activities that could equally be described under the heading of research, action research, risk assessment, or disease surveillance. We also consider how a better understanding of patterns and trends in substance use can help inform the development of local substance-use prevention activities. Our argument in the first part is that an understanding of the broader epidemiological situation represents an essential element for informing the design of programmes at both the national and local levels. Beyond this however, there is evidence to suggest that substance-use epidemiology as a practical accomplishment can be incorporated into local systems in which the collection and interpretation of data can be an important element for designing, targeting, and evaluating prevention activities. In short, these approaches can help put the evidence into evidence-based substance-use prevention programmes.

The topic of this book is the application of prevention science to substance-use prevention and this not only means basing prevention programmes on evidence of efficacy and effectiveness but also ensuring that they are informed by the epidemiology and aetiology of substance use. As already noted the term substance use is shorthand for a complex set of behaviours and associated outcomes which not only cut across both health and social domains but can also interact. This is one of the reasons that understanding prevalence (including incidence) and patterns and trends in substance use is so crucial to effective prevention programming. Our understanding of effectiveness for example is built on studies of specific populations with specific target outcomes. To be useful we have to match this knowledge with an understanding of patterns of substance use and their geographical and temporal prevalence, distribution, and determinants. Similarly the aetiology of substance use and associated problems informs our understanding of what constitutes high-risk and vulnerable populations and individuals. Identifying the extent to which these are present in local areas, and then using this information to inform the development and targeting of interventions, is therefore a crucial element of putting evidence-based prevention into practice. To some extent a valid criticism of historical prevention practice is that while monitoring has been used for programme evaluation purposes it has not always been integral to the planning, design, and targeting of interventions. We would argue that given the complexity of patterns of substance-use consumption and their dynamic nature, a failure to integrate epidemiological information, at least at the system level, into prevention programming, risks implementation of interventions that may be inappropriate, ineffective, or even counterproductive.

A strong argument can be made that epidemiological monitoring information is essential for understanding local substance-use problems and this understanding is crucial to shaping how prevention and other responses are included and articulated within a national and local strategy. Correspondingly in most comprehensive modern substance-use prevention strategies, monitoring and information is included as a pillar or a cross-cutting element usually with a commitment to using this information for informing the design and targeting of appropriate responses. Local prevention initiatives are usually developed within the context of a national or state perspective, and national monitoring exercises are themselves based on data collected at a local level. Thus a structural, if somewhat weak, link will usually exist between local prevention and epidemiological monitoring in most countries. Within this overall context however it is possible for information collected at the local level to be used to inform the delivery of prevention within that area.

Clear arguments can be made regarding the advantages of using local monitoring data to support substance-use prevention interventions. While programmes may often have a national lead and be rolled out across settings, their implementation largely takes place in communities, close to the information sources harnessed by city-level systems. This has a number of implications, all of which suggest that both national and local initiatives will benefit from drawing on sources that provide a local situational analysis and firm empirical foundation for the establishment of prevention responses. A central factor is the timeliness and hence increased relevance of local data, as compared with national epidemiological output, which necessarily requires additional steps of collation and dissemination adding sometimes significant time delays to the information production. Reduced tiers of bureaucracy can be particularly important when the emphasis is on rapid identification of new trends and potentially risky or harmful behaviours. In addition to enhanced reporting speed allowing increased service responsiveness to identified problems, local monitors will also allow for differentiated description and understanding of the local- and city-level threats and problems individual localities face. By comparison, national data fails to take into account regional and local variation in these problems and misses the granularity and different focuses required by programmes implemented in varied jurisdictions. Finally, local monitoring is likely to promote local ownership of substance use-related problems and the solutions they require. In many respects a virtual circle can be established involving data providers, planners, and responders to these issues. Engagement of central players, for example local outreach and treatment services, in monitoring activity with built-in feedback loops, regular reporting, etc. can establish and reinforce community support and collaboration to address issues that emerge. And in some cases the buy-in is made more valuable by the fact that agencies providing data are also those responding to clients and they will benefit if their routine statistics can be set in context, and validated by reports from other local players. It is worth emphasising that the use of local monitoring data as a basis for interventions can be a win-win for both national- and community-level operators. The local tailoring of responses that local data allows also ensures that national-level agencies are in receipt of a rich and more complex countrywide picture of patterns of substance use and harms.

Linking Local Data and Prevention: Interplay and Iterative Process

The relation and potential interaction between local data and the planning, selection, and implementation of prevention interventions and policies is a complex one, with data having a function in the identification of new trends and developments and even acting as a source for programme content. Prevention interventions are primarily implemented at the school, local community, or city level—only rarely are national audiences the target of campaigns or initiatives. As such, they are often instigated in response to local problems, and a knowledge of local issues, including substance-use prevalence and harms, is central and will underpin effective interventions. In this respect, local substance use-related data may be utilised in the establishment of local strategies and responses and can increase the understanding of the context or setting in which interventions are to be implemented, allowing tailoring, adaptation, and interpreting programmes to meet local needs and circumstances. Importantly, information may be available to help prioritise the most pressing problems, their contours and severity, as well as any new and emerging trends to be addressed. Certain data may be particularly useful for establishing a pre-intervention baseline, and to check for post-intervention changes.

The task of prevention planning potentially benefits in numerous ways from the utilisation of local epidemiological data. Perhaps the most recognised approach is the undertaking of local and community needs assessments as a prelude or aid to developing substance-use prevention plans and services. As a starting point for local substance-use prevention strategies, needs assessments are typically accompanied by mapping of existing service provision and gap analysis—forming the basis, justification, and starting point for subsequent activities. Available routine data and statistics, combined with user and professional surveys and consultations, are common elements used in this process, which can help inform decisions and priorities as well as inform what level of intervention is required—individual, group, or community and universal, selective, or indicated or all levels of intervention.

Similarly, when used to inform prevention planning, local data can support the identification of risk groups, vulnerable neighbourhoods, and targets for early intervention. In concrete terms, local community- and city-level action plans and strategies may draw on a range of epidemiological information, while associated baseline data and performance measures may utilise for example local survey data and indicators of substance use-related harm.

Local data has been central in certain jurisdictions to the development of risk indexes for local communities, where the establishment of specific measures of substance use-related vulnerability, risk, and protection has been used to establish the severity of local problems, identify the priorities for action, as well as allow comparison with other localities in the geographical area. In addition to local authority planning, community-based health and social care agencies may fruitfully draw on analysis of local substance-use problems and issues, for example substance use-related crime hotspots and clusters of overdoses, to inform their organisational development plans, and identify the optimum allocation of limited resources.

Local substance use-related data on the situation and problems can provide both important contextual detail for those implementing prevention interventions and content for the programmes themselves. An in-depth understanding of demographics, cultural, religious, and linguistic issues is likely to prove key for the successful implementation of a manual-based programme into a new locality. Success factors for programme transfer will involve tailoring to the needs of local target groups, and an informed process will be more likely to engender success. And many programmes will benefit from the inclusion of local information as part and parcel of this tailoring process. This may involve incorporation of facts and data, for example school survey prevalence figures, to clarify and correct perceptions of levels of substance use. Environmental programmes involving alcohol-serving training may draw on local information on substance use-related crime, drink driving, and hospital admissions in the city to inform the intervention.

Increasingly important in the fast-changing substance-use landscape is the systematic use of indicators to inform on the availability and use of new psychoactive substances, and emerging substance-use trends. In this context, reports from local data providers including forensic institutes, criminal justice agencies, and emergency health workers may be channelled rapidly to inform of newly identified substances or adverse health events. Sometimes local sources may be networked into national or even international signal detection or early warning systems. Alternatively, data may be analysed in the context of city-level monitors, capable of reporting on substance use-related trends over time. Local monitoring data used in this way provide the information necessary for early intervention and more timely public health and prevention responses.

Approaches to Information Collection: A Critical Overview

A range of epidemiological tools can help understand local patterns of substance *use*, in particular adult population surveys, student and school surveys, target group studies, capture recapture, treatment data, wastewater monitoring, key informant surveys, drug tests from the criminal justice system, and drink or drug driving data. Sources useful to understand harms include acute emergencies, syringe exchange, HIV and hepatitis C diagnoses, overdose, and other drug-related deaths. And insights into drug markets can be obtained from examining drug seizures, prices for 'street' drugs, arrests, sales of alcohol and medications, and prescribing data.

Importantly, these data are largely collected for purposes that are not related to substance-use prevention activity, so contextualisation, analysis, and data triangulation may be required to make sense of data and render them fully useful.

Understanding Patterns and Trends in Substance Use

A range of locally available data sources can be used to help understand patterns and trends in substance use, all with strengths and weaknesses and requiring careful interpretation. However, when they are taken together and triangulated, these data can nonetheless give some useful insight into local problems. By using a variety of indicators in combination, none of which is sufficient on its own, they can provide a more accurate picture of substance use in a given population. Discussing these data with community stakeholders is also important to gain an understanding of what the substance-use issues are and identifying intervention points. The central issue is that of finding a balance between the need for comparable data and the need to develop data collection methods that are sensitive to local cultures and contexts. Below we focus on surveys, indirect methods for data collection, and use of treatment data; however in addition, data from ad hoc research studies and more qualitative information from interviews with key informants such as substance-use researchers, law enforcement, healthcare providers and social workers, and substance users themselves can all contribute to the local information base on substance-use patterns and trends.

School and General Population Surveys

Two main approaches are used to provide data to comment directly on substance use (prevalence)—surveys and statistical models. Both provide basic information to help to understand patterns of use, risk perceptions, social and health correlates, and consequences of use of psychoactive substances. These focus primarily on the general and school populations where a relatively high degree of standardisation in data collection has been achieved and representative probabilistic samples are used.

Ideally, surveys will be repeated at regular intervals using similar methodologies to allow for identification of changes in prevalence and patterns of use and with sample sizes large enough to allow for analysis of the main subgroups identified in the population. At a minimum, data should be reported on period prevalence (lifetime, last year, and last month) of different psychoactive substances to include tobacco, alcohol, marijuana, opiates such as heroin, etc. Surveys are subject to a range of sampling and non-sampling errors common to the method being used. Furthermore, despite considerable improvement in comparability over time, differences still exist in methodologies used by various countries, reporting intervals vary, and cultural and contextual factors may result in differences in response and non-response bias.

School surveys typically collect data in classrooms through anonymous questionnaires on the use of alcohol and a range of psychoactive substances. School surveys are inexpensive and easy to conduct. These surveys are particularly useful because they target adolescents who are a high-risk group for substance use. In school populations, the target age of students surveyed can substantially influence the results. Furthermore, in many countries the children most at risk of using drugs do not attend school for various reasons, while in the developing world education is not often universal, or is limited to early years of schooling. Therefore generalisations from the results of school surveys to the wider population of young people need to be made with some caution (Hibell et al., 2012).

General population surveys of substance use allow for direct measurement of substance use and patterns of use for each individual under study at national and regional levels. These surveys provide direct population estimations of substance use and other parameters such as potential determinants and eventual consequences of use (health or social) and attitudes and risk perceptions. In addition, if national surveys produce reliable and valid information, they will also allow an informed comparative analysis on the prevalence and patterns of use in different countries and regions, providing broader perspectives for policy responses in different social and cultural contexts.

General population surveys are usually cross-sectional studies, collecting data at one point in time, and therefore they do not allow strict causal inference to be derived (e.g., social deprivation causes substance use) (Hartnoll et al., 1989). To obtain data on such relationships longitudinal surveys may be considered, although these require greater resources than cross-sectional surveys. There may also be place for occasional or one-off surveys focusing on a particular issue or exploring a key hypothesis. Although some surveys include very detailed questions to users, usually there are limitations on the number of questions that can be asked in a general survey (amounts used, details on substance use, risk assessment and management, etc.).

Targeted Surveys and Modelling

Targeted surveys among selected groups with high prevalence of use (e.g. young offenders, homeless groups, or attendees at clubs or festivals), using specific sampling and data collection methods, can provide detailed information from users, particularly regarding the initiation of use, that is valuable for the development and evaluation of specific interventions.

It is well known that surveys may underestimate substance use in certain hidden and/or vulnerable populations, such as heroin or crack cocaine users, or injectors, and are considered a poor tool for reporting on low prevalence and stigmatised behaviours. To address this, prevalence estimates based on statistical models may be used. Common approaches include targeted surveys, indirect methods, estimates from statistical modelling, capture-recapture, multiplier methods, multivariate indicator methods, and ethnographic methods. In addition, new methods are being developed in this area such as city-level wastewater monitoring (EMCDDA, 2008, 2017b) which can provide a useful complement to survey data and syringe residue testing (Nefau et al., 2015) which may support results coming from other methods estimating injecting substance use.

Substance-Use Treatment Data

Data on those entering substance-use treatment programmes may be used as a proxy indicator for the characteristics of those experiencing substance problems in the population and offers a perspective on the organisation and uptake of treatment. A distinction can be made between those entering treatment for the first time and those returning to treatment. This is because the characteristics of those who have never been in treatment before are considered likely to be more representative of new cases and thus more helpful for identifying new trends than the numbers of those who have already been in contact with treatment services (Griffiths, Mounteney, Lopez, Zobel, & Götz, 2012).

The purpose is to obtain reliable information on the number and characteristics of problem substance users presenting for treatment. Such information on the number and profile of treated problem substance users and their patterns of use can help in:

- Providing a measure of treatment demand
- Providing an indicator of trends in problem substance use
- Identifying populations who might benefit from prevention and early intervention
- Planning and evaluating services for substance users
- Estimating prevalence, when used alongside other datasets
- Providing opportunities for the integration of prevention interventions into treatment settings, such as those that focus on parenting skills

Monitoring the characteristics of people seeking substance-use treatment is influenced by the availability of such treatment services and factors such as court-mandated treatment. The numbers actually taken on for treatment might just reflect the capacity of services, whereas the number requesting help is more likely to reflect demand. Treatment demand can also be considered a lagged indicator, as there tends to be a considerable delay between initial substance use and application for treatment.

Understanding Substance-Related Harm

Substance use is one of the major causes of avoidable mortality among young people in Europe and more industrialised countries, both directly through overdose and indirectly through drug-related diseases, accidents, violence, and suicide. Data regarding drug-related deaths can supplement and deepen insight into substance-use patterns and trends, notably as an indicator of the overall health impact of substance use and the components of impact, to identify risk patterns of use and to potentially identify new risks (Hickman & Taylor, 2005).

Data on substance use-related deaths can be explored via population-based statistics on deaths directly attributable to the use of these substances (drug-induced deaths, poisonings, or overdose) and also through the estimations of the overall and cause-specific mortality among problem substance users (through mortality cohort studies), which also pick up on infectious diseases, injuries and violence, suicides, and other causes of death. This data complements routine statistics and provides information on the overall and cause-specific mortality rate based on a cohort of substance users, usually in contact with drug treatment services. Data are derived from existing routine statistical systems and registries cover the whole population either at national, regional, or local level. Interpreting overdose data is complicated by a range of factors, including systematic underreporting in some countries and process-induced delays in reporting.

With regard to substance use-related morbidity and mortality as a result of infectious disease, the data refer principally—but not only—to cases of human immunodeficiency virus (HIV) and hepatitis C virus (HCV) infections. Two main data sources are available on this topic. Notification data from annual HIV case reports, where route of transmission is known, are collected in some areas. In addition, studies and ongoing surveillance exercises conducted among people who inject drugs and who are tested for HIV and/or hepatitis B and C may be available. Interpreting study data in this area is complicated by the challenges of sampling and underreporting.

Additionally, data may be available from hospital emergency rooms, and on ambulance call-outs in some localities. This data can be usefully analysed and provide insights into patterns and trends into acute substance use-related harms (Euro-DEN, 2015).

obligatory for countries that are signatories to the UN drug control conventions, this data set is generally relatively robust at the international level. Nonetheless, seizure data are problematic to interpret because they are heavily influenced by large volume seizures, most of which relate to drugs in transit rather than being reflective of local drug consumption trends (Griffiths & Mounteney, 2010). At the 'user' level, the number of seizures is more significant than quantities seized. The significance of quantities seized is questionable, unless considered in conjunction with other market indicators. In reality, both the number and size of drug seizures depend to a large extent on the priorities and resources of the enforcement agencies, and a single large seizure can distort figures. Police arrests are also used as an indicator of trends in substance use. Yet, once again, their utility is questionable unless police practices and priorities are taken into account.

Understanding Local Markets

In addition to information on use and harms, at the local level, quantitative data from law enforcement, criminal justice, and forensic science sources are also generally available. The most comprehensive data sets are in the areas of number and volume (of drug seizures), the price and purity or potency of retail-level drugs, and the number of substance use-related offences. The interpretation of these data is complicated by many factors, which include national policies and national and local policing priorities and data quality issues.

For supply-related drug interdiction efforts, intelligence and law enforcement authorities monitor trends on drug seizures and arrests for drug-related offences, as well as market price and purity information. Seizures of illicit drugs, in particular the total amounts seized, tend to be used to monitor the illicit drug market, which in turn is assumed to reflect to a certain extent levels of consumption. Methodological approaches vary, as does the quality of the information available, with data on price and purity being generally poor or unavailable. Because reporting on the number and quantity of illicit drugs seized is

Information as a Key Element to Informing Local Prevention Activities: A Systems Approach

There are many different models addressing prevention objectives in local systems; however they all have a number of common components. While addressing and informing different aspects of prevention systems they all draw on a range of local data sources and have a multidisciplinary nature. We summarise four such systems below.

Local Information Systems with a Drug Alert Function (England)

In 2016, Public Health England produced guidance to local authorities to support the establishment of local drug information systems (LDIS), to help assess intelligence and issue public health alerts on new and/or novel, potent, adulterated, or contaminated drugs (PHE, 2016). In part this initiative has been geared towards preventing inaccurate media reports and scares of new drug-related phenomena, which are rarely confirmed by toxicology tests and may sometimes be counterproductive to public health messages intended to reduce substance-related harms and deaths. The advocated local drug information systems have a primary drug alert function, including sharing and assessing information, and issuing warnings and facilitating the rapid dissemination of high-quality information to those able to implement key policy and practice responses.

The LDIS model is intended to respond to immediate risk, to be a low-cost, low-maintenance, and multidisciplinary system that uses existing local expertise and resources. In terms of scope, the LDIS model is intended to respond to dangerous, new and/or novel, potent, adulterated, or contaminated substances regardless of their legal status, including psychoactive or performance- and image-enhancing substances. Practically speaking the LDIS has a designated local coordinator, and a multidisciplinary panel with a suitable level of expertise in relevant disciplines (medical, policing, pharmacology, drug specialists) to assist in the alert process. The system is supported by and interacts with a professional interactive online information network of local professionals who share information, and expertise. Network membership is likely to differ from area to area, but comprises a mix of professionals from a range of relevant backgrounds including from health and social services, law enforcement, and trading standards.

Local Needs Assessments to Inform National Prevention Resource Allocation (Portugal)

In 2009, the Portuguese Ministry of Health established the Operational Plan of Integrated Responses (PORI) as a core component in the national drug demand reduction plan (EMCDDA, 2017c). PORI established an intervention framework targeted at drug demand reduction which is managed nationally but targeted and organised at the local/regional level. As a first phase, national workshops were held and local professionals were trained in adapted rapid assessment techniques. Back in their communities the trained experts undertook needs assessments bringing together local stakeholders from different agencies, and exploring local drug-related problems requiring a demand reduction response. Needs assessments drew on the range of available data monitoring sources including where available local surveys and routine data as well as key informant information.

Within the PORI programme, the most vulnerable Portuguese localities were mapped in order to prioritise which areas would receive resource and intervention allocation. In total 163 localities were identified for the development of integrated intervention responses across a range of demand reduction levels (prevention, treatment, harm and risk reduction, and reintegration). In 2011 some 62 integrated prevention projects were implemented in different localities across the country, covering nearly 56,400 people, mainly through awareness raising, information activities, and educational interventions.

Prevention Responses Informed by a National Network of City Drug Monitors (US, CEWG)

Established in 1976, the Community Epidemiology Working Group (CEWG) is comprised of a group of epidemiology experts from sentinel cities across the United States which meets twice a year to share information from a range of local monitoring sources (Sloboda & Kozel, 2003). The primary source of local monitoring data used is reports from city agencies (hospitals, treatment, and law enforcement). These provide a primarily quantitatively based picture of the drug situation in their cities.

Among the CEWG aims are two areas of particular relevance to prevention interventions, namely defining emergent substance-use trends and examining the time-space relationship of substance-use patterns. New drugs detected through the CEWG included crack cocaine in the 1980s, Rohypnol in the 1990s, and OxyContin in the 1990s (Sloboda, 2005). Members were able to check back in their localities and document the use and spread of these substances and any associated health problems. In addition, this network is also able to identify new ways of using substances and emerging user populations, such as the spread of methamphetamine use. Information from this network of city monitors could be fed to both public health and law enforcement agencies informing the development of education and prevention activities in response to these new trends. The CEWG has remained a model for similar national or local data collection systems worldwide.

An Integrated Approach to Local Monitoring and Prevention (Norway)

The Bergen Clinics Foundation established a city-level drug monitor, the Bergen Earlier Warning System or BEWS in 2001, providing six monthly bulletins on substance-related trends and developments (Mounteney & Leirvag, 2004). As its name suggests, the monitor aims to provide early alerts of new and emerging drug trends to allow early intervention and rapid responses to problems before they develop and spread. BEWS draws on and analyses around 50 independent data sources for its biannual reporting, including routine statistics, surveys, key informant panels, and rapid assessments. In the past, the monitor has been central in the identification of emerging issues and trends including the misuse of opioid medicines, emergence of synthetic cannabinoids and GHB/GBL, and related problems in the city. A unique feature of the system is its ability to trigger in-depth rapid assessments of specific topics, where concerns are raised by multiple signals arising from the monitoring data. Notable examples include a rapid assessment implemented to explore findings from BEWS suggesting a new cohort of young opioid users in the city and an assessment of the shape, size, and implications of GHB use. The advantages of linking the local monitoring with rapid assessment are clear, as together these approaches are capable of flagging a new trend, exploring its contours and developing a local response with the involvement of local players (Mounteney & Utne Berg, 2008). The added value of rapid assessment approaches, which of themselves and without exception will also be drawing on and analysing epidemiological results and archival data, is that they incorporate a planning and intervention stage, and are thus action focused.

A central component of the BEWS system is a city-level school survey, which has been conducted regularly and which focuses on substance use and related issues among the general student population. As mentioned earlier, student surveys are a valuable source in themselves for establishing needs and local baselines for universal prevention interventions, and in Bergen this data was additionally analysed in tandem with a comparable survey of students with truancy problems, to establish parameters for selective prevention input for this known risk group of young people (Mounteney, Haugland, & Skutle, 2010).

Conclusions

Prevention interventions are typically implemented at the community or city level, often in response to specific localised concerns or problems. Monitoring local trends can provide important information on the nature of the local problems including insights into prevalence, harms, and markets which are important elements in the establishment of relevant and targeted strategies and responses.

For prevention science, selecting appropriate interventions based on the local epidemiology and aetiology, that is to say on the evidence of the situation, context, and problems to be addressed, is a prerequisite for success. With regard to implementation of prevention science programmes, the use of local- and city-level substance-related data can play a number of important roles. While national-, regional-, or state-level data may provide a backdrop, it is clear that local data is needed for relevant and timely interventions to be established. It can help to understand the context and setting within which interventions occur; facilitate the adaptation and tailoring of programmes to meet local needs and circumstances; highlight current, new, and emerging substance trends that may need to be addressed; and allow the establishment of a pre-intervention baseline and support the evaluation of post-intervention effects.

Systematic use of monitoring data alongside the professional expertise generated by human networks can form the bedrock for effective programmes—drawing on and supported by local knowledge generation, management, and dissemination systems. The contemporary substance-use problems experienced by young people and communities are dynamic, rapidly evolving, and complex. Successful prevention programming at the community level will need to engage local communities, be adept at configuring general learning to local needs, and make needed adjustments over time reflecting the changing nature of local problems and the need to target a range of new behaviours.

References

European Drug Emergencies Network (Euro-DEN). (2015, March). *Final report of the European Drug Emergencies Network (Euro-DEN)*. Luxembourg: Office for Official Publications of the European Committee.

European Monitoring Centre for Drugs and Drug Addiction (EMCDDA). (2008). Insights 9. *Assessing illicit drugs in wastewater, potential and limitations of a new monitoring approach*. Luxembourg: Office for Official Publications of the European Committee.

European Monitoring Centre for Drugs and Drug Addiction (EMCDDA). (2017a). *European drug report 2017: Trends and developments*. Luxembourg: Publications Office of the European Union.

European Monitoring Centre for Drugs and Drug Addiction (EMCDDA). (2017b). Perspectives on drugs *Wastewater analysis and drugs: a European multi-city study*. Lisbon: European Monitoring Centre for Drugs and Drug Addiction.

European Monitoring Centre for Drugs and Drug Addiction (EMCDDA). (2017c). *Portugal, country drug report 2017*. Luxembourg: Publications Office of the European Union.

Griffiths, P., & Mounteney, J. (2010). Drug trend monitoring. In P. G. Miller, J. Strang, & P. M. Miller (Eds.), *Addiction research methods*. Oxford: Wiley-Blackwell.

Griffiths, P., Mounteney, J., Lopez, D., Zobel, F., & Götz, W. (2012). Addiction research centres and the nurturing of creativity. Monitoring the European drug situation: The ongoing challenge for the European monitoring Centre for Drugs and Drug Addiction. *Addiction, 107*, 254–258.

Hartnoll, R., Avico, U., Ingold, F., Lange, K., Lenke, L., O'Hare, A., & de Roij-Motshagen, A. (1989). A multi-city study of drug misuse in Europe. *UNODC Bulletin, 41*, 3–27.

Hibell, B., Guttormsson, U., Ahlstrom, S., Balakireva, O., Bjarnason, T., & Kokkevi, A. (2012). *The 2011 ESPAD report: Substance use among students in 36 European countries*. Stockholm: The Swedish Council for Information on Alcohol and Other Drugs (CAN); European Monitoring Centre for Drugs and Drug Addiction (EMCDDA); Council of Europe.

Hickman, M., & Taylor, C. (2005). Indirect methods to estimate prevalence. In Z. Sloboda (Ed.), *Epidemiology of drug abuse* (pp. 113–132). New York: Springer.

Mounteney, J., Haugland, S., & Skutle, A. (2010). Truancy, alcohol use and alcohol related problems in secondary school pupils in Norway. *Health Education Research, 25*, 945–954.

Mounteney, J., & Leirvag, S.-E. (2004). Providing an earlier warning of emerging drug trends: The føre var system. *Drugs: Education, Prevention and Policy, 11*, 449–471.

Mounteney, J., & Utne Berg, E. (2008). Youth, risk and rapid assessment: A new model for community social work assessment? *European Journal of Social Work, 11*, 221–236.

Nefau, T., Charpentier, E., Elyasmino, N., Duplessy-Garson, C., Levi, Y., & Karolak, S. (2015). Drug analysis of residual content of used syringes: A new approach for improving knowledge of injected drugs and drug user practices. *International Journal of Drug Policy, 26*, 412–419.

Public Health England (PHE). (2016). *Public Health England annual report and accounts 2015 to 2016*. Open Government License, London.

Sloboda, Z. (2005). Defining and measuring drug abusing behaviors. In Z. Sloboda (Ed.), *Epidemiology of drug abuse* (pp. 3–14). New York: Springer.

Sloboda, Z., & Kozel, N. (2003). Understanding drug trends in the United States of America: The role of the Community Epidemiological Work Group as part of a comprehensive drug information system. *Bulletin on Narcotics, 1&2*, 41–51.

United Nations Office on Drugs and Crime (UNODC). 2016. *World drug report*. United Nations Publication Office, Vienna.

The Importance of Mediation Analysis in Substance-Use Prevention

Holly P. O'Rourke and David P. MacKinnon

Introduction

Mediation analysis is important because it provides a way to investigate practical and theoretical questions about how and why prevention programming is successful. Theory-based approaches to substance-use prevention help researchers specify which components or elements of a prevention program that are intended to reduce substance use and promote health actually are related to the programs' short-, intermediate-, and long-term outcomes (Amaro, Blake, Schwartz, & Flinchbaugh, 2001; Astbury & Leeuw, 2010; Chen, 1990; Jacobs, Sisco, Hill, Malter, & Figueredo, 2012; Moos, 2007a, 2007b; Rogers & Weiss, 2007; Sussman, 2001). These components target the constructs within the prevention program logic model that define the desired change process that should take place. These targeted constructs are mediators. Mediators are selected based on behavior change theory, and prior empirical research on the correlates and etiology of substance use. The rationale is that if a program changes a mediator, it will also change substance use because the mediator causes substance use (MacKinnon & Dwyer, 1993). Mediation analysis is the statistical method used to test the hypothesized links from the program to the mediator to the outcome. As noted by many prevention researchers, mediation analysis is a valuable tool that can help explain the process by which a prevention program reduces substance-use outcomes (Botvin, 2000; Cuijpers, 2002; Donaldson et al., 1996; Dwyer et al., 1989; Fairchild & MacKinnon, 2009; Kisbu-Sakarya, MacKinnon, & O'Rourke, 2015; MacKinnon, 1994, 2008; MacKinnon & Dwyer, 1993; MacKinnon, Taborga, & Morgan-Lopez, 2002; MacKinnon, Weber, & Pentz, 1989; McCaul & Glasgow, 1985; Stephens et al., 2009).

Some examples of mediators in substance-use programs are the following:

- A school-based smoking prevention program in Italy increases students' refusal skills for tobacco, which then decreases smoking (Carreras, Bosi, Angelini, & Gorini, 2016).
- A prevention program designed for female high school athletes increases knowledge of the harmful effects of steroids, and increased knowledge then decreases intentions to use steroids (Ranby et al., 2009).
- A school-based substance-use prevention program (the "unplugged" program) decreases positive attitudes about substance use,

H. P. O'Rourke (✉)
T. Denny Sanford School of Social and Family Dynamics, Arizona State University, Tempe, AZ, USA
e-mail: holly.orourke@asu.edu

D. P. MacKinnon
Psychology Department, Arizona State University, Tempe, AZ, USA
e-mail: davidpm@asu.edu

increases substance-use refusal skills, and changes perceptions of peer substance use, which all in turn decrease substance use (Giannotta, Vigna-Taglianti, Galanti, Scatigna, & Faggiano, 2014).

This chapter first discusses the theories that inform mediation in substance-use prevention and practical reasons for testing mediation. We then provide a brief review of mediators in the development and evaluation of substance-use prevention programs. Next, we describe how mediators differ from other variables that influence the relation between prevention programs and outcomes and explain statistical methods for examining mediators. We end by suggesting future directions for mediation analysis that further illustrate the importance of mediators in substance-use prevention.

Theoretical Mediation Model

Rohrbach (2014) and others (Bartholomew & Mullen, 2011) underscore that most evidence-based substance-use prevention interventions are based on theory and empirical evidence that provide an understanding of the environmental and behavioral determinants of behavior related to substance use, and that describe the potential mechanisms for producing change in the outcome or behavior of interest. Intervention developers use these theories to build models for the determinants associated with substance use that are amenable to change by intervention activities. These models also help specify hypotheses about how determinants will interact over time to lead to the desired outcomes such as reduced intentions to use psychoactive substances and actual use. In substance-use prevention research, many theoretical perspectives have guided program development such as social learning (Bandura, 1977), theory of planned behavior (Fishbein & Ajzen, 1975), biology, environmental influences, epidemiology, and developmental theory, and also extensive prior empirical literature demonstrating relations between mediators and outcomes (Chassin, Curran, Hussong, & Colder, 1996; Chassin, Pillow, Curran, Molina, & Barrera, 1993; Conrad, Flay, & Hill, 1992; Flay, 1985; Flay, Phil, Hu, & Richardson, 1998; Kisbu-Sakarya et al., 2015; MacKinnon, Taborga, et al., 2002; Rogosch, Chassin, & Sher, 1990; Sher, Walitzer, Wood, & Brent, 1991; Sloboda et al., 2009; Stephens et al., 2009).

There are two primary theoretical models for statistical mediation analysis corresponding to the relation of the intervention to the mediator called action theory (also called manipulation theory) and conceptual theory (also called treatment or recidivism theory) for the relation between the mediator and the outcome (Chen, 1990; Lipsey, 1993; MacKinnon, 2008; MacKinnon, Taborga, et al., 2002). Note that action theory in mediation analysis solely refers to the theory of how the intervention changes the mediator. This notion of action theory differs from the general notion of action theory in prevention science, which typically refers to the general actions of community intervention. For mediation, it refers to the actions of the intervention to change the mediator. Action theory also provides information on the strength of program components needed to influence the hypothesized mediators. Conceptual theory refers to the formulation of hypotheses about causes of substance-use outcomes. In other words, conceptual theory provides the rationale for the choice of the mediators targeted by the prevention program.

Figure 15.1 shows action and conceptual theory for the single-mediator model. Action theory informs the a path, the effect of a substance-use prevention program on the targeted mediator, and conceptual theory informs the b path, the effect of the mediator on the substance-use outcome. A goal of mediation analysis is to estimate the a and b path coefficients, thereby providing a statistical test of each theory, and a way to understand why and how a program achieved or did not achieve effects on an outcome variable. With more than one mediator, there are action and conceptual theory coefficients for each mediator. In summary, the mediation model is important in substance-use prevention because it provides information on action theory and conceptual theory that would not be available in a model examining only the program effect on an outcome.

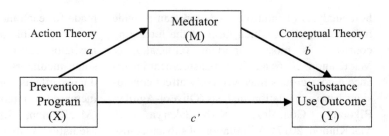

Fig. 15.1 Single-mediator model and action and conceptual theories (Kisbu-Sakarya et al., 2015)

It is helpful to place the mediation model in the context of the widely used logic model in prevention science. There are two types of logic models. The first logic model specifies the logical relations between the resources, activities, and outcomes of prevention programming (Millar, Simeone, & Carnevale, 2001; Weiss, 1972). The second logic model graphically depicts the relationship between a prevention program, specified mechanisms of change, and behavioral or health outcomes targeted by the program (Bartholomew & Mullen, 2011). Action theory in the mediation analysis context is an important part of the *logic model of the problem*, relating the components of a prevention program to determinants of health behavior. Conceptual theory is also known as the *logic model of change*, because it specifies the causal pathway from the determinants of change to the health outcomes of interest.

Practical Implications of the Theoretical Mediation Model

In addition to the core theoretical role of mediating variables in prevention of substance use, there are practical reasons for examining mediators (Judd & Kenny, 1981; MacKinnon, 1994; MacKinnon et al., 1991; MacKinnon & Dwyer, 1993; McCaul & Glasgow, 1985). When studies include measures of mediators, the measurement and analysis of the mediators and their relation to the intended outcome can provide information as to whether the prevention program first achieved the desired change in the mediator (action theory) and then whether the change in the mediator was related to the outcome of interest (conceptual theory). A significant effect of the prevention program on the targeted mediators provides information on whether a program changed the construct it was designed to change (MacKinnon, 1994, 2011; MacKinnon & Dwyer, 1993). If a prevention program that targets substance use through the mediator (e.g., refusal skills) does not change the mediator, that program component must be reviewed and revised to assure that refusal skills are significantly affected in future programs. Reasons for finding a nonsignificant effect of a prevention program on the mediator include low statistical power, inadequate measurement, and low dosage of the intervention such as from poor implementation. Planning based on statistical power calculations is as important for mediation analysis as for testing the overall program effect on the outcome. Several publications now describe approaches to determine the sample size necessary for adequate power to detect mediated effects (Fritz & MacKinnon, 2007; O'Rourke & MacKinnon, 2015; Thoemmes, MacKinnon, & Reiser, 2010). Lack of a program effect on the mediator suggests that the dose of the intervention targeting the mediator may need enhancement such as by adding additional components targeting that mediator. Inadequate implementation of program components may also lead to lack of program effects on mediators. If a program does not change a putative mediator, this could also indicate that the measurement of the mediator is unreliable or not valid. For example, if a prevention program does not have a significant effect on beliefs, it could be that a more reliable and valid measure of beliefs is needed to detect mediated effects. Of course, measurement of the mediator may be adequate but the program did not, in fact, change the mediating variable. Measurement of mediators has recently received more research attention, including some recent work that suggests how analysis of multiple mediators can provide information about which facet of the mediating construct is most important (Gonzalez & MacKinnon, 2016) and how measurement invariance across groups may adversely affect conclusions from a mediation analysis (Olivera-Aguilar, Rikoon, Gonzalez, Kisbu-Sakarya, & MacKinnon, 2017). A limitation of substance-use research in general is that there is not extensive psychometric literature on measures of mediating variables. Overall, the test of the action theory link in mediation analysis is very important because if a program does not change a putative mediator, the program is not likely to change the outcome (McCarthy, Bolt, & Baker, 2007).

A statistically significant relation of the mediator to the outcome is expected based on prior theory and empirical research. The mediator was selected for change in the program because of this hypothesized causal relation. If the observed relation of the mediator to the outcome is not statistically significant, then the theoretical and empirical basis of the program is questionable suggesting program revisions. Other reasons for the lack of a relation between the mediator and the outcome (as described above) include poor measurement of the mediator and/or outcome, and lack of statistical power. It is also possible that intervention effects on the outcome could emerge later or that the mediator was not essential in influencing the outcome (MacKinnon, 2008; MacKinnon & Dwyer, 1993).

In summary, even when the mediated effect is not statistically significant, mediation analysis provides critical insight about the prevention program by providing information on action and conceptual theory of the intervention. For example, mediation analysis provides information on *why* the program failed; that is, whether the program did not change the mediator (an action theory failure), the mediator was not related to the outcome (a conceptual theory failure), or both occurred. As a result, it is important to conduct mediation analysis whether or not there is a statistically significant effect of the program on the outcome variable because it provides information about the action and conceptual theory links in the mediation model. In practice, decisions are made for each mediator targeted by the program so it is possible that there is evidence for some mediators and not others. It is also possible that some mediators may actually have counterproductive effects, for example, changing a mediator increased intentions to use substance (MacKinnon, Krull, & Lockwood, 2000). Mediation analysis improves program efficiency by identifying ineffective program components that could be removed to reduce costs.

Mediators in Substance-Use Prevention

In substance-use prevention, an independent variable (X) is often a binary variable that represents random assignment to either a prevention program or comparison group, a mediator (M) represents a measure of the mechanism by which the prevention program achieves its effects, and an outcome (Y) is a substance-use measure. Historically, mediators have been used in substance-use prevention to develop programs based on variables that were related to the substance-use outcomes in prior theory and empirical research. As discussed above, ideally researchers have an a priori hypothesis about how the program will influence the outcome through the mediator (MacKinnon, 2008). For example, the Midwestern Prevention Project was designed to reduce student substance use by changing social norms, perceptions and beliefs about substance use, and intentions to use (MacKinnon et al., 1991). Project MYTRI (Mobilizing Youth for Tobacco-Related Initiatives in India) was designed to reduce adolescent smoking by increasing knowledge about the negative effects of tobacco use, changing beliefs about social consequences, and changing normative beliefs about tobacco use (Harrell Stigler, Perry, Smolenski, Arora, & Reddy, 2011).

Modern substance-use prevention programs commonly target one or more putative mediators that have emerged from the literature. Both psychological and behavioral mediators are targeted to prevent substance use (Kisbu-Sakarya et al., 2015). These mediators are often interrelated and can be categorized by their environmental context and risk or protective status. Mediators are typically either risk factors or protective factors (Hansen, 2002). Examples of protective factors are prosocial behaviors and problem-solving skills (Mason et al., 2009); examples of risk factors are aggression (DeGarmo, Eddy, & Reid, 2009) and susceptibility to peer pressure (Weichold, Tomasik, Silbereisen, & Spaeth, 2016). Several groups of mediators have commonly been investigated in substance-use prevention, as described next.

Social influence variables are important mediators of substance use (Cuijpers, 2002; MacKinnon, Taborga, et al., 2002). These mediators are especially important during the sensitive period of adolescence, when peer relations play an influential role in engagement in risky behaviors. Many substance-use prevention programs have targeted social influence mediators such as peer pressure or negative peer association (Henry, 2008; Weichold et al., 2016), perceptions of peer influence (Longshore, Ellickson, McCaffrey, & St. Clair, 2007; Orlando, Ellickson, McCaffrey, & Longshore, 2005), and norms (Giannotta et al., 2014; Harrell Stigler et al., 2011; Lewis Bate et al., 2009). Also related to social influence, school engagement has been examined as a protective mediator of substance use (Gonzalez et al., 2014; Wenzel, Weichold, & Silbereisen, 2009).

Parenting is important during childhood and adolescence (Sandler, Schoenfelder, Wolchik, & MacKinnon, 2011). Parent factors such as consistent and nurturing parenting style can have cascading effects through early adolescent behavior on adolescent substance use (Sitnick, Shaw, & Hyde, 2014). In later adolescence, parental behaviors such as monitoring (Vermeulen-Smit et al., 2014) and parental beliefs, attitudes, and rules about substance use (Koning, Maric, MacKinnon, & Vollebergh, 2015; Özdemir & Koutakis, 2016; Vermeulen-Smit et al., 2014) play a mediating role in the prevention of adolescent substance use. The family context is also important leading to targeting family relationships (Fang & Schinke, 2014) and family problem-solving (DeGarmo et al., 2009) mediators of substance use.

Cognitive mediators such as beliefs about substance-use consequences are also often targeted to reduce substance-use behaviors (Harrell Stigler et al., 2011; Longshore et al., 2007; Orlando et al., 2005). Additional cognitive mediators are intentions (Longshore et al., 2007; Stephens et al., 2009), knowledge about health effects or consequences (Bühler, Schröder, & Silbereisen, 2008; Harrell Stigler et al., 2011; Lewis Bate et al., 2009), and self-efficacy, or the belief in one's ability to succeed in specific situations (Fang & Schinke, 2014; Harrell Stigler et al., 2011; Longshore et al., 2007; Orlando et al., 2005).

Another set of important mediators of substance use focuses on self-regulation of behavior. Such mediators include self-control (Koning et al., 2015; Koning, van den Eijnden, Verdurmen, Engels, & Vollebergh, 2013), problem-solving (DeGarmo et al., 2009), and substance-use refusal techniques (Carreras et al., 2016; Epstein & Botvin, 2008; Giannotta et al., 2014). Table 15.1 summarizes these common mediators of substance-use prevention programs.

In summary, mediators have played a central role in substance-use prevention because of their importance in designing interventions and implications for theory testing. Because of the importance of mediators, a substantial amount of work has been devoted to developing statistical methods to most accurately test for mediating mechanisms for different research designs. The next section provides an overview of these developments.

Statistical Mediation Analysis

Third Variable Effects

Adding a third variable to the relation between program and outcome can result in different types of relationships besides mediation, such as moderation and confounding (MacKinnon, 2008) as summarized in Fig. 15.2. A third variable (Z) can be related to the program (X), the outcome (Y), or both. When Z is related to Y such that both the randomized programs X and Z have an effect on Y, Z is a covariate. When a covariate, Z, is

Table 15.1 Common mediators in substance-use prevention research

Mediator type			
Social influence	Parental factors	Cognitive factors	Behavior regulation
• Peer pressure/ association • Perceptions of peer influence • Norms • School engagement	• Parental monitoring • Parental rule setting • Parental beliefs/attitudes about alcohol use • Family dynamics	• Beliefs about consequences • Intentions to use substances • Knowledge about health effects/consequences • Self-efficacy	• Self-control • Problem-solving • Refusal skill techniques

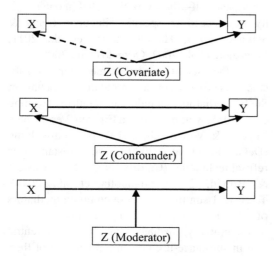

Fig. 15.2 Covariate, confounder, and moderator diagrams

related to Y, including it in a model will generally result in better prediction of Y, as more variability in Y is explained than if only X were a predictor. However, when Z is also related to X (e.g., in a nonrandomized study) such that the inclusion of Z in a model alters the relationship between X and Y, Z is a confounding variable. The predictors X and Z may be somewhat related, but as long as Z does not affect X's relation to Y, it is a covariate and not a confounder in the statistical analysis. In some situations, including a third variable Z will affect the relation between X and Y such that the X to Y relationship differs at different levels of Z; such a variable is a moderator.

To distinguish a mediator (M) from other third variables, mediators are defined by their intermediate position in the causal chain between X and Y (Cook & Campbell, 1979). For a variable to be considered a mediator, X must cause M, and then M must cause Y (MacKinnon, 2008). A mediator differs from a covariate or a confounder in that the mediator is intermediate in a causal sequence from X to M to Y. A mediator differs from a moderator in that a moderator is not intermediate in a causal sequence but affects the strength of the relation between X and Y. More discussion of third variable effects can be obtained in other publications (Elwert & Winship, 2014; MacKinnon, 2008; Valente, Pelham, Smyth, & MacKinnon, 2017).

The Single-Mediator Model

In this chapter, we use the following example of a substance-use prevention program to describe mediation scenarios. Imagine that a substance-use prevention program (X, a binary variable where participants are randomized to treatment or control) is designed to change substance-use refusal skills (M), which will then decrease substance use (Y). The following three regression equations map onto Fig. 15.3, using notation in MacKinnon (2008):

$$Y = i_1 + cX + e_1 \qquad (15.1)$$

$$Y = i_2 + c'X + bM + e_2 \qquad (15.2)$$

$$M = i_3 + aX + e_3 \qquad (15.3)$$

In the above equations, c is the effect of X on Y, or *total effect*, and in our example this is the program effect on the substance-use outcome if we excluded refusal skills (the mediator) from the model entirely. The total effect, c, is shown in the top model in Fig. 15.3. In the bottom model in

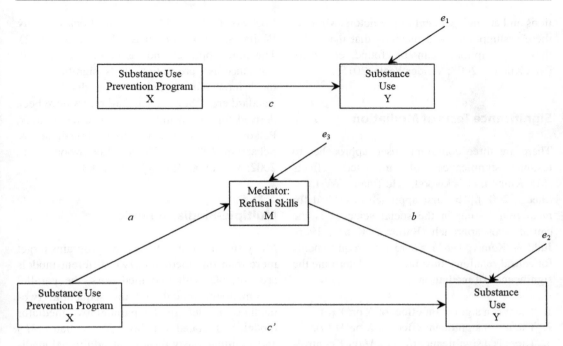

Fig. 15.3 Bivariate and single-mediator models for a substance-use prevention program example (MacKinnon, 2008)

Fig. 15.3, a is the effect of X on M (the effect of the program on refusal skills), b is the effect of M on Y controlling for X (the effect of refusal skills on substance-use controlling for the program), and c' is the effect of X on Y controlling for M or *direct effect* (the effect of the program on substance-use controlling for refusal skills). The parameters e_1, e_2, and e_3 represent the residuals. The intercepts for the equations are i_1, i_2, and i_3 and are not shown in the figure. Although both the total effect c and the direct effect c' represent the effect of X on Y (or the program effect), c' is the partial program effect controlling for the mediator.

Using these effects, for a single-mediator model using ordinary least squares (OLS) regression the mediated effect (also known as the indirect effect) can be defined in two ways. The mediated effect is often represented as the product of the a and b paths ab, or the difference between the total and direct effects $c - c'$. The total effect c is equal to the mediated effect ab plus the direct effect c', such that $ab = c - c'$ and $c = ab + c'$. The product of coefficients ab is equal to the difference $c - c'$ except in special cases, for example in logistic regression with binary Y (MacKinnon, Warsi, & Dwyer, 1995). Using our example, if substance use were measured as a binary variable (0 = never used alcohol or drugs, 1 = have used alcohol or drugs) and logistic regression was conducted, then ab would not equal $c - c'$.

The theory underlying the use of the ab mediation measure is that mediation occurs when X significantly influences M (a) and M significantly influences Y (b). A mediated effect is fully mediated when c' is zero, and ab is nonzero and statistically significant. Partial mediation occurs when c' is nonzero and there is a mediated effect. In our example, partial mediation would occur when the program significantly changed substance use through refusal skills (ab), and the program effect on substance-use controlling for refusal skills (c') was also significant. This method of estimating the mediated effect as ab or $c - c'$ has several assumptions (MacKinnon, 2008) including that the form of the causal relation between X, M, and Y is linear; no important variables that affect the relations are omitted; the model variables X, M, and Y are measured with adequate reliability and validity; and errors are independent across equations and are independent of predictors. More on these assumptions, and methods that may relax these assumptions, can be found elsewhere (MacKinnon, 2008; VanderWeele, 2015).

Significance Tests of Mediation

There are three commonly used approaches to testing significance of mediated effects (MacKinnon, Lockwood, Hoffman, West, & Sheets, 2002). The first approach described for mediation testing in the social sciences is the causal steps approach (Baron & Kenny, 1986; Judd & Kenny, 1981) where four requirements for causal relations must be met to determine the significance of mediation:

1. There is a significant effect of X on Y (c).
2. There is a significant effect of X on M (a).
3. There is a significant effect of M on Y controlling for X (b).
4. There is no significant effect of X on Y when controlling for M (c').

The fourth condition is not required for a partially mediated effect. Recent research has shown that the Baron and Kenny causal steps test has low statistical power to detect effects due to the first requirement of a significant c path (Fritz & MacKinnon, 2007; MacKinnon, Lockwood, et al., 2002; O'Rourke & MacKinnon, 2015; Shrout & Bolger, 2002). For this reason, in prevention research it is important to test for mediation even when the total effect c is not significant (O'Rourke & MacKinnon, 2018). Another causal steps approach, the test of joint significance, tests the a and b paths separately for significance to determine mediation such that if both paths are significant, mediation is present (Mackinnon, Lockwood, et al., 2002). The second approach to significance testing in mediation is the product of coefficients approach, which tests for significance using the mediated effect ab divided by its standard error (Sobel, 1982) in a z-test, or calculating asymmetric confidence intervals for ab using programs such as PRODCLIN and RMediation (MacKinnon, Fritz, Williams, & Lockwood, 2007; MacKinnon, Lockwood, & Williams, 2004; Tofighi & MacKinnon, 2011). The third approach, not as commonly used in substance-use prevention, tests significance of the difference in coefficients $c - c'$ divided by its standard error. Several standard errors have been derived for use in this significance test (Clogg, Petkova, & Shihadeh, 1992; Freedman & Schatzkin, 1992; MacKinnon, Lockwood, et al., 2002; McGuigan & Langholtz, 1988).

Multiple-Mediator Models

Many substance-use prevention programs target more than one mediator. Two different models are possible with two mediators, the parallel two-mediator model and the sequential two-mediator model. In the parallel two-mediator model, X is related to Y through a mediator (M_1) and simultaneously through an additional mediator (M_2), meaning each mediator has its own specific effects within the model. Building on our single mediator example, suppose we designed our substance-use prevention program so that a component of the program would increase substance-use refusal skills (M_1), while another component of the program would simultaneously increase self-control (M_2). Refusal skills and self-control may each work separately to decrease substance use. The following equations represent the parallel two-mediator model (MacKinnon, 2008):

$$Y = i_1 + c'X + b_1M_1 + b_2M_2 + \varepsilon_1 \quad (15.4)$$

$$M_1 = i_2 + a_1X + \varepsilon_2 \quad (15.5)$$

$$M_2 = i_3 + a_2X + \varepsilon_3 \quad (15.6)$$

In these equations, c' is the program effect on substance-use controlling for both mediators. For the a paths, a_1 is the effect of the program on refusal skills, and a_2 is the effect of the program on self-control. For the b paths, b_1 is the effect of refusal skills on substance-use controlling for self-control and the program, and b_2 is the effect of self-control on substance-use controlling for the other predictors.

Because the two mediators influence the relation between X and Y separately, there are two types of mediated effects in this model. The specific mediated effects are the product of the a and b paths, a_1b_1 and a_2b_2. The sum of the specific mediated effects is the total mediated effect, $a_1b_1 + a_2b_2$. The total mediated effect would be the mediated effect of the program on substance use through each of the parallel mediators, refusal skills and self-control. In the parallel two-mediator model, the total effect c is equal to the direct effect c' plus the total mediated effect, $a_1b_1 + a_2b_2 = c - c'$. Although there is no straightforward causal steps method for testing significance of mediation in the parallel two-mediator model, the product of coefficients method can be used to assess significance of the total mediated effect by dividing $a_1b_1 + a_2b_2$ by its standard error (MacKinnon, 2008). More accurate bootstrap confidence intervals can also be calculated for total and specific mediated effects (MacKinnon et al., 2004).

In the sequential two-mediator model, also referred to as the three-path mediator model (Taylor, MacKinnon, & Tein, 2008), two mediators (M_1 and M_2) intervene between X and Y. If we build on our single-mediator model example again, suppose we designed our program such that the program changed beliefs about substance use (M_1), which then *in turn* changed attitudes about substance use (M_2), which then *in turn* decreased substance use (Y). Equations for the sequential two-mediator model are as follows, using notation from MacKinnon (2008) and Taylor et al. (2008):

$$Y = i_1 + b_4 X + b_3 M_2 + b_6 M_1 + \varepsilon_1 \quad (15.7)$$

$$M_1 = i_2 + b_1 X + \varepsilon_2 \quad (15.8)$$

$$M_2 = i_3 + b_2 M_1 + b_5 X + \varepsilon_3 \quad (15.9)$$

In these equations, b_1 is the effect of the program on beliefs, b_2 is the effect of beliefs on attitudes controlling for the program, and b_3 is the effect of attitudes on substance-use controlling for the other predictors. The b_4 path is the *direct effect* of program on substance-use controlling for the other predictors (analogous to c' in the other models discussed in this chapter). The b_5 path is the effect of the program on attitudes controlling for beliefs, and b_6 is the effect of beliefs on substance-use controlling for the other predictors.

The sequential two-mediator model contains several different effects of X on Y. First, there is the direct effect of X on Y (b_4). Additionally, three effects form the total mediated effect: the three-path mediated effect ($b_1b_2b_3$), the two-path mediated effect passing through M_1 (b_1b_6), and the two-path mediated effect passing through M_2 (b_5b_3). The total mediated effect of X on Y is the sum of those three effects, $b_1b_2b_3 + b_1b_6 + b_5b_3$. As in the two previous models, the total mediated effect is equal to the difference between the total and direct effects, $b_1b_2b_3 + b_1b_6 + b_5b_3 = c - b_4$. The three-path mediated effect, $b_1b_2b_3$, is usually of interest in significance testing for the sequential two-mediator model. The three-path mediated effect is usually tested with the joint significance test, the product of coefficients method, or bootstrapping methods (MacKinnon, Lockwood, et al., 2002; Taylor et al., 2008).

Mediated Effect Sizes

Recent developments in effect sizes for mediation have allowed researchers to determine how large their mediated effects are, independent of sample size. If analysis of a prevention program focuses separately on action theory (a path) and conceptual theory (b path), researchers can use single effect size measures such as correlation coefficients or standardized regression coefficients separately for the a and b paths. Mediation effect sizes can be examined in two ways: individual path effect sizes (for a and b paths) and effect sizes for the mediated effect ab (MacKinnon, 2008). Several effect size measures exist for the single-mediator model (MacKinnon, 2008; Miočević, O'Rourke, MacKinnon, & Brown, 2018; Preacher & Kelley, 2011).

The R^2 effect size measure is the portion of variance in Y that is explained by the mediated effect (Fairchild, MacKinnon, Taborga, & Taylor, 2009). The proportion mediated describes the proportion of the total effect of X on Y that is mediated and is calculated as $ab/(ab + c')$. The ratio mediated compares the magnitude of the mediated effect with the direct effect of X on Y (c'), and is calculated as ab/c'. Two additional effect size measures for mediation are calculated using standard deviations of variables in the mediation model. The partially standardized mediated effect standardizes the mediated effect ab by the standard deviation of Y, and the fully standardized mediated effect standardizes ab or by the standard deviations of both X and Y (Cheung, 2009; MacKinnon, 2008). The fully standardized effect size would be useful in substance-use prevention studies with nonrandomized predictors, for example parental alcohol use (Chassin, Pillow, Curran, Molina, & Barrera, 1993). Recent methodological work on effect sizes for mediation has shown that the partially and fully standardized effect size measures have the best trade-off in terms of bias, variability, interpretability, power, and Type I error (Miočević et al., 2018). The proportion and ratio mediated effect size measures may be biased, especially at smaller sample sizes.

Future Directions for Mediation in Substance-Use Prevention

Over the last 30 years, mediation analysis has become increasingly important in substance-use prevention research. Though overall program effects on outcomes are often the primary concern in prevention research, mediation analysis can extract important additional information from substance-use studies beyond tests of program effects. Several areas of future development in substance-use prevention research are particularly relevant for mediation analysis.

Prevention programs are now being delivered in new formats with technology-based research, such as social media, ecological momentary assessment using smartphones (Baraldi, Wurpts, MacKinnon, & Lockhart, 2014), online program delivery, and increased knowledge through Massive Online Open Courses (MOOCS). Mediators provide a way to examine program mechanisms in any of these formats, but it is not clear if the same mediating mechanisms are present across different formats. Given substance-use theory, the same important mediating process operating in traditional prevention delivery settings (for example, schools) should apply in other domains, such as on social media platforms. Future research will help determine whether putative mechanisms can be more successfully targeted by new methods of program delivery in substance-use prevention.

One noteworthy limitation of the general study of mediators is measurement. Researchers often use different measures to examine a single mediating mechanism, and generally there are not accepted guidelines for measuring these constructs. Though there have been considerable developments in measures of outcomes (for example, the Patient-Reported Outcomes Measurement Information System (PROMIS) database; Cella et al., 2010), more research is needed on accurate and appropriate measurement of mediators in prevention research and other areas of research as well.

In conclusion, mediators will continue to be integral to substance-use prevention research for theoretical and practical reasons. Focus on mediators provides a framework for developing, evaluating, and improving substance-use prevention programs. Mediation analysis provides a way to test the theory upon which prevention programs are based and improves prevention programs by identifying critical ingredients that change substance use.

References

Amaro, H., Blake, S. M., Schwartz, P. M., & Flinchbaugh, L. J. (2001). Developing theory-based substance abuse prevention programs for young adolescent girls. *The Journal of Early Adolescence, 21*, 256–293.

Astbury, B., & Leeuw, F. L. (2010). Unpacking black boxes: Mechanisms and theory building in evaluation. *American Journal of Evaluation, 31*, 363–381.

Bandura, A. (1977). Self-efficacy: Toward a unifying theory of behavioral change. *Psychological Review, 84*, 191–215.

Baraldi, A. N., Wurpts, I. C., Mackinnon, D. P., & Lockhart, G. (2014). Evaluating mechanisms of behavior change to inform and evaluate technology-based interventions. In L. A. Marsch, S. E. Lord, & J. Dallery (Eds.), *Behavioral healthcare and technology: Using science-based innovations to transform practice* (pp. 187–199). New York: Oxford University Press.

Baron, R. M., & Kenny, D. A. (1986). The moderator-mediator variable distinction in social psychological research: Conceptual, strategic, and statistical considerations. *Journal of Personality and Social Psychology, 51*, 1173–1182.

Bartholomew, L. K., & Mullen, P. D. (2011). Five roles for using theory and evidence in the design and testing of behavior change interventions. *Journal of Public Health Dentistry, 71*, s20–s33.

Botvin, G. J. (2000). Preventing drug abuse in schools: Social and competence enhancement approaches targeting individual-level etiologic factors. *Addictive Behaviors, 25*, 887–897.

Bühler, A., Schröder, E., & Silbereisen, R. K. (2008). The role of life skills promotion in substance abuse prevention: A mediation analysis. *Health Education Research, 23*, 621–632.

Carreras, G., Bosi, S., Angelini, P., & Gorini, G. (2016). Mediating factors of a school-based multi-component smoking prevention intervention: The LdP cluster randomized controlled trial. *Health Education Research, 31*, 439–449.

Cella, D., Riley, W., Stone, A., Rothrock, N., Reeve, B., Yount, S., … on behalf of the PROMIS Cooperative Group. (2010). Initial item banks and first wave testing of the Patient-Reported Outcomes Measurement Information System (PROMIS) network: 2005–2008. *Journal of Clinical Epidemiology, 63*, 1179–1194.

Chassin, L., Curran, P. J., Hussong, A. M., & Colder, C. R. (1996). The relation of parent alcoholism to adolescent substance use: A longitudinal follow-up study. *Journal of Abnormal Psychology, 105*, 70–80.

Chassin, L., Pillow, D. R., Curran, P. J., Molina, B. S., & Barrera, M., Jr. (1993). Relation of parental alcoholism to early adolescent substance use: A test of three mediating mechanisms. *Journal of Abnormal Psychology, 102*, 3–19.

Chen, H. T. (1990). *Theory-driven evaluations*. Newbury Park, CA: Sage.

Cheung, M. W. (2009). Comparison of methods for constructing confidence intervals of standardized indirect effects. *Behavior Research Methods, 41*, 425–438.

Clogg, C. C., Petkova, E., & Shihadeh, E. S. (1992). Statistical methods for analyzing collapsibility in regression models. *Journal of Educational Statistics, 17*, 51–74.

Conrad, K. M., Flay, B. R., & Hill, D. (1992). Why children start smoking cigarettes: Predictors of onset. *Addiction, 87*, 1711–1724.

Cook, T. D., & Campbell, D. T. (1979). *Quasi-experimentation: Design and analysis for field settings*. Boston, MA: Houghton Mifflin.

Cuijpers, P. (2002). Effective ingredients of school-based drug prevention programs: A systematic review. *Addictive Behaviors, 27*, 1009–1023.

DeGarmo, D. S., Eddy, J. M., & Reid, J. B. (2009). Evaluating mediators of the impact of the Linking the Interests of Families and Teachers (LIFT) multimodal preventive intervention on substance use initiation and growth across adolescence. *Prevention Science, 10*, 208–220.

Donaldson, S. I., Sussman, S., MacKinnon, D. P., Severson, H. H., Glynn, T., Murray, D. M., & Stone, E. J. (1996). Drug abuse prevention programming: Do we know what content works? *American Behavioral Scientist, 39*, 868–883.

Dwyer, J. H., Mackinnon, D. P., Pentz, M. A., Flay, B. R., Hansen, W. B., Wang, E. Y. I., & Johnson, C. A. (1989). Estimating intervention effects in longitudinal studies. *American Journal of Epidemiology, 130*, 781–796.

Elwert, F., & Winship, C. (2014). Endogenous selection bias: The problem of conditioning on a collider variable. *Annual Review of Sociology, 40*, 31–53.

Epstein, J. A., & Botvin, G. J. (2008). Media resistance skills and drug skill refusal techniques: What is their relationship with alcohol use among inner-city adolescents? *Addictive Behaviors, 33*, 528–537.

Fairchild, A. J., & MacKinnon, D. P. (2009). A general model for testing mediation and moderation effects. *Prevention Science, 10*, 87–99.

Fairchild, A. J., MacKinnon, D. P., Taborga, M. P., & Taylor, A. B. (2009). R^2 effect-size measures for mediation analysis. *Behavior Research Methods, 41*, 486–498.

Fang, L., & Schinke, S. P. (2014). Mediation effects of a culturally generic substance use prevention program for Asian American adolescents. *Asian American Journal of Psychology, 5*, 116–125.

Fishbein, M., & Ajzen, I. (1975). *Belief, attitude, intention, and behavior: An introduction to theory and research*. Reading, MA: Addison-Wesley.

Flay, B. R. (1985). Psychosocial approaches to smoking prevention: A review of findings. *Health Psychology, 4*, 449–488.

Flay, B. R., Phil, D., Hu, F. B., & Richardson, J. (1998). Psychosocial predictors of different stages of cigarette smoking among high school students. *Preventive Medicine, 27*, A9–A18.

Freedman, L. S., & Schatzkin, A. (1992). Sample size for studying intermediate endpoints within intervention trials or observational studies. *American Journal of Epidemiology, 136*, 1148–1159.

Fritz, M. S., & MacKinnon, D. P. (2007). Required sample size to detect the mediated effect. *Psychological Science, 18*, 233–239.

Giannotta, F., Vigna-Tagliati, F., Galanti, M. R., Scatigna, M., & Faggiano, F. (2014). Short-term mediating factors of a school-based intervention to prevent youth substance use in Europe. *Journal of Adolescent Health, 54,* 565–573.

Gonzalez, N. A., Wong, J. J., Toomey, R. B., Millsap, R., Dumka, L. E., & Mauricio, A. M. (2014). School engagement mediates long-term prevention effects for Mexican American adolescents. *Prevention Science, 15,* 929–939.

Gonzalez, O., & MacKinnon, D. P. (2016). A bifactor approach to model multifaceted constructs in statistical mediation analysis. *Educational and Psychological Measurement, 78,* 5–31.

Hansen, W. B. (2002). Program evaluation strategies for substance abuse prevention. *The Journal of Primary Prevention, 22,* 409–436.

Harrell Stigler, M., Perry, C. L., Smolenski, D., Arora, M., & Reddy, K. S. (2011). A mediation analysis of a tobacco prevention program for adolescents in India: How did project MYTRI work? *Health Education & Behavior, 38,* 231–240.

Henry, K. L. (2008). Low prosocial attachment, involvement with drug-using peers, and adolescent drug use: A longitudinal examination of mediational mechanisms. *Psychology of Addictive Behaviors, 22,* 302–308.

Jacobs, W. J., Sisco, M., Hill, D., Malter, F., & Figueredo, A. J. (2012). Evaluating theory-based evaluation: Information, norms, and adherence. *Evaluation and Program Planning, 35,* 354–369.

Judd, C. M., & Kenny, D. A. (1981). *Estimating the effects of social interventions.* New York: Cambridge University Press.

Kisbu-Sakarya, Y., MacKinnon, D. P., & O'Rourke, H. P. (2015). Statistical models of mediation for drug program evaluation. In L. M. Scheier (Ed.), *Handbook of adolescent drug use prevention: Research, intervention strategies, and practice* (pp. 459–478). Washington, DC: American Psychological Association.

Koning, I. M., Maric, M., MacKinnon, D. P., & Vollebergh, W. A. M. (2015). Effects of a combined parent–student alcohol prevention program on intermediate factors and adolescents' drinking behavior: A sequential mediation model. *Journal of Consulting and Clinical Psychology, 83,* 719–727.

Koning, I. M., van den Eijnden, R. J. J. M., Verdurmen, J. E. E., Engels, R. C. M. E., & Vollebergh, W. A. M. (2013). A cluster randomized trial on the effects of a parent and student intervention on alcohol use in adolescents four years after baseline: No evidence of catching-up behavior. *Addictive Behaviors, 38,* 2032–2039.

Lewis Bate, S., Stigler, M. H., Thompson, M. S., Arora, M., Perry, C. L., Reddy, S., & MacKinnon, D. P. (2009). Psychosocial mediators of a school-based tobacco prevention program in India: Results from the first year of project MYTRI. *Prevention Science, 10,* 116–128.

Lipsey, M. W. (1993). Theory as method: Small theories of treatments. In L. B. Sechrest & H. G. Scott (Eds.), *Understanding causes and generalizing about them* (pp. 5–38). San Francisco, CA: Jossey-Bass.

Longshore, D., Ellickson, P. L., McCaffrey, D. F., & St. Clair, P. A. (2007). School-based drug prevention among at-risk adolescents: Effects of ALERT. *Health Education & Behavior, 34,* 651–668.

MacKinnon, D. P. (1994). Analysis of mediating variables in prevention intervention studies. In A. Cazares & L. A. Beatty (Eds.), *Scientific methods for prevention intervention research: NIDA research monograph 139* (DHHS Pub. No. 94-3631, pp. 127–153). Washington, DC: Superintendent of Documents, U. S. Government Printing Office.

MacKinnon, D. P. (2008). *Introduction to statistical mediation analysis.* Mahwah, NJ: Erlbaum.

MacKinnon, D. P. (2011). Integrating mediators and moderators in research design. *Research on Social Work Practice, 21,* 675–681.

MacKinnon, D. P., & Dwyer, J. H. (1993). Estimating mediated effects in prevention studies. *Evaluation Review, 17,* 144–158.

MacKinnon, D. P., Fritz, M. S., Williams, J., & Lockwood, C. M. (2007). Distribution of the product confidence limits for the indirect effect: Program PRODCLIN. *Behavior Research Methods, 39,* 384–389.

MacKinnon, D. P., Johnson, C. A., Pentz, M. A., Dwyer, J. H., Flay, B. R., Hansen, W. B., & Wang, E. (1991). Mediating mechanisms in a school-based drug prevention program: One year effects of the Midwestern Prevention Project. *Health Psychology, 10,* 164–172.

MacKinnon, D. P., Krull, J. L., & Lockwood, C. M. (2000). Equivalence of the mediation, confounding, and suppression effect. *Prevention Science, 1,* 173–181.

MacKinnon, D. P., Lockwood, C. M., Hoffman, J. M., West, S. G., & Sheets, V. (2002). Comparison of methods to test mediation and other intervening variable effects. *Psychological Methods, 7,* 83–104.

MacKinnon, D. P., Lockwood, C. M., & Williams, J. (2004). Confidence limits for the indirect effect: Distribution of the product and resampling methods. *Multivariate Behavioral Research, 39,* 99–128.

MacKinnon, D. P., Taborga, M. P., & Morgan-Lopez, A. A. (2002). Mediation designs for tobacco prevention research. *Drug and Alcohol Dependence, 68,* S69–S83.

MacKinnon, D. P., Warsi, G., & Dwyer, J. H. (1995). A simulation study of mediated effect measures. *Multivariate Behavioral Research, 30,* 41–62.

MacKinnon, D. P., Weber, M. D., & Pentz, M. A. (1989). How do school-based drug prevention programs work and for whom? *Drugs & Society, 3*(1–2), 125–144.

Mason, W. A., Kosterman, R., Haggerty, K. P., Hawkins, J. D., Redmond, C., Spoth, R. L., & Shin, C. (2009). Gender moderation and social developmental mediation of the effect of a family-focused substance use preventive intervention on young adult alcohol abuse. *Addictive Behaviors, 34,* 599–605.

McCarthy, D. E., Bolt, D. M., & Baker, T. B. (2007). The importance of how: A call for mechanistic research in tobacco dependence treatment studies. In T. B. Baker, R. Bootzin, & T. A. Treat (Eds.), *Psychological clinical science: Recent advances in theory and practice: Integrative perspectives in honor of Richard M. McFall* (pp. 133–163). New York: Lawrence Earlbaum Associates.

McCaul, K. D., & Glasgow, R. E. (1985). Preventing adolescent smoking: What have we learned about treatment construct validity? *Health Psychology, 4*, 361–387.

McGuigan, K., & Langholtz, B. (1988). *A note on testing mediation paths using ordinary least-squares regression.* Unpublished note.

Millar, A., Simeone, R. S., & Carnevale, J. T. (2001). Logic models: A systems tool for performance management. *Evaluation and Program Planning., 24*, 73–81.

Miočević, M., O'Rourke, H. P., MacKinnon, D. P., & Brown, C. H. (2018). Statistical properties of four effect-size measures for mediation models. *Behavior Research Methods, 50*, 285–301.

Moos, R. H. (2007a). Theory-based active ingredients of effective treatments for substance use disorders. *Drug and Alcohol Dependence, 88*, 109–121.

Moos, R. H. (2007b). Theory-based processes that promote the remission of substance use disorders. *Clinical Psychology Review, 27*, 537–551.

O'Rourke, H. P., & MacKinnon, D. P. (2015). When the test of mediation is more powerful than the test of the total effect. *Behavior Research Methods, 47*, 424–442.

O'Rourke, H. P., & MacKinnon, D. P. (2018). Reasons for testing mediation in the absence of an intervention effect: A research imperative in prevention and intervention research. *Journal on Studies of Alcohol and Drugs, 79*, 171–181.

Olivera-Aguilar, M., Rikoon, S. H., Gonzalez, O., Kisbu-Sakarya, Y., & MacKinnon, D. P. (2017). Bias, Type I error rates, and statistical power of a latent mediation model in the presence of violations of invariance. *Educational and Psychological Measurement, 78*, 460–481.

Orlando, M., Ellickson, P. L., McCaffrey, D. F., & Longshore, D. L. (2005). Mediation analysis of a school-based drug prevention program: Effects of project ALERT. *Prevention Science, 6*, 35–46.

Özdemir, M., & Koutakis, N. (2016). Does promoting parents' negative attitudes to underage drinking reduce adolescents' drinking?: The mediating process and moderators of the effects of the Örebro Prevention Programme. *Addiction, 111*, 263–271.

Preacher, K. J., & Kelley, K. (2011). Effect size measures for mediation models: Quantitative strategies for communicating indirect effects. *Psychological Methods, 16*, 93–115.

Ranby, K. W., Aiken, L. S., MacKinnon, D. P., Elliot, D. L., Moe, E. L., McGinnis, W., & Goldberg, L. (2009). A mediation analysis of the ATHENA intervention for female athletes: Prevention of athletic-enhancing substance use and unhealthy weight loss behaviors. *Journal of Pediatric Psychology, 34*, 1069–1083.

Rogers, P. J., & Weiss, C. H. (2007). Theory-based evaluation: Reflections ten years on: Theory-based evaluation: Past, present, and future. *New Directions for Evaluation, 114*, 63–81.

Rogosch, F., Chassin, L., & Sher, K. J. (1990). Personality variables as mediators and moderators of family history risk for alcoholism: Conceptual and methodological issues. *Journal of Studies on Alcohol, 51*, 310–318.

Rohrbach, L. A. (2014). Design of prevention interventions. In Z. Sloboda (Ed.), *Defining prevention science* (pp. 275–291). Boston, MA: Springer.

Sandler, I. N., Schoenfelder, E. N., Wolchik, S. A., & MacKinnon, D. P. (2011). Long-term impact of prevention programs to promote effective parenting: Lasting effects but uncertain processes. *Annual Review of Psychology, 62*, 299–329.

Sher, K. J., Walitzer, K. S., Wood, P. K., & Brent, E. E. (1991). Characteristics of children of alcoholics: Putative risk factors, substance use and abuse, and psychopathology. *Journal of Abnormal Psychology, 100*, 427–448.

Shrout, P. E., & Bolger, N. (2002). Mediation in experimental and nonexperimental studies: New procedures and recommendations. *Psychological Methods, 7*, 422–445.

Sitnick, S. L., Shaw, D. S., & Hyde, L. W. (2014). Precursors of adolescent substance use from early childhood and early adolescence: Testing a developmental cascade model. *Development and Psychopathology, 26*, 125–140.

Sloboda, Z., Stephens, R. C., Stephens, P. C., Grey, S. F., Teasdale, B., Hawthorne, R. D., … Marquette, J. F. (2009). The adolescent substance abuse prevention study: A randomized field trial of a universal substance abuse prevention program. *Drug and Alcohol Dependence, 102*, 1–10.

Sobel, M. E. (1982). Asymptotic confidence intervals for indirect effects in structural equation models. In S. Leinhardt (Ed.), *Sociological methodology* (pp. 290–312). Washington, DC: American Sociological Association.

Stephens, P. C., Sloboda, Z., Stephens, R. C., Teasdale, B., Grey, S. F., Hawthorne, R. D., & Williams, J. (2009). Universal school-based substance abuse prevention programs: Modeling targeted mediators and outcomes for adolescent cigarette, alcohol, and marijuana use. *Drug and Alcohol Dependence, 102*, 19–29.

Sussman, S. (Ed.). (2001). *Handbook of program development for health behavior research and practice.* Thousand Oaks, CA: Sage.

Taylor, A. B., MacKinnon, D., & Tein, J.-Y. (2008). Test of the three-path mediated effect. *Organizational Research Methods, 11*, 241–269.

Thoemmes, F., MacKinnon, D. P., & Reiser, M. R. (2010). Power analysis for complex mediational designs using Monte Carlo methods. *Structural Equation Modeling, 17*, 510–534.

Tofighi, D., & MacKinnon, D. P. (2011). RMediation: An R package for mediation analysis confidence intervals. *Behavior Research Methods, 43*, 692–700.

Valente, M. J., Pelham, W., Smyth, H., & MacKinnon, D. P. (2017). Confounding in statistical mediation analysis: What it is and how to address it. *Journal of Counseling Psychology, 64*, 659–671.

VanderWeele, T. (2015). *Explanation in causal inference: Methods for mediation and interaction.* New York, NY: Oxford University Press.

Vermeulen-Smit, E., Mares, S. H. W., Verdurmen, J. E. E., Van der Vorst, H., Schulten, I. G. H., Engels, R. C. M. E., & Vollebergh, W. A. M. (2014). Mediation and moderation effects of an in-home family intervention: The "In control: No alcohol!" pilot study. *Prevention Science, 15*, 633–642.

Weichold, K., Tomasik, M. J., Silbereisen, R. K., & Spaeth, M. (2016). The effectiveness of the life skills program IPSY for the prevention of adolescent tobacco use: The mediating role of yielding to peer pressure. *The Journal of Early Adolescence, 36*, 881–908.

Weiss, C. H. (1972). *Evaluation research: Methods for assessing program effectiveness.* Englewood Cliffs, NJ: Prentice-Hall, Inc.

Wenzel, V., Weichold, K., & Silbereisen, R. K. (2009). The life skills program IPSY: Positive influences on school bonding and prevention of substance misuse. *Journal of Adolescence, 32*, 1391–1401.

Subgroup Analysis: "What Works Best for Whom and Why?"

Ferdinand Keller

Introduction

The chapter starts with an introductory example using main results from two large randomized trials to evaluate substance use prevention programs. Basic questions are explored such as: Is the program equally effective for boys and girls, or is it effective for baseline users of alcohol although no overall beneficial effect could be confirmed? The next section looks at how subgroups can be defined and introduces the distinction between manifest (= directly observable) and latent (= not directly observable) variables. Then, statistical approaches for conducting subgroup analyses are presented. The focus will be on mainly newer methods taking into account the multilevel structure of data, mediation and moderation approaches, and the testing of the interaction effect as gold standard in biostatistics. Special emphasis is given to models using latent variables such as latent class analysis (LCA) and growth mixture models (GMM). Exploratory subgroup analysis has been enhanced considerably by applying these so-called mixture models (LCA and GMM are just two specific methods of the family of mixture models). They help in identifying potential differences in outcome that might exist in a population, and to estimate treatment effects for previously unknown subgroups.

Despite this pool of advantageous new methods, some basic (intrinsic) risks in subgroup analyses remain. Two major issues for the appraisal of subgroup findings are introduced: (a) is there an overall significant effect in the trial, and (b) is the subgroup analysis preplanned (= confirmatory analysis) or use primarily for exploratory purposes. These subjects set the framework for a proper interpretation of subgroup results. In particular, the problem of finding false-positive results arises, but, conversely, it may also falsely be concluded that an intervention is not effective in a subgroup (false-negative result). Some examples from the literature are given to illustrate potential pitfalls. Finally, strategies for dealing with the risks and limitations of subgroup analysis are discussed (i.e., meta-analysis, statistical adjustment of error rates, and some recent methods), and some agreed-upon recommendations for reporting of results are provided.

Why Subgroup Analysis?

Subgroup analysis can help in detecting differential response to an intervention and is often used to evaluate the effectiveness for specific subgroups. Consider as an illustrating example the results of two large randomized trials that were designed to evaluate the effectiveness of

F. Keller (✉)
Department of Child and Adolescent Psychiatry and Psychotherapy, University Hospital Ulm, Ulm, Germany
e-mail: Ferdinand.keller@uniklinik-ulm.de

universal school-based substance abuse prevention programs with comparable preventive interventions applied to same-aged populations. One is the U.S. Adolescent Substance Abuse Prevention Study (ASAPS) (Sloboda et al., 2009) and the other the EU-DAP study (EUropean Drug Addiction Prevention trial) (Faggiano et al., 2010). The overall findings of these two interventions varied across programs. A full summary of the results is beyond the scope of this chapter, but there were differences with regard to alcohol use that may serve as an initial focus for the present topic. In the 18-month follow-up of EU-DAP, persisting beneficial program effects were found for episodes of drunkenness (Faggiano et al., 2010). In ASAPS follow-up, no beneficial effects on alcohol use were found (Sloboda et al., 2009). Several questions arise consequently for further analyses: Is there a beneficial effect for a specific subgroup within the ASAPS sample (despite the missing overall effect), e.g., for baseline users of alcohol? For EU-DAP: Is the (overall significant) intervention also effective in specific subgroups, e.g., in male and female students alike?

More generally, Bloom and Michalopoulos (2013) propose three types of research questions that may motivate subgroup analyses:

– how widespread are the effects of an intervention?
– is the intervention effective for a specific subgroup?
– is the intervention effective for any subgroup?

Definition and Types of Subgroups

Subgroup analysis is usually defined as an analysis in which the intervention effect is evaluated in a defined subset of the participants in a trial, or in complementary subsets, such as by sex or in age categories. Subgroups can be characterized by manifest (= directly observable) or latent (= not directly observable) variables.

In application to prevention research, subgroups can be defined in many different ways and Bloom and Michalopoulos (2013) suggest defining subgroups in terms of several characteristics:

- Demographic variables (age, gender, educational background, etc.)
- Risk factors (past smoking, drinking, drug abuse, etc.)
- Current health status or severity of a problem/disease which is to be treated by the intervention

In larger studies, subgroups may also be built according to geographic location or site (county, state; hospital, school). More recently, new kinds of variables are available for statistical analyses, in particular genetic and epigenetic predictors (Latendresse, Musci, & Maher, 2018). It should be emphasized that subgroup analyses should not be based on all variables that are available in the data set, but should be motivated by the underlying theory of change of the intervention program. The theory should also provide guidance to determine factors that explain variation in responsiveness to the intervention as well as moderators and mediators of impact.

Characteristics like those listed above are considered directly observable and they are called manifest variables in statistical terminology. Many characteristics are, however, not directly observable, but are inferred from indicators such as items of questionnaires or by other types of assessment instruments. Examples are ample in the social sciences, e.g., personality factors or intelligence components are considered to be latent constructs. Examples in prevention science are that not everyone involved in a targeted intervention responds equally to the intervention due to a (unknown) combination of variables (Nylund-Gibson & Hart, 2014), or a persons' attitude towards alcohol or drug use. Such variables are termed latent variables. Both manifest and latent variables are often used to model heterogeneity, i.e., to explain quantitative or qualitative differences in a population. Understanding the heterogeneity among individuals within a targeted population, or, vice versa, uncovering the way individuals are similar, ultimately provides the opportunity to understand outcomes and to design better treatment measures and intervention efforts (Nylund-Gibson & Hart, 2014).

Latent subgroups may also be defined longitudinally, i.e., by the responsiveness to an intervention or by trajectories in outcome across the observation period. Examples are the course of aggressive behavior across school grades (Petras, Masyn, & Ialongo, 2011) or the degree of delinquent behavior during adolescence (Jones & Nagin, 2007). These "definitions," however, are based on probabilistic assignment of individuals to their most likely class and emerge only during the study. Since group membership is not known at baseline and, therefore, stratified randomization of treatment assignment to the subgroups is not possible, this type of subgroup is usually not included in "pure" subgroup analysis recommendations. Nonetheless, heterogeneity in the developmental course and subgroup differences can be hypothesized and used for confirmatory analyses of the trial.

Statistical Approaches for Conducting Subgroup Analysis

Subgroup Analysis with Manifest Variables

For the analysis of subgroups defined by manifest variables, several statistical approaches have been proposed. In a simplifying manner, two main approaches could be distinguished: (1) hierarchical (or multilevel) linear models for longitudinal designs and (2) the mediation and moderation approach. Both model families are discussed only briefly below, since they cover a wide range of potential models and an extensive introduction is beyond the scope of this chapter. Furthermore, mediational models are addressed in a special chapter in this book (O'Rourke and MacKinnon). Finally, (3) the addition of interaction terms to the statistical model in question as the recommended method in biostatistics is introduced and discussed.

1. Hierarchical (or multilevel) linear models are often applied in the social sciences. They correct for clustering (e.g., students nested in classes, classes nested in schools, or, in the longitudinal case, observations within persons and with explaining covariates added) and provide correct p-values for this type of nested data. They also overcome some limitations of "classical," well-known techniques such as repeated measures ANOVA, in allowing for missing data and unequal time spaces between observations (Hox, 2010; Singer & Willett, 2003; Verbeke & Molenberghs, 2000).

2. Another well-known and applied approach is mediation and moderation analysis. Fairchild and MacKinnon (2014) in their introduction to these methods target the same question as the title of this chapter when they discuss these models "with the ultimate goals of identifying the active ingredients of these programs and to address the question what works for whom under what conditions" (p. 538). Advantages of the mediation-moderation approach are its potential to inform about the effectiveness of program components and thus to refine curriculum development and implementation strategies. Fairchild and MacKinnon (2014) provide a comprehensive introduction into the mediation model and the moderation model, and also their combination. For example, they found in the evaluation of a worksite wellness program that outcome was moderated by part-time versus full-time work status. A mediation model was then used to explain this difference, and it could be shown that full-time workers were getting more exposure to program-related social norms at the work place, contributing to their larger program effect. If mediators are also measured repeatedly during a trial, they can be incorporated in various types of longitudinal structural equation mediation models to determine the active components of a program. Goldsmith et al. (2017) provide a tutorial how to fit and interpret various longitudinal mediation models, based on a trial of rehabili-

tative treatments for chronic fatigue syndrome as a motivating example. Wang and Ware (2013) also show the opportunities of moderator analyses in detecting subgroup effects. Schochet, Puma, and Deke (2014) provide a formal introduction into subgroup analysis within the regression context and Cordova et al. (2014) give a conceptual overview over statistical models that aim to identify those pathways through which prevention interventions work.

3. In biostatistics, there is agreement that the appropriate way to examine whether a treatment effect differs between subgroups is to test for an interaction effect between treatment and subgroup (Brookes et al., 2004; Rothwell, 2005; Schulz, Altman, Moher, & CONSORT Group, 2010). (In the social sciences, the question of interest whether the treatment effect varies among the levels of a baseline factor is often referred to as moderator analysis). Separate analyses of the treatment effect within each subgroup are not recommended since such multiple comparisons increase the risk of obtaining false-positive results. Conversely, subgroup-specific comparisons result in smaller data sets and thus reduced power to detect a true treatment effect (false-negative finding).

The test of the interaction effect revealed to be quite reliable; simulation studies have shown that the interaction test performed well (Brookes et al., 2001). When there was no true overall treatment effect, the percentage of false-positive overall tests remained at 5%; in the presence of a true overall effect, the percentage of tests that were (correctly) significant reflected the power of the data set (Brookes et al., 2004). These authors also show how power goes down in subgroup analyses. Regarding power of the interaction test, a trial with 80% power for the overall effect had only 29% power to detect an interaction effect of the same magnitude. For interactions of this size to be detected with the same power as the overall effect, sample sizes need to be inflated fourfold (Brookes et al., 2004). Given this lack of power for the interaction test in the analysis of a trial (that is usually powered only for the main effect), failure to find a significant interaction does not show that the treatment effect seen overall applies to all individuals (Wang & Ware, 2013).

Subgroup Analysis with Latent Variables

If one is interested in detecting unknown subpopulations defined by a *set* of indicators within the study sample who respond differently to the intervention, identification of subpopulations based on mixture models is well suited. The basic idea behind mixture modeling lies in assuming that the observed values of variables (e.g., means, frequencies in cross-tables, regression coefficients, trajectories) are not the same for all persons in the sample, but are different for subgroups within the sample. In other words, and narrowed down to the case of latent class analysis (LCA), one assumes that the overall population heterogeneity with respect to a set of manifest (categorical) variables results from the existence of two or more distinct homogeneous subgroups, or latent classes, of individuals (Masyn, 2013). Over the last two decades, several variations of mixture modeling have been developed, and the models can be grouped according to whether the latent variable is considered categorical or continuous, and whether analysis of a cross-sectional or a longitudinal design is intended (c.f. Muthén, 2002; Nylund-Gibson & Hart, 2014).

Most applications of these mixture models in prevention science seem to use a categorical latent variable to describe population heterogeneity. An example of LCA is provided by Lanza and Rhoades (2013, see below in Section "Recent Strategies"). Conventional regression analysis can be made more flexible by regression mixture analysis where latent classes in the data can be identified and regression parameter estimates can vary between latent classes. Van Horn et al.

(2009) use regression mixture analysis to capture differential effects of family resources on children's academic outcomes and Ding (2006) provides a worked-through example of this method where differential relationships between children's math achievement, children's math self-concept, and teacher's rating are analyzed.

LCA can be extended to the longitudinal case, called latent transition analysis (LTA—e.g., Collins & Lanza, 2010). In longitudinal studies with continuous outcome variables, especially with more than three assessment points, it is favorable to identify latent classes with the latent class growth model (LCGM) proposed by Nagin (Jones & Nagin, 2007; Nagin, 1999) or in a more general form, the so-called growth mixture models (GMM—Muthén and Muthén, 2000; Pickles & Croudace, 2010). GMM are conducted to estimate the number of latent classes with the same trajectory, the size of the latent classes, and to attribute individuals to these trajectory classes which are characterized by different courses over time. For example, Petras et al. (2011) examined the impact of two universal preventive interventions in first grade on the growth of aggressive/disruptive behavior in grades 1–3 and 6–12. They modeled growth trajectories for each of the two time periods separately, and then associated the latent trajectory classes of aggressive/disruptive behavior across the two time periods using a latent transition model. Subsequently, it was tested whether the interventions had direct effects on trajectory class membership in the two time periods and whether the interventions affected the transition between periods. One of the findings was that males in the intervention condition were significantly more likely than control males to transition from the high trajectory class in grades 1–3 to a low class in grades 6–12.

A challenge of these methods lies in the problem that the number of latent classes is unknown and must be estimated by comparing various statistical criteria such as goodness of fit and information criteria (Petras & Masyn, 2010; Wright & Hallquist, 2014; Muthén, 2003). The trajectory groups cannot be prespecified (and are therefore not known at baseline), but it is usually attempted to relate the latent classes that emerge in the GMM to baseline characteristics or consequences of change, e.g., relate the course of aggressive behavior trajectories in school to records of violent and criminal behavior as young adults (cf. Petras & Masyn, 2010). An excellent introduction with applications in Mplus syntax (Muthén and Muthén, 1998–2012) is given in Jung and Wickrama (2008).

The mixture model approach is mostly used in an exploratory manner and seems especially promising in prevention science since most subgroup analyses are conducted for universal intervention programs. It helps to gain more information on heterogeneity in the sample and to transfer and integrate the findings into substantive theories. The cost for making use of these very flexible methods is that they are (primarily) data-driven and hypotheses based on the findings should be subjected to further testing. There has also been extended discussion about how to find the "correct" number of latent classes and whether the classes represent "real" entities or more statistical artifacts (see Masyn, 2013; Muthén, 2003). Unfortunately, some of these issues cannot be solved by means of replication since a new sample will give a similar distribution with similar ambiguities about the characteristics of the population distribution (Petras & Masyn, 2010).

In principle, approaches like hierarchical (or multilevel) linear models and especially moderator/mediator models deal with relations (covariance) between *variables* and are called variable-oriented, while LCA/GMM deal with *individuals*, called person-oriented approach. Both look at the same data matrix (one on the "columns," the other on the "rows") and are equivalent, but have their advantages depending on the research question (Masyn, 2013; Muthén & Muthén, 2000). Advantage of the person-oriented approach is the identification of previously unknown groups of persons (latent classes) which is usually not possible in the variable-oriented approach (the distinguishing combination(s) of moderator variables had to be known).

Risks and Limitations of Subgroup Analysis

The second part of this chapter details some risks and problems that arise when applying and interpreting subgroup analysis. Let us refer back to the questions from the introductory example, e.g., it was asked whether the intervention in EU-DAP was effective for boys and for girls. Indeed, the effectiveness of the program was examined according to sex, and a significant association between the program and a lower prevalence of all behavioral outcomes was found among boys, but not among girls (Vigna-Taglianti et al., 2009). The researchers state as a limitation that there was not enough power in the study for subgroup analyses, which had an impact on the precision of the estimates. Thus, it may be likely that no significant effect was found for a specific subgroup (here: females), because there was not sufficient statistical power to detect the effect, and it is falsely assumed that this subgroup received no benefit from the intervention. This type of error is called false-negative or (in statistics) type II error. On the other hand, testing for subgroup differences in the ASAPS study might reveal a significant effect for a specific subgroup, but it may be a statistical artifact caused by performing many statistical tests and thus increasing the chance of finding a (spurious) significant effect. This type of error is called false-positive or type I error. Furthermore, many statisticians would question the validity of such post-hoc subgroup differences in the absence of an overall significant effect (here: no significant overall effect on alcohol use in ASAPS).

More generally, proper interpretation of subgroup differences demands consideration of various prerequisites, in particular the number of statistical tests performed, whether they are testing preplanned hypotheses or are exploratory, and whether the intervention effect is significant in the full sample of the trial.[1]

In case of a positive overall effect in a study, further subgroup analysis is justified and can be used to detect differential response to an intervention. The general research question then is "Do the treatment effects vary among the levels of a baseline factor?" (Wang, Lagakos, Ware, Hunter, & Drazen, 2007, p. 2189), e.g., for males and females, for different ethnicities, or for varying levels of illness at baseline. However, as indicated above, in these applications of subgroup analysis there is the risk of false-negative results.

In the case where no overall effect is found in a study, the situation gets more complicated. Since usually much time, effort, and money have been invested in conducting large prevention program studies with randomized control groups or quasi-experimental designs, the question arises whether the tested program is effective for specific subgroups within the study population (although there is no significant effect on the overall study population). In general, statisticians would reject these further analyses (except for conducting exploratory analyses that have to be confirmed in future studies) and would call this approach as "rescuing a failed trial" or "exercises in pure data dredging." Applied scientists, on the other hand, may argue that a difference in effectiveness for subgroups is valid if there are good reasons to explain the difference. Prevention scientists/practitioners may argue as well, based on their experience while planning and conducting the prevention programs, that a subgroup difference may be valid. Unfortunately, almost all subgroup differences seem explainable post-hoc, and there are numerous examples where these effects turned out later to be false-positive (see the example from biotech research below).

Besides the question whether there is a significant overall effect in the trial, another distinction is important for statistical analysis and interpretation of subgroup findings: were the analyses

---

[1] A special situation arises in some universal prevention trials where it is not expected to find an overall effect, but only for a specific subgroup. For technical and/or ethical reasons, however, it is not possible to apply targeted prevention to this subgroup. For example, Petras et al. (2011) evaluated the program Good Behavior Game in school classes and expected that the impact on aggressive behavior was concentrated among high aggressive boys. Usually, though, overall effects are reported in universal prevention, and the effect sizes of the full trial are included in meta-analysis.

exploratory or confirmatory? Confirmatory analyses provide an appropriate basis to assess how strongly the study's prespecified central hypotheses are supported by the data. Exploratory analyses, on the other hand, examine relationships within the data to identify outcomes or subgroups for which impacts may exist. The goal of these exploratory analyses is to generate hypotheses that could be subject to more rigorous future examination. Overall, the strength of evidence based on confirmatory findings is higher than that based on exploratory findings, and this difference should be made clear to one's reader (Bloom & Michalopoulos, 2013).

Biostatisticians have especially criticized that exploratory analyses testing many subgroup differences increase the risk of false-positive results and may produce spurious findings. This problem is known under different names, e.g., alpha-error inflation, multiple testing problem, or as multiplicity in biomedical guidelines. Most statistical textbooks provide a formal treatment of the problem of multiple testing. The following excurse is based on Schochet (2008).

For example, a difference between two treatment groups is to be explored, and a t-test is applied for testing the significance of the difference. Suppose that the null hypothesis is true for each test and that the tests are independent. Then, the chance of finding at least one spurious impact is $1 - (1 - alpha^N)$, where alpha is the percentage of type I errors and N is the number of tests, e.g., if several outcomes or, equivalently, subgroups are tested. If the alpha error is set at 5%, the probability of making at least one type I error is 10% if two tests are conducted, and 23% if five tests and 40% if ten tests are conducted.

Thus, the more subgroup analyses are performed the higher the chance to find significant subgroup differences. Therefore, guidelines have been developed for statistical analyses in pharmacological trials as well as recommendations for interpreting and reporting estimates of intervention effects for subgroups of a study sample. These guidelines have become very strict and it is unlikely that any conclusion of treatment efficacy based solely on exploratory subgroup analyses would be accepted in the absence of a significant overall effect (EMA—ICH E9, 2006). However, there is also the risk of false-negative results in subgroup analysis, i.e., the finding that a particular subgroup does not benefit from an intervention program or gets even worse. Such findings may also be chance findings or a consequence of low power to detect true effects.

The examples presented in the next section show some false-positive as well as false-negative findings that were from minor up to major importance. Because no good examples from substance use research seem available, they come from medical science. Furthermore, problems with post-hoc findings in subgroups have been recognized much earlier in medical science, in particular in pharmacological treatment studies, than in prevention research. Therefore, exploratory findings in, e.g., cardiology have meanwhile been subject to replications, and it could be determined whether reproducibility could be achieved. Several elaborated reviews of these results have been compiled, biostatisticians have developed consensus on the process and requirements of statistical analysis, and finally guidelines have been published for planning and presenting the results of investigations (see below).

Example: subgroups with false-positive finding

Differentiation according to the severity of illness is a common practice in doing exploratory analyses of trials (especially if there is no overall significant effect), e.g., one is interested in whether the intervention is effective at an early stage of the disease or at an advanced stage or in both. Major erroneous findings seem not to exist in prevention science, at least they are not referenced in respective articles. Therefore, a striking example from biotech research where personal and financial consequences have been dramatic may illustrate the potential danger of a post-hoc subgroup interpretation that was prematurely communicated as a scientific result and turned out later to be false-positive. The following summary is based on an article by David Brown in the *Washington Post (September 23,* 2013*);* c.f. also Hodgson (2016).

The biotech company InterMune sought approval to market its drug for a more common ailment, idiopathic pulmonary fibrosis (IPF). In all, 330 patients were randomly assigned to get either interferon gamma-1b or placebo injections. Disease progression or death occurred in 46 percent of those on the drug and 52 percent of those on placebo. That was not a significant difference ($p = 0.08$). However, when looking into subgroups it turned out that people with mild to moderate cases of the disease had a dramatic difference in survival: only 5% of those taking the drug died, compared with 16% of those on placebo. The p-value was 0.004.

The company announced in a press release that the drug *"Reduces Mortality by 70% in Patients with Mild to Moderate Disease."* This statement had severe consequences for the CEO (6 months of home confinement and partial exclusion from working).

InterMune run another trial (planned sample: 826 patients at 81 hospitals) in order to maximize the chance of getting clear-cut results. It enrolled only people with mild to moderate lung damage. And it failed. A little more than a year into the study, more people on the drug had died (15%) than people on placebo (13%).

Besides the personal consequences for the CEO, the more interesting thing for science is that the findings of exploratory subgroup analyses (i.e., a positive treatment effect in mild/moderate illness) should be clearly distinguished from confirmed results. The example also underscores the importance of replication studies.

Examples: subgroups with no or negative finding

Rothwell (2005) warns that we must also be cautious in focusing on subgroups with an apparent neutral or negative trend. As mentioned above, the correct statistical analysis is not to test the significance of the treatment effect in every subgroup, but whether the effect differs between the subgroups, i.e., the interaction effect treatment × subgroup has to be examined.

The following examples taken from Rothwell (2005) illustrate complications on various levels of interpretability of the findings:

1. In a trial on the treatment of severe stenosis, carotid endarterectomy was significantly beneficial. A subgroup analysis according to day of birth revealed that there was no significant effect for patients born on the weekend and on Tuesday and Thursday. Significant effects emerge for Monday, Wednesday, and Friday. These differences in effectiveness were due to chance; there was no subgroup × treatment effect interaction ($p = 0.83$).
2. In a large trial on the effectiveness of Aspirin vs. Placebo in acute myocardial infarction, the study result was highly significant in favor of Aspirin ($p < 0.0001$). In subsequent subgroup analyses, the zodiac signs of the patients were considered and Aspirin was ineffective in patients born under zodiac signs of Libra and Gemini, but was beneficial in all other zodiac signs. The subgroup treatment effect interaction seems $p = 0.01$ (estimated by Rothwell), but there is no explanation of this result (Libra and Gemini are not adjacent on the Zodiac) and Rothwell concludes that a more appropriate test of the interaction effect would "undoubtedly be nonsignificant" (Rothwell, 2005, p. 182).
3. However, Rothwell provides further examples where highly significant interaction effects occur by chance indicating that some subgroups have no benefit. One comes from the stenosis trial explained above, where different benefits were observed according to month of birth of the patient (interaction $p < 0.001$), but the differences could not be explained by any other plausible variable.
4. While these examples are more or less curious and had no practical consequences for treatment decisions, others were more damaging. Rothwell (2005) reports the observation in a large Canadian study in the 1970s that aspirin was effective in preventing stroke and death in men but not in women (interaction $p = 0.003$). Thus, women were considered not to benefit from aspirin and were undertreated for at least a decade, until subsequent studies and meta-analyses showed effectiveness in both groups.

These examples have shown that some of the differential results can easily be falsified if the correct statistical test (= test of interaction effect) is applied (example 1). Others are more difficult to reject, but finally will be rejected, usually because there is no rational explanation for a subgroup finding (example 2), and even others like the gender difference in the effectiveness of aspirin (example 4) can only be overcome by replication in subsequent trials and by combining their outcomes in meta-analyses. Thus, the best test of the validity of subgroup-specific effects is reproducibility in other trials, since interaction effects may yield spurious results because of alpha error (examples 3 and 4).

Risk-Benefit Considerations

Beyond the methodological and statistical problems in determining the effectiveness of a program, a risk not to be neglected is the potential harm of prevention programs. For example, Sloboda et al. (2009) found moderate iatrogenic effects for the subgroup of baseline nonusers of alcohol in the ASAPS study.

Usually, prevention interventions are not considered to be harmful, at least in the context of universal prevention programs (in selected intervention programs, there is the risk of labeling and stigmatization). However, there are hints that iatrogenic effects emerge in universal substance prevention programs. Another example for negative consequences caused by a prevention program is the evaluation of the National Youth Anti-Drug Media Campaign (1998–2004) in the USA (Hornik, Jacobsohn, Orwin, Piesse, & Kalton, 2008). The campaign followed three large, nationally representative cohorts of adolescents over four time-points. The evaluation results revealed that the campaign had no overall effect on marijuana use or other outcome variables. Furthermore, there were hints for promarijuana effects in time-lagged analyses, i.e., unfavorable lagged exposure effects. Based on these results and further analyses of the campaign, Burkhart and Simon (2015) discuss the important ethical concern that an increasing intention to use cannabis (and even actual use) occurred in some subgroups that previously had little interest in the drug. The analysis found evidence that these effects were due to an increase in the perceived popularity and prevalence of marijuana use through the campaign. Mass media campaigns may have iatrogenic effects—by increasing normative beliefs, resulting in higher intentions to use (Burkhart & Simon, 2015).

In addition to the problem of actual harm, there is the general problem that use of an ineffective treatment can be highly detrimental if this prevents the use of a more effective alternative (Rothwell, 2005). Faggiano, Giannotta, and Allara (2014) provide further examples of unexpected or counterintuitive effects in prevention research and some possible explanations.

Strategies against Chance Findings

Replication and Meta-Analysis

There is general agreement that the best test of validity of subgroup-treatment effect interactions is not significance but reproducibility in other trials (Rothwell, 2005; or, more generally, Cohen, 1994). In prevention science, replication studies to confirm findings are also considered an important scientific principle for improving our knowledge. In the first "standards of evidence" in prevention science provided by Flay and colleagues in 2005 it was recognized that exact replication in which the same intervention is tested on a new sample from the same population, delivered in the same way to the same kinds of people with the same training as in the original study, is rare (Gottfredson et al., 2015, p. 908). However, almost a contradiction, replication studies are much more likely to be for the purpose of testing *variations* in the intervention or of generalizing results to *different* settings or populations than for ruling out chance findings (Gottfredson et al., 2015).

If a sufficient number of studies on a topic are available, meta-analysis is a promising way to see patterns of effects for subpopulations across trials. Borenstein and Higgins (2013) recommend the use of meta-analysis because it allows the researcher to compare the treatment effect in different subgroups, even if these subgroups appear in separate studies. They also discuss several statistical issues related to this procedure (e.g., selection of a statistical model, statistical power for the comparison). Concerning the field of cardiovascular disease prevention and treatment, Rao et al. (2017) made a recent statement on the methodological standards for meta-analyses. Their paper also outlines some emerging methods, specifically network analysis (i.e.: test and relate several treatment conditions which have not been tested in the same trial) or Bayes methods which permit the incorporation of evidence from a variety of sources and prior knowledge.

Other statistical methods for pooling results have been proposed as well. Brown et al. (2013) present three data-sharing strategies for combining information across trials. Besides the standard meta-analysis with no sharing of data, they discuss the integrative data analysis for moderator effects where (in contrast to traditional meta-analysis) all the individual level data are combined into one dataset. The third strategy uses parallel data analysis where each of the respective trial research groups conduct analysis on their own data, following standardized analysis protocols. Results of these analyses done in parallel are then combined into a synthesis. Brown et al. (2013) conclude that the last two methods, integrative data analysis and parallel data analyses, share advantages over traditional methods available in meta-analysis.

Finally, suffice to say, results of this accumulation of empirical knowledge by these data analytic strategies should be viewed in parallel with substantive theory development and theoretically grounded research questions to move those results to a confirmatory framework and to design subsequent studies accordingly.

Statistical Techniques

In a specific trial or study, however, interpretation has to be based on currently available empirical results. Several statistical solutions have been proposed to protect against false-positive subgroup findings. Probably the most popular approach is Bonferroni correction where the level of significance is adjusted to the number of tests conducted. However, this approach yields conservative bounds on type I error and, hence, has low power (Schochet, 2008). This author (based on meetings by a 13-member Expert Advisory Panel) offers an overview of some modified and sometimes more powerful versions of the Bonferroni method and discusses advantages and limitations (c.f. also Bloom & Michalopoulos, 2013; Wang & Ware, 2013). In particular, strategies for dealing with multiplicity must strike a reasonable balance between testing rigor, i.e., to adjust downward the alpha level, and statistical power, i.e., the chance of finding truly effective interventions in subgroups (Schochet, 2008).

In addition to computing such formal adjustments, there may be cases where the overall picture seems straightforward. In the study on the effects of an antidrug media campaign on adolescents, Hornik et al. (2008) performed 80 subgroup analyses in the final set of analyses, and they found 20 significant effects, with 19 of those in a pro-marijuana direction. Thus, they conclude that there is "an overriding pattern of unfavorable lagged exposure effects" (p. 2232). In contrast, only three of 80 (= 3.7%) subgroup analyses revealed significant effects for contemporaneous associations and they were therefore considered as chance findings.

More generally, Bloom and Michalopoulos (2013) propose four main approaches to minimize the risk of revealing spuriously significant results due to multiple hypothesis testing:

1. Distinguish between confirmatory and explanatory findings
2. Minimize the number of confirmatory hypothesis tests
3. Create an omnibus hypothesis test
4. Make adjustments to multiple tests

Recent Strategies

Other strategies beyond "simple subgroup testing" have been proposed and used as well. In many medical publications, variables that are identified in previous research or in hypothesis-generating analyses are combined into a composite index. Patients are categorized according to a "risk score" based on their profile considering multiple prognostic or predictive characteristics.

In psychometrics, it is well known that unidimensionality of scores must be confirmed, e.g., by confirmatory factor analysis (CFA) or even by testing the strict assumptions of the Rasch model in the item response theory (IRT) context. In addition, there might be higher-order interactions in variables used for subgrouping which are not captured by these analyses. Therefore, it seems preferable to make less demanding assumptions for establishing sum scores and use qualitative differences between groups of persons. A well-elaborated approach to find previously unknown classes of persons on the basis of several categorical characteristics and combinations thereof is latent class analysis (LCA—see Nylund-Gibson and Hart (2014) for a comprehensive introduction into LCA in prevention science, and Masyn (2013) for a general overview).

The LCA strategy to reduce the risk of many tests was proposed and applied by Lanza and Rhoades (2013) in a prevention context. They used six variables with binary coding each (e.g., household poverty, single-parent status, peer alcohol use) and applied LCA to identify a small set of underlying subgroups characterized by multiple dimensions, which may differ in their response to treatment. The LCA revealed five latent subgroups that represent key patterns: Low Risk, Peer Risk, Economic Risk, Household and Peer Risk, and Multi-Contextual Risk. A comparison of these five subgroups concerning outcome is feasible, while a combination of the six variables would have led to $2^6 = 64$ different subgroups. A similar approach was taken by Bühler, Seemüller, and Läge (2014) where initial illness severity was not taken as a sum score but LCA was conducted to identify different types of depression on the symptom level and treat them as separate groups in the longitudinal analysis. Instead of reducing the number of response patterns by latent variables, the identification of "types" (and "anti-types") has also been proposed on the manifest level by means of configuration frequency analysis (c.f. Stemmler, 2014).

It should be added that many have commented on the dangers of subgroup analysis (Foster, Taylor, & Ruberg, 2011), but there has been little serious investigation of methodologies for proper identification of subgroups other than the above-mentioned statistical adjustments for alpha error. Foster et al. propose a method, referred to as "virtual twins," that involves predicting response probabilities for treatment and control "twins" for each subject. The difference in these probabilities is then used as the outcome in a classification or regression tree, which can potentially include any set of the covariates. Another recent proposition is to use a Bayesian approach for identifying patient subgroups within the subgroup of patients that showed positive treatment effects (Schnell, Tang, Offen, & Carlin, 2016). The authors propose a *credible subgroup* method to identify two bounding subgroups for the benefiting subgroup: one for which it is likely that all members simultaneously have a treatment effect exceeding a specified threshold, and another for which it is likely that no members do.

Finally, yet importantly, it should be emphasized that drawing valid conclusions regarding subgroups is an issue to be addressed at the planning stage. Stratified randomization of treatment assignment might be considered to ensure sufficient representation in the subgroups of interest (Wang & Ware, 2013).

Recommendations for Reporting Subgroup Findings

In general, incomplete reporting of the interventions tested and the methods used for conducting a trial has often been a problem in scientific reporting, and therefore, numerous guidelines across different fields have been proposed. One of the best known for reporting parallel group randomized trials is the Consolidated Standards of Reporting Trials (CONSORT—Schulz et al., 2010). The CONSORT guideline was developed by biomedical researchers and is therefore not broad enough to cover all aspects relevant for reporting in prevention science (Gottfredson et al., 2015). A new CONSORT extension for randomized controlled trials in social and psychological research (CONSORT—SPI) has been announced, but has not yet been released.

Independently from these extensions, standards for reporting are quite comparable in their main requests. CONSORT (Schulz et al., 2010, Table 1) demand as information concerning ancillary analyses when reporting a randomized trial: "Results of any other analyses performed, including subgroup analyses and adjusted analyses, distinguishing pre-specified from exploratory." Gottfredson et al. (2015, p. 909) follow CONSORT in stating: "…should include the elements identified in …CONSORT… or extension of these guidelines" (p. 908). In addition, results must be reported for every targeted outcome that has been measured in an efficacy study, regardless of whether they are positive, nonsignificant, or negative.

Specifically for "subgroup issues," recommendations are analogous and follow the same conventions. Rothwell (2005, p. 177) proposes that "all subgroup analyses that were done should be reported—i.e., not only the number of subgroup variables but also the number of different outcomes analysed by subgroup, different lengths of follow-up etc." Wang et al. (2007, p. 2193) recommend (among other points) the following:

- present subgroup results in the abstract only if the subgroup analyses were based on a primary study outcome, if they were prespecified, and if they were interpreted in light of the totality of prespecified subgroup analyses undertaken.
- avoid overinterpretation of subgroup differences. Be properly cautious in appraising their credibility, acknowledge the limitations, and provide supporting or contradictory data from other studies, if any.

With regard to prevention science, nonetheless, there are still challenges around reporting and interpreting subgroup findings, and there was no consensus around a number of critical issues in the expert meeting (Supplee, Kelly, MacKinnon, & Yoches Barofsky, 2013).

Conclusions

This chapter intended to give a broad conceptual introduction into the current status of subgroup analysis. It aimed at presenting the many opportunities provided by recently developed statistical approaches for subgroup analysis, be it confirmatory or exploratory, but also presents the potential risks of subgroup analysis.

The scientific background for this chapter is guided by placing an emphasis on methodological principles and the consequences of increasing regulatory constraints demanded by federal agencies like the Food and Drug Administration in the United States or the European Medicines Agency, in reaction to publication bias concerning study results, and in-transparent and selective reporting of significant outcome differences. These requirements are helpful for the evaluation of effectiveness and efficacy within a regulatory framework.

On the other hand, statistical concerns about mining the data may have been overemphasized and may present barriers to progress in understanding the effects of interventions. Furthermore, the prominence of adhering to the p-value as the definite criterion for decision-making seems sometimes too arbitrary or overly rigid (besides the widely observed misunderstanding and misuse of statistical inference). That issue was criticized not only by social scientists (e.g., Cohen, 1994) but also by statisticians themselves over the past few decades (see the statement of the American Statistical Association (Wasserstein & Lazar, 2016)).

In conclusion, many advanced statistical techniques are available. However as emphasized often in this chapter, there is a need for the development of strong theories in prevention science that would guide subgroup analyses that need to be considered during any study's planning phase. Thus, confirmatory tests are not conducted enough during exploratory research. However, it is recommended that all the new methods be used in an exploratory way to increase knowledge, but their findings should be distinguished clearly from confirmatory results and ALL exploratory findings should be reported, in order to bring them finally (via pooling of results with meta-analysis or integrated data analysis) to a confirmatory framework. Proper inference requires full reporting and transparency (Wasserstein & Lazar, 2016). In a single trial, the limitations of subgroup analysis should be acknowledged.

Acknowledgements I gratefully acknowledge thoughtful comments and suggestions provided by Hanno Petras, Zili Sloboda and Anke de Haan on an earlier version of this chapter.

References

Bloom, H. S., & Michalopoulos, C. (2013). When is the story in the subgroups? Strategies for interpreting and reporting intervention effects for subgroups. *Prevention Science, 14*, 179–188.

Borenstein, M., & Higgins, J. P. T. (2013). Meta-analysis and subgroups. *Prevention Science, 14*, 134–143.

Brookes, S. T., Whitley, E., Egger, M., Davey Smith, G., Mulheran, P. A., & Peters, T. J. (2004). Subgroup analyses in randomized trials: Risks of subgroup-specific analyses; power and sample size for the interaction test. *Journal of Clinical Epidemiology, 57*, 229–236.

Brookes, S. T., Whitley, E., Peters, T. J., Mulheran, P. A., Egger, M., & Davey Smith, G. (2001). Subgroup analyses in randomised controlled trials: Quantifying the risks of false-positives and false-negatives. *Health Technology Assessment, 5*, 1–56.

Brown, C. H., Sloboda, Z., Faggiano, F., Teasdale, B., Keller, F., Burkhart, G., … the Prevention Science and Methodology Group. (2013). Methods for synthesizing findings on moderation effects across multiple randomized trials. *Prevention Science, 14*, 144–156.

Brown, D. (2013, September 23). The press-release conviction of a biotech CEO and its impact on scientific research. *Washington Post*.

Bühler, J., Seemüller, F., & Läge, D. (2014). The predictive power of subgroups: An empirical approach to identify depressive symptom patterns that predict response to treatment. *Journal of Affective Disorders, 163*, 81–87.

Burkhart, G., & Simon, R. (2015). Prevention strategies and basics. In N. el-Guebaly et al. (Eds.), *Textbook of addiction treatment: International perspectives* (pp. 115–141). Milan: Springer.

Cohen, J. (1994). The earth is round ($p < .05$). *American Psychologist, 49*, 997–1003.

Collins, L. M., & Lanza, S. T. (2010). *Latent class and latent transition analysis: With applications in the social, behavioral, and health sciences*. Hoboken, NJ: Wiley.

Cordova, D., Estrada, Y., Malcolm, S. N., Huang, S., Brown, C. H., Pantin, H., & Prado, G. (2014). Prevention science: An epidemiological approach. In Z. Sloboda & H. Petras (Eds.), *Defining prevention science* (pp. 1–23). New York, NY: Springer.

Ding, C.S. (2006). Using regression mixture analysis in educational research. *Practical Assessment, Research & Evaluation, 11*(11). Retrieved February 2, 2018, from http://pareonline.net/getvn.asp?v=11&n=11

European Medicines Agency. (2006). ICH Topic E 9 Statistical Principles for Clinical Trials. Retrieved February 1, 2018, from http://www.ema.europa.eu/docs/en_GB/document_library/Scientific_guideline/2009/09/WC500002928.pdf

Faggiano, F., Giannotta, F., & Allara, E. (2014). Strengthening prevention science to ensure effectiveness of intervention in practice: Setting up an international agenda. In Z. Sloboda & H. Petras (Eds.), *Defining prevention science* (pp. 597–613). New York, NY: Springer.

Faggiano, F., Vigna-Taglianti, F., Burkhart, G., Bohrn, K., Cuomo, L., Gregori, D., …, Galanti, M.R. & the EU-Dap Study Group. (2010). The effectiveness of a school-based substance abuse prevention program: 18-month follow-up of the EU-dap cluster randomized controlled trial. *Drug and Alcohol Dependence, 108*, 56–64.

Fairchild, A. J., & MacKinnon, D. P. (2014). Using mediation and moderation analysis to enhance prevention research. In Z. Sloboda & H. Petras (Eds.), *Defining prevention science* (pp. 537–555). New York, NY: Springer.

Foster, J. C., Taylor, J. M. G., & Ruberg, S. J. (2011). Subgroup identification from randomized clinical trial data. *Statistics in Medicine, 30*, 2867–2880.

Goldsmith, K. A., MacKinnon, D. P., Chalder, T., White, P. D., Sharpe, M., & Pickles, A. (2017). Tutorial: The practical application of longitudinal structural equation mediation models in clinical trials. *Psychological Methods, 23*, 191–207.

Gottfredson, D. C., Cook, T. D., Gardner, F. E. M., Gorman-Smith, D., Howe, G. W., Sandler, I. N., & Zafft, K. M. (2015). Standards of evidence for efficacy, effectiveness, and scale-up research in prevention science: Next generation. *Prevention Science, 16*, 893–926.

Hodgson, J. (2016). When biotech goes bad. *Nature Biotechnology, 14*, 284–291.

Hornik, R., Jacobsohn, L., Orwin, R., Piesse, A., & Kalton, G. (2008). Effects of the national youth anti-drug media campaign on youths. *American Journal of Public Health, 98*, 2229–2236.

Hox, J. (2010). *Multilevel analysis: Techniques and applications* (2nd ed.). New York, NY: Routledge.

Jones, B. L., & Nagin, D. S. (2007). Advances in group-based trajectory modeling and a SAS procedure for estimating them. *Sociological Methods Research, 35,* 542–571.

Jung, T., & Wickrama, K. A. S. (2008). An introduction to latent class growth analysis and growth mixture modeling. *Social and Personality Psychology Compass, 2*(1), 302–317.

Lanza, S. T., & Rhoades, B. L. (2013). Latent class analysis: An alternative perspective on subgroup analysis in prevention and treatment. *Prevention Science, 14,* 157–168.

Latendresse, S. J., Musci, R., & Maher, B. S. (2018). Critical issues in the inclusion of genetic and epigenetic information in prevention and intervention trials. *Prevention Science, 19,* 58–67.

Masyn, K. (2013). Latent class analysis and finite mixture modeling. In T. Little (Ed.), *The Oxford handbook of quantitative methods in psychology* (Statistical analysis) (Vol. 2, pp. 551–611). New York, NY: Oxford University Press.

Muthén, B. O. (2002). Beyond SEM: General latent variable modeling. *Behaviormetrika, 29,* 81–117.

Muthén, B. O. (2003). Statistical and substantive checking in growth mixture modeling. *Psychological Methods, 8,* 369–377.

Muthén, B. O., & Muthén, L. (2000). Integrating person-centered and variable-centered analyses: Growth mixture modeling with latent trajectory classes. *Alcoholism: Clinical and Experimental Research, 24,* 882–891.

Muthén, L. K., & Muthén, B. O. (1998–2012). *Mplus user's guide* (7th ed.). Los Angeles, CA: Muthén & Muthén.

Nagin, D. S. (1999). Analyzing developmental trajectories: A semiparametric, group-based approach. *Psychological Methods, 4,* 139–157.

Nylund-Gibson, K., & Hart, S. H. (2014). Latent class analysis in prevention science. In Z. Sloboda & H. Petras (Eds.), *Defining prevention science* (pp. 493–511). New York, NY: Springer.

Petras, H., & Masyn, K. (2010). General growth mixture analysis with antecedents and consequences of change. In A. Piquero & D. Weisburd (Eds.), *Handbook of quantitative criminology* (pp. 69–100). New York, NY: Springer.

Petras, H., Masyn, K., & Ialongo, N. (2011). The developmental impact of two first grade preventive interventions on aggressive/disruptive behavior in childhood and adolescence: An application of Latent Transition Growth Mixture Modeling. *Prevention Science, 12,* 300–313.

Pickles, A., & Croudace, T. (2010). Latent mixture models for multivariate and longitudinal outcomes. *Statistical Methods in Medical Research, 19,* 271–289.

Rao, G., Lopez-Jimenez, F., Boyd, J., D'Amico, F., Durant, N. H., Hlatky, M. A., … Wessel, J. (2017). Methodological standards for meta-analyses and qualitative systematic reviews of cardiac prevention and treatment studies: A scientific statement from the American Heart Association. *Circulation, 136,* e172–e194.

Rothwell, P. M. (2005). Subgroup analysis in randomised controlled trials: Importance, indications, and interpretation. *Lancet, 365,* 176–186.

Schnell, P. M., Tang, Q., Offen, W. W., & Carlin, B. P. (2016). A Bayesian credible subgroups approach to identifying patient subgroups with positive treatment effects. *Biometrics, 72,* 1026–1036.

Schochet, P. Z. (2008). *Technical methods report: Guidelines for multiple testing in impact evaluations* (NCEE 2008-4018). Washington, DC: National Center for Education Evaluation and Regional Assistance, Institute of Education Sciences, U.S. Department of Education. Retrieved February 2, 2018, from http://ncee.ed.gov

Schochet, P. Z., Puma, M., & Deke, J. (2014). *Understanding variation in treatment effects in education impact evaluations: An overview of quantitative methods* (NCEE 2014–4017). Washington, DC: U.S. Department of Education, Institute of Education Sciences, National Center for Education Evaluation and Regional Assistance, Analytic Technical Assistance and Development. Retrieved February 1, 2018, from http://ies.ed.gov/ncee/edlabs

Schulz, K.F., Altman, D.G., Moher, D., & CONSORT Group. (2010). *CONSORT 2010 statement: Updated guidelines for reporting parallel group randomised trials.* Retrieved February 1, 2018, from http://www.consort-statement.org/downloads/consort-statement

Singer, J. D., & Willett, J. B. (2003). *Applied longitudinal data analysis.* New York, NY: Oxford University Press.

Sloboda, Z., Stephens, R. C., Stephens, P. C., Grey, S. F., Teasdale, B., Hawthorne, R. D., … Marquette, J. F. (2009). The adolescent substance abuse prevention study: A randomized field trial of a universal substance abuse prevention program. *Drug and Alcohol Dependence, 102,* 1–10.

Stemmler, M. (2014). *Person-centered methods: Configural frequency analysis (CFA) and other methods for the analysis of contingency tables.* Heidelberg: Springer.

Supplee, L. H., Kelly, B. C., MacKinnon, D. P., & Yoches Barofsky, M. (2013). Introduction to the special issue: Subgroup analysis in prevention and intervention research. *Prevention Science, 14,* 107–110.

Van Horn, M. L., Jaki, T., Masyn, K., Ramey, S. L., Smith, J. A., & Antaramian, S. (2009). Assessing differential effects: Applying regression mixture models to identify variations in the influence of family resources on academic achievement. *Developmental Psychology, 45*(5), 1298–1313.

Verbeke, G., & Molenberghs, M. (2000). *Linear mixed models for longitudinal data* (2nd ed.). New York: Springer.

Vigna-Taglianti, F., Vadrucci, S., Faggiano, F., Burkhart, G., Siliquini, R., Galanti, M. R., & EU-Dap Study Group. (2009). Is universal prevention against youths' substance misuse really universal? Gender specific effects in the EU-Dap school-based prevention trial.

Journal of Epidemiology and Community Health, 63, 722–728.
Wang, R., Lagakos, S. W., Ware, J. H., Hunter, D. J., & Drazen, J. M. (2007). Statistics in medicine: Reporting of subgroup analyses in clinical trials. *New England Journal of Medicine, 357,* 2189–2194.
Wang, R., & Ware, J. H. (2013). Detecting moderator effects using subgroup analysis. *Prevention Science, 14,* 111–120.
Wasserstein, R. L., & Lazar, N. A. (2016). The ASA's statement on p-values: Context, process, and purpose. *The American Statistician, 70,* 129–133.
Wright, A. G. C., & Hallquist, M. N. (2014). Mixture modeling methods for the assessment of normal and abnormal personality, part II: Longitudinal models. *Journal of Personality Assessment, 96,* 269–282.

Adaptive Intervention Designs in Substance Use Prevention

Kelly L. Hall, Inbal Nahum-Shani, Gerald J. August, Megan E. Patrick, Susan A. Murphy, and Daniel Almirall

Introduction

Despite the growing evidence supporting substance use treatment and prevention programs, there is considerable heterogeneity in outcomes within both individual and family-based intervention models, and no one type of intervention model can be expected to work optimally for all individuals (Waldron & Turner, 2008). There is room for improvement, and intervention approaches that account for individual differences should be explored. Increasingly, substance use prevention researchers are calling for a "personalized" approach to more effectively address the heterogeneity in baseline characteristics among at-risk populations, as well as the heterogeneity in response to intervention (Kranzler & McKay, 2012; *National Institute of Mental Health Strategic Plan for Research*, 2015).

Adaptive preventive interventions provide one approach to personalization. An *adaptive preventive intervention* (Collins, Murphy, & Bierman, 2004) is a replicable intervention design that uses prespecified decision rules, baseline individual characteristics, and during-intervention information about an individual to make dynamic preventive intervention decisions. In other words, an adaptive preventive intervention is a sequence of individually tailored decision rules that specify whether, how, when, and based on which measures to alter the dosage, type, or delivery of intervention components at critical decision points over time. In an adaptive preventive intervention, baseline characteristics, such as demographics, biomarkers, or baseline risk for long-term substance use disorder, may inform initial preventive intervention decisions. In addition, during-intervention variables, such as changes in intervention engagement, changes in the individual's family situation, changes in the individual's risk status, or any new information that may arise about an individual as a result of previous intervention, may be used to make subsequent preventive intervention decisions. Intervention type or dosage may be altered as a result (August, Piehler, & Bloomquist, 2014; Stormshak & Dishion, 2009; Tebes et al., 2007). Such adaptive preventive interventions have shown promise in the prevention of substance use disorders (August et al., 2014; Collins et al., 2004; Connell, Dishion, Yasui, & Kavanagh, 2007), as well as in the treatment of substance use disorders (Breslin et al., 1998; Kranzler & McKay, 2012; McKay, 2009; Waldron & Turner, 2008) and in other areas (Almirall & Chronis-Tuscano, 2016; Marlowe et al., 2008).

Adaptive preventive interventions provide an alternative to "one-size-fits-all" interventions. For example, a one-size-fits-all universal alcohol use prevention intervention might assign all high school sophomores in a community to a series of three online alcohol use prevention modules. These modules might provide some level of benefit to most students, but some students, such as those displaying risk factors for alcohol abuse, will require additional intervention. An adaptive preventive intervention, in contrast, might begin by providing all high school sophomores the three online alcohol use modules and monitoring students for subsequent risk status. Then, based on this information, those students displaying risk for alcohol abuse are assigned to a more comprehensive intervention, while those students not displaying risk for alcohol abuse continue to be monitored for subsequent risk status. In this hypothetical example, the intervention is modified based on dynamic information about the participants following the initial prevention effort.

Contributions and Outline of this Chapter

This chapter contributes to substance use prevention science in two ways. The first contribution is to illustrate different types of adaptive preventive interventions and describe how they fit within the universal, selective, and indicated prevention framework, a three-fold classification of prevention programs based on the risk classification of the population served. Four examples will be presented to illustrate how adaptive preventive interventions can be designed to target one or multiple risk classifications, using decision rules to systematically transition individuals within or between universal, selective, or indicated prevention interventions.

The first example, based on recent work by August et al. (2014), is designed to transition youth identified by law enforcement as juvenile offenders from selective to indicated prevention in order to reduce conduct disorder, recidivism, and substance use problems. The second example, based on work proposed by Megan Patrick and colleagues at the University of Michigan, is designed to transition college students from universal to indicated prevention in order to prevent binge drinking. The third example is the Family Check-Up program (Stormshak & Dishion, 2009), which transitions middle school students from universal, to selective, and then to indicated prevention, in order to prevent substance abuse. The fourth example describes one of the many interventions within the Fast Track program, an adaptive prevention intervention for a home-visitation schedule, where only selective interventions are used (Bierman, Nix, Maples, Murphy, & Group, 2009).

The second contribution of this chapter is to illustrate the use of sequential multiple assignment randomized trials (SMART) design as a potentially useful tool for addressing open scientific questions that prevention scientists might confront when developing an adaptive preventive intervention. We describe the design of two SMART studies that aim to develop adaptive preventive interventions for preventing long-term substance use disorder, one among first-time juvenile offenders and the other among freshmen college students. For each study, we describe its rationale and the primary and secondary scientific questions it seeks to address.

Given the growing interest in using data to develop empirically based adaptive preventive interventions (August et al., 2014), our hope is that this chapter will motivate the development of new and creative approaches to adaptive preventive interventions so as to improve the lives of greater numbers of individuals or families at risk for substance use disorders.

Motivations for Making a Preventive Intervention Adaptive

Modifying an intervention based on dynamic information about an individual (including response to initial or previous intervention) is a potentially valuable decision-making tool in substance abuse prevention programs for the following reasons:

First, the same prevention intervention might not address or reduce risk status in the same way for all individuals, given that individuals and families served by these programs often vary widely in their risk trajectories as well as their responses to treatment (Allen et al., 1997; Dishion et al., 2014; Winters, 1999). While some participants might respond well to an intervention, it may be ineffective or frustrating for others. In an adaptive preventive intervention, we can identify and take early action with those people for whom a given prevention intervention is not beneficial.

Second, not all individuals adhere to or actively engage in preventive interventions, and intervention fatigue is common (Heckman, Mathew, & Carpenter, 2015). Such nonadherence or disengagement may occur for various reasons, and is a particular problem in prevention programs, where individuals are not typically help-seekers because they do not believe they are at risk (Spoth, Guyll, & Day, 2002). Interventions can be burdensome for some people, such as interventions that individuals perceive as time-consuming, disruptive, or frustrating. Other factors, such as boredom, major events in participants' lives, feelings that they do not "need" an intervention, and stigmatization from peers, can also jeopardize adherence. Hence, it is important to identify signs of burden, stigma, or intervention fatigue and modify the intensity or nature of the intervention to address these conditions (Ennett et al., 2011; Ingoldsby, 2010; Marlatt & Donovan, 2005).

Third, the primary mechanisms driving at-risk patterns can change over time as a function of developmental and contextual transitions (Armeli, Todd, & Mohr, 2005; Dvorak, Pearson, & Day, 2014; Radomski, Read, & Bowker, 2015). Even the best baseline screening assessment, one that perfectly addresses a participant's initial needs, may not necessarily predict during-intervention changes in risk or onset of risk behaviors that indicate the need for a subsequent change in intervention. For example, while social norms are a major driver of at-risk drinking while in college, stressful experiences might be the primary mechanism driving drinking as individuals transition out of college and into the workforce (Read, Wood, Kahler, Maddock, & Palfai, 2003). Hence, in the course of the transition from college to work, different types or dosages of intervention may be needed to ameliorate at-risk behaviors. The monitoring schedule (e.g., how frequently risk is assessed) could also be adapted to time-varying fluctuations in risk.

Finally, in many settings, there may be a concern over monetary cost. Many preventive interventions are expensive, while resources are limited (Spoth et al., 2002). Adaptive preventive interventions can potentially alleviate some of this cost burden by providing individuals the level of intervention they need—but no more (Collins et al., 2004). In some cases, it is cost-effective to consider a stepped-up approach whereby the least intensive interventions are offered first, followed by more costly interventions only for those who need them. This is the typical "stepped-care model" (Sobell & Sobell, 2000). In other cases, it may be more cost-effective in the long run to begin with a costlier intervention, at least for the highest risk individuals or families, and then consider stepping down to less expensive interventions for individuals or families who show improvement.

All of the reasons given above provide justification for how an adaptive preventive intervention approach can improve outcomes in the prevention of substance use disorders for greater numbers of individuals, and potentially in a more efficient and cost-effective way.

Adaptive Preventive Interventions and the Universal, Selective, and Indicated (USI) Prevention Framework

An adaptive preventive intervention is designed to guide and formalize the process of sequential preventive intervention decision-making. An adaptive preventive intervention governs this process with decision rules (i.e., decision guides), which are stated prior to beginning the intervention. Decision rules use information about participants to suggest when it is best, for example, to begin or conclude an intervention, to switch interventions, or to adjust dosage.

All adaptive preventive interventions include the five intervention components listed below. In two of the four example adaptive preventive interventions in this chapter, these components are specified.

1. Intervention decision points
2. Intervention options (or components) at each decision point
3. Tailoring variables (individual characteristics that are associated with intervention response)
4. Decision rules used to link the value of the tailoring variables with intervention options at each point
5. Proximal and distal outcomes

As with most interventions, adaptive preventive interventions should be designed to be replicable (Becker & Curry, 2008). This replicability ensures that the adaptive preventive intervention can be utilized by clinicians in practice, as well as by other intervention scientists who might want to improve upon it. To ensure replicability, all of the above components are specified and operationalized prior to the use of the adaptive preventive intervention in practice or in a study.

As with most behavioral interventions, all adaptive preventive interventions are, by definition, multicomponent interventions (Collins, Chakraborty, Murphy, & Strecher, 2009; Collins, Nahum-Shani, & Almirall, 2014) because they involve transitions between different intervention components (e.g., monitoring schedules, intervention types, durations, or dosages).

The Universal, Selective, and Indicated (USI) Prevention Framework

Health practitioners and prevention scientists have long understood that preventive interventions are most effective when they are appropriately matched to their target population's level of risk (Stormshak, Dishion, Light, & Yasui, 2005). The concept of universal, selective, and indicated (USI) prevention interventions, which is generally well accepted in the prevention science literature, provides a broad framework for classifying preventive interventions in terms of risk level and the scope of the population being served (Gordon, 1983). This framework is useful in clarifying the differing objectives of various prevention interventions and matching these objectives to the needs of the target population.

Universal prevention interventions target general population groups without reference to those at particular risk. Examples include schoolwide interventions provided to all students at a school or health information interventions provided to all patients who visit a physician's office (Gottfredson & Wilson, 2003). Some members of such groups could benefit from universal prevention efforts, yet for other individuals, e.g., those who are at higher risk, such efforts might be helpful but not provide sufficient intensity.

Selective prevention interventions target subgroups of the population at higher-than-average risk. This high risk derives from exposure to health-compromising biological or experiential factors, such as living with a substance abusive parent, loss of a close relative or friend, or affiliations with deviant peers. An example of a selective prevention intervention is a positive-development after-school program for high-risk urban students (Tebes et al., 2007). By targeting specific risk factors, these interventions can reach large groups of individuals likely to be at elevated risk.

Indicated prevention interventions target individuals or families who display early problem behaviors that place them at heightened risk for problem escalation, health-compromising behavior, or disorder development. Examples of indicated interventions include individual counseling or family interventions for youth who are at the early stages of problem behavior but not yet diagnosable for mental health or substance use disorder (Kumpfer, Alvarado, & Whiteside, 2003). These prevention interventions can provide targeted, high-intensity support to those individuals who need it most.

The following four examples demonstrate how adaptive preventive interventions operate within or across the universal, selective, and indicated interventions framework. For each of the first two examples, we explicitly describe the five components that make up the adaptive preventive intervention, and we explain how each adaptive preventive intervention spans two of the three USI classification categories for prevention interventions. The latter two examples are drawn from the existing prevention science literature: one is an adaptive preventive intervention that spans all three levels of the USI framework, and the other is an adaptive preventive intervention that is confined to a single level of the framework. Together, these examples illustrate the diversity of adaptive preventive interventions.

At this point, our goal is to provide example adaptive preventive interventions, rather than describe *studies* which evaluate (or test components of) these adaptive preventive interventions. Later in this chapter, we discuss two novel studies that motivated the first two example adaptive preventive interventions. For this reason, our focus below is on the first two examples, which we describe in greater detail.

Example 1: An Adaptive Preventive Intervention Which Transitions from Selective to Indicated

In this example, an adaptive preventive intervention is used to guide the transition between selective and indicated intervention components. This adaptive preventive intervention, one of four embedded in a larger study by August et al. (2014), was designed for a culturally diverse group of 13–17-year-old participants identified by law enforcement as early-stage juvenile offenders, with the ultimate goal of preventing the escalation and progression of serious conduct problems, including use and abuse of illicit substances. This group varied widely in ethnic background, gender, and risk of reoffending. The adaptive preventive intervention involves an empirically validated intervention program called *Teen Intervene* ("TI"; Winters & Leitten, 2007). TI can be delivered with varying intensity and duration, conforming to either brief or extended formats (more on this below), and it is delivered by counselors in 1-h sessions. It is a youth-centered program that includes elements of motivational interviewing, goal-setting, and self-change. The sessions strive to boost the youth's problem recognition and interest in change by raising awareness of the problem, placing responsibility for change with the youth, and negotiating responsible goals. In addition, there is a focus on managing impulsive behaviors and making responsible decisions that anticipate potential consequences.

Figure 17.1 illustrates the example adaptive preventive intervention. In the first stage, all participants are enrolled in a "brief" version of TI which consists of three sessions, completed whenever the participant's schedule allows, within a maximum time span of 3 months. The three sessions are led by a diversion counselor and are 60 min each. At the conclusion of the initial stage, youth are assessed for response status using a multidimensional risk-assessment measure—described below—that encompasses persistence of conduct problems, functional impairment, and deviant peer affiliations. In the second stage of the adaptive preventive intervention, "responders" are stepped down to monitoring only, while "non-responders" are stepped up to the *TI-Extended* intervention program for five additional 60-min sessions.

This intervention contains all of the above-specified elements of adaptive preventive interventions. There are two decision points, at decision points 1 and 2 in Fig. 17.1. These represent points where participants are assessed and intervention is assigned. Decision point 1 is upon entry into the intervention following referral from law enforcement. Decision point 2 is after three sessions of *TI-Brief*, which must be completed within 3 months. At decision point 1, there

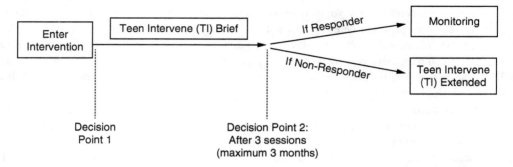

Fig. 17.1 An adaptive preventive intervention in conduct problems prevention for first-time juvenile offenders (August et al., 2014)

is only one intervention option: *TI-Brief*. At decision point 2, there are two intervention options, *TI-Extended* or monitoring.

Following the three sessions of *TI-Brief*, participants are classified as responders or non-responders based on a risk score derived from several tailoring variables. For example, youth are identified as non-responders if they showed evidence of any *one* of the following criteria: (a) conduct problems >1 standard deviation above the mean as rated by parents on the Behavioral Assessment System for Children (BASC-2 [T-Score > 60]; Reynolds, Kamphaus, & Vannest, 2011), (b) impaired functioning as rated by counselors on the Child and Adolescent Functional Assessment Scale (CAFAS [T-Score > 60]; Hodges & Wotring, 2000), or (c) elevated exposure to deviant peer influences on the Friendship Scale (T-Score > 60; Child and Family Center, 2013a, 2013b). The decision rule at decision point 2 then suggests that responders are discontinued from TI-Brief and monitored for maintenance, while non-responders are provided with TI-Extended.

Proximal outcomes for this adaptive preventive intervention include many of the variables assessed in the responder/non-responder measure, such as whether substance and alcohol usage, truancy, and peer affiliations improve following intervention. Distal outcomes, on the other hand, are the behaviors the intervention is designed to ultimately prevent: in this case, substance use disorder and additional criminal offending.

This example adaptive preventive intervention can be conceptualized as one that guides the transition between selective and indicated preventive interventions for substance use disorder. The initial three-session *TI-Brief* (stage 1) is a *selective* intervention for substance use disorder. The fact that the youth have participated in early criminal activities may reflect a vulnerability for substance use disorder. Further, the vast majority of these youth live in economically disadvantaged and high crime neighborhoods, which represent risk factors for subsequent substance use. This population may have a significantly higher risk of longer-term substance use problems; however, not all of these youth will have substance use disorder. That is, this group likely contains a combination of lower and higher risk individuals. Many of them will benefit from a preventive intervention with selective intervention components for substance use disorder such as *TI-Brief*. However, it will not be apparent at program entry (prior to *TI-Brief*) whether a participant has clear prodromal signs related to a substance use disorder. Hence, in addition to providing a low level of intervention intended to have positive preventive effects, the first-stage intervention also serves a diagnostic purpose by eliciting information, via the response versus nonresponse measure, which is used to determine whether additional (indicated) intervention is needed. If additional intervention is required, the participant will be "stepped up" to the indicated intervention—in this case, five additional sessions of more targeted counseling with additional emphasis on substance use disorder.

Example 2: An Adaptive Preventive Intervention Which Transitions from Universal to Indicated

As a second example, we present a proposed adaptive preventive intervention developed by Megan Patrick and colleagues at the University of Michigan. It begins with a universal approach to preventing and monitoring alcohol use among a general pool of college freshmen of all risk levels (see Patrick, Lee, & Neighbors, 2014), and then transitions students identified as heavy drinkers to an indicated intervention.

There are two decision points in this example, at the beginning and end of the first semester of college as illustrated in Fig. 17.2. At decision point 1, 1st-year college students receive a web-based personalized normative feedback (PNF) intervention prior to the beginning of classes. This decision rule is not tailored—all students receive the PNF intervention. PNF, which provides feedback about students' accuracy of their perceived norms of peer substance use and provides protective behavior strategies, is considered a universal intervention because it is designed for all types of college students, regardless of alcohol use or consequences. This intervention is low cost and easy to distribute widely (via web-based interface optimized for viewing on mobile devices), making it an attractive option to deliver to large cohorts of students. The PNF intervention also includes a low-burden, technology-based monitoring component, whereby students are asked via text message once per month during the course of the semester to report number of "binge drinking" episodes in the past month, where binge drinking is defined for females as consuming four or more drinks in a row and for males as consuming five or more drinks in a row.

Decision point 2 occurs at the end of the first semester of college. At decision point 2, students are classified as "heavy drinkers" or "non-heavy drinkers" based on frequency of binge drinking using their text message responses. If they average more than two episodes of binge drinking per month, they are classified as heavy drinkers. The decision rule suggests that non-heavy drinkers receive no further intervention, while heavy drinkers are provided Web-based Brief Alcohol Screening and Intervention for College Students (BASICS; Dimeff, 1999). BASICS provides a more intense intervention—an indicated intervention—for those students who are showing signs of alcohol abuse.

Proximal outcomes for this adaptive preventive intervention include frequency of binge drinking, while distal outcomes include long-term health consequences (e.g., symptoms of alcohol use disorders).

As an example, consider a student who received Web-based PNF before her 1st week of class and, upon assessment, was classified as a non-heavy drinker. This student is not provided further intervention. The results of her end-of-semester assessment did not indicate that more intense and time-consuming BASICS intervention—the indicated intervention—was necessary.

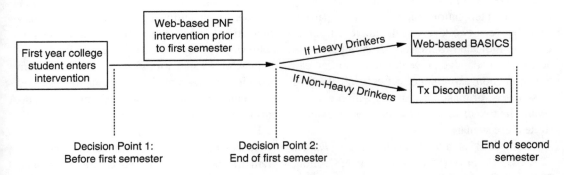

Fig. 17.2 An adaptive preventive intervention for preventing heavy alcohol use in 1st-year college students (proposed by Patrick et al., based on an intervention designed by Patrick, Lee, & Neighbors, 2014)

Table 17.1 Summary of the five components of the adaptive preventive interventions described in examples 1 (August et al., 2014) and 2 (Patrick et al.)

Component	Example 1: Early-Stage Juvenile Offenders	Example 2: Alcohol Use in College Students
Decision points	(1) At intervention entry, and (2) after three sessions of *TI-Brief*	(1) Prior to beginning the first semester of college, and (2) directly following the first semester
Intervention options	One option in stage 1: *TI-Brief*. Two options in stage 2: *TI-Extended* or monitoring	One option in stage 1: *Web-based PNF*. Two options in stage 2: *Web-based BASICS* or treatment discontinuation
Tailoring variables	Conduct problems, impaired functioning, and deviant peer influences, as measured through scores on BASC-2, CAFAS, and Friendship Scales	Frequency of binge drinking
Decision rules	At decision point 1: all participants assigned to *TI-Brief* At decision point 2: classified as a "non-responder" and assigned to *TI-Extended* if: (a) >1 standard deviation above the mean on BASC-2 (b) T-score > 60 on Friendship Scale, *OR* (c) T-score > 60 on CAFAS Otherwise, assigned to monitoring	At decision point 1: all participants assigned to *Web-Based PNF* At decision point 2: classified as a "heavy drinker" and assigned to *Web-based BASICS* if average more than 2 occasions of binge drinking (4/5+ drinks for females/males in a row) per month Otherwise, assigned to treatment discontinuation
Distal and proximal outcomes	Proximal: substance and alcohol use, truancy, and peer affiliations Distal: substance use disorder or additional criminal behaviors	Proximal: frequency of binge drinking Distal: long-term health consequences, such as alcohol use disorders

Table 17.1 summarizes the five intervention components of the adaptive preventive interventions described in examples 1 and 2.

Examples 3 and 4: An Adaptive Preventive Intervention that Spans the USI Framework, and an Adaptive Preventive Intervention that is Only Selective

The above examples illustrate an approach by which an intervention might transition participants between two levels of the universal, selective, and indicated framework. It is important to note that an adaptive preventive intervention can also transition participants between all three of these levels, or make adaptations within a single level. The two examples provided below demonstrate these scenarios.

Example 3 is a component of the *Family Check-Up Program* (FCU; Stormshak & Dishion, 2009). FCU offers a sequence of universal, selective, and indicated components for children and families in the school context, with the aim of preventing substance use, family management deficits, deviant peer affiliations, and problem behavior at school (Stormshak & Dishion, 2009). For the universal component, a family resource center is made available to all families whose children attended the school. A selective "Family Check-Up" program is provided to families whose children were at moderate to high risk but not currently demonstrating serious behavior problems. The Family Check-Up is a series of three meetings with parents or caregivers which includes goal-setting, assessments of family interaction, and motivational interviewing. Following Family Check-Up, the families of students who began demonstrating serious problem behaviors are assigned to a menu of indicated interventions, which include trainings with parents on family management skills.

Example 4 is the *Fast Track Program* (Bierman et al., 2009). *Fast Track*, a multicomponent program designed to prevent conduct problems among high-risk children, contains an adaptive preventive intervention component which is selective.

Children at risk for serious conduct problems are identified at school entry and provided with multicomponent prevention services such as group trainings, academic tutoring, and family interventions.

One of Fast Track's components is a home visiting program designed to promote parental functioning, where families are visited by clinicians, or "family coordinators," over a multiyear period. Family coordinators help foster a positive home environment by reinforcing behavior management skills taught in parenting classes and helping parents to practice these skills.

All students receiving the home visits have been identified during first grade as being at elevated risk for antisocial behaviors and conduct problems. Thus, the home visiting program is a selective intervention. During the 1st year, in the first stage of the home visiting intervention, all families receive biweekly home visits. At the end of the 1st year, family coordinators assess parental functioning and family need (based on ratings of variables such as parental warmth, physical punishment, and stressful life events) and adjust the frequency of home visits accordingly. In second and third grade, then, families receive either weekly, biweekly, or monthly home visits based on the assessment of parental functioning and need. This second phase is still selective, as the goal is to prevent students from developing serious conduct problems. While some families display lower levels of functioning than others, all still have children at risk for these behaviors. Thus, the Fast Track home visit program serves as an example of an adaptive preventive intervention that adapts its intervention components *within* a single level of the USI framework, rather than transferring its participants between levels of the framework.

Common Scientific Questions in the Development of an Adaptive Preventive Intervention

Adaptive preventive interventions, such as those described above, attempt to deliver the appropriate type or amount of intervention, at the right times, to improve outcomes in the longer term, such as to reduce the risk of substance use.

Designing such interventions raises several scientific questions, as it is often not clear how best to put together the components of an adaptive preventive intervention, or which (of various) adaptive preventive intervention designs will lead to the best outcomes. Here, we review some of these questions in the context of the first two examples described above.

There are questions concerning how best to begin an adaptive preventive intervention. In the previously discussed study of juvenile offenders (August et al., 2014), for example, researchers might wonder whether *Teen Intervene-Brief* is truly the best initial selective intervention for first-time juvenile offenders. Perhaps proximal and distal outcomes would be improved if the intervention included both youth and their parents at the first stage. An alternative brief intervention that includes families, such as a brief intervention drawing from *Everyday Parenting* ("EP"; Dishion, Stormshak, & Kavanagh, 2011), might provide superior results for certain youth. EP includes both youth and parents and addresses three broad areas of effective parenting practices and family skill-building presented in modular format. The first module, "Positive Behavior Support," is devoted to monitoring and supervision of adolescent activities, whereabouts, and peer relations; reinforcing positive behavior; and using a behavior change plan. The second module, "Healthy Limit Setting," focuses on specifying clear rules and expectations. The third module, "Communication and Problem Solving," is geared toward enhancing parent-youth interactions, including discussion of pertinent teen topics such as peers, dating, and alcohol/substances. The "brief" version of EP, in comparison to the brief version of TI, might be more effective initially.

There are questions concerning the costs-versus-benefits of starting with one intervention component versus another. For example, example 2 above begins with a relatively lower-cost, lower-burden three-session *TI-Brief* intervention for early-stage juvenile offenders. Here, providers "step up" to a more indicated intervention only for those participants that demonstrate higher risk. Alternatively, providers could begin with a relatively higher-cost, higher-burden indicated intervention and then "step down" to a lower-intensity selective intervention for participants who show sufficient improvement.

There are questions concerning the initial timing of the intervention. In the above-described Patrick et al. adaptive preventive intervention, for example, the Web-based PNF for college alcohol use is delivered prior to the 1st day of the first semester of college. Is this truly the best time to deliver this initial intervention? Researchers might wish to investigate whether it would be more salient to provide the Web-based PNF a few weeks into classes or even later into the first semester, after some college students have had the opportunity to experience consequences from drinking.

There are questions concerning how best to monitor individuals or families for signs of nonresponse (or response) in order to guide subsequent intervention. Recall that a critical component of an adaptive preventive intervention is the monitoring of participants (e.g., assessing response/nonresponse, or adherence/nonadherence) using a predetermined measure. Often, however, there are questions as to the most cost-effective or least burdensome approach to doing this. For example, in cases where monitoring and assessment are potentially burdensome, researchers might ask whether face-to-face monitoring is necessary. Perhaps less intensive methods, such as brief telephone checkups, interactive voice response (IVR) calls, or text message-based monitoring, could be equally effective. Such questions are important because different approaches to monitoring might elicit different kinds of information, and this information is critical for tailoring the next step in treatment.

For monitoring to occur, researchers must first establish which features they are monitoring—that is, how the response/nonresponse measure will be defined. Thus, there are questions concerning which features or indicators to use as tailoring variables for guiding subsequent intervention decisions. This question is a particular challenge in prevention, as prevention is initiated prior to the onset of a disorder. Thus, often, there are no clinical features resulting directly from the disorder (e.g., symptoms or functional impairments) that can be used to guide subsequent intervention decisions. Instead, in prevention, change in *risk trajectory* is often used to make subsequent decisions. Examples of variables that might be included in a substance use risk trajectory measure include changes in association with substance-using peers, attitudes toward substance use, knowledge of the norms of substance use, and expectations of benefits derived from substance use. The risk trajectory measure may also combine these variables with level of adherence or engagement with the intervention. A major challenge in prevention is which of these measures, or which combination of these measures, should be used to tailor subsequent intervention decisions.

Sequential Multiple Assignment Randomized Trials

A Sequential Multiple Assignment Random Trial (SMART) is a multistage randomized trial design that can be used to address important questions at multiple points in the development of an adaptive preventive intervention. In a SMART, participants may be randomized to different intervention options at multiple points throughout the trial. Data obtained from a SMART is then used to design an adaptive preventive intervention by answering questions such as those given above.

Note that in the example adaptive preventive interventions described in the previous section, participants are not randomized. In contrast, a SMART is not an adaptive intervention, but rather a randomized trial design that provides data for informing the construction of appropriate decision rules for those interventions (Collins et al., 2014). Motivated by the first two example adaptive preventive interventions above, we now describe two SMART designs and the types of questions they are intended to answer.

Example 1: SMART Design to Develop an Adaptive Preventive Intervention Which Transitions from Selective to Indicated

Earlier in this chapter, an example was presented of an adaptive preventive intervention that transitioned first-time juvenile offenders from a selective to an indicated intervention (Fig. 17.1). This adaptive preventive intervention was one of four embedded within a SMART conducted by August et al. (2014). Figure 17.3 illustrates this SMART in full.

The overarching goal of the study is to develop an adaptive preventive intervention for preventing future conduct disorder and substance use among a heterogeneous population of youth (13–17 years old) identified by law enforcement as early-stage juvenile offenders. The SMART design was motivated by two key scientific questions:

1. How do we best begin an adaptive preventive intervention for youth at risk of substance use disorder: with a brief parent-centered approach (*Everyday Parenting-Brief*) or a brief youth-centered approach (*Teen Intervene-Brief*)? That is, which of these two interventions should be offered initially?
2. How do we best extend intervention for participants who—after three sessions of either *Everyday Parenting-Brief* or *Teen Intervene-Brief*—are non-responders to the initial intervention? Is it best to extend intervention using the intervention used initially (continuation approach), or is it best to provide an extended version of the opposite intervention in the second stage (switch approach)?

To address these questions, the investigators designed a two-stage SMART. In the first stage of the study, participants were randomized to *Teen Intervene-Brief* or *Everyday Parenting-Brief*. After three sessions on initial intervention, response/nonresponse status was determined using the multidimensional risk-assessment tool described in Section Example 1: An Adaptive Preventive Intervention Which Transitions from Selective to Indicated. At the conclusion of the initial stage, "responders" were stepped down and monitored, while "non-responders" were re-randomized to extended versions of one of the intervention programs for five additional 60-min sessions.

The rationale for this SMART stems from the previously discussed scientific questions: both youth-centered and parent-centered approaches are available for intervening with these youth. *Teen Intervene* is a youth-centered approach, while *Everyday Parenting* is a parent-centered approach, and both have been shown to be effective. However, initially providing both a youth-centered *and* a parent-centered intervention to all youth identified by law enforcement as early-stage offenders is not feasible. Practically, we must begin with one or the other, but it is unknown which is best. Furthermore, for youth identified as non-responders at the end of initial intervention, it is unknown whether providing an extended version of the same intervention or of a different intervention is superior. For example, it may be that nonresponding youth who are not engaged in the initial intervention method would benefit from extended intervention that takes a markedly different approach.

There are four adaptive preventive interventions embedded within this SMART. They differ in terms of the presence and sequencing of the *Teen Intervene* and *Everyday Parenting* interventions. Table 17.2 extracts and compares these four adaptive preventive interventions.

In addition to providing data on the primary research questions described above, this SMART can be used to compare longitudinal outcomes—conduct problems, impaired functioning, and deviant peer influences, as described above—between the four embedded adaptive preventive interventions. The results from these analyses could be used to determine which (or which set) of the four adaptive preventive interventions is clearly best or worse for preventing future conduct disorders and substance use for first-time juvenile offenders. For guidance on how to conduct these analyses, see Nahum-Shani et al. (2012a).

The SMART can also be used to collect and analyze information that could potentially be

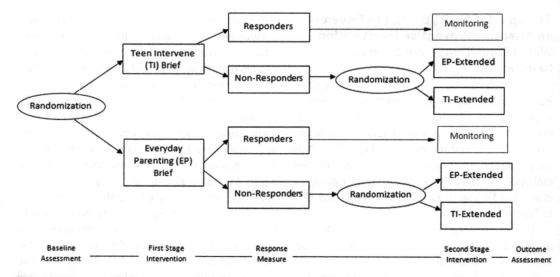

Fig. 17.3 SMART design for an adaptive preventive intervention pilot study in adolescent conduct problems prevention (August et al., 2014). There are four adaptive preventive interventions embedded within this study, represented by the four combinations of interventions that branch through this decision tree

used for tailoring variables (i.e., the SMART can be used to provide empirical support for adaptive preventive interventions that are more individually tailored than those provided in Table 17.2). For example, the SMART could be used to explore whether adherence or engagement to initial intervention (*TI-Brief* or *EP-Brief*) is important in deciding whether to extend the same intervention or switch to the opposite intervention in the second stage among non-responders. For guidance on how to conduct these analyses (which are extensions of moderators analysis to the time-varying setting), see Nahum-Shani et al. (2012b).

Example 2: SMART Design for an Adaptive Preventive Intervention Which Transitions from Universal to Indicated

In Section "Motivations for Making a Preventive Intervention Adaptive", an adaptive preventive intervention was described that administered a preventive intervention to college freshmen prior to the start of their first semester, and later assigned those identified as "heavy drinkers" to the Web-based BASICS intervention (Fig. 17.2). However, what if introducing the intervention prior to the beginning of the semester was not optimal? What if those identified as "heavy drinkers" require a more intensive intervention? To address these considerations, a SMART study was proposed by Patrick et al. (Fig. 17.4). The motivating scientific questions for this study include:

1. What is the optimal timing for introducing a universal substance use prevention module to 1st-year college students?
2. What is the best second-stage selective intervention for those identified as heavy drinkers? Should the BASICS intervention be administered in-person (in-person BASICS) or via the computer (Web-BASICS)?

Each of the adaptive preventive interventions examined in this study begin with a universal approach to preventing and monitoring alcohol use among college students, and then aim to transition students to effective indicated interventions based on need.

The study design is as follows: Initially, a sample of 1st-year college students would be randomized to receive a universal web-based personalized normative feedback (PNF) intervention

Table 17.2 The four adaptive preventive interventions embedded in the August et al. SMART

#	Adaptive preventive intervention	Stage 1	Stage 2
1	Youth-only sequence	TI-Brief	Monitoring (step-down for youth exhibiting a positive response to initial *TI-Brief*)
			TI-Extended (step-up for youth exhibiting nonresponse)
2	Youth skills then parent support sequence	TI-Brief	Monitoring (step-down for youth exhibiting a positive response to initial *TI-Brief*)
			EP-Extended (step-up and *switch* to parenting intervention for youth exhibiting nonresponse)
3	Parent-only support sequence	EP-Brief	Monitoring (step-down for youth exhibiting a positive response to initial *EP-Brief*)
			EP-Extended (step-up for youth exhibiting nonresponse)
4	Parent support then youth sequence	EP-Brief	Monitoring (step-down for youth exhibiting a positive response to initial *EP-Brief*)
			TI-Extended (step-up and *switch* to youth-only intervention for youth exhibiting nonresponse)

at one of three times throughout the first semester: prior to classes beginning, in the 1st few weeks of the semester, or near mid-term exams. At the end of the first semester, following assessment for frequency of binge drinking, non-heavy drinkers receive no further intervention, while heavy drinkers are re-randomized to one of two versions of Brief Alcohol Screening and Intervention for College Students (BASICS): Web-BASICS, which students complete online, or in-person BASICS, which is delivered by trained university staff. BASICS provides a more intense intervention—an indicated intervention—for those students who show signs of alcohol abuse. Data collection for research purposes would be completed using web-based surveys administered throughout the academic year.

There are six adaptive preventive interventions embedded in this study, described in Table 17.3. For example, a student might be randomized to receive Web-based PNF at Week 4. Upon assessment, at the end of the first semester, this student is classified as a heavy drinker and is re-randomized to receive In-Person BASICS. Because he is classified as a heavy drinker, a selective intervention is provided.

Data from this SMART could be used to compare longitudinal outcomes between the six adaptive preventive interventions embedded in the study. It could also be used to identify variables, such as gender, major, or extracurricular activities, that might act as additional tailoring variables.

Note that, although all of the example SMARTs described in this section make comparisons in the context of interventions that have already been shown to be evidence-based (e.g., PNF and BASICS in the college alcohol use study), this is not a requirement for SMARTs. For example, a recent SMART among minimally verbal children with autism investigated the effectiveness of a speech-generating device, which prior to that study had not yet been tested in any full-scale randomized trial (Kasari et al., 2014).

Discussion and Conclusion

Adaptive preventive interventions provide a guide for sequencing the provision of preventive interventions in an individualized way. In the substance use prevention field, with its often widely heterogeneous populations, such individualization could be especially valuable, because it could lead to sequences of interventions responsive to the changing context, engagement, and risk of participants. Adaptive preventive interventions could be designed to target multiple risk classifications, using decision rules to systematically transition individuals across universal, selective, and indicated preventions.

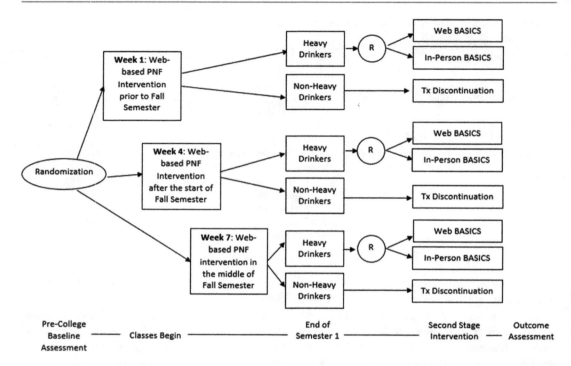

Fig. 17.4 SMART design for an adaptive preventive intervention pilot study for preventing heavy alcohol use in 1st-year college students (Patrick et al.)

Scientists face various scientific questions when conducting research on adaptive preventive interventions. In this book chapter, we focused on the use of SMART studies as one potentially useful type of randomized trial design; as we describe, SMARTs can be used to answer questions concerning the development of high-quality adaptive preventive interventions. However, SMART studies are not the only type of randomized trial design that can be used to conduct research about adaptive preventive interventions. For example, consider the example SMART shown in Fig. 17.4 concerning college drinking. If the researchers did not have a question about the optimal timing for introducing a universal substance use prevention module to 1st-year college students and only had a question concerning how best to intervene with a student identified as a heavy drinker, then the randomized trial design would different from a SMART. Rather, it would be a singly randomized trial where all college students are offered the universal intervention at some point in the fall semester and then only students identified as heavy drinkers are randomized to Web BASICS versus In-person BASICS.

A common misconception about SMARTs is that a very large sample size is needed to have adequate statistical power. As with any type of randomized trial design, the minimum sample size required depends on the primary aim of the SMART; it is not always the case that sample size required for a SMART is larger than the sample size required of a standard trial design answering the same (or a similar) scientific question. Based on the current body of SMARTs that are either finished or still in the field, sample sizes for SMARTs have ranged from $N = 61$ (Kasari et al., 2014) to $N = 1000$ (Fu et al., 2017). There are now a number of easy-to-use sample size calculators for SMARTs (See Penn State Methodology Center resources: https://methodology.psu.edu/downloads).

Researchers might also worry about multiple comparisons testing with a SMART. As with any randomized trial, multiple-comparison adjustments are required when primary aim comparisons are made on multiple outcome measures, or

Table 17.3 The six adaptive preventive interventions embedded in the Patrick et al. SMART

#	Adaptive preventive intervention	Stage 1	Stage 2
1	Pre-semester PNF plus Web-BASICS	Web-based PNF at Week 1	Web-BASICS (for heavy drinkers)
			Tx Discontinuation (for non-heavy drinkers)
2	Pre-semester PNF plus In-Person BASICS	Web-based PNF at Week 1	In-Person BASICS (for heavy drinkers)
			Tx Discontinuation (for non-heavy drinkers)
3	Early-semester PNF plus Web-BASICS	Web-based PNF at Week 4	Web-BASICS (for heavy drinkers)
			Tx Discontinuation (for non-heavy drinkers)
4	Early-semester PNF plus In-Person BASICS	Web-based PNF at Week 4	In-Person BASICS (for heavy drinkers)
			Tx Discontinuation (for non-heavy drinkers)
5	Mid-semester PNF plus Web-BASICS	Web-based PNF at Week 7	Web-BASICS (for heavy drinkers)
			Tx Discontinuation (for non-heavy drinkers)
6	Mid-semester PNF plus In-Person BASICS	Web-based PNF at Week 7	In-Person BASICS (for heavy drinkers)
			Tx Discontinuation (for non-heavy drinkers)

when the primary aim involves multiple comparisons (e.g., two or more pairwise comparisons). SMARTs are no different in this respect. SMARTs differ from standard trial designs in that there are multiple randomizations, but multiple randomizations alone do not necessitate a multiple-comparison adjustment. For example, the SMART described in Fig. 17.4 might be sized to detect the effect of Web-BASICS versus In-Person BASICS among college students who are heavy drinkers after the initial substance use prevention program (a single comparison), but also have other randomized comparisons (as secondary aims) that are not included as comparisons for purposes of the sample size calculation.

Another concern that is commonly raised about SMARTs has to do with intervention dropout, nonadherence, or disengagement and the (in)ability to re-randomize a participant who drops out of intervention. For example, in the context of the example SMART in Fig. 17.4, one concern might be how to categorize a college student as a heavy drinker (or not) if the student disengages from the (monitoring) intervention, e.g., does not provide the information needed to make the assessment. However, closer examination reveals that this concern is not about the SMART design, but rather is a concern with the adaptive preventive intervention itself. Indeed, if the study were, for example, a conventional 2-arm randomized trial of the adaptive preventive intervention versus business as usual, it would be equally important to prespecify an intervention plan for how to continue to monitor or intervene with individuals who are showing early signs of dropout or have dropped out of intervention. A key idea here is that the response/nonresponse assessment that is often used in SMARTs to determine whether the participant will be re-randomized is not a research assessment but is, rather, an intervention assessment (see Almirall, Lizotte, & Murphy, 2012 for more details).

One direction for future substantive and methodological work concerns the use of group-level prevention programs. In this chapter, we focused solely on adaptive preventive interventions that guide the sequencing of individual-level interventions and intervention components. However, often in prevention, interventions are provided to *groups* of individuals, such as school- or classroom-based prevention programs (Agabio et al., 2015; Wasserman et al., 2015). Adaptive preventive interventions could also be used to guide the sequencing of and transition between different cluster-level interventions or from cluster to individual interventions (Kilbourne et al., 2014; Necamp, Kilbourne, & Almirall, 2017).

For example, the Fast Track study also includes a universal prevention program for elementary school classrooms, where teachers are provided with weekly consultations on classroom behavior management (Bierman et al., 2009). Following the PATHS: Promoting Alternative Thinking Strategies curriculum (Greenberg, Kusche, Cook, & Quamma, 1995), which is designed to help children understand and discuss emotions, the initial universal prevention was group based in that it was offered to all students in their classroom at once. The classroom-based universal prevention was followed by selective prevention for the group of students within the cluster who, because of their risk status, needed a more intensive one-on-one intervention. Some individuals within the classroom would never be offered the individualized selective intervention, whereas others would receive both the cluster and the individual prevention interventions.

Adaptive preventive interventions have the potential to reduce waste, increase compliance, enhance intervention potency, and reduce negative effects of inappropriate intervention dosages. In the substance use prevention field, adaptive preventive interventions, and the use of randomized trials (such as SMART) to inform their development, can better serve the needs of those at risk for substance use.

References

Agabio, R., Trincas, G., Floris, F., Mura, G., Sancassiani, F., & Angermeyer, M. C. (2015). A systematic review of school-based alcohol and other drug prevention programs. *Clinical Practice and Epidemiology in Mental Health, 11*, 102–112. https://doi.org/10.1111/j.1465-3362.2012.00517.x

Allen, J. P., Mattson, M. E., Miller, W. R., Tonigan, J. S., Connors, G. J., Rychtarik, R. G., & Cooney, N. L. (1997). Matching alcoholism treatments to client heterogeneity: Project MATCH posttreatment drinking outcomes. *Journal of Studies on Alcohol, 58*(1), 7–29. https://doi.org/10.15288/jsa.1997.58.7

Almirall, D., Lizotte, D. J., & Murphy, S. A. (2012). Comment on "evaluation of viable dynamic treatment regimes in a sequentially randomized trial of advanced prostate cancer". *Journal of the American Statistical Association, 107*(498), 509–512.

Almirall, D., & Chronis-Tuscano, A. (2016). Adaptive interventions in child and adolescent mental health. *Journal of Clinical Child & Adolescent Psychology, 45*(4), 383–395.

Armeli, S., Todd, M., & Mohr, C. (2005). A daily process approach to individual differences in stress-related alcohol use. *Journal of Personality, 73*(6), 1–30. https://doi.org/10.1111/j.1467-6494.2005.00362.x

August, G. J., Piehler, T. F., & Bloomquist, M. L. (2014). Being "SMART" about adolescent conduct problems prevention: Executing a SMART pilot study in a juvenile diversion agency. *Journal of Clinical Child & Adolescent Psychology, 4416*(9), 1–15. https://doi.org/10.1080/15374416.2014.945212

Becker, S. J., & Curry, J. F. (2008). Outpatient interventions for adolescent substance abuse: A quality of evidence review. *Journal of Consulting and Clinical Psychology, 76*(4), 531–543. https://doi.org/10.1037/0022-006X.76.4.531

Bierman, K. L., Nix, R. L., Maples, J. J., Murphy, S. A., & Group, C. P. P. R. (2009). Examining clinical judgement in an adaptive intervention design: The fast track program. *Journal of Consulting and Clinical Psychology, 74*(3), 468–481. https://doi.org/10.1037/0022-006X.74.3.468.Examining

Breslin, F. C., Sobell, M. B., Sobell, L. C., Cunningham, J. A., Sdao-Jarvie, K., & Borsoi, D. (1998). Problem drinkers: Evaluation of a stepped-care approach. *Journal of Substance Abuse, 10*(3), 217–232.

Child and Family Center. (2013a). *FCU Caregiver Questionnaire: Adolescence (11–17)*. Eugene. Retrieved from http://fcu.cfc.uoregon.edu

Child and Family Center. (2013b). *FCU Youth Questionnaire: Adolescence (11–17)*. Eugene. Retrieved from http://fcu.cfc.uoregon.edu

Collins, L. M., Chakraborty, B., Murphy, S. a., & Strecher, V. (2009). Comparison of a phased experimental approach and a single randomized clinical trial for developing multicomponent behavioral interventions. *Clinical Trials (London, England), 6*(1), 5–15. https://doi.org/10.1177/1740774508100973

Collins, L. M., Murphy, S. A., & Bierman, K. L. (2004). A conceptual framework for adaptive preventive interventions. *Prevention Science, 5*(3), 185–196. https://doi.org/10.1016/j.surg.2006.10.010.Use

Collins, L. M., Nahum-Shani, I., & Almirall, D. (2014). Optimization of behavioral dynamic treatment regimens based on the sequential, multiple assignment, randomized trial (SMART). *Clinical Trials, 11*(4), 426–434. https://doi.org/10.1177/1740774514536795

Connell, A. M., Dishion, T. J., Yasui, M., & Kavanagh, K. (2007). An adaptive approach to family intervention: Linking engagement in family-centered intervention to reductions in adolescent problem behavior. *Journal of Consulting and Clinical Psychology, 75*(4), 568–579. https://doi.org/10.1037/0022-006X.75.4.568

Dimeff, L. A. (1999). *Brief alcohol screening and intervention for college students (BASICS): A harm reduction approach*. New York: Guilford Press.

Dishion, T. J., Brennan, L. M., Shaw, D. S., McEachern, A. D., Wilson, M. N., & Jo, B. (2014). Prevention of problem behavior through annual family check-ups in early childhood: Intervention effects from home to early elementary school. *Journal of Abnormal Child Psychology, 42*(3), 343–354. https://doi.org/10.1007/s10802-013-9768-2

Dishion, T. J., Stormshak, E. A., & Kavanagh, K. (2011). *Everyday parenting: A therapist's guide for supporting family management practices.* Champaign, IL: Research Press.

Dvorak, R. D., Pearson, M. R., & Day, A. M. (2014). Ecological momentary assessment of acute alcohol use disorder symptoms: Associations with mood, motives, and use on planned drinking days. *Experimental and Clinical Psychopharmacology, 22*, 285–297.

Ennett, S. T., Haws, S., Ringwalt, C. L., Vincus, A. A., Hanley, S., Bowling, J. M., & Rohrbach, L. A. (2011). Evidence-based practice in school substance use prevention: Fidelity of implementation under real-world conditions. *Health Education Research, 26*(2), 361–371. https://doi.org/10.1093/her/cyr013

Fu, S. S., Rothman, A. J., Vock, D. M., Lindgren, B., Almirall, D., Begnaud, A., ... Joseph, A. M. (2017). Program for lung cancer screening and tobacco cessation: Study protocol of a sequential, multiple assignment, randomized trial. *Contemporary Clinical Trials, 60*, 86–95. https://doi.org/10.1016/j.cct.2017.07.002

Gordon, R. S. (1983). An operational classification of disease prevention. *Public Health Reports, 98*(2), 107–109. https://doi.org/10.2307/4627374

Gottfredson, D. C., & Wilson, D. B. (2003). Characteristics of effective school-based substance abuse prevention. *Prevention Science: The Official Journal of the Society for Prevention Research, 4*(1), 27–38.

Greenberg, M. T., Kusche, C. a., Cook, E. T., & Quamma, J. P. (1995). Promoting emotional competence in school-aged children: The effects of the PATHS curriculum. *Development and Psychopathology, 7*(1), 117–136. https://doi.org/10.1017/S0954579400006374

Heckman, B. W., Mathew, A. R., & Carpenter, M. J. (2015). Treatment burden and treatment fatigue as barriers to health. *Current Opinion in Psychology, 5*, 31–36. https://doi.org/10.1016/j.copsyc.2015.03.004

Hodges, K., & Wotring, J. (2000). Client typology based on functioning across domains using the CAFAS: Implications for service planning. *Journal of Behavioral Health Services & Research, 27*(3), 257–270. https://doi.org/10.1007/BF02291738

Ingoldsby, E. M. (2010). Review of interventions to improve family engagement and retention in parent and child mental health programs. *Journal of Child and Family Studies, 19*(5), 629–645. https://doi.org/10.1007/s10826-009-9350-2

Kasari, C., Kaiser, A., Goods, K., Nietfeld, J., Mathy, P., Landa, R., & Almirall, D. (2014). Communication interventions for minimally verbal children with autism: A sequential multiple assignment randomized trial. *Journal of the American Academy of Child & Adolescent Psychiatry, 53*(6), 635–646.

Kilbourne, A. M., Almirall, D., Eisenberg, D., Waxmonsky, J., Goodrich, D. E., Fortney, J. C., ... Thomas, M. R. (2014). Adaptive Implementation of Effective Programs Trial (ADEPT): Cluster randomized SMART trial comparing a standard versus enhanced implementation strategy to improve outcomes of a mood disorders program. *Implementation Science, 9*(1), 132. https://doi.org/10.1186/s13012-014-0132-x

Kranzler, H. R., & McKay, J. R. (2012). Personalized treatment of alcohol dependence. *Current Psychiatry Reports, 14*(5), 486–493. https://doi.org/10.1007/s11920-012-0296-5

Kumpfer, K. L., Alvarado, R., & Whiteside, H. O. (2003). Family-based interventions for substance use and misuse prevention. *Substance Use & Misuse, 38*(11–13), 1759–1787. https://doi.org/10.1081/JA-120024240

Marlatt, G. A., & Donovan, D. M. (2005). *Relapse prevention: Maintenance strategies in the treatment of addictive behaviors.* New York: Guilford Press.

Marlowe, D. B., Festinger, D. S., Arabia, P. L., Dugosh, K. L., Benasutti, K. M., Croft, J. R., & McKay, J. R. (2008). Adaptive interventions in drug court: A pilot experiment. *Criminal Justice Review, 33*(3), 343–360.

McKay, J. R. (2009). Treating substance use disorders with adaptive continuing care. *American Psychological Association.*

Nahum-Shani, I., Qian, M., Almirall, D., Pelham, W. E., Gnagy, B., Fabiano, G. A., & Murphy, S. A. (2012a). Experimental design and primary data analysis methods for comparing adaptive interventions. *Psychological Methods, 17*(4), 457.

Nahum-Shani, I., Qian, M., Almirall, D., Pelham, W. E., Gnagy, B., Fabiano, G. A., & Murphy, S. A. (2012b). Q-learning: A data analysis method for constructing adaptive interventions. *Psychological Methods, 17*(4), 478.

National Institute of Mental Health. (2015). National Institute of Mental Health Strategic Plan For Research (NIH Publication No. 15-6368). Bethesda, MD: U.S. Government Printing Office.

Necamp, T., Kilbourne, A., & Almirall, D. (2017). Comparing cluster-level dynamic treatment regimens using sequential, multiple assignment, randomized trials: Regression estimation and sample size considerations. *Statistical Methods in Medical Research, 26*(4), 1572–1589.

Patrick, M. E., Lee, C. M., & Neighbors, C. (2014). Web-based intervention to change perceived norms of college student alcohol use and sexual behavior on Spring Break. *Addictive Behaviors, 39*(3), 600–606. https://doi.org/10.1016/j.addbeh.2013.11.014

Radomski, S. A., Read, J. P., & Bowker, J. C. (2015). The role of goals and alcohol behavior during the transition out of college. *Psychology of Addictive Behaviors, 29*, 142–153.

Read, J. P., Wood, M. D., Kahler, C. W., Maddock, J. E., & Palfai, T. P. (2003). Examining the role of drinking motives in college student alcohol use and problems. *Psychology of Addictive Behaviors, 17*(1), 13.

Reynolds C. R., Kamphaus R. W., & Vannest K. J. (2011). Behavior Assessment System for Children (BASC). In: J. S. Kreutzer, J. DeLuca, B. Caplan (Eds.),

Encyclopedia of Clinical Neuropsychology (pp. 366–371). New York, NY: Springer.

Sobell, M. B., & Sobell, L. C. (2000). Stepped care as a heuristic approach to the treatment of alcohol problems. *Journal of Consulting and Clinical Psychology, 68*(4), 573.

Spoth, R. L., Guyll, M., & Day, S. X. (2002). Universal family-focused interventions in alcohol-use disorder prevention: Cost-effectiveness and cost-benefit analyses of two interventions. *Journal of Studies on Alcohol, 63*(2), 219–228.

Stormshak, E. A., & Dishion, T. J. (2009). A school-based, family-Centered intervention to prevent substance use: The family check-up. *The American Journal of Drug and Alcohol Abuse, 35*(4), 227–232. https://doi.org/10.1080/00952990903005908

Stormshak, E. A., Dishion, T. J., Light, J., & Yasui, M. (2005). Implementing family-centered interventions within the public middle school: Linking service delivery to change in student problem behavior. *Journal of Abnormal Child Psychology, 33*(6), 723–733. https://doi.org/10.1007/s10802-005-7650-6

Tebes, J. K., Feinn, R., Vanderploeg, J. J., Chinman, M. J., Shepard, J., Brabham, T., ... Connell, C. (2007). Impact of a positive youth development program in urban after-school settings on the prevention of adolescent substance use. *Journal of Adolescent Health, 41*(3), 239–247. https://doi.org/10.1016/j.jadohealth.2007.02.016

Waldron, H. B., & Turner, C. W. (2008). Evidence-based psychosocial treatments for adolescent substance abuse. *Journal of Clinical Child and Adolescent Psychology, 37*(1), 238–261. https://doi.org/10.1080/15374410701820133

Wasserman, D., Hoven, C. W., Wasserman, C., Wall, M., Eisenberg, R., Hadlaczky, G., ... Carli, V. (2015). School-based suicide prevention programmes: The SEYLE cluster-randomised, controlled trial. *The Lancet, 385*(9977), 1536–1544. https://doi.org/10.1016/S0140-6736(14)61213-7

Winters, K. C. (1999). Treating adolescents with substance use disorders: An overview of practice issues and treatment outcome. *Substance Abuse, 20*(4), 203–225. https://doi.org/10.1080/08897079909511407

Winters, K. C., & Leitten, W. (2007). Brief intervention for drug-abusing adolescents in a school setting. *Psychology of Addictive Behaviors, 21*(2), 249.

Ethical Issues in Substance-Use Prevention Research

Celia B. Fisher and Rimah Jaber

Introduction

An estimated 27 million people aged 12 and older are current users of illicit drugs in the United States, of which 21.5 million have a substance-use disorder (SUD). Addiction is a primary chronic disease of brain reward, motivation, memory, and related circuitry in which individuals pursue reward and/or relief through substance use and behaviors (American Society of Addiction Medicine, 2011). Although marijuana remains the most illegally used drug in the United States, addiction to opioids (heroin and prescription pain relievers) caused 10,574 of the 18,893 overdose deaths in 2014, and was the leading cause of accidental death in the United States (Center for Behavioral Health Statistics and Quality [CBHSQ], 2015; Center for Disease Control and Prevention, 2015; NIDA, 2015a, 2015b). In the United States, combined abuse of tobacco, alcohol, and illicit drug use costs substance users, their families, and society more than $700 billion annually in public costs associated with crime, associated health problems, and lost work productivity (CBHSQ, 2015; NIDA, 2011). According to a 2013 survey, first-time drug use in the United States most often occurs during adolescence with about 7800 new uses per day (NIDA, 2015a, 2015b) (accessed 11/29/18). Over half of youth surveyed (54.1%) were under the age of 18 with drug use highest in the late teens and early 20s. The survey also found that about 22.7% of people between the ages of 12 and 20 use alcohol with 14.2% partaking in binge drinking. In addition, early alcohol use has been shown to be a marker of risk for alcohol-use disorder (AUD) in both African-American and European-American youth with an average age of 17.6 (Sartor et al., 2016).

Vulnerable populations bear the largest burden of illicit drug use and addiction. Racial and ethnic minorities in the United States disproportionately suffer from the social burdens and health disparities associated with substance use including poverty, high-crime neighborhoods, under- or unemployment, and inadequate health social services (Buka & Kington, 2001; Carliner, Delker, Fink, Keyes, & Hasin, 2016; Davey-Rothwell, Siconolfi, Tobin, & Latkin, 2015; Fisher, 2004; Lê Cook & Alegría, 2011). For example, according to most recent data from the National Survey on Drug Use and Health (CBHSQ, 2015), American-Indians and Alaska Natives experience the highest rate of illegal substance use and comorbid mental disorders compared to other US groups. The rate of illegal drug use among African-Americans and Hispanic/Latino/a population aged 12 and older, while somewhat lower, continues to be higher than in the general population (CBHSQ, 2015). Recent

C. B. Fisher (✉) · R. Jaber
Center for Ethics Education, Fordham University, Bronx, NY, USA
e-mail: fisher@fordham.edu; rjaber@fordham.edu

public attention has also turned to substance-abuse problems including fatal heroin overdoses among white ethnic populations in areas characterized by decreasing employment (Adams, Kirzinger, & Martinez, 2012; Case & Deaton, 2015). In a 2013 survey (NIDA, 2015a, 2015b) 6.5 million Americans aged 12 or older reported using prescription drugs non-medically in the month prior to collection of survey data including pain relievers, tranquilizers, stimulants, and sedatives with 1.9 million claiming dependence or abuse of pain relievers.

Research Risks and Benefits

Based on the principle of beneficence, federal regulations for human subject protections require that research have a favorable ratio of benefit to risk (DHHS, 2017). That is, the study must be designed such that the potential benefits of the research will be maximized and potential harms to participants minimized. The development of effective prevention programs relies on the identification of psychological, social, environmental, and systemic factors associated with the onset of substance use and substance-use dependence. Researchers engaged in the critical task of generating survey data upon which substance-use scientific theory, prevention services, public opinion, and policies may be based are faced with the formidable responsibility of ensuring that their procedures meet accepted scientific standards of research practice while protecting participant rights and welfare (Fisher, 1999, 2003).

Research on Predictors of Substance Use and Abuse

Factors influencing substance use and substance-use disorders are identified through epidemiological, survey, interview, and other methods that collect information from participants about their own and family history of substance use, personality characteristics such as impulsivity, as well as the bidirectional relationship between substance use and high-risk behaviors including unprotected sexual encounters and violence. Investigators often encounter roadblocks to the conduct of scientifically valid and socially valuable research as a result of IRB risk/benefit assessments that overestimate participant risk and risk protections required (Shah, 2004). This is particularly true for research involving adolescents where IRB decisions are often based on the empirically unsupported assumption that surveys or interviews on substance use and other related health-compromising behaviors may harm adolescents or encourage youth to engage in such behaviors (Fendrich, Lippert, & Johnson, 2007; Fisher, 2002, 2003; Langhinrichsen-Rohling, Arata, O'Brien, Bowers, & Klibert, 2006). This often results in institutional barriers to the quality and conduct of socially critical prevention research (Fisher, Brunquell et al., 2013; Mustanski, 2011; Wendler et al., 2005).

Whether participants perceive these questions to be relevant or harmful to their everyday experiences is often overlooked when investigators and IRB members rely solely on their own moral compass to calculate the risk-benefit balance of survey-derived data. In the absence of data on participant concerns, investigators and IRB members risk over- or underestimating the probability and magnitude of harm posed by such studies (Fisher, 1999, 2004, 2015). In addition, participant wariness of research risks when unknown and left unaddressed can have a negative impact on recruitment. For example, Fisher (2003) found that a majority of parents and teenagers in a multiethnic sample disagreed with the claim advanced by some IRBs that the use of adolescent drug use surveys encourages the behaviors it seeks to understand. Most expressed optimism is that surveys might improve public policies aimed at drug prevention and endorsed the value of surveys for helping individual participants, their parents, and schools understand and prevent adolescent drug use and suicide. At the same time, many respondents were skeptical about the validity of youth reports, the value of surveys that fail to consider the impact of government policies and neighborhood factors on drug use, and investigator motives to ascertain the truth about youth problems (Fisher, 2003; Fisher & Wallace, 2000).

Responses also indicated apprehension about participant distress and privacy violations in reaction to questions about health-compromising behaviors.

Such perceptions should encourage scientists working with similar populations to empirically examine post-experimental distress in reaction to youth survey participation, develop debriefing procedures to adequately address any distress that might arise, and discuss these concerns with prospective participants and their guardians during recruitment and informed consent. Participant views also strongly suggest that the extent to which survey findings accurately reflect participant substance-use attitudes and behaviors that can be successfully applied to prevention programs in real-world setting depends on whether they believe the study is relevant to their life experiences, have faith in the investigators' integrity, and believe the research will adequately address the causes and nature of substance use in real-world contexts.

Group Stigmatization and Social-Political Influences on Substance-Use Research

Several government panels have identified psychological and social vulnerability in research as procedures that intentionally or not disvalue participants, their interests, or their contributions to society fostering embarrassment or shame (National Commission, 1979; National Bioethics Advisory Committee, , 2001; National Research Council, 2014). Recruitment of individuals who are assumed to be at risk for substance-use disorders because of their socioeconomic status, race/ethnicity, or sexual orientation or gender identity can have the unintended effect of exacerbating internalized stigma or feelings of hopelessness in resisting health-compromising substance use (Fisher, 2004). It can also have a negative effect on family coherence and community status when children are recruited to participate in longitudinal studies of the developmental trajectory of substance use based on the documented substance-use disorders of their parents or older siblings.

Sociopolitical influences on substance use and abuse: Communities suffering from social and economic challenges due to poverty, lack of quality education, unequal access to health care, and unequal treatment within the healthcare system are most vulnerable to factors associated with substance use (Cargill & Stone, 2005; Fisher, 2004). The National Institute on Drug Abuse's *Strategic Plan:* , 2016–2020 has committed to addressing health disparities in research through the study of SUDs in minority populations and the support of health equity in research. Although, as illustrated in this volume, the field of substance-use prevention science has made great strides in conceptualizing, operationalizing, and empirically disentangling multilevel effects on substance use, challenges remain in identifying empirical and practical ways to address the pervasive influence of social, economic, and political macro-systems on substance use and abuse. Although balancing risks and benefits of research participation is a standard practice in all research, it is especially important for vulnerable or minority populations because there is little literature on if and/or how underserved they are (Slomka, McCurdy, Ratliff, Timpson, & Williams, 2008).

Economic and political concerns such as crime, welfare dependency, and health care often determine funding for substance-use prevention research and thus dictate the nature of studies that will be conducted. This way of identifying areas that should be targeted for public health investigations often excludes from the decision-making process people who are most at risk for substance-use dependency and related health-compromising behaviors (Fisher, 1999, 2004), and may produce participant protections that are neither lax, harmful, nor overly protective and inflexible in a way that diminishes beneficial research (Mastrioanni & Kahn, 2001).

Prevention scientists have long debated whether consideration of the practical consequences of research should be considered a threat to scientific progress and academic freedom or a hallmark of scientific responsibility (Fisher & McCarthy, 2013; Sarason, 1984; Zuckerman,

1990). In their classic article on social justice and prevention science, Albee and Ryan-Finn (1993) argued that the biological and tertiary approaches to prevention characteristic of the time had the unintended effect of maintaining an inequitable social order by focusing on individual risks and remedies rather than environmental conditions that foster oppression and inequity.

In recent years Prilleltensky and his colleagues (Prilleltensky, 2003; Prilleltensky & Nelson, 2002) have called for scientists to incorporate notions of oppression (systematic exclusion of and discrimination toward groups) and liberation (resistance to and recovery from oppression) into prevention research designs by incorporating knowledge of the sources, experiences, and consequences of oppression, the power dynamics operating at the psychological and institutional levels, and ways to address systemic inequities that sustain health disparities. From this perspective, the success of substance-use prevention science requires the design of studies that not only consider the influences of individual, family, and peer contexts but also include policy analysis that takes into account and attempts to change the pervasive and distal sociocultural sources and influences of oppression substance use and misuse (Fisher, Busch-Rossnagel, Jopp, & Brown, 2012).

Boundary Challenges in Ethnographic and Community Research

Researchers conducting ethnographic research exploring individual, family, and social influences on substance use often immerse themselves into the lives of participants for extended periods of time. This can result in confusion over personal and professional boundaries of responsibility (Fisher, 2011). Similarly, community-based research often engages members of the participant community as frontline staff which can also lead to questions of professional and personal obligation.

Ethnographic research: In ethnographic and participant observation research on the sequelae of substance use and abuse, the relationship between researchers and participants creates a supportive network for participants, as well as access to health care and services otherwise not available (Fisher, Fried, Desmond, Macapagal, & Mustanski, 2017). These methods can empower participants by placing value on their expertise, knowledge, and personal experience for the sake of helping others. On the other hand, investigators may feel pressure to give into participant requests for advice, become a witness to illegal behaviors (e.g., obtaining or selling alcohol or drugs to underage youth) or feeling pressured to provide money and resources over what is allocated for participation in the research (Singer et al., 1999). Consequently, multiple relationships due to unclear personal/professional boundaries can create complex ethical tensions related to coercion, exploitation, confidentiality, and other harms as well as invalidate the data collected (Fisher, 2004; Marshall et al., 2012).

There has been a paucity of research on ethical challenges of conducting ethnographic research on substance-use prevention. However, studies on the perspectives of economically marginalized adults engaged in street drug use can help inform the ethical challenges faced by investigators conducting in vivo prevention research. For example, Fisher (2011) developed a scenario depicting a researcher who had over the course of a year conducted monthly interviews with a group of women who use drugs about their child-rearing challenges. The interviews were conducted in the neighborhood, often on the streets, and the investigator had built strong trusting bonds with the participants. In the scenario, the investigator was asked to hide a participant's drugs during a surprise police raid who feared her child would be taken away if she was arrested. Fisher asked an ethnically diverse sample of male and female adults currently using illegal substances to comment on the ethics of whether the investigator should hide the drugs. Some respondents thought that the investigator had a responsibility to hide the drugs based on the idea that over the course of time the researcher and participant were likely to have become "friends." However, contrary to expectations, most respondents believed that the researcher should refuse to hide the drugs. Drawing on the principles of fidelity and fiduciary responsibility, they expressed their belief that investigators should maintain a professional code of ethics that prohibits engaging in illegal activities and that to do otherwise would jeopardize participants' confidence in the researcher's professionalism. This type of study highlights the importance of establishing and sustaining professional boundaries during intensive ethnographic research to preserve not only scientific integrity but also continued trust in participant populations.

Moral Stress Among Frontline Staff

In community-based substance-use prevention research involving economically marginalized populations frontline research staff have direct contact with participants who lack adequate economic, educational, and health resources (Fisher, 2013). For these studies frontline staff are often hired because they are members of the communities being studied with special relationships and expertise with this population. To date, there has been little empirical examination of how frontline researchers perceive the effectiveness of research procedures in their real-world application and the stress they may experience when adherence to scientific procedures appears to conflict with participant protections.

A recent study administered psychometrically validated instruments to examine moral distress and its relationship to ethical conduct, institutional research, and ethics climate among 275 frontline staff members involved in community-based survey, prevention, and intervention substance-use research (Fisher, True, Alexander, & Fried, 2013). Moral stress was defined as feelings of frustration, anxiety, and job burnout as a consequence of implementing research procedures staff believed were ethically inadequate to meet the needs of participants. Overall, frontline staff members' commitment to work, producing valid data, and protecting the rights and well-being of participants created tensions with their supervisors as well as the implementation of research. Many felt that inclusion and exclusion criteria did not reflect the actual life experience of research participants. Others felt they had to recruit ineligible participants to meet their supervisor's pressure for "numbers." Over half the participants had high scores on the moral stress scale and over one-third associated this with job demands, and feelings of frustration (i.e., not being able to provide adequate referrals), and burnout. Concerns about implementing protections of subjects were frequent including the danger of participants not understanding consent or risks of exploitation when monetary payments were offered. Frontline researchers who evidence a strong commitment to their role in the research process and who perceive their organizations as committed to research ethics and staff support experienced lower levels of moral stress. However, those who were distrustful of the research enterprise frequently grappled with moral practice dilemmas and reported higher levels of moral stress.

The nature of community-based substance-use research places frontline staff in daily contact with social injustices experienced by the marginalized populations with whom they work and the real-world constraints on the implementation of research ethics procedures, the external validity of research protocols, and the harms and goods of participation to individual participants (Fisher, True et al., 2013). These results strongly suggest that principal investigators implement organizational strategies for reducing moral stress and enhancing the responsible conduct of research. As recommended by Fisher and her colleagues (Fisher, True et al., 2013) such strategies can include during the design stage drawing on frontline staff expertise in the challenges facing community-based research including informed consent preparedness, barriers to recruitment, practical limitations of inclusion/exclusion criteria, and expectations regarding services. Once the study begins it can also include regular debriefing sessions for staff to recognize the reality of and help reduce moral stress and to provide counseling when needed, especially for staff who are in successful recovery, who may be at risk for relapse through their constant engagement with participants in the drug-using community.

Informed Consent

Consent to participate in research must be informed, voluntary, and rational (Belmont Report, 1979). The informed component of consent requires that prospective participants are provided all pertinent information needed to make a reasoned choice about whether they wish to participate in a study. Although informed consent is a standard requirement for conducting research, ensuring that individuals are providing informed, rational, and voluntary consent raises challenges. Age, lack of education or familiarity with research procedures and terminology, health risk behaviors, and comorbid mental health disorders associated with substance-use risk can compromise consent understanding (Fisher et al., 2008; Levy, 2016; Regmi et al., 2016). For example, investigators and institutional review boards (IRBs) are often concerned that impulsivity and risk-taking often associated with substance-use risk may compromise a reasoned participation choice even if prospective participants are cognitively competent at the time of consent (Cohen, 2002). A recent study, however, argued that this assumption is flawed and stigmatizing and provided evidence that in the absence of withdrawal or intoxication, a majority of patients with SUDs had the capacity to provide autonomous consent (Moran-Sanchez, Luna, Sanchez-Munoz, Aguilera-Alcaraz, & Perez-Carceles, 2016).

Federal regulations require that investigators and IRBs consider consent as an ongoing process. Planned re-consent procedures are particularly important in longitudinal studies examining the developmental correlates of substance use and abuse as well as for prevention trials in which some participants may demonstrate substance use or disorders during or at the end of the prevention trial. For example, adolescents' assent capacity and attitudes toward participation research may change over the course of a multiyear substance-use study. Moreover, youth may also not be aware that their participation continues to be voluntary from year to year. Respecting youth's developing autonomy rights thus requires re-consent procedures tailored to their increased maturity. In addition, across the course of substance-use prevention trials it will be expected that some participants will engage in substance use and may reach levels of alcohol or drug dependency. These participants may come to testing sessions with transitive cognitive impairments based on intoxication or withdrawal and standard re-consent procedures are a valuable tool to ensure the continued rationale and voluntary nature of consent.

Deciding whether to participate in a randomized substance-use prevention trial must be based on comprehension and acceptance of research risk, an understanding of random assignment, as well as a healthy skepticism of potential personal benefits. A newly emerging concern regarding informed consent for prevention trials is "preventive misconception." Preventive misconception has been defined as the overestimation of personal protection that is afforded by enrollment in a preventive intervention trial (Ott, Alexander, Lally, Steever, & Zimet, 2013). This relatively new concept grew out of empirical research on "therapeutic misconception" in clinical trials. Appelbaum, Roth, and Lidz (1982) coined the term to describe two common but incorrect beliefs held by participants regarding randomized clinical trials: (1) that their individualized needs will be taken into account in condition assignment and (2) that there is a high probability that they will benefit from research participation (see also Appelbaum, Lidz, & Grisso, 2004). These misconceptions may be due to poorly implemented informed consent, underestimation of risks or dispositional optimism on the part of a participant, and different cognitive "mindsets" for planned actions compounded by therapeutic mistrust in underserved or marginalized populations (Fisher et al., 2008; Jansen, 2014). How can investigators minimize preventive misconception? One strategy is to develop educational efforts during informed consent aimed at improving comprehension of research procedures and reducing confusion about differences between preventive research and preventive. While clear and culturally sensitive informed consent dialogues are essential first steps, they cannot remedy misconceptions based upon mistrust of the investigator who is providing the information, nor pessimism about healthcare outcomes in general. This suggests that in addition to educational efforts, investigators need to anticipate and effectively address the personal and collective history of research abuse or health disparities that some populations may have experienced.

Consent in Ethnographic Studies

In comparison to epidemiological research and prevention trials, ethnographic, observational studies are inherently exploratory and less restrictive. The open-ended nature of these designs can make it difficult to anticipate the exact nature of information that may be gained through participant–investigator interactions. Specifically the focus on discovering emergent themes in qualitative research means that investigators do not always know beforehand stressful content or privacy and confidentiality issues that may emerge during the course of research. In some cases, individuals in substance-use studies have been found to be surprisingly open when discussing illegal activities, a finding which investigators have attributed to participants' desire to share their own narratives (Sandberg & Copes, 2012). However others have reported that participants did raise questions about law enforcement involvement and requested assurance that sensitive information obtained in the study did not reach police (Small, Maher, & Kerr, 2014).

To meet these challenges, during the initial informed consent investigators should include a description about the type of information if any (e.g., child abuse, drug overdose, threats of violence in school-based research) they are legally or ethically required to report. They should alert the prospective participant to this possibility during informed consent, monitor verbal or behavioral information during the course of the interviews, and remind the participant about confidentiality protections and limitations when unexpected issues arise (Fisher, 2004; Fisher, et al., 2017; Fisher & Goodman, 2009). If a new direction of inquiry emerges that might be in conflict with participants' confidentiality expectations, this should be identified and the participant given the opportunity to re-consent. In observational field studies involving drug use or other illegal behaviors, an agreement can be reached during informed consent about which activities will and will not be asked or witnessed (Fisher, 2009; Singer et al., 1999).

Child Assent and Waiver of Guardian Permission for Adolescent Substance-Use Research

In *law* and ethics, guardian permission is required to protect children from consent vulnerabilities related to immature cognitive skills, lack of emotional preparedness and experience in clinical or research settings, and actual or perceived power differentials between children and adults (Fisher & Vacanti-Shova, 2011; Koocher & Henderson, 2012). Out of respect for children's developing autonomy, federal regulations (DHHS, 2017) require the informed assent of children capable of providing assent. Investigators conducting substance-use prevention studies involving children and adolescents should be familiar with the growing body of empirical data on the development of children's understanding of the nature of research and with rights-related concepts such as confidentiality and voluntary assent or dissent (Bruzzese & Fisher, 2003; Chenneville, Sibille, & Bendell-Estroff, 2010; Condie & Koocher, 2008; Daniels & Jenkins, 2010; Field & Behrman, 2004; Gibson, Stasiulis, Gutfreund, McDonald, & Dade, 2011; Koelch et al., 2009; Unguru, 2011). There are instances when guardian permission for health-related research is not required or possible for children younger than 18 years of age. For example, *emancipated minor* is a legal status conferred on persons who have not yet attained the age of legal competency (as defined by state law) but are entitled to treatment as if they have such status by virtue of assuming adult responsibilities, such as self-support, marriage, or procreation. *Mature minor* is someone who has not reached adulthood (as defined by state law) but who, according to state law, may be treated as an adult for certain purposes (e.g., consenting to psychological assessment, or treatment for drug abuse, or emotional disorders).

There are other instances in which adolescents will refuse to participate in substance-use surveys and other types of behavioral risk research if guardian permission is required (Fisher, True, et al., 2013). This is especially true for studies examining substance use and related health-compromising behaviors among LGBT youth who fear family rejection if guardian permission reveals their sexual orientation or gender identities to parents (Fisher, Arbeit, Dumont, Macapagal, & Mustanski, 2016; Fisher & Mustanski, 2014; Mustanski & Fisher, 2016). Under federal regulations (DHHS, 2017). The production of scientifically informed and adolescent-appropriate approaches to substance-use prevention approaches is hindered when guardian permission requirements prohibit participation from youth most vulnerable to substance use and abuse. Under these circumstances guardian permission can be waived if research meets the requirements of Common Rule (DHHS, 2017) that (i) the research involves no more than minimal risk to the subjects; (ii) the research could not practicably be carried out without the waiver; (iii) the research involves using identifiable information; (iv) the research could not be practicably carried out without identifiers; (v) the waiver will not adversely affect the rights and welfare of the subjects; and (vi) whenever appropriate the participants (or their legal representative) will be provided with additional pertinent information after participation. To meet these requirements investigators need to demonstrate to their IRBs that informed consent procedures are age appropriate, tailored to the adolescent participants' developmental level, and include consent-enhancing educative material to ensure understanding of research procedures and participant research rights, especially their right to refuse or withdraw from participation. Having a consent advocate can also ensure that youth rights are protected (Fisher et al., 2017).

At the same time guardian permission should never be waived for investigator convenience or solely for reasons of cost or speed or other expedient measures if doing so it weakens protection of subjects' rights and welfare. Too often investigators view parents' reluctance to permit their children to participate in research as a legitimate reason to claim that the research could not be feasibly carried out without the waiver, especially when recruitment is focused on economically and socially marginalized youth populations. Empirical data suggests that parental reluctance in these populations is based on the failure of investigators to justify the real-world validity of their studies or to counter experimental mistrust in these populations. Thus investigators should draw on community advisory boards to understand such reluctance and use such knowledge to increase sensitivity to and understanding of the research, recruitment, and consent procedures within that population (Fisher et al., 2013).

Informed Consent for Online Research

The absence of direct, in-person contact for online survey research on correlates of substance use and abuse raises concerns regarding verification of identity and legal age and ensuring comprehension. Comprehension can be addressed by quizzes embedded in consent information, and documentation of consent can be obtained through a check box indicating agreement with consent information or through electronic signatures when necessary. In some cases, the posted recruitment information can include a link for the potential participant to permit a member of the research team to contact them by phone to conduct screening, validate age and other inclusion criteria, and obtain consent/assent and guardian permission if required, and informed consent. For all online research the consent process should include explanations of how data are stored, maintained, disseminated, and disposed (Fisher et al., 2017). In addition, to ensure the voluntary nature of participation, consent should clarify how individuals can withdraw from participation once they have begun the survey, whether they are free to leave some items unanswered, and whether compensation for participation is dependent on completing part of all of the survey.

Consent for research conducting on social media sites: Facebook is a powerful platform for social science research that allows for selective recruiting through targeted advertising and mining of vast stores of data about individuals and potentially members of their social networks. Although informed consent may not be required for research involving Facebook profile and other information approved by the user for public posting, it is required for studies that utilize the Facebook platform for the collection of survey, focus group, or other forms of data collected specifically for research purposes. Informed consent for research involving the collection of nonpublic Facebook data should include clear details on the nature of information that will be extracted, who will have access to the data, *and* how participants can best use Facebook privacy options to limit investigator access to non-research-related data and to preclude members of their social network from being aware of their participation in a study (Fisher et al., 2017). The Facebook pages of users who consent to participation will also contain comments and pictures of Facebook friends and others who are not participants. Kosinski, Matz, Gosling, Popov, and Stillwell (2015) suggest that such nonparticipant data could be used without consent if collected in the aggregate (without identification) for the purpose of extracting knowledge about consenting participants, such as their popularity or social activity.

Other forms of online research on substance-use attitudes and descriptions of behaviors do not require informed consent because information is obtained from public chat rooms or from games utilizing virtual representations such as avatars. According to Fisher et al. (2017) such research can be considered naturalistic observation as long as the investigator does not interact with or otherwise influence the nature of individuals' responses and the Internet personae cannot be linked with personal identifiers. When conducting naturalistic observation on any of these sites, investigators must ensure that existing law or privacy policies associated with the terms of the host site do not explicitly preclude the use of data for research purposes. Other criteria for determining whether information to be collected online requires informed consent include sites in which a password is required to join a chat room to discuss substance use or other socially sensitive topics. According to Fisher et al. (2017) a conservative ethical approach to this question is to follow the published privacy/confidentiality policy at the site that can be assumed to reflect the shared privacy priorities of the members such as those of Alcoholics Anonymous (see also the DHHS Secretary's Advisory Committee on Human Research Protections (DHHS, 2013).

Confidentiality

Prevention studies on substance often elicit sensitive information about illegal use of substances, behaviors, family and peer relationships, and mental health. Such information is necessary to generate critical knowledge about the correlates, sequelae, and personal and social mediators of substance use and abuse. Obtaining such information raises unique confidentiality and disclosure concerns. First, surveys on the use, purchase, or selling of illicit drugs or distribution of alcohol or cigarettes to underage youth may uncover information that if revealed could place participants, their family members, friends, or others in social, physical, economic, or legal jeopardy. Similarly, although prevention programs may initially target school-aged participants or nonclinical populations who are at risk for but not engaged in substance use or substance-use dependence, outcome measures especially with long-term follow-up must include recognition that collecting data on the acquisition of most addictive substances or underage purchase of alcohol involves illegal activity and that some may over the course of a study engage in sex work, illegal distribution of addictive substances, or behaviors that place their health and physical safety in danger.

Second, baseline and follow-up measures whether for inclusion or exclusion criteria often reveal information about serious psychological (e.g., suicidality) or medical (HIV status or toxic drug dose administration) problems of which the participant (or the guardians of underage youth) may or may not be aware. For example, a study of youth (aged 6–12.9) with manic symptoms found that 34.9% over the age of 9 used alcohol at least once with 11.9% regular users; 30.1% used drugs with 16.2% regular users; and predictors of regular alcohol and drug use included parental marital status in addition to stress life events (Horwitz et al., 2017).

Finally, investigators often uncover aspects of participants' behaviors that pose a serious danger to known others such as a planned gang hit, an impulsive participant obtaining a gun, or while intoxicated keeping sexual partners naïve about their highly contagious sexually transmitted diseases (Fisher & Goodman, 2009).

The confidentiality risks and reporting obligations of community-based prevention scientists working with high-risk populations are less clear than the ethical obligations of those working in clinical settings where assessment and intervention are expected (Cooper & McNair, 2015). Consequently, for nonintervention prevention research, the selection of ethically appropriate confidentiality procedures and guidelines for disclosing confidential information must be fitted to (a) the probability and the magnitude of harm if confidentiality is or is not protected; (b) the validity of the potential harm assessment; and (c) the availability of social, service, or legal systems to support the confidentiality or disclosure decision (Fisher, 1994, 2003; Fisher & Goodman, 2009).

Certificate of Confidentiality

Two common research approaches to protect participant privacy are the Certificate of Confidentiality (CoC) and use of quasi-anonymity techniques. A Certificate of Confidentiality under 301[d] of the Public Health Service Act provides investigators with immunity from government or civil order to disclose identifying information contained in research records (https://humansubjects.nih.gov/coc/index). Although a CoC can protect researchers from having to release data in response to a subpoena, it does not prevent researchers from disclosing confidential information if they believe it is a moral imperative (Fisher et al., 2017). If investigators who have acquired a CoC intend to make certain voluntary disclosures to protect the research participant or others from harm, the consent form should detail the types of information that will be disclosed. For these reasons, once participants understand the limitations of a CoC they may underreport, compromising the validity of data. Quasi-anonymity is a method that ensures participants' names and study identification numbers are stored separately from other research information (Beatty, Chase, & Ondersma, 2014). A study comparing the two methods found that quasi-anonymity increased overall disclosure of sensitive information including drug and alcohol use, while CoCs only appeared to increase disclosure of drug use and facilitated self-reporting (Beatty et al., 2014).

Although the CoC is presumed to offer strong privacy protections, case law has been variable on the extent of protection offered (State of North Carolina v. Bradley, 2006; Wolf et al., 2012) and future cases may rest on whether a defendant's constitutional rights are privileged over statutory protections offered by the CoC, especially within the context of government's increasingly broad legal powers to obtain confidential information since 9/11 (Beskow, Dame, & Costello, 2008). In addition to acquiring a CoC, researchers collecting sensitive data for populations who are at higher risk for court or government requests for information should consider additional data protections, including de-identification or destruction of data as soon as scientifically feasible and in accord with record-keeping responsibilities, and describing such protections during informed consent (Fisher et al., 2017).

Geospatial Mapping

Utilizing mobile phones and other new technologies to collect geographic data identifying "hot spots" for use of illicit drugs and "health service deserts" is a relatively new methodology for gaining insights into the role of environmental influences on drug use (Conners et al., 2016; Hallett & Barber, 2014). However, geospatial mapping also raises unique confidentiality concerns. For example, in a recent study Rudolph, Bassi, and Fish (Rudolph, Bazzi, & Fish, 2016) found that participants in geo-mapping studies of street drug use expressed privacy and safety concerns associated with the collection of information on the specific locations in which illegal drug transactions take place as well as the potential negative repercussions of such procedures for friends and family also involved in these transactions. Use of mobile phone technology approaches to investigate social influences on underage drinking and illicit drug use may raise similar confidentiality and data validity issues (Meisel, Clifton, MacKillop, & Goodie, 2015; Philip, Ford, Henry, Rasmus, & Alan, 2016). For example, mobile phone diary keeping has become a popular means of identifying situational factors influencing substance use. These types of methodologies' ethical procedures should include directly addressing during recruitment and informed consent the extent and limits of confidentiality when data is collected via the mobile phone, asking participants about their safety and confidentiality concerns, and providing training on how they can protect the confidentiality of data entered into their phones while out in the field.

Disclosure of Confidential Information

Substance-use prevention research often involves the discovery of previously unidentified problems of which the participant or their guardians are unaware (e.g., cognitive deficits) or serious social (e.g., victimization) or mental health disorders (e.g., depression) that may require immediate attention. Scientists have typically been reluctant to disclose information about participants uncovered during nonintervention research because (a) assessments designed to evaluate differences between groups may lack diagnostic validity for individual participants; (b) taking action to help participants (e.g., making referrals for treatment) can threaten the internal validity of a research design (especially longitudinal designs), betray the trust of participants, or jeopardize recruitment; and (c) disclosing information can create harmful or stressful consequences for participants (Fisher, 2003; Fisher & Goodman, 2009; Fisher, Higgins-D'Allesandro, Rau, Kuther, & Belanger, 1996).

When investigators are licensed practitioners and thus mandatory reporters there may be situations in which the decision to disclose may be more clear-cut, such as in instances of reported child abuse. However, prevention scientists often face less clear-cut disclosure decisions. Fisher and Goodman (2009) have outlined the following key considerations for investigators deciding whether they should disclose confidential information gained during nonintervention studies. The first step is to draw on extant empirical data to anticipate the types of behavior or information that might require disclosure of confidential information within the participant population. Second, investigators should determine whether the assessment instruments to be used while valid for testing hypotheses about aggregate populations have sufficient predictive power to conclude whether an individual is at imminent risk of harm to self or others. Third, investigators should familiarize themselves with relevant state or local reporting laws (for example in a few states all citizens and/or researchers specifically are listed as mandated reporters). Fourth, they should identify availability of legal and social services if a referral is most appropriate. Fifth, once a confidentiality and disclosure policy is determined, investigators should train research staff on procedures necessary to identify, evaluate, and report information that requires disclosure and inform prospective participants of this policy during informed consent. Final steps include monitoring staff implementation of the disclosure policy, evaluating the positive or negative outcomes of the policy, and modifying procedures if necessary.

Monetary Incentives for Research Participation

The use of monetary incentives for participation in substance-use prevention research has prompted debate on its efficacy and ethicality (Ritter, Fry, & Swan, 2003; Seddon, 2005). Selecting noncoercive compensation for research participation helps ensure that participation is voluntary, that research burdens are not borne unequally by economically disadvantaged populations, and that these populations have the opportunity to participate in research that may improve future substance-use and prevention programs (Fisher et al., 2017). Compensation for effort, time, and travel is permitted under federal regulations if the nature or the amount does not encourage individuals to lie or conceal information that would disqualify them from the research or lure them into procedures they would otherwise choose to avoid.

The central features of current ethical debate regarding the use of monetary incentives as a recruitment technique have focused on (1) whether or not it is ethical for researchers to provide monetary incentives when they may be used to support drug use in high-risk populations and (2) whether or not monetary incentives distort the ability of adolescent or adult members of economically marginalized populations to give voluntary and uncoerced participation consent (Buchanan et al., 2002; Dickert & Grady, 1999; Emanuel, 2005; Festinger et al., 2005; Fisher, 2004; Fry & Dwyer, 2001; Slomka et al., 2008). Although these concerns constitute major misgivings on the part of ethics scholars and institutional review boards, very little research has directly addressed them.

Some forms of research do not require extensive recruitment and retention incentives, while others, such as studies involving marginalized populations at greatest risk for substance use and abuse, have low rates of recruitment and retention (Festinger & Dugosh, 2012b; VanderWalde & Kurzban, 2011). For example, recent studies have found concerns about confidentiality and fear of law enforcement involvement were barriers to research participation for people who use drugs (Barratt, Norman, & Fry, 2007; Souleymanov et al., 2016). Although not documented, similar concerns may emerge among participants in preventive intervention studies in which outcome measures may detect illegal drug use or other illegal activities (e.g., alcohol-associated delinquency or violence). Since monetary compensation can be an important motive for an individual's decision to participate, investigators must ensure that it is neither an undue inducement nor considered a benefit in the evaluation of research procedure risks and benefit (DHHS, 2017; Fisher et al., 2017). Economically marginalized research participants often consider participation in paid research studies as a source of income, understand the time spent in the study as "work," and may feel frustrated and "ripped off" if the compensation provided is not monetary (Cooper & McNair, 2015). On the one hand, inadequate incentives can skew sampling by discouraging individuals with less economic resources from participating or result in an unfair burden to those who suffer from economic disparities. On the other hand, excessive compensation as a recruitment technique can compromise voluntary consent and jeopardize internal validity if it encourages participants to lie about substance-use histories that would make them ineligible for participation.

Although it has been repeatedly demonstrated that monetary payments are effective in both increasing recruitment and decreasing participation attrition, institutional review boards are often hesitant to approve such incentives for studies involving vulnerable and the revised Common Rule specifically defines research vulnerability in terms of "the possibility of coercion or undue influence" (DHHS, 2017). As a result, investigators are often required to provide lower magnitude, noncash incentives (Festinger & Dugosh, 2012a; Fisher, 2004). However, studies demonstrate that participants at risk for or who use addictive substances generally use payments in a responsible and safe manner. For example, Festinger et al. (2005) found that while increasing amounts of monetary incentives were effective in preventing study attrition among drug-using participants, they led to neither drug use nor higher rates of self-reported coercion. Fisher (2003) found that the majority of adolescents and parents from diverse ethnic and economic settings thought it was fair to pay teens for time spent answering surveys on substance use, although teens more than parents thought payments might prevent participants from complaining if they thought the investigator did something wrong.

IRBs often suggest that investigators "protect" vulnerable participants from unwise use of monetary incentives by providing food or other types of coupons that restrict what the participant can purchase. Some have argued that store coupons in lieu of monetary payments further stigmatize and reinforce economic disadvantages and violate the principle of respect by assuming that members of this vulnerable population are incapable of making good or responsible decisions for themselves or (Davidson & Page, 2012; Fisher, 2004; Oransky, Fisher, Mahadevan, & Singer, 2009; Seddon, 2005). Moreover, substituting food store coupons may violate principles of fairness since participants from economically marginalized populations who have received such compensation informally report that they often sell these coupons below market value and find noncash coupons or vouchers patronizing offensive and misguided use (Oransky et al., 2009). Other studies have indicated that participants used cash and check payments to purchase household items and to cover living expenses such as bills and transportation, while gift cards were generally used on nonessentials such as gifts and luxury items (Festinger & Dugosh, 2012a). These data suggest that when community consultation identifies a fair market price for research participation the use of food or other restricted coupons is not an ethical substitute for cash payments.

Identifying Fair Versus Coercive Incentives

The question of research incentives and compensation remains paradoxical. Different economic and cultural circumstances may lead to varying perceptions of a research incentive and compensation as fair or coercive. At the same time, fairness and justice entitle all persons to equal compensation for equal levels of participation in a particular research project (Fisher et al., 2017). Financial concerns are often a barrier to research participation in economically distressed communities. Taking time off from work to participate in research may be an economic burden for individuals who earn an hourly wage or work double shifts to support their families (Fisher et al., 2002). Consulting with members of the population who will be recruited for research participation about different types of research compensation can help investigators and their IRBs determine the extent to which cash or nonmonetary compensation is fair or coercive. The different socioeconomic and cultural lenses through which participants judge fair compensation versus coercion are valuable sources for solving ethical dilemmas and determining fair and just behavior in substance use research (Fisher, 2004). Emanuel (2005) has argued that incentives should be defined as coercive only when they distort people's reasoning abilities to such an extent that they undertake something that exposes them to unreasonable risks that they would not take if they were sober and reasoning clearly. With this in mind, decisions regarding fair and respectful compensation for participation in substance-use prevention studies require a combination of effective strategies for ensuring that research risks are minimal and reasonable, consent procedures are tailored to the developmental and educational level of prospective participants, and levels of compensation are considered fair and non-excessive by members of or advocates for the population under study and (Oransky et al., 2009).

Conclusion

Research is critical to the construction and evaluation of fair and effective social policies that will help prevent substance-use disorders and related health-compromising behaviors. In substance use research, life circumstances that increase participants' research vulnerability can include a combination of demographic, social, and health characteristics. For example, comorbid mental disorders, lower levels of education, or intoxication, cravings, or withdrawal can compromise informed consent. Social stigma or membership in violent social networks can exacerbate research risks not present in other populations. Engagement in behaviors to obtain illicit drugs or undocumented immigration status can lead to legal risk if recruitment or geospatial mapping procedures do not take such risks into account. Finally, lack of economic resources and healthcare disparities can make participants more susceptible to exploitation.

In what Fisher has described as goodness-of-fit ethics, research vulnerability is defined in terms of a susceptibility to research harms that is not solely determined by participant characteristics that society views as disadvantageous, but by the degree to which participant welfare is dependent on the specific actions of scientists within a specific experimental context (Fisher, 2003, 2004, 2015; Fisher & Goodman, 2009; Fisher & Ragsdale, 2006; Masty & Fisher, 2008). From this perspective, protecting the "vulnerable" research participant is a moral obligation that emerges from the research design itself rather than a charitable inclination of scientists as moral agents to protect those who are intrinsically vulnerable (Fisher, 1999).

The goodness-of-fit framework for substance-use prevention science presents an opportunity to correct biases and misperceptions. The model assumes that adequate ethical decision-making requires more than slight modifications to traditional ways of conducting science. Rather it necessitates critical reflection about potential modifications in research goals and design that can enhance scientific validity, participant protections, and social value (Fisher, 1997; Fisher & Ragsdale, 2006). The goodness-of-fit perspective shifts judgments regarding ethical procedures away from an exclusive focus on assumed participant vulnerabilities to (a) an examination of those aspects of the research setting that are creating or exacerbating research vulnerability and (b) consideration of how the design and ethical procedures can be modified to best advance science and participant and social welfare (Fisher, 2015).

Goodness-of-fit ethics is essentially optimistic in its view that research vulnerability is not predetermined. It posits that even for persons whom society views as most vulnerable, research risks and harms can be minimized by understanding not only participants' problems but also their personal and social network strengths (Fisher & Goodman, 2009). This understanding of population resilience contributes to fitting research designs in ways that maximize opportunities for participant autonomy and welfare.

The development of ethical procedures should not stand in isolation from the values, fears, and hopes that participants bring to the research enterprise. Conceptualizing participants and members of their communities as important resources for illuminating ethical issues and solutions can help fit participant protections to the unique challenges that emerge when such vulnerabilities are the focus of study. The goodness-of-fit framework assumes that engaging participants in dialogue about the responsible conduct of research presents an opportunity to correct biases and misperceptions that arise when research ethics decision-making is restricted to the perspectives of investigators, IRB members, and regulators (Dubois et al., 2011; Fantuzzo, McWayne, & Childs, 2006; Fisher, 1999, 2003; Fisher, 2015; Fisher & Ragsdale, 2006). Finally, as with all ethical endeavors, creating participant-fitted ethical practices provides scientists with opportunities for moral growth. It pushes us to envision research ethics as a process that draws on our knowledge as scientists of the human condition and our responsiveness to others as members of society to discover new means of meeting our obligations as scientists and citizens.

Acknowledgement The writing of this chapter was partially supported by a grant from the National Institutes on Drug Abuse of the National Institutes of Health under award number R25 DA031608-011 (PI Celia. B. Fisher).

References

Adams, P. F., Kirzinger, W. K., & Martinez, M. E. (2012). Summary health statistics for the U.S. population: National Health Interview Survey. National Center for Health Statistics. *Vital and Health Statistics, 10*(259), 2013.

Albee, G., & Ryan-Finn, K. (1993). An overview of primary prevention. *Journal of Counseling & Development, 72*(2), 115–123.

American Society of Addiction Medicine. (2011). *Public policy statement: Definition of addiction.*

Retrieved from http://www.asam.org/quality-practice/definition-of-addiction

Appelbaum, P. S., Lidz, C. W., & Grisso, T. (2004). Therapeutic misconception in clinical research: Frequency and risk factors. *IRB, 26,* 1–8.

Appelbaum, P. S., Roth, L. H., & Lidz, C. (1982). The therapeutic misconception: Informed consent in psychiatric research. *International Journal of Law and Psychiatry, 5,* 319–329.

Barratt, M. J., Norman, J. S., & Fry, C. L. (2007). Positive and negative aspects of participation in illicit drug research: Implications for recruitment and ethical conduct. *International Journal of Drug Policy, 18,* 235–238.

Beatty, J. R., Chase, S. K., & Ondersma, S. J. (2014). A randomized study of the effect of anonymity, quasi-anonymity, and certificates of confidentiality on postpartum women's disclosure of sensitive information. *Drug and Alcohol Dependence, 134,* 280–284.

Belmont Report. (1979). *The Belmont Report: Ethical principles and guidelines for the protection of human subjects of research.* Retrieved February 1, 2017, from hhs.gov/ohrp/humansubjects/guidance/belmont.html

Beskow, L. M., Dame, L., & Costello, J. (2008). Certificates of confidentiality and the compelled disclosure of research data. *Science, 14,* 1054–1055. https://doi.org/10.1126/science.1164100

Bruzzese, J. M., & Fisher, C. B. (2003). Assessing and enhancing the research consent capacity of children and youth. *Applied Developmental Science, 7,* 13–26. https://doi.org/10.1207/S1532480XADS0701_2

Buchanan, D., Khoshnood, K., Stopka, T., Shaw, S., Santelices, C., & Singer, M. (2002). Ethical dilemmas created by the criminalization of status behaviors: Case examples from ethnographic field research with injection drug users. *Health Education & Behavior, 29,* 30–42.

Buka, S., & Kington, R. (2001). Health disparities among racial and ethnic populations: Theoretical frameworks and conceptual models guiding the research. Differential drug use, HIV/AIDS, and related health outcomes among racial and ethnic populations: A knowledge assessment workshop, NIDA, Bethesda, MD April 26–27.

Cargill, V. A., & Stone, V. E. (2005). HIV/AIDS: A minority health issue. *The Medical Clinics of North America, 89,* 895–912.

Carliner, H., Delker, E., Fink, D. S., Keyes, K. M., & Hasin, D. S. (2016). Racial discrimination, socioeconomic position, and illicit drug use among US Blacks. *Social Psychiatry and Psychiatric Epidemiology, 51,* 551. https://doi.org/10.1007/s00127-016-1174-y

Case, A., & Deaton, A. (2015). Rising morbidity and mortality in midlife among white non-Hispanic Americans in the 21st century. *Proceedings of the National Academies of Sciences, 112,* 15708–15083.

Center for Behavioral Health Statistics and Quality. (2015). *Behavioral health trends in the United States: Results from the 2014 National Survey on Drug Use and Health* (HHS Publication No. SMA 15-4927, NSDUH Series H-50). Retrieved from http://www.samhsa.gov/data/OriginatingOffice

Center for Disease Control and Prevention, National Center for Health Statistics, National Vital Statistics System, Mortality File. (2015). *Number and age-adjusted rates of drug-poisoning deaths involving opioid analgesics and heroin: United States, 2000–2014.* Atlanta, GA: Center for Disease Control and Prevention. Retrieved from http://www.cdc.gov/nchs/data/health_policy/AADR_drug_poisoning_involving_OA_Heroin_US_2000-2014.pdf

Chenneville, T., Sibille, K., & Bendell-Estroff, D. (2010). Decisional capacity among minors with HIV: A model for balancing autonomy rights with the need for protection. *Ethics & Behavior, 20*(2), 83–94.

Cohen, P. J. (2002). Untreated addiction imposes an ethical bar to recruiting addicts for non-therapeutic studies of addictive drugs. *Journal of Law, Medicine & Ethics, 30,* 73–81.

Condie, L., & Koocher, G. P. (2008). Clinical management of children's incomplete comprehension of confidentiality limits. *Journal of Child Custody: Research, Issues, and Practices, 5*(3–4), 161–191.

Conners, E. E., West, B. S., Roth, A. M., Meckel-Parker, K. G., Kwan, M. P., Magis-Rodriguez, C., ... Brouwer, K. C. (2016). Quantitative, qualitative and geospatial methods to characterize HIV risk environments. *PLoS One, 11*(5), e0155693. https://doi.org/10.1371/journal.pone.0155693

Cooper, J. A., & McNair, L. (2015). Simplifying the complexity of confidentiality in research. *Journal of Empirical Research on Human Research Ethics, 10*(1), 100–102.

Daniels, D., & Jenkins, P. (2010). *Therapy with children: Children's rights, confidentiality and the law* (2nd ed.). Thousand Oaks, CA: Sage.

Davey-Rothwell, M. A., Siconolfi, D. E., Tobin, K. E., & Latkin, C. A. (2015). The role of neighborhoods in shaping perceived norms: An exploration of neighborhood disorder and norms among injection drug users in Baltimore, MD. *Health & Place, 33,* 181–186.

Davidson, P., & Page, K. (2012). Research participation as work: Comparing the perspectives of researchers and economically marginalized populations. *American Journal of Public Health, 102*(7), 1254–1259.

Department of Health and Human Services. (2017). 45CFR46 protection of human subjects subpart A. *Federal Register* Vol. 82, No. 12/Thursday, January 19, 2017/Rules and Regulation.

Department of Health and Human Services Secretary's Advisory Committee on Human Research Protections (SACHRP). (2013). *Attachment B: Considerations and recommendations concerning Internet research and human subjects research regulations with revisions.* Retrieved from http://www.hhs.gov/ohrp/sachrp/commsecbytopic/Internet%20Research/may20,2013,attachmentb.html

Dickert, N., & Grady, C. (1999). What's the price of a research subject? Approaches to payment for research participation. *New England Journal of Medicine, 341,* 198–203.

Dubois, J. M., Bailey-Burch, B., Bustillos, D., Campbell, J., Cottler, L., Fisher, C. B., ... Stevenson, R. D. (2011). Ethical issues in mental health research: The case for community engagement. *Current Opinion in Psychiatry, 24*(3), 208–214. https://doi.org/10.1097/YCO.0b013e3283459422

Emanuel, E. J. (2005). Undue inducement: nonsense on stilts? *The American Journal of Bioethics, 5,* 9–13.

Fantuzzo, J., McWayne, C., & Childs, S. (2006). In J. E. Trimble & C. B. Fisher (Eds.),. The handbook of ethical research with ethnocultural populations and communities *Scientist-community collaborations: A dynamic tension between rights and responsibilities.* Thousand Oaks, CA: Sage.

Fendrich, M., Lippert, A. M., & Johnson, T. P. (2007). Respondent reactions to sensitive questions. *Journal of Empirical Research on Human Research Ethics, 2*(3), 31–37.

Festinger, D., & Dugosh, K. (2012a). Improving the informed consent process in research with substance-abusing participants. In A. Chapman (Ed.), *Genetic Research on Addiction: Ethics, the Law, and Public Health* (pp. 41–60). Cambridge: Cambridge University Press. https://doi.org/10.1017/CBO9781139058971.005

Festinger, D. S., & Dugosh, K. L. (2012b). Paying substance abusers in research studies: Where does the money go? *The American Journal of Drug and Alcohol Abuse, 38,* 43–48.

Festinger, D. S., Marlowe, D. B., Croft, J. R., Dugosh, K. L., Mastro, N. K., Lee, P. A., et al. (2005). Do research payments precipitate drug use or coerce participation? *Drug and Alcohol Dependence, 78,* 275–281.

Field, M. J., & Behrman, R. E. (Eds.). (2004). *Ethical conduct of clinical research involving children.* Washington, DC: National Academies Press.

Fisher, C. B. (1994). Reporting and referring research participants: Ethical challenges for investigators studying children and youth. *Ethics & Behavior, 4,* 87–95. https://doi.org/10.1207/s15327019eb0402_2

Fisher, C. B. (1997). A relational perspective on ethics-in-science decision making for research with vulnerable populations. IRB: Review of Human Subjects Research, 19, 1–4. (Reprinted in Research ethics: Text and readings, by D. R. Barnbaum & M. B. Kent, Eds., 2001, New York: Prentice-Hall.). DOI: https://doi.org/10.2307/3564120.

Fisher, C. B. (1999). Relational ethics and research with vulnerable populations. In Reports on research involving persons with mental disorders that may affect decision-making capacity (Vol. 2, pp. 29–49). Commissioned Papers by the National Bioethics Advisory Commission. Rockville, MD: National Bioethics Advisory Commission. Retrieved October 26, 2009, from http://www.bioethics.gov/reports/past_commissions/nbac_mental2.pdf.

Fisher, C. B. (2002). A goodness-of-fit ethic of informed consent. *Fordham Urban Law Journal, 30,* 159–171.

Fisher, C. B. (2003). Adolescent and parent perspectives on ethical issues in youth drug use and suicide survey research. *Ethics & Behavior, 13*(4), 303–332.

Fisher, C. B. (2004). Ethics in drug abuse and related HIV risk research. *Applied Developmental Science, 8*(2), 90–102.

Fisher, C. B. (2009). *Decoding the ethics code: A practical guide for psychologists* (2nd ed.). Thousand Oaks, CA: Sage.

Fisher, C. B. (2011). Addiction research ethics and the Belmont principles: Do drug users have a different moral voice? *Substance Use and Misuse, 46*(6), 728–741.

Fisher, C. B. (2015). Enhancing the responsible conduct of sexual health prevention research across global and local contexts: Training for evidence-based research ethics. *Ethics & Behavior, 25*(2), 87–96.

Fisher, C. B., Arbeit, M. R., Dumont, M. S., Macapagal, K., & Mustanski, B. (2016). Self-consent for HIV prevention research involving sexual and gender minority youth: Reducing barriers through evidence-based ethics. *Journal of Research on Human Research Ethics, 11,* 3–14. https://doi.org/10.1177/1556264616633963

Fisher, C. B., Brunquell, D. J., Hughes, D. L., Liben, L. S., Maholmes, V., Plattner, S., ... Sussman, E. J. (2013). Preserving and enhancing the responsible conduct of research involving children and youth: a response to proposed changes in federal regulations. *Social Policy Report, 27*(1), 3–15.

Fisher, C. B., Busch-Rossnagel, N. B., Jopp, D. S., & Brown, J. L. (2012). Applied developmental science, social justice and socio-political wellbeing. *Applied Developmental Science, 16*(1), 54–64.

Fisher, C. B., Fried, A. L., Desmond, M., Macapagal, K., & Mustanski, B. (2017). Facilitators and barriers to participation in PrEP HIV prevention trials involving adolescent and emerging adult transgender men and women. AIDS Education and Prevention, 29(3), 205–217. doi:10.1521/aeap.2017.29.3.205 PMC5768197

Fisher, C. B., & Goodman, S. J. (2009). Goodness-of-fit ethics for non-intervention research involving dangerous and illegal behaviors. In D. Buchanan, C. B. Fisher, & L. Gable (Eds.), *Research with high-risk populations: Balancing science, ethics, and law* (pp. 25–46). Washington, DC: APA Books.

Fisher, C. B., Higgins-D'Allesandro, A., Rau, J. M. B., Kuther, T., & Belanger, S. (1996). Referring and reporting research participants at risk: Views from urban adolescents. *Child Development, 67,* 2086–2099.

Fisher, C. B., Hoagwood, K., Boyce, C., Duster, T., Frank, D. A., Grisso, T., ... Zayas, L. H. (2002). Research ethics for mental health science involving ethnic minority children and youths. *American Psychologist, 57*(12), 1024–1040.

Fisher, C. B., & McCarthy, E. L. (2013). Ethics in prevention science involving genetic testing. *Prevention Science, 14*(3), 310–318.

Fisher, C. B., & Mustanski, B. (2014). Reducing health disparities and enhancing the responsible conduct of research involving LGBT youth. *Hastings Center Report, 5*, 28–31.. Retrieved from http://www.ncbi.nlm.nih.gov/pmc/articles/PMC4617525

Fisher, C. B., Oransky, M., Mahadevan, M., Singer, M., Mirhej, G., & Hodge, G. D. (2008). Marginalized populations and drug addiction research: Realism, mistrust and misconception. *IRB: Ethics & Human Research, 30*, 1–9.

Fisher, C. B., & Ragsdale, K. (2006). A goodness-of-fit ethics for multicultural research. In J. Trimble & C. B. Fisher (Eds.), *The handbook of ethical research with ethnocultural populations and communities* (pp. 3–26). Thousand Oaks, CA: Sage.

Fisher, C. B., True, G., Alexander, L., & Fried, A. L. (2013). Moral stress, moral practice and ethical climate in community-based drug use research: Views from the frontline. *American Journal of Bioethics: Primary Research., 4*(3), 27–38.

Fisher, C. B., & Vacanti-Shova, K. (2011). The responsible conduct of psychological research: An overview of ethical principles, APA Ethics Code standards, and federal regulations. In M. Gottlieb, M. Handelsman, L. VandeCreek, & S. Knapp (Eds.), *Handbook of ethics in psychology* (Vol. 2, pp. 335–370). Washington, DC: APA Publications.

Fisher, C. B., & Wallace, S. A. (2000). Through the community looking glass: Re-evaluating the ethical and policy implications of research on adolescent risk and psychopathology. *Ethics & Behavior, 10*(2), 99–118. https://doi.org/10.1207/S15327019EB1002_01

Fisher, C. B. (2013). Confidentiality and disclosure in non-intervention adolescent risk research. *Applied Developmental Science, 17*(2), 88–93.

Fry, C., & Dwyer, R. (2001). For love or money? An exploratory study of why injecting drug users participate in research. *Addiction, 96*, 1319–1325.

Gibson, B. E., Stasiulis, E., Gutfreund, S., McDonald, M., & Dade, L. (2011). Assessment of children's capacity to consent for research: A descriptive qualitative study of researchers' practices. *Journal of Medical Ethics: Journal of the Institute of Medical Ethics, 37*(8), 504–509.

Hallett, R. E., & Barber, K. (2014). Ethnographic research in a cyber era. *Journal of Contemporary Ethnography, 43*, 306–330. https://doi.org/10.1177/0891241613497749

Horwitz, S. M., Storfer-Isser, A., Young, A. S., Youngstrom, E. A., Taylor, H. G., Frazier, T. W., … Findling, R. L. (2017). Development of alcohol and drug use in youth with manic symptoms. *Journal of the American Academy of Child and Adolescent Psychiatry, 56*(2), 149–156.

Jansen, L. A. (2014). Mindsets, informed consent, and research. *Hastings Center Report, 44*(1), 25–32.

Koelch, M., Singer, H., Prestel, A., Burkert, J., Schulze, U., & Fegert, J. M. (2009). "… because I am something special" or "I think I will be something like a guinea pig": Information and assent of legal minors in clinical trials—Assessment of understanding, appreciation and reasoning. *Child and Adolescent Psychiatry and Mental Health, 3*(1), 2.

Koocher, G. P., & Henderson, D. J. (2012). Treating children and adolescents. In S. J. Knapp, M. C. Gottlieb, M. M. Handelsman, L. D. VandeCreek, S. J. Knapp, M. C. Gottlieb, & L. D. VandeCreek (Eds.), *APA handbook of ethics in psychology* (Vol. 2. Practice, teaching, and research, pp. 3–14). Washington, DC: American Psychological Association.

Kosinski, M., Matz, S. C., Gosling, S. D., Popov, V., & Stillwell, D. (2015). Facebook as a research tool for the social sciences: Opportunities, challenges, ethical considerations, and practical guidelines. *American Psychologist, 70*(6), 543–556.

Langhinrichsen-Rohling, J., Arata, C., O'Brien, N., Bowers, D., & Klibert, J. (2006). Sensitive research with adolescents: Just how upsetting are selfreport surveys anyway? *Violence and Victims, 21*(4), 425–444.

Lê Cook, B., & Alegría, M. (2011). Racial-ethnic disparities in substance abuse treatment: The role of criminal history and socioeconomic status. *Psychiatric Services, 62*(11), 1273–1281.

Levy, N. (2016). Addiction, autonomy, and informed consent: On and off the garden path. *Journal of Medicine and Philosophy, 41*, 56–73.

Marshall, Z., Nixon, S., Nepveux, D., Vo, T., Wilson, C., Flicker, S., … Proudfoot, D. (2012). Navigating risks and professional roles: Research with lesbian, gay, bisexual, trans, and queer people with intellectual disabilities. *Journal of Empirical Research on Human Research Ethics, 7*(4), 20–33. https://doi.org/10.1525/jer.2012.7.4.20

Mastrioanni, A., & Kahn, J. (2001). Swinging on the pendulum: Shifting view of justice in human subjects research. *Hastings Center Report, 31*, 21–28.

Masty, J., & Fisher, C. B. (2008). A goodness of fit approach to parent permission and child assent pediatric intervention research. *Ethics & Behavior, 13*, 139–160.

Meisel, M. K., Clifton, A. D., MacKillop, J., & Goodie, A. S. (2015). A social network analysis approach to alcohol use and co-occurring addictive behavior in young adults. *Addictive Behaviors, 51*, 72–79.

Moran-Sanchez, I., Luna, A., Sanchez-Munoz, M., Aguilera-Alcaraz, B., & Perez-Carceles, M. D. (2016). Decision-making capacity for research participation among addicted people: A cross-sectional study. *BMC Medical Ethics, 17*(1), 3. https://doi.org/10.1186/s12910-015-0086-9

Mustanski, B. (2011). Ethical and regulatory issues with conducting sexuality research with LGBT adolescents: A call to action for a scientifically informed approach. *Archives of Sexual Behavior, 40*(4), 673–686.

Mustanski, B., & Fisher, C. B. (2016). HIV rates are increasing in gay/bisexual teens: IRB barriers to research must be resolved to bend the curve. *American Journal of Preventive Medicine.* https://doi.org/10.1016/j.amepre.2016.02.026

National Bioethics Advisory Commission. (2001). *Ethical an policy issues in research involving human participants*. Bethesda, MD: National Bioethics Advisory Commission.

National Commission. (1979). *The Belmont report: Ethical principles and guidelines for the protection of human subjects of research*. Washington, DC: Department of Health, Education and Welfare.

National Institute on Drug Abuse; National Institutes of Health; U.S. Department of Health and Human Services. (2016). *Strategic plan in reducing health disparities*. Retrieved from https://www.drugabuse.gov/about-nida/2016-2020-nida-strategic-plan

National Research Council. (2014). *Proposed revisions to the common rule for the protection of human subjects in research in the Behavioral and social sciences*. Washington, DC: National Academies Press.

NIDA. (2011). *Trends & statistics*. Retrieved from https://www.drugabuse.gov/related-topics/trends-statistics

NIDA. (2015a). *Nationwide trends*. Retrieved from https://www.drugabuse.gov/publications/drugfacts/nationwide-trends

NIDA. (2015b). *Opioids*. Retrieved from https://www.drugabuse.gov/drugs-abuse/opioids

Oransky, M., Fisher, C. B., Mahadevan, M., & Singer, M. (2009). Barriers and opportunities for recruitment for nonintervention studies on HIV risk: Perspectives of street drug users. *Substance Use & Misuse, 44*, 1642–1659.

Ott, M. A., Alexander, A. B., Lally, M., Steever, J. B., & Zimet, G. D. (2013). Preventive misconception and adolescents' knowledge about HIV vaccine trials. *Journal of Medical Ethics, 39*, 765–771.

Philip, J., Ford, T., Henry, D., Rasmus, S., & Alan, J. (2016). Relationship of social network to protective factors in suicide and alcohol use disorder intervention for rural Yup'ik Alaska native youth. *Psychosocial Intervention, 25*, 45–54.

Prilleltensky, I. (2003). Understanding, resisting, and overcoming oppression: Toward psychopolitical validity. *American Journal of Community Psychology, 31*, 195–202.

Prilleltensky, I., & Nelson, G. (2002). *Doing psychology critically: Making a difference in diverse settings*. New York, NY: Palgrave Macmillan.

Regmi, P. R., Aryal, N., Kurmi, O., Pant, P. R., van Teijlingen, E., & Wasti, S. P. (2016). Informed consent in health research: Challenges and barriers in low-and middle-income countries with specific reference to Nepal. *Developing World Bioethics, 17*, 84–89. https://doi.org/10.1111/dewb.12123

Ritter, A. J., Fry, C. L., & Swan, A. (2003). The ethics of reimbursing injecting drug users for public health research interviews: What price are we prepared to pay? *International Journal of Drug Policy, 14*(1), 1–3.

Rudolph, A. E., Bazzi, A. R., & Fish, S. (2016). Ethical considerations and potential threats to validity for three methods commonly used to collect geographic information in studies among people who use drugs. *Addictive Behaviors, 61*, 84–90.

Sandberg, S., & Copes, H. (2012). Speaking with ethnographers: The challenges of researching drug dealers and offenders. *Journal of Drug Issues, 43*, 176–197.

Sarason, S. B. (1984). If it can be studied or developed, should it be? *American Psychologist, 39*(5), 477–485.

Sartor, C. E., Jackson, K. M., McCutcheon, V. V., Duncan, A. E., Grant, J. D., Werner, K. B., & Bucholz, K. K. (2016). Progression from first drink, first intoxication, and regular drinking to alcohol use disorder: A comparison of African American and European American youth. *Alcoholism, Clinical and Experimental Research, 7*, 1515–1523.

Seddon, T. (2005). Paying drug users to take part in research: Justice, human rights and business perspectives on the use of incentive payments. *Addiction Research and Theory, 13*, 101–109.

Shah, S. (2004). How do institutional review boards apply the federal risk and benefit standards for pediatric research? *JAMA, 291*(4), 476.

Singer, M., Marshall, P. L., Trotter, R. T. II, Schensul, J. J., Weeks, M. R., Simmons, J. E., & Radda, K. E. (1999). *Ethics, ethnography, drug use, and AIDS: Dilemmas and standards in federally funded research. Integrating cultural, observational, and epidemiological approaches in the prevention of drug abuse and HIV/AIDS*. National Institute on Drug Abuse, NIH Pub. No. 99-4565. Rockville, MD: NIDA, pp. 198–222.

Slomka, J., McCurdy, S., Ratliff, E. A., Timpson, S., & Williams, M. L. (2008). Perceptions of risk in research participation among underserved minority drug users. *Substance Use & Misuse, 43*(11), 1640–1652.

Small, W., Maher, L., & Kerr, T. (2014). Institutional ethical review and ethnographic research involving injection drug users: A case study. *Social Science & Medicine, 104*, 157–162. https://doi.org/10.1016/j.socscimed.2013.12.010

Souleymanov, R., Kuzmanović, D., Marshall, Z., Scheim, A. I., Mikiki, M., Worthington, C., & Millson, P. (2016). The ethics of community-based research with people who use drugs: Results of a scoping review. *BMC Medical Ethics, 17*(1), 25.

State of North Carolina v. Bradley (2006) 179 NC App 551, 634 SE2d 258.

Unguru, Y. (2011). Making sense of adolescent decision-making: Challenge and reality. *Adolescent Medicine: State of the Art Reviews, 22*(2), 195–206, vii–viii.

VanderWalde, A., & Kurzban, S. (2011). Paying human subjects in research: Where are we, how did we get here, and now what? *Journal of Law, Medicine & Ethics, 39*(3), 543–558.

Wendler, D., Kington, R., Madans, J., Van Wye, G., Christ-Schmidt, H., Pratt, L. A., ... Emanuel, E. (2005). Are racial and ethnic minorities less willing to participate in health research? *PLoS Medicine, 3*(2), e19.

Wolf, L. E., Dame, L. A., Patel, M. J., Williams, B. A., Austin, J. A., & Beskow, L. M. (2012). Certificates of confidentiality: Legal counsels' experiences with and perspectives on legal demands for research Data. *Journal of Empirical Research on Human Research Ethics, 7*(4), 1–9.

Zuckerman, M. (1990). Some dubious premises in research and theory on racial differences: Scientific, social, and ethical issues. *American Psychologist, 45*(12), 1297–1303.

Part IV

Emerging Areas

Creating Persuasive Substance-Use Prevention Communications: The EQUIP Model

William D. Crano, Eusebio M. Alvaro, and Jason T. Siegel

Creating Persuasive Substance-Use Prevention Communications: The EQUIP Model

Media-based campaigns designed to discourage use of psychoactive substances have not fared well. Although notable prevention successes have been reported, they are not common (e.g., Derzon & Lipsey, 2002; Head, Noar, Innarino, & Harrington, 2013). Recent failures of large-scale, comprehensive prevention campaigns have given rise to doubts among policymakers about the elemental effectiveness of media-based psychoactive substance-use (PSU) prevention efforts, and research does little to assuage these doubts (e.g., Hornik, Jacobsohn, Orwin, Piesse, & Kalton, 2008). For example, mass media prevention campaigns were either not carried out or cut back in more than one-third of the 30 countries involved in the European Monitoring Center for Drugs and Drug Addiction (n.d.). In a comprehensive review of the evidence-based literature on media-based PSU prevention campaigns, the United Nations Office on Drugs and Crime (UNODC) stated, "in combination with other prevention components, [media campaigns] can prevent tobacco use (reporting median reduction of 2.4 per cent) … no significant findings were reported for alcohol abuse, and only weak findings with regard to drug use" (UNODC, 2015, p. 27; but see Derzon & Lipsey, 2002; Snyder & Hamilton, 2002).

The UNODC's (2015) review noted several features that appeared to enhance the effects of media-based PSU prevention efforts, but these factors were rarely studied in the meta-analyses, which typically contrasted only campaign presence or absence. Among others, these factors include identifying a specific target group; basing messages on established theory and thorough formative research; achieving widespread and frequent exposure; targeting parents in preventing adolescent PSU; and providing credible information about normative use rates, which often are widely overestimated (Crano, Gilbert, Alvaro, & Siegel, 2008; Martens et al., 2006). Review of media-based PSU prevention studies revealed that few studies met even some of these recommendations (Crano, Siegel, & Alvaro, 2012).

Given media's (and media campaigns') less than sterling record of success, questions regarding its utility and advisability in PSU prevention efforts may appear well founded. However, we believe the cause of the media's apparent futility as instruments of PSU prevention has been misidentified. To accept the assessment that the media cannot effectively deliver preventive information is to ignore the fact that the media are merely vehicles through which persuasive communications are

W. D. Crano (✉) · E. M. Alvaro · J. T. Siegel
Department of Psychology, Claremont Graduate University, Claremont, CA, USA
e-mail: william.crano@cgu.edu; Eusebio.Alvaro@cgu.edu; jason.siegel@cgu.edu

delivered. We argue that it is not the media that have failed as instruments of prevention, but rather the messages the media have conveyed. A pen that does not write may be deemed worthless, but the judgment is premature if the pen has not been filled with ink. Similarly, judgments of the media as ineffectual purveyors of preventive information are premature if the messages they deliver are not persuasive. The medium is *not* the message; it is merely a mechanism through which the message is transported (apologies to McLuhan, 1964). Failure of media-based prevention efforts may be the result of the (ineffective) messages, the very heart of all persuasion campaigns, rather than the medium through which the messages are delivered. This chapter is designed to prompt a more measured judgment of media "failures," and to describe a middle-range prototype, the EQUIP model of message development, that may materially enhance the effectiveness of future media-based PSU prevention campaigns.

Persuasion and Message-Based PSU Prevention

The UNODC (2015) suggested crucial reasons why media-based PSU prevention attempts have not lived up to expectations. Although some well-planned, well-intentioned, and comprehensive efforts (e.g., the National Youth Anti-drug Media Campaign) largely anticipated the proffered advice—to target a specific audience, use established theory, achieve wide exposure, and attack exaggerated usage norms—the fundamental components of any persuasion campaign, the messages that constituted its "deliverables," would not be deemed persuasive by many with even an elementary knowledge of the science of persuasion. The focus on the persuasiveness of messages is intentional, because successful media- or communication-based prevention almost inevitably involves persuasion, and persuasion almost always involves overcoming receivers' resistance to the appeal (Crano, Alvaro, Tan, & Siegel, 2017; Crano & Prislin, 2006), except in rare instances in which a PSU prevention communication involves only information about a substance unknown to the targeted group, and hence is not designed to *change* attitudes but to *inform* (e.g., "WARNING!!! Newly available street heroin has been cut with fentanyl. It is responsible for ten deaths in the city in the past week."). In a nutshell, we hold that message-based prevention failures usually involve a failure of the persuasiveness of the communications, not the mechanism used to deliver them.

The Less than Optimal Choice of Theory

The UNODC's advice to base media prevention approaches on established theory is eminently sensible, but the established theories that have been used to realize this directive operate at a level largely uninformative of the proper design of persuasive appeals. Consider the major theories used to guide research in prevention. These include, among others, Ajzen and Fishbein's (2005) theory of planned behavior, the health belief model (Rosenstock, 1974), social learning theory (Bandura, 1974), the transtheoretical (stages of change) model (DiClemente & Prochaska, 1982), and social norms theory (Perkins & Berkowitz, 1986). These theories point to some of the factors linked to PSU, but they operate at a level that is removed from the mechanics involved in constructing the persuasive messages designed to affect these factors, a fundamental of message-based prevention. The models operate at or near the abstract level of "grand theory" (Mills, 1959; Parsons, 1937/1968), and thus provide only Delphic advice on the means needed to develop persuasive PSU prevention messages. Their guidance is well taken. They recommend factors theoretically linked to attitude and behavior change, and variables that interrupt the progression from abstinence to initiation to consistent use; but they are *not* informative with respect to the specifics of message construction; they tell us what to do, but not how to do it.

Consider Ajzen's (1991) theory of planned behavior (TPB), a model with considerable explanatory power, one of whose key propositions stresses the importance of subjective norm perceptions in influencing behavioral intentions, and hence behavior. Using the TPB as guidance, a researcher may find that substance use is perceived as normative in a targeted population, and as such is a powerful predictor of intentions. The conclusion obviously is to focus on changing norms. But how is this to be done? How should messages be developed to maximize persuasion? The theory begs the question.

Creating an Optimal Model of Message Development

Merton (1994, p. 13) persuasively argued "for 'theories of the middle range' as mediating between gross empiricism and grand speculative doctrines." Middle-range theories provide more explicit and actionable advice about the construction and arrangement of the basic building blocks of persuasive communications (Merton, 1991), which are required if we are to mount serious PSU prevention research. Consistent with Merton's views, we believe that media-oriented PSU prevention models should integrate the tenets of grand theory approaches with fundamental ideas about the ways in which the theories may be realized in the design of actionable research. It is one thing to have a grand theory that specifies the variables critical in persuasion, and quite another to have a usable model that specifies how these variables can be realized. We propose just such an approach, the EQUIP model of persuasive communication development. It appeals to and integrates the pioneering work of Lasswell (1948, 1951) and his influential and informative communication "formula" with Hovland and associates' message-learning theory (Hovland, Janis, & Kelley, 1953) and McGuire's (1985) communication-persuasion model.

The Unique Role of Resistance in Persuasion

Before discussing the origins and development of the EQUIP model in detail, we must consider the role of resistance in persuasion. In our view, message-based persuasion presupposes receivers' resistance except under the most trivial of circumstances, which typically involve beliefs that are not vested or self-relevant (Crano, 2001, 2010). In contentious contexts in which established attitudes are held, persuasive communications must be designed to overcome the resistance that arises inevitably from attempts to change these beliefs. The greater the perceived importance and hedonic relevance of the attitude, the more difficult it is to change. In this scheme, messages designed solely to inform audiences about the dangers of an unfamiliar substance (e.g., "Avoid RP32, a new substance on the city's streets that has killed seven people in the past week.") would not completely satisfy our definition of a *persuasive* communication, at least for most audiences, who would have no established attitude about the substance, and thus little reason to resist information recommending its avoidance—unless, of course, the message receiver had developed a mindset to resist any prevention-relevant communications (Crano et al., 2012; Tormala & Petty, 2004).

The EQUIP Model of Persuasive Message Development

EQUIP is an acronym for a communication design model that outlines evidence-based message features expected to maximize the likelihood of successful persuasion. It is based on insights of the mid-level theories of Lasswell, Hovland, and McGuire, whose unique but complementary views have influenced persuasion research for decades.

Lasswell. The view of the communication process variables that must be considered in creating a communicative appeal was expressed by Lasswell (1948) in a single, if complex, question that requires we understand "*Who* says *what* to *whom*, and with what *effect*?" His question is useful because it prompts researchers to be mindful of specific features involved in the persuasion process: the communication source (the *who*), message content and delivery medium (the *what*), and message target (*to whom*) when assessing a communication's persuasive outcome (*with what effect?*). These are key elements of any persuasive message, and they must be considered when developing effective appeals.

Hovland. The message-learning theory of Hovland and colleagues is complementary to Lasswell's formula, if considerably more involved. It prescribes the requirements a communication must satisfy if it is to be persuasive. According to Hovland et al. (1953), a persuasive communication must raise a question in the mind of the receiver (e.g., "Are you certain that prescription opioids are not dangerous?"), it must answer the question ("Prescription opioids can be as addictive and as dangerous as street heroin."), it must offer some incentive to overcome receivers' reluctance to accept the proffered answer ("Some of the world's leading experts in human physiology agree."), and ideally it should present an explicit or implicit conclusion ("Therefore, according to a comprehensive study published by renowned scientists from the Johns Hopkins Bloomberg School of Public Health, this substance and its derivatives should be avoided unless prescribed by a physician for a specific problem."). Combined with Lasswell's formula, Hovland provides a useful framework for message-based persuasion. Of central importance to our view of persuasion is that Hovland's approach recognizes that persuasive contexts almost inevitably involve resistance, else why bother with questioning established beliefs and developing methods to overcome it.

McGuire. Following Hovland, the communication-persuasion model of McGuire (1985) designates crucial input variables to be considered, along with the mediating and outcome variables that affect the ways these factors operate. McGuire's input variables are congruent with Hovland and Lasswell's formulas, and include source ("who"), message ("what": content and medium), target (to "whom"), and focus of the communication (e.g., marijuana, heroin, amphetamines, gambling, overeating). Its outcome variables include, among others, attention, understanding, and attitude change. McGuire's distinction differentiates among evaluative outcomes. It suggests, for example, that if attitude change is the research focus, a message that merely attracts attention (e.g., "This is your brain on drugs …") is likely to disappoint.

The insights of Lasswell, Hovland, and McGuire provide the foundation for the development of a theory of message construction that has long been called for in communication and persuasion research, often promised, and rarely realized. Complexities involved in the design of persuasive messages have stymied systematic message development in prevention science. Arguably, the factors that must be controlled when designing effective messages, along with their many combinations, have seriously retarded progress. An organizing model is needed, integrating the working parts of the persuasion process, alerting researchers to critical and theoretically requisite features of persuasive communication, and ensuring that they are not ignored. Ideally, this model would incorporate insights from "grand" theories, and build on them with the EQUIP, a middle-range theory detailing ways in which their insights might be tested.

Components of the EQUIP Model

The EQUIP model of message development was designed to highlight and take advantage of the features deemed necessary by the three foundational middle-range models of Lasswell, Hovland, McGuire in creating persuasive communications. To meet the requirements of the EQUIP, the communication must Engage receivers, Question their established belief, Undermine or destabilize the belief, Inform the receiver of a superior alternative, and Persuade the receiver to accept this alternative. Each of these interacting requisites should be met if the communication is to have maximal effect.

Engage

Capture and maintain attention. The first and most obvious feature of the Engage requirements is to capture message receivers' attention to the persuasive communication. If it does not engage the audience, the communication cannot be expected to initiate the attitude-change process. The Engage function involves two distinct but related processes. The message must attract audience members' attention (Groenendyk & Valentino, 2002) and be sufficiently engaging to ensure that attention is maintained throughout the message's presentation (Wyer & Shrum, 2015). An interesting realization of the Engage principle is found in a brief ad developed in the Truth's anti-smoking campaign (https://www.thetruth.com/the-facts/fact-190):

FORMALDEHYDE IS FOUND IN CIGARETTE SMOKE. IT'S ALSO USED TO PRESERVE DEAD ANIMALS.

The opening line of the ad was meant to draw attention. We believe it succeeded for most readers. The attention probably persisted during the short time it took readers to process its brief appeal, which was followed by a citation of research from the National Cancer Institute. It was devised to cause young people to avoid or quit tobacco use, and presented information that probably surprised most of its young audience. It did not fulfill all of the EQUIP functions, but paired with the Truth brand may have succeeded in motivating many to learn more, and perhaps reconsider the desirability of tobacco use.

Content or Executional Variables. This attention-inducing example relies on message content to engage message receivers. Engagement is fostered by the content of what is said or written. This can be an effective and common approach. However, noncontent *executional features* also can engage targeted audience. Executional features include color (the Truth ad used alternating green and white print), and in video presentations the number or rapidity of cuts, music, movement, vividness, flashy graphics, topical relevance, etc. (see Ophir, Brennan, Maloney, & Cappella, 2017).

Attractiveness. The source of a communication also may be considered a significant executional element. Attractive sources are likely to garner more attention, which may augment message effects if their message is strong (Petty & Cacioppo, 1986). Attractiveness appears to affect explicit and implicit evaluations (Smith & De Houwer, 2014). Attractiveness can be a disadvantage, however, as enhanced message elaboration may lead message receivers to recognize its weaknesses. The ideal parlay involves attractive message sources paired with strong messages, which the EQUIP is designed to enable.

Source-statement incongruity. Attention also must be paid to the interaction between message sources and message content. Messages contrary to those expected to emanate from a communication source often have been found to be more believable, and hence persuasive, than those judged as consistent with the source's established position (Koeske & Crano, 1968).

This tactic is found in a bright orange poster ad from the Truth campaign, which stated,

WE ♥ SMOKERS, followed by, "**Heck, we love everybody. Our philosophy isn't anti-smoker or pro-smoker. It's not even about smoking. It's about the tobacco industry manipulating their products, research and advertising to secure replacements for the 1,200 customers they "lose" every day in America. You know, because they die."**

The unexpectedness of the ad's opening line was meant to capture attention, owing to the unfavorable normative status of smokers in the United States. The follow-on text presented arguments with a high degree of irony (appealing to adolescents), and delivered the ad's preventive material. The unexpectedness of the communication neutralized the perception of its manipulative intent, thereby enhancing its effect (Briñol, Rucker, & Petty, 2015).

Expectancy violations. The unexpectedness of a communication also affects its persuasiveness. Expectancy violation theory (EVT) holds that violating the expected tone and content of a communication can augment or diminish its effect (Burgoon, Dillard, & Doran, 1983). In persuasion, an expectancy violation disrupts the normal conversational conventions by adopting an unexpected position, or using irony or unexpectedly extreme or mild language. Such language usages violate expectancies resulting in more persuasive ads, probably via the same cognitive pathways operative in source-statement incongruity effects (Siegel & Burgoon, 2002).

Self-relevance, or vested interest of the message. Whereas message features discussed to this point may effectively garner attention, topics that affect the receiver's vested interest can motivate receivers to elaborate a communication. If the message is strong, enhanced elaboration will foster acceptance, because enhanced elaboration exposes the message's strong or weak points (Petty, Wegener, & Fabrigar, 1999). Considerable research has shown that the vested interest construct operates as a significant moderator of attitude-behavior consistency across a range of behaviors (De Dominicis et al., 2014; Donaldson, Siegel, & Crano, 2016; Lehman & Crano, 2002). With strong messages of the type that can be developed through careful adherence to the requirements of the EQUIP model, intense message elaboration favors a positive persuasive outcome.

To engage an audience, then, researchers should consider using one or another of the following theory and evidence-based recommendations: Draw on message content or executional variables to capture and maintain attention. Pair expected sources with unexpected positions (source-statement incongruity). Positively violate receivers' expectancies regarding the language used in a substance prevention message (language expectancy violation). And ensure messages that are perceived by receivers are important and self-relevant (vested interest).

Question

The function of EQUIP's Question phase is to reduce a receiver's certainty in the validity of the attitude that is the focus of the persuasive appeal. Hovland et al.'s (1953) middle-range persuasion theory holds that to induce attitude change, a communication must raise a question in the receiver's mind about the validity of an established belief. In EQUIP, raising a question about an established attitude is not designed to change the belief, but rather to introduce a degree of uncertainty about it. Youth vary in the certainty with which they hold their different attitudes. Youth may be ambivalent, holding both positive ("Using marijuana will make me seem more grown up.") and negative beliefs ("Using marijuana might result in my being expelled from school.") about the advisability of using a substance. Inducing and capitalizing on uncertainty could prove a useful stage in the attitude-change process.

Uncertainty also may play a positive role in one's broader belief system. Attitudes, especially complex attitudes, are linked structurally in the cognitive network to related beliefs, often resulting in relations among attitudes that are not internally consistent or logical (Crano & Lyrintzis, 2015). One might, for example, applaud one's political party's economic plans, detest its stand on same-sex marriage, and be indifferent to party members' sometimes overindulgent use of gin. Inducing reflection or doubt regarding the validity of the attitudes that comprise the structure is sufficient for the Question phase of the EQUIP. With Festinger (1957) and most other consistency theorists (Abelson et al., 1968), we assume that holding valid attitudes is an important human need. Raising questions about an attitude's validity should lower resistance to change.

Normative Consensus and Meta-Cognitive Theory

Attitudes held with high certainty are assumed to enjoy normative consensus ("everyone believes this"). Assumed consensus is positively associated with the self-relevance of the attitude (Crano, 1983). That assumed normative consensus bolsters beliefs also is a central tenet of Tormala and colleagues' meta-cognitive model of attitude resistance and change (Barden & Tormala, 2014; Tormala & Petty, 2004), which postulates that attitudes are more easily changed if the certainty with which they are held is reduced by a persuasive message. In prevention applications, attitude certainty is strengthened when the individual weathers an influence attempt, and the more powerful the resisted attack, the greater the certainty gain. The implication of the meta-cognitive model is that failed persuasion attempts lessen the likelihood that future persuasive efforts will succeed.

In summary, the function of the Question phase of the EQUIP model is to introduce in the individual a degree of uncertainty about the correctness of a critical attitude. Attitudes vary in the extent to which they are thought to be consensual. If the assumed consensus surrounding an attitude is weakened or brought into question, it becomes more susceptible to change. This enhancement of susceptibility does not necessarily result in attitude change; rather, its readiness to change is heightened. Conversely, unsuccessful attempts at attitude change strengthen resistance to subsequent persuasive communications.

Undermine

Developing communications that raise questions about the validity of an attitude is a necessary requisite of the EQUIP model, but merely raising doubts, a natural outcome of the attack on assumed consensus, usually is not sufficient to cause change. The EQUIP model requires that the persuasive message not only raise doubt about a belief's validity, but provide a credible alternative to the destabilized attitude, a reason to abandon the attitude and adopt a new position. Successful undermining capitalizes on the weakened attitude brought about by the attack on consensus surrounding the original belief. By providing arguments that confirm the legitimacy of the doubt that was raised, and providing a credible alternative, the Undermine process legitimizes the doubts introduced in the Question phase, and promotes attitude change (e.g., see Crano, Gorenflo, & Shackelford, 1988; Crano & Sivacek, 1984).

The Question and Undermine phases of the EQUIP go hand in hand. The first of the two processes weakens the consensus surrounding a belief, and the second takes advantage of this weakened attitude to posit an alternative, which resolves some or all of the unpleasant cognitive inconsistencies generated by the Question. Merely questioning a position may not be sufficient to change a belief. Questioning is necessary to initiate the change process, but successful attitude change is more likely when a viable alternative position is made apparent in the Undermine phase.

Inform

Once a person is engaged with a persuasive communication and induced to question the validity of an established belief through the Question and Undermine processes, the destabilized attitude should be replaced or overlaid with one that is congruent with the position of the message source. This requires provision of topic-relevant information, as attitudes based on greater knowledge are stronger, more enduring, and more predictive of behavior (Fabrigar, Petty, Smith, & Crites, 2006). In the context of PSU prevention, evidence suggests that this information should focus on attitudes that influence use, and misconceptions about the effects of the substance under consideration; it should not disparage or threaten the user. Too often, the physical harms of the PSU are the sole focus of a persuasive communication. Audiences often perceive such messages as unrealistic. Such communications are resisted strongly.

Research on dual-process models of attitude change has stressed the importance of strong messages in persuasion (e.g., Petty & Cacioppo, 1986). The EQUIP model is designed to provide the basis to facilitate constructing such messages. A central issue involves the information contained in the message. In most cases, this information should be evidence based. It should not be based on opinion or hearsay, or on easily dismissed platitudes. Nor should it fly in the face of the audience's experience, for example, arguing that methamphetamines can be immediately addictive is true, but this is not an inevitable outcome. Thus, many view campaigns based on this threat as false, and we have learned that rejected persuasive communications make the acceptance of later ones less likely.

When developing the Inform feature of the EQUIP, it is important to ensure that the PSU prevention argument is not immediately rejected by those whose experience belies its apparent truth. Further, threatening harms that might occur in the distant future is not likely to prove effective, nor is it useful to present information about the dangers of a substance that are well known and widely accepted. These mistakes represent wasted opportunities, as many substance users are cognizant of the dangers of their behavior; however, this is not to say that they respond well to threats (Maddux & Rogers, 1983). Calls for campaigns focusing on issues other than the physical harms of PSU are based on such findings (Halpern-Felsher, Biehl, Kropp, & Rubinstein, 2004). In promising research, Siegel, Alvaro, Lac, Crano, and Alexander (2008) found that information focusing on social (vs. physical) harms facilitated inhalant prevention efforts. A challenge to be overcome is that factors predicting PSU in one group may not be predictive in another.

Vested Interest

General principles of self-interest in persuasion may facilitate selection and development of information to maximize influence (Crano, 1995; Johnson et al., 2014). A primary informational goal is to provide evidence that PSU is not in the immediate or long-term self-interest of the audience members. Donaldson et al. (2016) found that the harms of PSU (or the benefits of avoidance) were most effective when the prevention messages focused on proximal outcomes. The benefits of abstinence projected into the distant future seem to have little effect on perceived self-interest, and hence on behavior (Crano & Prislin, 1995; Siegel et al., 2008).

In addition to the immediacy of the consequences communicated in the prevention message, its salience also should be considered. A persuasive communication will have a stronger effect on attitudes and actions if it is presented in a way that renders it salient when the potential for usage arises. Salience of PSU prevention is enhanced if it is a common topic of informed discussion in the respondent population (Prislin, 1988). Frequency of presentation of a message bolsters its salience, although salience alone is not sufficient to induce change.

Certainty of outcomes of PSU or their avoidance also can be a positive factor in prevention. Many positive outcomes of adolescent PSU avoidance have been established—they include, among others, better school and job performance, and lower likelihood of car accidents, unintended pregnancies, or arrests in later life. These features can prove powerful inducements for abstinence or cessation, if presented with strong evidence and without exaggeration or unrealistic threat. However, knowing that one should avoid a substance and knowing how to do so involve different cognitions and behaviors. This is a prime reason why many prevention programs fail (Nancy Regan's "Just say no" and the original DARE campaign come to mind: see Donaldson, 2002; Lilienfeld & Arkowitz, 2014). Failure to provide the means necessary for targeted individuals to call to mind PSU prevention information may be a prime reason for the lack of clear effects of many media-based prevention campaigns.

In summary, the information provided in a persuasive communication can have a critical effect not only on its likelihood of success, but also on the likelihood of iatrogenic responses occurring in the event of persuasive failure. Decisions concerning the specific approach to be adopted in delivering a persuasive appeal are crucial, but the specifics of the delivered information are just as important. The general recommendation derived from the past 30 years of dual-process model research is that strong messages should be used if the audience is carefully elaborating (i.e., thinking about, considering) the communication. Strong messages are viewed as having a clear basis in evidence rather than opinion, and are presented in a logical and understandable fashion. A communication's effectiveness is enhanced if it contains novel and actionable information. Information that is already well known is unlikely to have much impact.

Fear-arousing communications, long-standing staples of prevention campaigns, focus on the threats posed by PSU. These communications can prove effective if they adhere to precise guidelines. They must maintain credibility, and not exaggerate threats in terms of either severity or receivers' susceptibility. They must be presented by a highly credible source, who must provide specific advice about behaviors that can alleviate the threatened negative outcomes of use. If any of these elements is missing, the chance of persuasive failure is greatly increased. If these requisites cannot be satisfied, fear appeals should be avoided.

The information presented in a persuasive communication will be most effective if it engages the vested interest of the audience members. Discussing physiological effects that a substance user does not care about will not foster close message elaboration. In short, to ensure attention to a persuasive communication, ensure that audience members recognize that they are vested in the likely outcomes of their behaviors. At the same time, avoid setting expectations about the use of a substance that may be readily disproved or dismissed. Promised outcomes should comport with experienced reality to avoid message rejection and subsequent strengthening of the attitude that was the target of persuasion. Long-term outcomes of use of a substance are easy to relegate as inconsequential; thus, persuasive communications focused on avoiding near-term outcomes may prove more effective, even if they are less serious than long-term effects.

Persuade

As a group, the preceding elements of the EQUIP model—Engage, Question, Undermine, and Inform—set the stage for prevention. They are designed to highlight features that should guide development of persuasive communications that render message targets more accepting of its arguments. There remains a need to enact the final EQUIP element—to persuade. A compelling communication is required after satisfying the earlier features of the EQUIP if it is to be accepted, thereby changing an established attitude. Ideally, this changed attitude also will affect behavioral intentions and subsequent behaviors.

To this point in the EQUIP cycle, intended targets of persuasion have been engaged by a communication, led to question current beliefs, exposed to communicative elements designed to undermine those beliefs, and provided with new information relevant to establishing new attitudes that discourage PSU. However, receivers have not yet been induced to accept this new information and the concomitant beliefs, intentions, and actions that follow from it. Two key considerations for implementers of the final EQUIP element include the need to motivate acceptance, and to mitigate resistance, or counterargumentation, allowing for a reasonably open-minded elaboration of the PSU persuasive prevention communication.

Motivation plays a central role in persuasion. At a minimum, receivers must be encouraged to consider the position advocated in a persuasive communication. What is the impetus to process and perhaps accept this new information, thereby modifying a currently held attitude? Motivating factors include holding valid beliefs (Festinger, 1957), holding beliefs congruent with those of significant others (e.g., holding prescriptively normative beliefs: Ajzen, 1991), maintaining attitudinal congruence with one's behavior (e.g., attitude-behavior consistency: Crano, 1997, 2000; Donaldson et al., 2016; Fabrigar, Wegener, & MacDonald, 2010), and being consistent with one's values (e.g., Deci & Ryan, 2002, 2010). These are but some of the factors motivating acceptance of new information and attitude change.

In mitigating counterargumentation, considerable evidence dating to Hovland et al.'s (1953) early research supports what Gilbert (1991) called the *Spinozan* perspective, which assumes that comprehension of new information and its acceptance "are not clearly separable psychological acts, but rather that comprehension includes acceptance of that which is comprehended" (p. 107). Only after initial acceptance of a communication—an automatic response in the Spinozan framework—is the truth value of the information examined critically. This position accords with Grice's (1975, 1978) maxims that conversations follow principles of cooperation and mutual understanding, which specify, among others, the norm that apposite, truthful, and relevant messages are exchanged between communicants in the course of normal social interaction.

Subsequent rejection of accepted information is predicated on a resource-heavy message evaluation process that follows the initial tendency to accept the message. The initial communication is accepted to the extent that the evaluation process is interrupted, forestalled, or judged unnecessary. To reject new or incoming information involves a follow-on contemplative process of counterargumentation after its initial (automatic) acceptance. Thus, a key objective of persuasion is to defuse or circumvent resistance at least until after the initial cognitive elaboration of the message, thereby enhancing the likelihood that new information, initially and tentatively accepted, is not rejected upon subsequent consideration. Forestalling the process of counterargumentation is a central feature of most persuasive techniques, and is a logical outgrowth of the Spinozan perspective.

Gruder and associates (1978) reported strong research that indirectly supports the Spinozan orientation. In their experiment, participants read a strong communication that argued in favor of a 4-day workweek. Immediately at the end of the message, which was formatted as a glossy magazine article to enhance its credibility, half the subjects read a "Note from the Editor" that discounted the basic premise of the article, stating that the information it contained had been found to be false. Immediate posttest measurement revealed that those in the discounting condition were significantly less persuaded by the article than were those who had not received the disclaimer. However, a second posttest administered 6 weeks afterwards showed no differences between the groups. Over the intervening weeks, both groups' attitudes toward the 4-day workweek had become more favorable, but the attitudes of subjects whose communication was discounted grew significantly more favorable. After the 6-week delay, their scores were indistinguishable from those of the non-discounted subjects.

These results are consistent with a Spinozan interpretation, which holds that the group in the discounting condition had read the communication with an open mind, and had accepted the information as presented. Immediately thereafter, they learned that the information was false. They reasonably rejected the communication upon immediate attitude measurement, but the damage had been done. The message had been accepted initially as true, if we are to believe Grice and Spinoza. Its gist was not undone by a subsequent process of counterargumentation because the editor's discounting mitigated the need for this resource-heavy cognitive investment. However, as time passed, the discounting cue faded and became dissociated from the message, and what remained was the initially accepted information. Given the discounting cue, the heavy lifting of counterargumentation became unnecessary, and this induced cognitive laziness discouraged participants from closely revisiting the message. Thus, the message originally accepted as true was adopted. This research focuses our attention on the critical nature of counterargumentation, and the ways in which the process can be deactivated, the central issue in persuasion. These results inform our understanding and application of the EQUIP. As cognitive misers, when lacking sufficient motivation, we favor avoiding cognitive effort. This economy is bought at a price: We cannot outsource counterargumentation.

Elements of Persuasive Communications

Earlier, we introduced three orientations that guided development of the EQUIP model. Of these, Lasswell's (1948; Lasswell & Leites, 1949) model supplies instructive insights regarding specific elements that should be considered when developing communications that persuade, the final phase of the EQUIP model. Lasswell's maxim, *Who* says *what* to *whom*, and with what *effect*, points precisely to these fundamental and essential features of persuasive messages.

The Source ("Who")

The very act of communicating presupposes a communicator—a source encoding and delivering a message to an intended receiver. In PSU prevention campaigns, a source may be clearly manifest or left implied. In the former instance, the source is identifiable and its characteristics open to examination and judgment. Receivers can use visual and auditory cues to assess source features such as attractiveness, similarity, status, and expertise. In the case of implied sources, the absence of visual and sometimes identifiable auditory cues renders source characteristics to be inferred. In either case, perceptions of a message source can influence message acceptance. The phrase "perceptions of a message source" is intended, as it is the receiver's perceptions of source characteristics that determine their impact. Consider a characteristic such as "attractiveness." There is considerable support for the proposition that attractive sources are more persuasive than unattractive ones, but attractiveness is in the eye of the beholder. Formative research should be used to determine the most effective ways to operationalize source constructs for the predefined targets of persuasion.

It is important to distinguish manifest from implied sources. Whereas a message developer may manipulate features of a manifest source, those of an implied source can be difficult to control. A useful standard for message developers is to maintain as much control as possible over message creation, delivery, and interpretation. Thus, a strong case can be made for the use of explicit, rather than implied, message sources. In the absence of an explicitly identified source, receivers are left to speculate about its characteristics and motives. Given a counter-attitudinal message, it is unlikely that these attributions will be unilaterally favorable.

Credibility and Trustworthiness

Although orthogonal to the message, different features of the communication context can enhance communication effects. At least in part, source factors operate by enhancing engagement. Source features also may operate as heuristic cues that interact with content to enhance message strength (Ziegler & Diehl, 2003). A useful method of engaging an audience in message-based communication involves attributing a message to a source of high credibility. From Hovland's classic work on source credibility (Hovland et al., 1953) to more contemporary studies (e.g., Smith, De Houwer, & Nosek, 2013), research indicates clearly that message sources

perceived as expert (i.e., as having the capacity to deliver valid information) or trustworthy (i.e., one whose persuasive appeals are not conditioned on personal gain) are more likely to persuade than sources who do not share these attributes.

The dual-process models of persuasion that have inspired considerable research in social psychology emphasize the audience's close elaboration of communications as a prerequisite for persistent attitude change (Petty & Cacioppo, 1986). Arguably, credible message sources should excite greater message elaboration and less resistance. Thus, sources of high expertise and trustworthiness are more likely to persuade than those lacking these features.

Matching

Matching is concerned with the isomorphism of source and intended audience on noticeable features deemed important by receivers. Features commonly used in matching include age, gender, race or ethnicity, and social status. When matching, the aim is that receivers recognize, consciously or not, that the source is similar to them. In primary prevention campaigns addressing adolescent PSU, messages often feature sources that are peers of the intended audience; if the campaign involves an in-person presentation at a school or some other community setting, it is easy to select the appropriate source. However, most campaigns do not have this advantage, and thus the source might not match the intended receivers. With youth, it generally is assumed that younger audience will attend to sources somewhat older than they are; they are not likely to be influenced by younger message sources.

Risk or Usage Status

Message receivers at different stages of substance usage are susceptible to different forms of persuasive communication. For example, in an experiment involving young adolescents, Crano, Siegel, Alvaro, and Patel (2007) found that resolute nonusers were uniformly more favorably disposed to a PSU communication than vulnerable (i.e., high risk) nonusers or users, and that difference held regardless of source status (adult or peer) or the target of the communication (in some of the experimental variations, the communication was apparently directed toward the parents of the subjects, even though it was presented only to the audience of young adolescents). Vulnerable nonusers (i.e., nonusers who would not definitely rule out future use) were more amenable to prevention communications attributed to slightly older peers. Unexpectedly, users were most favorably disposed to communications delivered by a young physician, perhaps because they were concerned about the physical consequences of their inhalant use. This research suggests that it is important to understand the motivations of the targeted group and to respond accordingly to enhance persuasion. It indicates that formative research must be carried out in advance of moving a prevention campaign to the field.

The Message (What and How is it said?). The dual-process *elaboration likelihood model* (ELM) of Petty and Cacioppo (1986) has been a mainstay of persuasion research for many years. A central assumption of the model is that for a message to attain the greatest effect, its receivers must be motivated to process it and possess the ability to do so. If both requirements are satisfied, the persuasive outcome of the process depends on the strength of the message. Message strength is a crucial factor in persuasion (Carpenter, 2015). However, the procedures that enhance message strength have not been articulated clearly in either social psychology or communication science. The EQUIP model was developed to remedy this shortcoming by specifying many of the critical factors implicated in developing strong communications. To be maximally effective, the content of a message should contain information the receiver wants or needs, and should be based on strong evidence. Message strength may reside in the eye of the beholder, but in general evidence-based arguments are more likely to persuade than appeals based on unsupported opinion.

Although the EQUIP's features have been discussed independently for purposes of clarity, they are highly interactive, and the interaction almost always involves features of the receiver (the "to whom" in Lasswell's equation). This reflects our view that tailoring persuasive messages to the specific vulnerabilities of the individual, or targeting a communication to groups of individuals, all of whom possess similar traits (e.g., sexual orientation, age, political concerns) is the most productive prevention approach. The EQUIP is not an automatic formula for creating unerringly persuasive messages. Rather, it is a model that facilitates creation of persuasive communications by highlighting variables that years of research have indicated as critically important in the persuasion process. In most cases, these variables operate interactively, requiring consideration of all of the EQUIP's factors that control the form of the message.

How a message is conveyed by its source also is an important feature of Lasswell's "What/How" question. Information can be conveyed via a known or visible source, in which case the many factors affecting source credibility can be brought into play. The extremity of language the source uses to present information also is an important factor. Crano et al. (2017) showed that adults' unexpectedly moderate language regarding PSU avoidance was significantly more influential than more extreme, demanding language when dealing with adolescent participants. These differences in message receptivity as a function of language extremity were not evident in adolescents' responses to fellow adolescents. The extremity of language used by one's adolescent peers may not be a deciding feature in PSU prevention message acceptance, but when adult sources convey prevention appeals to adolescents, moderation matters.

The audience (To Whom is it said?). Targeting a persuasive communication to features of its audience has been a fixture in marketing for decades. To attain maximal effects, the communication must be relevant to its intended audience, thereby encouraging attention. The Engage element of the EQUIP recognizes the importance of securing and maintaining an audience's attention to the persuasive appeal. Tailoring operates at a more sophisticated and fine-grained level than targeting in matching audience and communication features (Noar, Benac, & Harris, 2007). Tailoring is a process by which message variations are used to take advantage of specific, varying features (needs, vulnerabilities, etc.) of each individual in the receiver audience (Lustria et al., 2013). The communicator matches features of the message and receiver that in theory will incline the receiver to accept the appeal. Tailored communications are designed to appeal individually to each audience member, thereby enhancing message relevance and impact.

The outcome (with What Effect?). The final component of Lasswell's formula is concerned with the outcome of the communication and persuasion process. Obviously, the test of campaign effectiveness requires a clear measurement aim. What is the goal of the prevention campaign? Among other possibilities, it may be to change attitudes toward a substance, to inform, arouse fear, prevent initiation, change norms, reduce use, or encourage cessation. All of these possible outcomes, and more, are legitimate and all could appropriately frame the focus of a prevention campaign. It is the campaign designer's job to specify its goals well in advance of program initiation, and to design the persuasive interventions to maximize desired outcomes.

A Note on the Special Case of Media-Based Preventive *Communications*

Mounting an effective persuasion campaign is considerably facilitated to the extent that a clearly delineated evidence-based model provides strategic guidance for the organization of specific persuasion tactics, as well as the evaluation of their efficacy and effectiveness. We believe that the EQUIP provides such guidance. As a middle-range model of persuasive message development, EQUIP circumvents the vagaries inherent in grand theories—especially for those seeking guidance for real-world development and implementation of PSU prevention campaigns.

The EQUIP provides systematic guidance whose purpose is to enhance message persuasiveness. It is useful in any communication context, from small-group persuasive interactions to mass media presentations. However, introducing *media* into the equation requires considerations over and above those involved in effective message creation. Lazarsfeld argued that the mass media operated indirectly, its effects transmitted from authoritative media receivers to their *opinion followers,* whose interpretation, acceptance, or rejection of the media message was conditioned in part by the responses of the authoritative receiver (the *opinion leader*). According to Lazarsfeld, Berelson, and Gaudet (1944, p. 151), "Influences stemming from the mass media first reach 'opinion leaders' who, in turn, pass on what they [see] read and hear to those of their every-day associates for whom they are influential." In the *two-step flow of communication model,* persuasive mass media operate through opinion leaders, the "go-betweens who filter the flow of information and influence to their intimate associates" (Katz, 1994, p. ix). The leader's interpretations, rationalizations, or dissent influences followers' responses to media communications. Neglect of two-step flow logic may be one of the reasons for the outcomes commonly judged as mass media prevention failures. Lazarsfeld's model implies that opinion leaders should be the principal targets of persuasive prevention communications, not the mass public, the ultimate target of most persuasive campaigns. Ignoring go-betweens may weaken the communicative impact of even well-constructed (i.e., EQUIP-based) prevention messages. Misidentifying the target, even to a small degree, inevitably reduces a media campaign's effectiveness. By implication, failing to construct persuasive messages to influence opinion leaders, and which instead target the mass public, cannot result in messages of maximal effect. Misspecification of the appropriate targets in a test of a persuasive PSU prevention communication inevitably leads to construction of messages that miss the mark.

Concluding Considerations

The EQUIP model of message development is a new approach to a long-standing question, namely, how can we develop persuasive communications of maximal effect. This issue assumes great importance in considerations of PSU prevention, given the enormous costs brought on by the misuse of increasingly more powerful psychotropic substances that have become ever more available. PSU media prevention campaigns have a spotty record, at best. We have argued that this is a function, at least in part, of a failure to recognize that prevention fundamentally involves persuasion, and thus principles of persuasion must be invoked if we are to create successful preventive messages. This is a difficult road, but it need not be made even more difficult by ignoring the literature of more than a half-century's empirical research. The EQUIP is heavily dependent on this research, and promises to guide development of persuasive communications. EQUIP is a dynamic model that allows for the incorporation of new theory and research relevant to each of its five central features. Undoubtedly, new research may suggest better ways to move an audience, but the EQUIP seems a reasonable starting point.

By implication, the model highlights the kinds of messages that should *not* be a part of a persuasive PSU prevention communication or campaign. We believe that EQUIP provides one of the most promising methods to date of using the insights of some of the many fine theories of persuasion to facilitate PSU prevention. It specifies techniques that can serve as useful adjuncts to the grand theories whose general outlines orient the central goals of the research. Importantly, in so doing, the EQUIP moves the implications of persuasion theory into media applications. This model, and others to follow, hopefully, will allow us to realize the goal of PSU prevention, and will accelerate our efforts to communicate the positive features of substance avoidance and cessation persuasively.

References

Abelson, R. P., Aronson, E., McGuire, W. J., Newcomb, T. M., Rosenberg, M. J., & Tannenbaum, P. (1968). *Theories of cognitive consistency: A sourcebook.* Chicago, IL: Rand-McNally.

Ajzen, I. (1991). The theory of planned behavior. *Organizational Behavior and Human Decision Processes, 50,* 179–211.

Ajzen, I., & Fishbein, M. (2005). The influence of attitudes on behavior. In D. Albarracin, B. T. Johnson, & M. P. Zanna (Eds.), *The handbook of attitudes* (pp. 173–221). Mahwah, NJ: Erlbaum.

Bandura, A. (1974). Behavior theory and the models of man. *American Psychologist, 29,* 859–869.

Barden, J., & Tormala, Z. L. (2014). Elaboration and attitude strength: The new meta-cognitive perspective. *Social and Personality Psychology Compass, 8,* 17–29.

Briñol, P., Rucker, D. D., & Petty, R. E. (2015). Naïve theories about persuasion: Implications for information processing and consumer attitude change. *International Journal of Advertising: The Quarterly Review of Marketing Communications, 34,* 85–106.

Burgoon, M., Dillard, J. P., & Doran, N. E. (1983). Friendly or unfriendly persuasion: The effects of violations of expectations by males and females. *Human Communication Research, 10,* 283–294.

Carpenter, C. J. (2015). A meta-analysis of the ELM's argument quality × processing type predictions. *Human Communication Research, 41,* 501–534.

Crano, W. D. (1983). Assumed consensus of attitudes: The effect of vested interest. *Personality and Social Psychology Bulletin, 9,* 597–608.

Crano, W. D. (1995). Attitude strength and vested interest. In R. E. Petty & J. A. Krosnick (Eds.), *Attitude strength: Antecedents and consequences. The Ohio State University series in attitudes and persuasion* (Vol. 4, pp. 131–157). Hillsdale, NJ: Erlbaum.

Crano, W. D. (1997). Vested interest, symbolic politics, and attitude-behavior consistency. *Journal of Personality and Social Psychology, 72,* 485–491.

Crano, W. D. (2000). Milestones in the psychological analysis of social influence. *Group Dynamics: Theory, Research, and Practice, 4,* 68–80.

Crano, W. D. (2001). Directed social influence. In J. P. Forgas, K. D. Williams, & L. Wheeler (Eds.), *The social mind: Cognitive and motivational perspectives on social behaviour* (pp. 389–405). New York: Cambridge University Press.

Crano, W. D. (2010). Applying established theories of persuasion to problems that matter: On becoming susceptible to our own knowledge. In J. P. Forgas, J. Cooper, & W. D. Crano (Eds.), *The psychology of attitudes and attitude change.* New York, NY: Psychology Press.

Crano, W. D., Alvaro, E. M., Tan, C. N., & Siegel, J. T. (2017). Social mediation of persuasive media in adolescent substance prevention. *Psychology of Addictive Behaviors, 31,* 479–487.

Crano, W. D., Gilbert, C., Alvaro, E. M., & Siegel, J. (2008). Enhancing prediction of inhalant abuse risk in samples of early adolescents: A secondary analysis. *Addictive Behaviors, 33,* 895–905.

Crano, W. D., Gorenflo, D., & Shackelford, S. (1988). Overjustification, assumed consensus, and attitude change: Further investigation of the incentive-aroused ambivalence hypothesis. *Journal of Personality and Social Psychology, 55,* 12–22.

Crano, W. D., & Lyrintzis, E. (2015). Structure and change of complex political attitudes. In J. P. Forgas, K. Fiedler, & W. D. Crano (Eds.), *Social psychology and politics* (pp. 21–39). New York, NY: Psychology Press.

Crano, W. D., & Prislin, R. (1995). Components of vested interest and attitude-behavior consistency. *Basic and Applied Social Psychology, 17*, 1–21.

Crano, W. D., & Prislin, R. (2006). Attitudes and persuasion. *Annual Review of Psychology, 57*, 345–374.

Crano, W. D., Siegel, J. T., & Alvaro, E. M. (2012). The Siren's call: Mass media and drug prevention. In J. P. Dillard & L. Shen (Eds.), *The Sage handbook of persuasion: Developments in theory and practice* (2nd ed., pp. 296–313). Los Angeles, CA: Sage.

Crano, W. D., Siegel, J. T., Alvaro, E. M., & Patel, N. M. (2007). Overcoming adolescents' resistance to anti-inhalant messages. *Psychology of Addictive Behaviors, 21*, 516–524.

Crano, W. D., & Sivacek, J. (1984). The influence of incentive-aroused ambivalence on overjustification effects in attitude change. *Journal of Experimental Social Psychology, 20*, 137–158.

De Dominicis, S., Crano, W. D., Ganucci Cancellieri, U., Mosco, B., Bonnes, M., Hohman, Z., & Bonaiuto, M. (2014). Vested interest and environmental risk communication: Improving willingness to cope with impending disasters. *Journal of Applied Social Psychology, 44*, 364–374.

Deci, E. L., & Ryan, R. M. (2002). *Handbook of self-determination research*. Rochester, NY: University of Rochester Press.

Deci, E. L., & Ryan, R. M. (2010). *Self-determination*. New York, NY: John Wiley & Sons.

Derzon, J. H., & Lipsey, M. W. (2002). A meta-analysis of the effectiveness of mass-communication for changing substance-use knowledge, attitudes, and behavior. In W. D. Crano & M. Burgoon (Eds.), *Mass media and drug prevention: Classic and contemporary theories and research* (pp. 231–258). Mahwah, NJ: Erlbaum.

DiClemente, C. C., & Prochaska, J. O. (1982). Self-change and therapy change of smoking behavior: A comparison of processes of change in cessation and maintenance. *Addictive Behaviors, 7*, 133–142.

Donaldson, C., Siegel, J. T., & Crano, W. D. (2016). Predicting and preventing prescription stimulant misuse: Attitudes, intentions, and vested interest theory. *Addictive Behaviors, 53*, 101–107.

Donaldson, S. I. (2002). High-potential mediators of drug-abuse prevention program effects. In W. D. Crano & M. Burgoon (Eds.), *Mass media and drug prevention: Classic and contemporary theories and research* (pp. 215–230). Mahwah, NJ: Erlbaum.

European Monitoring Center for Drugs and Drug Addiction. (n.d.). *Perspectives on drugs: Mass media campaigns for the prevention of drug use in young people*. Retrieved July 4, 2016, from http://www.emcdda.europa.eu/attachements.cfm/att_212357_EN_EMCDDA_POD_2013_Mass%20media%20campaigns.pdf.

Fabrigar, L. R., Petty, R. E., Smith, S. M., & Crites, S. L., Jr. (2006). Understanding knowledge effects on attitude-behavior consistency: The role of relevance, complexity, and amount of knowledge. *Journal of Personality and Social Psychology, 90*, 556–577.

Fabrigar, L. R., Wegener, D. T., & MacDonald, T. K. (2010). Distinguishing between prediction and influence: Multiple processes underlying attitude-behavior consistency. In: C. R. Agnew, D. E. Carlston, W. G. Graziano, J. R. Kelly, (Eds.), *Then a Miracle Occurs: Focusing on Behavior in Social Psychological Theory and Research* (pp. 162–185). New York, NY: Oxford University Press.

Festinger, L. (1957). *A theory of cognitive dissonance*. Stanford, CA: Stanford University Press.

Gilbert, D. T. (1991). How mental systems believe. *American Psychologist, 46*, 107–119.

Grice, H. P. (1975). Logic and conversation. In P. Cole, & J. I. Morgan, (Eds.), *Syntax and Semantics, 3: Speech Acts* (pp. 41–58). New York, NY: Academic Press.

Grice, H. P. (1978). Further notes on logic and conversation. In J. E. Adler & L. J. Rips, (Eds.), *Reasoning: Studies of human inference and its foundations* (pp. 765–773). New York, NY: Cambridge University Press.

Groenendyk, E. W., & Valentino, N. A. (2002). Of dark clouds and silver linings: Exposure to issue over issue candidate advertising on persuasion, information retention, and issue salience. *Communication Research, 29*, 295–319.

Gruder, C. L., Cook, T. D., Hennigan, K. M., Flay, B. R., Alessis, C., & Halamaj, J. (1978). Empirical tests of the absolute sleeper effect predicted from the discounting cue hypothesis. *Journal of Personality and Social Psychology, 36*, 1061–1074.

Halpern-Felsher, B. L., Biehl, M. A., Kropp, R. Y., & Rubinstein, M. L. (2004). Perceived risks and benefits of smoking: Differences among adolescents with different expectancies and intentions. *Preventive Medicine, 39*, 559–567.

Head, K. J., Noar, S. M., Iannarino, N. T., & Harrington, N. G. (2013). Efficacy of text messaging-based interventions for health promotion: A meta-analysis. *Social Science & Medicine, 97*, 41.

Hornik, R., Jacobsohn, L., Orwin, R., Piesse, A., & Kalton, G. (2008). Effects of the National Youth Anti-Drug Media Campaign on Youth. *American Journal of Public Health, 98*, 2229–2236.

Hovland, C. I., Janis, I. L., & Kelley, H. H. (1953). *Communication and persuasion*. New Haven, CT: Yale University Press.

Johnson, I. M., Siegel, J. T., & Crano, W. D. (2014). Expanding the reach of vested interest in predicting attitude-consistent behavior. *Social Influence, 9*, 20–36.

Katz, E. (1994). Foreword, in G. Weimann, *The influentials: People who influence people* (p. ix). Albany, NY: State University of New York Press.

Koeske, G., & Crano, W. D. (1968). The effect of congruous and incongruous source-statement combinations on the judged credibility of a communication. *Journal of Experimental Social Psychology, 4*, 384–399.

Lasswell, H. D. (1948). The structure and function of communication in society. In L. Bryson (Ed.), *The communication of ideas: A series of addresses* (pp. 37–51). New York, NY: Institute for Religious and Social Studies.

Lasswell, H. D. (1951). *The political writings of Harold Lasswell. Psychopathology and politics. Politics: Who says what, how. Democratic character.* New York, NY: Free Press.

Lasswell, H. D., & Leites, N. (1949). *Language of politics; studies in quantitative semantics.* New York: G.W. Stewart.

Lazarsfeld, P. F., Berelson, B., & Gaudet, H. (1944). *The people's choice.* Oxford, England: Duell, Sloan & Pearce.

Lehman, B., & Crano, W. D. (2002). The pervasive effects of vested interest on attitude-criterion consistency in political judgment. *Journal of Experimental Social Psychology, 38*, 101–112.

Lilienfeld, S. O., & Arkowitz, H. (2014). Why "Just say no" doesn't work. *Scientific American.* Retrieved from http://www.scientificamerican.com/article/why-just-say-no-doesnt-work/

Lustria, M. L. A., Noar, S. M., Cortese, J., Van Stee, S. K., Glueckauf, R. L., & Lee, J. (2013). A meta-analysis of web-delivered tailored health behavior change interventions. *Journal of Health Communication, 18*, 1039–1069.

Maddux, J. E., & Rogers, R. W. (1983). Protection motivation and self-efficacy: A revised theory of fear appeals and attitude change. *Journal of Experimental Social Psychology, 19*, 469–479.

Martens, M., Page, J., Mowry, E., Damann, K., Taylor, K., & Cimini, M. (2006). Differences between actual and perceived student norms: An examination of alcohol use, drug use, and sexual behavior. *Journal of American College Health, 54*, 295–300.

McGuire, W. J. (1985). Attitudes and attitude change. In G. Lindzey & E. Aronson (Eds.), *Handbook of social psychology* (Volume II: Special fields and applications) (3rd ed.). New York, NY: Random House.

McLuhan, M. (1964). *Understanding media: The extensions of man.* New York, NY: Mentor.

Merton, R. K. (1991). *Introduction to sociology.* New York, NY: Harcourt Brace Jovonovich.

Merton, R. K. (1994). A life of learning. C.S. Haskins Lecture, American Council of Learned Societies. Retrieved July 11, 2016, from http://www.csudh.edu/dearhabermas/merton01.htm

Mills, C. W. (1959). *The sociological imagination.* Oxford, GB: Oxford University Press.

Noar, S. M., Benac, C. N., & Harris, M. S. (2007). Does tailoring matter? Meta-analytic review of tailored print health behavior change interventions. *Psychological Bulletin, 133*, 673–693.

Ophir, Y., Brennan, E., Maloney, E., & Cappella, J. N. (2017). The effects of graphic warning labels' vividness on message engagement and intentions to quit smoking. *Communication Research.* https://doi.org/10.1177/0093650217700226

Parsons, T. (1937/1968). *The structure of social actions.* Glencoe, IL: Free Press.

Perkins, H. W., & Berkowitz, A. D. (1986). Perceiving the community norms of alcohol use among students: Some research implications for campus alcohol education programming. *International Journal of the Addictions, 21*, 961–976.

Petty, R. E., & Cacioppo, J. T. (1986). *Communication and persuasion.* New York, NY: Springer.

Petty, R. E., Wegener, D. T., & Fabrigar, L. T. (1999). The elaboration likelihood model: Current status and controversies. *Annual Review of Psychology, 48*, 609–647.

Prislin, R. (1988). Attitude-behaviour relationship: Attitude salience and implications of behaviour. *Psychologische Beitrage, 30*, 129–138.

Rosenstock, I. M. (1974). Historical origins of the health belief model. *Health Education & Behavior, 2*, 328–335.

Siegel, J. T., Alvaro, E., Lac, A., Crano, W. D., & Alexander, S. (2008). Intentions of becoming a living organ donor among Hispanics: A theoretical approach exploring differences between living and non-living organ donation. *Journal of Health Communication, 13*, 80–99.

Siegel, J. T., Alvaro, E. M., Crano, W. D., Skendarian, J., Lac, A., & Patel, N. (2008). Influencing inhalant intentions by changing socio-personal expectations. *Prevention Science, 9*, 153–165.

Siegel, J. T., & Burgoon, J. K. (2002). Expectancy theory approaches to prevention: Violating adolescent expectations to increase the effectiveness of public service announcements. In W. D. Crano & M. Burgoon (Eds.), *Mass media and drug prevention: Classic and contemporary theories and research* (pp. 163–186). Mahwah, NJ: Erlbaum.

Smith, C. T., & De Houwer, J. (2014). The impact of persuasive messages on IAT performance is moderated by source attractiveness and likeability. *Social Psychology, 45*, 437–448.

Smith, C. T., De Houwer, J., & Nosek, B. A. (2013). Consider the source: Persuasion of implicit evaluations is moderated by source credibility. *Personality and Social Psychology Bulletin, 39*, 193–205.

Snyder, L. B., & Hamilton, M. A. (2002). A meta-analysis of U.S. health campaign effects on behavior: Emphasize enforcement, exposure, and new information, and beware the secular trend. In R. C. Hornik (Ed.), *Public health communication: Evidence for behavior change* (pp. 357–383). Mahwah, NJ: Erlbaum.

Tormala, Z. L., & Petty, R. E. (2004). Resisting persuasion and attitude certainty: A meta-cognitive analysis. In E. S. Knowles & J. A. Linn (Eds.), *Resistance and persuasion* (pp. 65–82). Mahwah, NJ: Erlbaum.

United Nations Office on Drugs and Crime. (2015). *International standards on drug use prevention.* Retrieved July 8, 2016, from www.unodc.org/unodc/en/prevention/prevention-standards.html

Wyer, R. S., & Shrum, L. J. (2015). The role of comprehension processes in communication and persuasion. *Media Psychology, 18*, 163–195.

Ziegler, R., & Diehl, M. (2003). Is politician A or politician B more persuasive? Recipients' source preference and the direction of biased message processing. *European Journal of Social Psychology, 33*(5), 623–637.

Use of Media and Social Media in the Prevention of Substance Use

20

David B. Buller, Barbara J. Walkosz, and W. Gill Woodall

Introduction

Despite rapid changes over the past three decades, mass media are one of the most potentially influential communication channels in modern societies. Nearly all adults and most children, even from an early age (Rideout, 2013), are connected in some way to mass media and media consumption is increasing. Nielsen estimated in 2014 that the average American household spent nearly 60 h a week consuming media ("The U.S. Digital Consumer Report," 2014). Messages in the media also reach individuals indirectly through interpersonal communication with acquaintances, friends, and family (sometimes information is received both directly and indirectly). Television remains the single most consumed form of media for adults ("The Total Audience Report: Q1 2016," 2016; "The U.S. Digital Consumer Report," 2014), the youngest children aged 0–8 (58% watched daily) and preadolescents aged 8–12 (62% watched daily), and is second only to listening to music among adolescents aged 13–17 (58% watched daily) (GfK Inc., 2015; Rideout, 2013). Radio is consumed by more Americans than any other single medium and is the second largest portion of their daily media mix ("The Total Audience Report: Q1 2016," 2016). Print media, while experiencing declines in the past two decades, has been revitalized by the Internet and advent of online news websites.

Several changes have occurred in the past 20 years that have revolutionized the media, derived from the advent of personal computers and digital networking technology. These changes have further expanded media's reach, broadened individuals' choice of content, shifted time and location of consumption ("The U.S. Digital Consumer Report," 2014), and provided the ability for individuals to contribute to the creation and delivery of content. The first change was the birth of the Internet in 1991 (Bryant, 2011). In the 25 years since that time, the media landscape has been transformed by a wide array of digital formats. By 2014, 87% of American adults used the Internet ("Internet User Demographics," 2014). While use remains lowest among Americans 65 or older, high school graduates, and the least affluent (<$30,000), a majority of all subgroups currently use the Internet.

With the Internet, the second change was the emergence of new media in which content is available on-demand. It includes but is not limited to social media (e.g., Facebook and Twitter), websites, online advertising, mobile apps, and streaming videos. These new media provide additional channels for prevention interventions that have the ability to positively impact public health and connect hard-to-reach populations (Burke-Garcia

D. B. Buller (✉) · B. J. Walkosz · W. G. Woodall
Klein Buendel, Inc., Golden, CO, USA
e-mail: dbuller@kleinbuendel.com;
bwalkosz@kleinbuendel.com; gwoodall@kleinbuendel.com

& Scally, 2014). Social media in particular allows individuals to actively participate in the development and distribution of prevention messages like never before (GfK Inc., 2015). Starting with forums, newsgroups, and blogs, social media are now comprised of a range of online services (e.g., Facebook, Twitter, Instagram, and Pinterest) on which individuals and organizations post, modify, share, and comment upon a variety of digital media content. As of 2015, 65% of American adults were using social networking sites (and most of them used it every day) ("The U.S. Digital Consumer Report," 2014), with use being highest among younger (90% of 18–29 year old adults use social media) and more educated adults, those with higher incomes, and adults living in suburban and urban areas (Perrin, 2015). Adolescents aged 13–17 are the most enthusiastic users of social media, with 71% using Facebook, 52% Instagram, 41% Snapchat, and 33% Twitter in 2015 and girls being more active on social media than boys (Lenhart, 2015). With its rise in popularity, many of the players in the traditional broadcast and print media have come to embrace the new media, producing a convergence that has blurred the lines between traditional and new media content. For instance, most newspapers now publish content both in hard copy newsprint and online. The major broadcast news and entertainment networks stream video content online, as well as distributing it over the air or on cable systems. Online media routinely re-post content from the traditional media. These practices are quickly rendering the distinction between traditional and new media obsolete.

A third change that has revolutionized the media environment is the introduction of mobile computing. Mobile computing has placed media devices connected to the vast international digital networks in the hands of many individuals, so they are nearly always connected to and engaged with the media wherever they may be, often across several platforms simultaneously ("The U.S. Digital Consumer Report," 2014). It is estimated that 92% of Americans owned a cell phone in 2015 and by 2016, 81% owned a smartphone and 58% a tablet computer (by comparison 73% owned desktop or laptop computers) ("Three Technology Revolutions," 2012; "The Total Audience Report: Q1 2016," 2016). Teens (aged 13–17) are the most connected generation. Nearly all teens (92%) go online daily and a quarter are almost constantly online (Lenhart, 2015) (spending 9 h daily using digital media) (GfK Inc., 2015). Mobile devices account for 46% of all screen time by teens. Preadolescents (aged 8–12) also spend considerable time with the media (i.e., 6 h a day) and 41% of their screen time is spent on mobile devices (GfK Inc., 2015). Among the millions of mobile apps for these devices are ones provided by major media corporations to deliver content typically delivered over broadcast media (e.g., video streaming services such as from Netflix, Hulu, and CNN) or on paper (e.g., news websites from established newspapers such as the New York Times and Wall Street Journal and from online news services such as Politico, BuzzFeed, and Huffington Post) and those for the most popular (e.g., Facebook and YouTube) and emerging (e.g., Instagram and Snapchat) social media ("The U.S. Digital Consumer Report," 2014). Streaming video on-demand continues to expand in popularity ("The Total Audience Report: Q1 2016," 2016) and has changed the times and locations where individuals receive televised media content.

In this chapter we consider the role of media in efforts to prevent substance use. Our focus is on evaluations of large media interventions and their influence, rather than smaller-scale studies that have explored narrowly focused issues such as short-term effects of alternative message formats. Given the often incremental and deliberate progress in science, it is not surprising that the published literature on the effectiveness of campaigns to prevent substance use in the convergent new media environment has lagged behind the media revolutions. Much of what we know about the role of media in substance use prevention comes from research that has relied on older media, with only limited research available on the potential influence of the newest online, social and mobile media. Thus, we will raise more questions about the influence of new media than provide conclusive answers and consider some of the challenges for conducting research on effects of large-scale substance use prevention interventions delivered over them. With the expanded role of individuals in the new media environment, we will consider the role of audience activity starting first with concept of audience exposure determined by selective attention, exposure, and retention, processes that have been described for decades in the media effects literature and moving on to discuss user-generated content in the new media.

Media Campaigns for Substance Use Prevention

Nature and Effectiveness of Media Campaigns

Large mass media campaigns have been conducted over the past 15 years aimed at preventing substance use, most often marijuana use, and subjected to careful evaluation primarily among adolescents. In the United States, one of the largest was the National Youth Anti-drug Media Campaign (NYADMC) by the Office of the National Drug Control Policy (ONDCP). Two versions of the campaign were conducted. The first, *My Anti-Drug,* focused on negative consequences of drug use, self-efficacy and normative beliefs about drug use or avoidance, and resistance skills. The second, *Above the Influence,* focused on bolstering resistance skill and autonomy and aspirations of youth as they related to consequences of using or avoiding drugs starting (Hornik & Jacobsohn, 2007; Hornik, Jacobsohn, Orwin, Piesse, & Kalton, 2008; Scheier, Grenard, & Holtz, 2011). The NYADMC campaigns delivered messages over broadcast media, primarily television. However, these campaigns by ONDCP also placed messages in print publications (e.g., magazines), in movie theater advertising, and over the Internet and established partnerships with community and professional groups and appealed to industries (i.e., media, entertainment, and sports) to help distribute the campaign messages (Hornik et al., 2008; Hornik & Jacobsohn, 2007). One similar campaign compared with the NYADMC *Above the Influence,* the *Be Under Your Own Influence* campaign, relied on in-school media and community-based efforts but similarly targeted youth's autonomy and aspirations (Slater, Kelly, Lawrence, Stanley, & Comello, 2011). A few smaller scale campaigns relying on mass media have been evaluated, such as a statewide campaign to prevent use of methamphetamine in Montana (Siebel & Mange, 2009) and a campus campaign to reduce alcohol and drug use in New Mexico (Miller, Toscova, Miller, & Sanchez, 2000). Several of the substance use prevention campaigns created messages based on scientific research on behavior change, communication, and disease prevention such as the Social Cognitive Theory, Theory of Reasoned Action, Self-regulation Theory, Health Belief Model, and the Sensation Seeking Targeting Prevention Approach and some submitted the messages to formative testing prior to launch (Miller et al., 2000; Palmgreen, Donohew, Lorch, Hoyle, & Stephenson, 2001; Scheier et al., 2011; Werb et al., 2011).

The mass media campaigns have been evaluated by two methods, using non-randomized observational designs assessing pre-post change before and after campaign implementation and randomized controlled trials comparing groups of teens who were exposed or not exposed to the campaign (Allara, Ferri, Bo, Gasparrini, & Faggiano, 2015; Werb et al., 2011). Generally speaking, the evaluations of these mass media campaigns have not found that they were broadly effective at altering drug use. Two recent meta-analyses found evidence that mass media campaigns have succeeded in reducing marijuana use only in a few studies and may have had the unintended impact of increasing marijuana use in other studies (Allara et al., 2015; Werb et al., 2011). One of the meta-analyses also showed very little effect of a mass media campaign to reduce the use of methamphetamine but the evaluation methods for this campaign in Montana have been criticized (Erceg-Hurn, 2008). Also, a comparison of methamphetamine use in Montana to use in other states showed no effect of the campaign on use of this drug (Anderson, 2010). Specifically considering the NYADMC campaigns, there was no change in marijuana use between 2000 and 2004 during the My Anti-drug campaign (Hornik et al., 2008; Hornik & Jacobsohn, 2007). Moreover, the campaign may have produced positive beliefs about marijuana use, leading to the speculation that it had a boomerang effect (Hornik et al., 2008; Hornik & Jacobsohn, 2007). However, the *Above the Influence* campaign showed favorable effects on adolescents in grades 8–9 in a school-based evaluation, while the effects of the mass media campaign may have overwhelmed any effects of the in-school and community intervention that also targeted messages to adolescents' autonomy and aspirations (both cognitions mediated the impact of the *Above the Influence* campaign) (Slater et al., 2011). An earlier evaluation of the in-school and community intervention was successful during the My Anti-drug mass media campaign, so it appears that the similarity in messaging in the mass media campaign, not the overall campaign per se, swamped the influence of the former (Slater et al., 2006). An evaluation of a campus campaign using print media found only small reductions in alcohol and drug use (Miller et al., 2000).

It is possible that the mass media campaigns have been effective with only certain subgroups of the population (Werb et al., 2011). One analysis suggested that the *Above the Influence* campaign was associated with lower marijuana use by girls in the eighth grade but not boys in eighth grade or adolescents in grades 10 or 12 (Carpenter & Pechmann, 2011). An evaluation of a mass media campaign to prevent methamphetamine use also found a reduction in past-year use among younger (12–17 years old) rather than older (18–24 years old) youth (Allara et al., 2015). Another analysis suggested that the campaign was effective with high sensation seeking adolescents (Palmgreen, Lorch, Stephenson, Hoyle, & Donohew, 2007). High sensation seeking has been associated with greater risk taking and more drug use (Stephenson, 2003), so the NYDAMC campaign targeted them with specific messaging, and use of messages with high sensation value in the campaign appeared to explain the expected positive effect on high sensation seekers (Palmgreen et al., 2007).

Further, the campaign did not reduce marijuana use in low sensation seekers. This replicated an earlier study that supported targeting television campaign messages to high sensation seekers (Palmgreen et al., 2001).

Several explanations have been offered for the inconsistent or lack of effects of mass media campaigns. One possibility is that the theories used to design the campaigns do not take into account the environmental, socio-demographic, and other factors, as well as cognitions and intentions that were targeted by that campaign, that influence the initiation of substance use (Werb et al., 2011). It may be that youth are already exposed to large numbers of messages from the media and other sources (e.g., school-based substance use education; advice from family and friends) arguing that they avoid substance use so the campaign messages lacked novelty (Hornik et al., 2008; Hornik & Jacobsohn, 2007). Communication from others also may mediate the influence of campaigns, potentially in unfavorable ways that produce pro-drug attitudes (David, Cappella, & Fishbein, 2006). It is also possible that messages advocating not to use psychoactive substances such as marijuana produced reactance in teens and holding pro-marijuana attitudes helped them re-establish their freedom of choice (Hornik et al., 2008). Increasing the number of messages related to substance use in the media may also have the unintended effect of creating the perception that many people use these substances and produced pressure to conform to the actions of peers (Hornik et al., 2008; Hornik & Jacobsohn, 2007). Media campaigns may be more effective when they reach teens before they make decisions about whether to use alcohol, tobacco, or other substances, which would explain why some campaigns seemed to have better effects on younger rather than older individuals (Allara et al., 2015; Carpenter & Pechmann, 2011). The emotional climate of puberty may make girls especially receptive to messages that advocate avoidance of substance use by preserving autonomy and supporting their aspirations for the future (Carpenter & Pechmann, 2011). Also, reductions in a campaign budget that result in lower exposure to campaigns could lower effectiveness (Carpenter & Pechmann, 2011).

Finally, some methodological weaknesses of the evaluations have been noted. These include biases in self-reports of marijuana and other substance use, reverse-causality bias recall measures of exposure, where those more interested in substance use at the outset of a campaign led to greater attention to anti-substance use messages, and lack of an untreated control group (Magura, 2012).

Role of Campaign Exposure

It is well established in decades of media effects research that audience activity determines media influence (Hawkins & Pingree, 1986; Kim & Rubin, 1997; Woodall, 1986). Audience members are selective in their choice of media and content within media (Zillman & Bryant, 1985). Selective exposure to media arises because people have limited capacity to process messages and in today's media environment, choices of media and media content are essentially endless, with messages competing across traditional broadcast and print media, online media, social media, and mobile media. Attention is driven by volitional processes (needs and motivations) and automatic cognitive orienting systems (Lang, 2000), as explained in the Cognitive Mediation Model (Beaudoin & Thorson, 2004; Eveland, 2001). Common motivations are interest, surveillance, and a desire to obtain information for future discussions with others. Exposure provokes attention and elaboration or message involvement and it is these information processing attributes that determine message effectiveness. However, users are selective in their attention to content within media and common behaviors such as scanning rather than carefully reading content can interfere with learning (Eveland & Dunwoody, 2002). Moreover, selective exposure means that people also can choose to avoid messages that do not interest them (Kim & Rubin, 1997). Finally, it is likely that memory for messages is short lived, meaning the effect of messages declines over time, which has been seen in media campaigns for both preventing drug and tobacco use (Carpenter & Pechmann, 2011; Farrelly, Davis, Haviland, Messeri, & Healton, 2005).

Large mass media campaigns have been conducted in ways to try to achieve sufficient exposure to affect the target audiences. This was accomplished often with paid placement of campaign messages in broadcast media with a certain level of frequency that should have achieved exposure among the target population. For example the NYADMC's *My Anti-drug* campaign intended to achieve an exposure level at least 2.5 advertisements per week (Hornik et al., 2008; Hornik & Jacobsohn, 2007). Common media metrics of exposure, i.e., gross (or total) rating points of each message (or total rating points) based on advertising buys, as well as recall of messages and logos in surveys of youth, have been used to assess this exposure (Palmgreen et al., 2007). Generally, the national campaigns succeeded in achieving relatively high levels of exposure among the intended audiences. For example, the *Above the Influence* version of the NYADMC exposed teens to approximately 1360 total rating points of advertising in 2006–2008, which translated into reaching all teens with approximately 13.6 messages per month (Carpenter & Pechmann, 2011). An evaluation of the *My Anti-drug* campaign in the NYADMC revealed the 94% of teens aged 9–18 who were nonusers of marijuana at baseline reported exposure to an anti-drug message (Hornik et al., 2008; Hornik & Jacobsohn, 2007). Likewise, the NYADMC *Above the Influence* campaign achieved recall of campaign messages among two-thirds of a sample of 14–16 year olds in mall intercept surveys and memory for the campaign logos among more than half of respondents (73% had definitely seen the campaign in a school-based evaluation) (Scheier et al., 2011; Slater et al., 2011). A time-series analysis found that reported exposure was associated with greater messages placed in the mass media, as indicated by increases in radio and television gross rating points (Palmgreen et al., 2007). Exposure to substance use campaign messages has been associated with a few social factors, including being a female (Scheier et al., 2011), an older teen (Scheier et al., 2011), and White or African American (compared to Hispanics) in some instances (Scheier et al., 2011), but some high exposure campaigns had few gender and age differences (Carpenter & Pechmann, 2011).

Exposure in some studies appeared to influence campaign effectiveness, but not in all studies. In one study, awareness of the *Above the Influence* campaign was associated with lower marijuana use by teens 14–16, mediated through anti-drug beliefs (Scheier et al., 2011) but in an evaluation of the earlier *My Anti-drug* version of the campaign exposure was not related to anti-drug cognitions (Hornik et al., 2008). Further, a time-series analysis assessing high and low sensation seekers also failed to show any relationship between message exposure and substance use (Palmgreen et al., 2007).

Given the fundamental nature of audience activity, it is also not surprising that selective exposure has been demonstrated in new media such as the Internet and social media. Low use of health websites appears common when implemented in community settings and often some immediate need, most commonly a real or potential health problem, seems to motivate this Internet use. Some topics or message formats in the media may be automatically attention getting. For example, website ads containing attributes such as animation and novelty may elicit an involuntary orienting response and improve their effects (Diao & Sundar, 2004; Lang, Borse, Wise, & David, 2002). Leads for online news stories that highlight conflict and agony produced more selective exposure than other frames, perhaps because people inherently orient to danger-conveying signals or empathic sensitivities (Zillman, Chen, Knobloch, & Callison, 2004). Social media messages that contain imagery may achieve more user engagement overall (both liking and sharing) while positive information promotes sharing and negative affect and crowdsourcing increases commenting (Rus & Cameron, 2016). We previously showed that messages highlighting the presence of new content on a website described as being created especially for the users increased logins (Woodall et al., 2007), which may be evidence that personalizing messages or creating messages with which individuals can identify increases attention to them (Cohen, 2001; Kreuter et al., 2007; McQueen, Kreuter, Kalesan, & Alcaraz, 2011).

Online and social media have added a new dimension to audience activity, namely the ability to contribute content to these media, often referred to as user-generated content. Also, these media promote interactivity both with the content and among other users. This interactivity has the potential to increase attention and involvement in the media content. Also, social aspects of social media may heighten the sense of individuation. Thus, new media format may produce a much more dynamic and engaging audience experience and elevate the relevance of media messages, and thus alter what it means to be exposed to substance use prevention campaigns.

New Media and Substance Use

The use of the Internet for substance use prevention continues to significantly increase with the emergence of new media platforms. These approaches include but are not limited to web- and social media-based interventions, mobile apps, and the dissemination of user-generated content on platforms such as *You Tube* and blogs. However, new media may play an undesirable role that runs counter to prevention. A body of evolving research suggests that new media may promote substance use as evidenced by the links between posted behaviors on social networking sites (Hanson, Cannon, Burton, & Giraud-Carrier, 2013) and substance use, through online industry marketing (e.g., online advertising) that mimics the influential nature of offline marketing, and the ongoing analysis of prevalence data (White et al., 2010) on sites that respectively promote prevention of substance use.

Web-Based Interventions

Web-based interventions were among the first to employ the Internet to promote behavior change, including substance use prevention. The benefits of these early interventions were to offer solutions to barriers associated with prevention campaigns such as access to special populations, stigma associated with face-to-face services, cost, anonymity, and real-time availability (Rooke, Copeland, Norberg, Hine, & McCambridge, 2013; Tait, Spijkerman, & Riper, 2013). However, while some success has been achieved with problematic alcohol use (Rooke et al., 2013) and tobacco cessation (Evans, 2016), web-based programs for substance use prevention remain at the preliminary stages of evaluation (Tait et al., 2013). For example, the Substance Abuse and Mental Health Services Administration (SAMHSA) has supported a number of web-based media campaigns for substance use prevention aimed at a range of targeted audiences (e.g., parents and teens). Only a few of these efforts have been systematically evaluated (Evans, 2016), but they do show promise (Newton, Han, Stewart, Ryan, & Williamson, 2011). A meta-analysis that examined the use of Internet and computer-based programs to reduce cannabis use identified a small but significant overall effect size ($g = 0.16$) with a number-needed-to-treat (NNT) of 11. Even though the effect size was smaller than that found for in-person interventions, the potential reach of Internet interventions could have significant public health impact. In an RCT designed for individuals who wanted to reduce their cannabis use, it was found that when compared to a website education-only program, a web-based intervention based on face-to-face treatment protocols reduced cannabis use frequency with a 43% reduction in smoking days per month, a finding similar to that found in the face-to-face interventions. Other outcomes, such as quantity of cannabis use, lower levels of cannabis dependence, and fewer symptoms of cannabis use, were partially supported (Rooke et al., 2013). Another intervention that tested a web-based counseling program (*Can Reduce*) with and without chat counseling with problematic/heavy users was effective (Schaub et al., 2013). In a family-focused program, Internet-delivered substance use prevention content for early adolescent Asian-American girls focused on improving mother-daughter communication and increasing maternal monitoring was delivered exclusively online, which was effective in lowering risk factors for substance use, enhancing individual skills and familial protective factors, and reducing substance uptake (Fang & Schinke, 2013).

Tobacco cessation and alcohol prevention programs delivered via the Internet have also met with some success. Quitlines, phone-based services that provided evidence-based counseling, have evolved to now include self-directed web-based counseling programs (45 states) with counseling (64%) (Rudie, 2016). Among ten free state Quitlines, the participants who selected the web-only versus a phone/web cessation program were younger, healthier smokers of higher socio-economic status who interacted more intensely with services in a single session but were less likely to re-engage or access NRT benefits (Nash, Vickerman, Kellogg, & Zbikowski, 2015). Online alcohol interventions have confirmed the acceptability of online screening and intervention providing a forum that far surpasses the reach of face-to-face interventions (Cloud & Peacock, 2001; Cunningham, Humphreys, & Koski-Jännes, 2000). A systematic review of online alcohol interventions in randomized controlled trials suggests that Internet interventions offer a feasible alternative for individuals with alcohol-related problems, especially for women and younger individuals who generally do not access traditional health services (White et al., 2010). The studies under review included those that evaluated the impact of brief personalized feedback and that investigated an online multi-module information/education program. The analysis concluded that regardless of program type the online interventions "appeared to bring about small but meaningful differential reactions in 10-gram alcohol units consumed, blood alcohol concentration levels, and a range of other alcohol-related measures." The potential for cost-effective delivery of these interventions has been somewhat effective while at the same time requiring more research with diverse populations as well as needing to ensure the transfer of the effective components of face-to-face interventions to technology platforms (White et al., 2010).

Social Media

Social media interventions have the potential to prevent substance use because they can easily disseminate information (Korda & Itani, 2011; Portnoy, Scott-Sheldon, Johnson, & Carey, 2008) and are now essential channels for engaging large populations, especially populations like young adults. Social media sites share common characteristics that allow each user to create accounts, connect to other users or groups, and provide the ability to comment and post photographs, videos, and other content (Kietzmann, Hermkens, McCarthy, & Silvestre, 2011), making the design of interventions across platforms feasible.

The selection of social media platforms for substance use programs can vary depending on the intent of the campaign as each type of social media has different suitability for types of interactions. For example, Facebook may be more suited to intermittent posts about health facts and engage more users; Twitter may be more suited to daily external links and news items (Moreno & Whitehill, 2014); and Pinterest and Instagram are suited for photos and visual information. However, it should be noted that the evolution of these different capacities and features across all of these social media sites and applications is ongoing, and that the particular strength in providing messages of different types to different audiences will change over time. Multiple social media platforms can be employed in a campaign, each with its own purpose, but regardless of the platform, social media have transformed audiences into active participants in public communication, as they routinely create and share personal stories and information. The information shared on social media from (perceived) knowledgeable peers can have a powerful impact (Walther, Pingree, Hawkins, & Buller, 2005; Walther, Tong, DeAndrea, Carr, & Van Der Heide, 2011). Medical and other practitioners, while afforded a modicum of credibility, are at times only on par with social media "friends" and sometimes are rated below them (Wang, Walther, Pingree, & Hawkins, 2008). While the accuracy of user-generated content is a concern, social media's transparency can allow practitioners to identify misinformation and correct it" (Chou, Prestin, Lyons, & Wen, 2013).

Unfortunately, the benefit of user-generated content and interactivity for health interventions at this time remains understudied (Chou et al., 2013), although by looking at substance use broadly, including alcohol and tobacco, the potential of social media in substance use prevention seems evident. Substance use prevention programs have primarily been implemented on Facebook. In a 2-year study that explored the use of a social networking site to change behavior, Facebook and text messages were utilized to reduce the use of alcohol by college students at festive events. The Facebook page, "Auvernight," employed mostly videos along with posters and slogans from other alcohol prevention campaigns and reminded participants of ways to reduce excessive alcohol consumption. The intervention showed a reduction in the association of alcohol and festive events among college students along with a declared reduction in alcohol consumption while partying (Flaudias et al., 2015) and supported the decision to use social networking to influence behavior.

The assessment of engagement and participation (the expanded nature of exposure in social media) is critical to inform our understanding of how to leverage these new media to facilitate behavior change. For example, the Smokefree Women Facebook page, an open access smoking cessation community, with over 27,000 likes, found that in a 13-month period, there were 875 posts and 4088 comments from approximately 4243 participants and 1088 comments from the moderator. Network visualization that assessed connections between participants and the role of the moderator found that participants interacted with each other in small hubs, with and without the moderator, suggesting that the network was robust to random attack (loss of a participant without regard to their position in the network) but sensitive to selective attack (loss of a specific member who are hubs of the network). However, the moderator emerged as a key to the hub and the network was severely affected by loss of the moderator. It was also clear that participant interaction was driven by posts on Facebook. Super participants or highly connected individuals served as centers of hubs and help to maintain person-to-person interaction (Albert, Jeong, & Barabási, 2000). Highly engaged participants offered support and advice while less engaged participants announced their status and sought cessation strategies. Likewise, more central and connected people appeared to be further along in their journey towards smoke-free status and less central users were at the beginning of their smoke-free journey (Cole-Lewis et al., 2016). Facebook has also been used as one component of a multimedia tobacco prevention campaign. The *Crush the Crave* (CTC) campaign for tobacco cessation included a Facebook page as part of their overall intervention, with over 100 posts promoting the campaign and smoking cessation. Users posted nearly 300 replies to the program posts, but most frequently to post with smoking cessation information; user engagement was most commonly associated with images. These findings suggest that social networking sites should be considered in substance use prevention campaigns to engage participants and improve exposure to campaign messages.

Challenges for Using Social Media in Substance Use Campaigns

The emergence of new media holds promise for future campaigns but also comes with a number of challenges and considerations. First, theories of social media impact are not well developed. To date, most of the research that has been conducted on social media and substance use has been descriptive and observational in nature. Moreno and colleagues have developed a Facebook Influence Model that identified key domains that explain the influence of Facebook on older adolescent users (Moreno, Kota, Schoohs, & Whitehill, 2013). The domains include (a) connection, related to peer influence, (b) comparison, aligned with social norms and modeling behavior, (c) identification that suggests you interact with the media based on who you are at that time and on who you want to be, and (d) the immersive Facebook experience that purports that Facebook has the ability to alter the experience of an individual on any given day, including moods and decisions. Theories of behavior change commonly used in prevention efforts address these domains and could be used to employ social media effectively in substance use campaigns. For example, Diffusion of Innovations Theory (DIT) and social network principles (Rogers, 2003) purport that (a) the elevated audience involvement in social media may increase dissemination and impact and (b) influence involves both delivering carefully crafted content by external change agents (e.g., experts) and spreading it among community members, especially by opinion leaders (i.e., knowledgeable others who have informal peer influence). Opinion leaders, or super participants (Cole-Lewis et al., 2016), can emerge on social media and stimulate collective action as people depend on them for information (Rogers, 2003), especially on issues that carry risk and uncertainty (Lenz, 1984; Pescosolido, 1992; Reagan & Collins, 1987). Content shared in social media can breed collective action as participants interpret and respond to it through a process of social comparison/identity (Erickson, 1988; Rogers, 2003; Turner, 1982; Turner & Killian, 1992). Users routinely compare themselves with social network members (Suls & Miller, 1977) and conform to avoid uncertainty (Festinger, 1954). They perceive themselves in abstract social categories and roles (e.g., female, friend, parent, healthy person) and create their collective identity in the group, stabilizing behavior changes (Turner, 1982; Turner & Killian, 1992). Likewise, Transportation Theory (TT) and research on persuasive narratives may explain that user-generated content in social media, such as comments or testimonials that often can contain personal stories, can be more powerful than conventional persuasive strategies (Reinhart & Feeley, 2007). TT (Green & Brock, 2000, 2002) holds that people are transported into narratives and often change their beliefs based on information, claims, or events depicted (Green, 2006) that conform to existing cognitive schemas (i.e., framework/concept that helps organize/interpret information) (Petraglia, 2007) that make narratives seem real. Persons identify with characters in a story, which increases social influence (Cohen, 2001; Slater, Buller, Waters, Archibeque, & LeBlanc, 2003). Narratives can shift normative beliefs about risks, including marijuana use (Bellis, Hughes, Dillon, Copeland, & Gates, 2007; Bellis, Hughes, & Lowey, 2002; Bellis, Hughes, Thomson, & Bennett, 2004; Benotsch et al., 2007; Eiser & Ford, 1995; Hughes et al., 2008; Ragsdale, Difranceisco, & Pinkerton, 2006; Tutenges & Hesse, 2008).

A second challenge is the development of effective methodologies to measure and assess the effects of emerging media (Burke-Garcia & Scally, 2014). Reporting standards that define intervention and participant characteristics need to be developed so that interventions can be compared and approaches that are efficacious and have high success can be determined (Pagoto et al., 2016). Also, research is needed to determine not only how to measure new concepts like engagement (hitting a "like" button, making a comment, or posting original content) but also to decide what qualifies as meaningful engagement that might result in changes in knowledge, behavior, or other key outcomes (Pagoto et al., 2016). The use of social analytics programs to extract data should also be considered as a means of analysis, especially for interventions with large numbers of participants over long periods of time (Pagoto et al., 2016). And determining how specific new media (e.g., Facebook, Twitter, Pinterest, Instagram, Snapchat) influence behavior may require unique assessment tools.

A third challenge for researchers is to determine how commercial online marketing strategies (e.g., digital ads) influence substance use (e.g., alcohol and marijuana) (Bierut, Krauss, Sowles, & Cavazos-Rehg, 2016) and how social marketing approaches can use similar strategies for prevention. In one case, online ad exposure was associated with confirmed visits to the *Tips* 2012 campaign site (TIPS from Former Smokers) and the results suggest that these ads may also cue audiences to seek other smoking cessation-related websites (Kim et al., 2016). Alcohol companies use a number of marketing strategies on Facebook including asking users to "like" their posts and to post content that displays brand use. Perhaps similar approaches could be used by prevention campaigns.

Fourth, research programs need to understand the use of multiple platforms that can be used for promotion. Media campaigns are now delivered across a variety of broadcast, print, and online media. Contents on Facebook, Twitter, Instagram, and YouTube are tailored for the social media site. This approach requires an understanding of both the audience and the content of unique social media sites. For example, based on recent social media data ("Reach of leading social media and networking sites used by teenagers and young adults in the United States as of February 2016," 2016), an intervention directed to teens may be more effective on a site like Facebook and Instagram than on Twitter or even Vine. Government organizations, such as the Centers for Disease Control and Prevention, have developed communication strategies that recommend the use of multiple sites in order to encourage engagement and ensure maximum exposure.

A fifth challenge is to determine how to best leverage and encourage user-generated media for substance use interventions. With the proliferation of YouTube, blogs, and personal Facebook and Instagram accounts, individuals are increasingly engaged in the creation of content. While studies have been conducted on how displays of risk-related behavior can influence social norms around that behavior, scant research has been conducted on how user-generated content can be used to promote substance use prevention. The development of interventions that encourage storytelling, hold video contests for intervention content, and invite posts about alternatives to substance use (e.g., other sensation seeking behaviors) is needed to identify effective methods that employ user-generated content.

Finally, the interactive nature of emerging media should be explored more fully (Moreno & Whitehill, 2014). While a few studies have encouraged interaction between participants, a greater understanding of how peers and experts communicate in social media is needed. For example, more research is needed on the content of communication about substance use on social networking sites and if any opportunities exist to confront and intervene on displays of substance use (Moreno & Whitehill, 2014). However, privacy settings must be recognized and respected in such instances and confidentially must be protected.

Influence of Internet Content on Substance Use

The monitoring of behavior and discourse on the Internet, especially on social media such as Facebook, Twitter, and YouTube, can inform public health practitioners and campaign planners about emerging substance use trends that may warrant prevention efforts and also suggest strategies to create effective campaigns. Infodemiology is a new field of study that examines the determinants and distribution of information on Internet channels, such as social networking sites (Eysenbach, 2009). This information could be used to develop prevention messages for campaigns. For example, messages that underscore the risk of teen use of marijuana such as addiction, cognitive impairments, and the dangers of driving while intoxicated (Cavazos-Rehg, Krauss, Grucza, & Bierut, 2014) could be employed in campaigns based on substance use information gleaned from social networking sites.

Exposure to information and making connections on social media may be important determinants of how behavior displayed online can provide modeling cues and influence social norms for substance use (Cabrera-Nguyen, Cavazos-Rehg, Krauss, Bierut, & Moreno, 2016). For example, teens using social networking sites were two times more likely to use marijuana, three times more likely to use alcohol, and five more times more likely to use tobacco (Casacolumbia, 2011). In one case, simply seeing a photo of someone using drugs on a social media site was associated with increased marijuana use (Casacolumbia, 2012).

The monitoring of social networks can identify trends among participants. A study of the social circles of those who misuse prescription medications on Twitter found that connections consisted mainly of other Twitter users who also discussed the misuse of prescription medications (Hanson et al., 2013). These connections have the potential to reinforce this negative behavior and normalize the misuse of prescription medications. In another case, the online reaction of drug users to the reformulation of OxyContin that was intended to present obstacles to use by non-oral routes of administration was reviewed (McNaughton et al., 2014). A systematic monitoring of nearly 20,000 posts to message boards suggested that the reformulation had an impact on the online discussions among drug users, resulting in reduced sentiment for the drug and emergence of manipulation-attempt recipes (e.g., oral, snorting, injecting, smoking, and rectal). The study demonstrated that an analysis of Internet-based discussions can inform the impact of reformulation on the substance use community and potentially identify a use-deterrent effect, such as a tamper resistant opioid formulation (McNaughton et al., 2014).

Marijuana use is promoted on social networking sites. Displays of dabbing, the extraction of oil from marijuana leaves and flowers, are easily found and accessed on YouTube. An analysis of 116 videos of persons dabbing had a total of 9,535,482 views, with 89% of the videos showing at least one person dabbing. Product reviews, instructions, and some cautionary messages were also provided. The popularity of these videos could potentially increase and normalize this potent form of marijuana use. Another study hypothesized that an understanding of the discourse on Twitter that encouraged marijuana use could inform the development of prevention messages. The study conducted a content analysis of tweets (over 2500 in more than 6 months) and the demographics of a pro-marijuana Twitter handle. The overwhelming majority of tweets were positive about marijuana and the majority of the followers were 19 years of age or younger (Cavazos-Rehg et al., 2014). An analysis of marijuana posts on Instagram identified over 2100 posts related to cannabis with the most common imagers being that of marijuana plants (e.g., buds/leaves), with less common images depicting concentrates, dabbing, and marijuana display ads.

The Internet is a source of information for use of other substances, too. Displays of alcohol use include but are not limited to texts, photographs, and videos talking about or displaying alcohol consumption as well as links to alcohol-related groups or companies (Egan & Moreno, 2011). An analysis of 70 YouTube videos related to alcohol intoxication had been viewed about a third of a billion times. Even though 86% of videos portrayed active intoxication, only 7% contained references to alcohol dependence, with videos that showed humor, games, attractiveness, and no intoxication or injury were rated most positively. Young adults exposure to peer behavior and alcohol advertising on social media are often associated with alcohol use (Jernigan & Rushman, 2014; Mundt, 2011) and a summary of this literature found significant associations between exposure to Internet-based alcohol-related content and intentions to drink and positive attitudes towards alcohol drinking among young adults (Gupta, Pettigrew, Lam, & Tait, 2016; Tait et al., 2015). Likewise, online marketing of alcohol includes advertisements, contests, promotion of branded events, interactive games, and invitations to drink (Nicholls, 2012). Alcohol-related sites do not verify age of users (Barry et al., 2015) and one study found that using fictitious underage profiles, users were able to successfully subscribe to 16 official YouTube channels sponsored by alcohol and beer companies demonstrating that their self-imposed restrictions for online advertising to minors were not being followed (Barry et al., 2015). Finally, one study (Huang, Kornfield, & Emery, 2016) found over 28,000 videos of e-cigarettes had been viewed over 100 million times, rated more than 380,000 times, and commented on more than 280,000 times. The use of these videos included brand marketing and the promotion of e-cigarettes as smoking cessation tools.

Conclusions

Unfortunately, mass media campaigns have not been very effective at impacting substance use. At best, the results of the largest campaigns have been mixed and there is some concern that the large NYADMC had a boomerang effect of increasing marijuana use. A number of concerns have been raised about the quality of the evaluations of campaigns (Scheier et al., 2011). However, there are also concerns that the theories underlying these campaigns were not capable of designing effective campaign messages or the campaigns did not reach individuals at young enough ages to influence substance use decisions before use began. The media environment has changed radically over the past 25 years such that any campaign conducted today will need to rely not only on traditional broadcast and print media but also on the new media, especially the social media that has come to dominate the media world of many adolescents and young adults. There are numerous challenges to deploying the social media in substance use campaigns that need future research to integrate behavioral theories with what we know about how individuals use and interact with media today. But, those challenges also represent tremendous opportunities both to better understand and more effectively impact many different groups and populations for the improvement of their health.

References

Albert, R., Jeong, H., & Barabási, A.-L. (2000). Error and attack tolerance of complex networks. *Nature, 406*(6794), 378–382.

Allara, E., Ferri, M., Bo, A., Gasparrini, A., & Faggiano, F. (2015). Are mass-media campaigns effective in preventing drug use? A Cochrane systematic review and meta-analysis. *BMJ Open, 5*(9), e007449.

Anderson, D. M. (2010). Does information matter? The effect of the Meth Project on meth use among youths. *Journal of Health Economics, 29*(5), 732–742.

Barry, A. E., Johnson, E., Rabre, A., Darville, G., Donovan, K. M., & Efunbumi, O. (2015). Underage access to online alcohol marketing content: A YouTube case study. *Alcohol and Alcoholism, 50*(1), 89–94.

Beaudoin, C. E., & Thorson, E. (2004). Testing the cognitive mediation model: The roles of news reliance and three gratifications sought. *Communication Research, 31*(4), 446–471.

Bellis, M. A., Hughes, K., & Lowey, H. (2002). Healthy nightclubs and recreational substance use. From a harm minimisation to a healthy settings approach. *Addictive Behaviors, 27*(6), 1025–1035.

Bellis, M. A., Hughes, K., Thomson, R., & Bennett, A. (2004). Sexual behaviour of young people in international tourist resorts. *Sexually Transmitted Infections, 80*(1), 43–47.

Bellis, M. A., Hughes, K. E., Dillon, P., Copeland, J., & Gates, P. (2007). Effects of backpacking holidays in Australia on alcohol, tobacco and drug use of UK residents. *BMC Public Health, 7*, 1.

Benotsch, E. G., Nettles, C. D., Wong, F., Redmann, J., Boschini, J., Pinkerton, S. D., Ragsdale K., Mikytuck, J. J. (2007). Sexual risk behavior in men attending Mardi Gras celebrations in New Orleans, Louisiana. *Journal of Community Health, 32*(5), 343–356.

Bierut, T., Krauss, M. J., Sowles, S. J., & Cavazos-Rehg, P. A. (2016). Exploring marijuana advertising on Weedmaps, a popular online directory. *Prevention Science, 18*, 183–192.

Bryant, M. (2011). 20 years ago today, the World Wide Web opened to the public. *Insider.* Retrieved from http://thenextweb.com/insider/2011/08/06/20-years-ago-today-the-world-wide-web-opened-to-the-public/

Burke-Garcia, A., & Scally, G. (2014). Trending now: Future directions in digital media for the public health sector. *Journal of Public Health, 36*(4), 527–534.

Cabrera-Nguyen, E. P., Cavazos-Rehg, P., Krauss, M., Bierut, L. J., & Moreno, M. A. (2016). Young adults' exposure to alcohol-and marijuana-related content on Twitter. *Journal of Studies on Alcohol and Drugs, 77*(2), 349–353.

Carpenter, C. S., & Pechmann, C. (2011). Exposure to the Above the Influence antidrug advertisements and adolescent marijuana use in the United States, 2006–2008. *American Journal of Public Health, 101*(5), 948–954.

Casacolumbia. (2011). National survey of American attitudes on substance abuse XVI: Teens and parents. Retrieved from http://www.casacolumbia.org/addiction-research/reports/national-survey-american-attitudes-substance-abuse-teens-parents-2011

Casacolumbia. (2012). National survey on American attitudes on substance abuse XVII: Teens. Retrieved from http://www.casacolumbia.org/addiction-research/reports/national-survey-american-attitudes-substance-abuse-teens-2012

Cavazos-Rehg, P., Krauss, M., Grucza, R., & Bierut, L. (2014). Characterizing the followers and tweets of a marijuana-focused Twitter handle. *Journal of Medical Internet Research, 16*(6), e157.

Chou, W. Y. S., Prestin, A., Lyons, C., & Wen, K. Y. (2013). Web 2.0 for health promotion: Reviewing the current evidence. *American Journal of Public Health, 103*(1), e9–e18.

Cloud, R. N., & Peacock, P. L. (2001). Internet screening and interventions for problem drinking: Results from the www.carebetter.com. *Alcoholism Treatment Quarterly, 19*(2), 23–44.

Cohen, J. (2001). Defining identification: A theoretical look at identification of audiences with media characters. *Mass Communication and Society, 4*(3), 245–264.

Cole-Lewis, H., Perotte, A., Galica, K., Dreyer, L., Griffith, C., Schwarz, M., ... Augustson, E. (2016). Social network behavior and engagement within a smoking cessation Facebook page. *Journal of Medical Internet Research, 18*(8), e205.

Cunningham, J. A., Humphreys, K., & Koski-Jännes, A. (2000). Providing personalized assessment feedback for problem drinking on the Internet: A pilot project. *Journal of Studies on Alcohol, 61*(6), 794–798.

David, C., Cappella, J. N., & Fishbein, M. (2006). The social diffusion of influence among adolescents: Group interaction in a chat room environment about antidrug advertisements. *Communication Theory, 16*(1), 118–140.

Diao, F., & Sundar, S. S. (2004). Orienting response and memory for web advertisements: Exploring effects of pop-up window and animation. *Communication Research, 31*(5), 537–567.

Egan, K. G., & Moreno, M. A. (2011). Alcohol references on undergraduate males' Facebook profiles. *American Journal of Men's Health, 5*(5), 413–420.

Eiser, J., & Ford, N. (1995). Sexual relationships on holiday: A case of situational disinhibition. *Journal of Social and Personal Relationships, 12*(3), 323–339.

Erceg-Hurn, D. M. (2008). Drugs, money, and graphic ads: A critical review of the Montana Meth Project. *Prevention Science, 9*(4), 256–263.

Erickson, B. H. (1988). The relational basis of attitudes. In B. Wellman & S. D. Berkowitz (Eds.), *Social structures: A network approach.* (pp. 99–121). Cambridge: Cambridge University Press.

Evans, W. D. (2016). *Social marketing research for global public health.* New York, NY: Oxford University Press.

Eveland, W. P. (2001). The cognitive mediation model of learning from the news. *Communication Research, 28*(5), 571–601.

Eveland, W. P., & Dunwoody, S. (2002). An investigation of elaboration and selective scanning as mediators of learning from the web versus print. *Journal of Broadcasting & Electronic Media, 46*(1), 34–53.

Eysenbach, G. (2009). Infodemiology and infoveillance: Framework for an emerging set of public health informatics methods to analyze search, communication and publication behavior on the Internet. *Journal of Medical Internet Research, 11*(1), e11.

Fang, L., & Schinke, S. P. (2013). Two-year outcomes of a randomized, family-based substance use prevention trial for Asian American adolescent girls. *Psychology of Addictive Behaviors, 27*(3), 788–798.

Farrelly, M. C., Davis, K. C., Haviland, M. L., Messeri, P., & Healton, C. G. (2005). Evidence of a dose-response relationship between "truth" antismoking ads and youth smoking prevalence. *American Journal of Public Health, 95*(3), 425–431.

Festinger, L. (1954). A theory of social comparison processes. *Human Relations, 7*(2), 117–140.

Flaudias, V., de Chazeron, I., Zerhouni, O., Boudesseul, J., Begue, L., Bouthier, R., ... Brousse, G. (2015). Preventing alcohol abuse through social networking sites: A first assessment of a two-year ecological approach. *Journal of Medical Internet Research, 17*(12), e278.

GfK Inc. (2015). *The common sense census.* Retrieved from https://www.commonsensemedia.org/the-common-sense-census-media-use-by-tweens-and-teens-infographic#

Green, M. C. (2006). Narratives and cancer communication. *The Journal of Communication, 56*(1), S163–S183.

Green, M. C., & Brock, T. C. (2000). The role of transportation in the persuasiveness of public narratives. *Journal of Personality and Social Psychology, 79*(5), 701–721.

Green, M. C., & Brock, T. C. (2002). In the mind's eye: Transportation-imagery model of narrative persuasion. In M. C. Green, J. J. Strange, & T. C. Brock (Eds.), *Narrative impact: Social and cognitive foundations* (pp. 315–341). Mahwah, NJ: Erlbaum.

Gupta, H., Pettigrew, S., Lam, T., & Tait, R. J. (2016). A systematic review of the impact of exposure to internet-based alcohol-related content on young people's alcohol use behaviours. *Alcohol and Alcoholism, 51*, 763–771. https://doi.org/10.1093/alcalc/agw050

Hanson, C. L., Cannon, B., Burton, S., & Giraud-Carrier, C. (2013). An exploration of social circles and prescription drug abuse through Twitter. *Journal of Medical Internet Research, 15*(9), e189.

Hawkins, R. P., & Pingree, S. (1986). Activity in the effects of television on children. In J. Bryant & D. Zillman (Eds.), *Perspectives on media effects* (pp. 233–250). Hillsdale, NJ: Lawrence Erlbaum and Associates.

Hornik, R., & Jacobsohn, L. (2007). The best laid plans: Disappointments of the National Youth Anti-Drug Media Campaign. *LDI Issue Brief, 14*(2), 1–4.

Hornik, R., Jacobsohn, L., Orwin, R., Piesse, A., & Kalton, G. (2008). Effects of the national youth anti-drug media campaign on youths. *American Journal of Public Health, 98*(12), 2229–2236.

Huang, J., Kornfield, R., & Emery, S. L. (2016). 100 million views of electronic cigarette YouTube videos and counting: Quantification, content evaluation, and engagement levels of videos. *Journal of Medical Internet Research, 18*(3), e67.

Hughes, K., Bellis, M. A., Calafat, A., Juan, M., Schnitzer, S., & Anderson, Z. (2008). Predictors of violence in young tourists: A comparative study of British, German and Spanish holidaymakers. *European Journal of Public Health, 18*(6), 569–574.

Internet User Demographics. (2014). Retrieved from http://www.pewinternet.org/data-trend/internet-use/latest-stats/

Jernigan, D. H., & Rushman, A. E. (2014). Measuring youth exposure to alcohol marketing on social networking sites: Challenges and prospects. *Journal of Public Health Policy, 35*(1), 91–104.

Kietzmann, J. H., Hermkens, K., McCarthy, I. P., & Silvestre, B. S. (2011). Social media? Get serious! Understanding the functional building blocks of social media. *Business Horizons, 54*(3), 241–251.

Kim, A., Hansen, H., Duke, J., Davis, K., Alexander, R., Rowland, A., & Mitchko, J. (2016). Does digital ad exposure influence information-seeking behavior online? Evidence from the 2012 Tips From Former Smokers National Tobacco Prevention Campaign. *Journal of Medical Internet Research, 18*(3), e64.

Kim, J., & Rubin, A. M. (1997). The variable of audience activity on media effects. *Communication Research, 24*(2), 107–135.

Korda, H., & Itani, Z. (2011). Harnessing social media for health promotion and behavior change. *Health Promotion Practice, 14*(1), 15–23.

Kreuter, M. W., Green, M. C., Cappella, J. N., Slater, M. D., Wise, M. E., Storey, D., … Woolley, S. (2007). Narrative communication in cancer prevention and control: A framework to guide research and application. *Annals of Behavioral Medicine, 33*(3), 221–235.

Lang, A. (2000). The limited capacity model of mediated message processing. *The Journal of Communication, 50*(1), 46–67.

Lang, A., Borse, J., Wise, K., & David, P. (2002). Captured by the world wide web: Orienting to structural and content features of computer-presented information. *Communication Research, 29*(3), 215–245.

Lenhart, A. (2015, April 9). *Teens, social media & technology overview 2015*. Retrieved from http://www.pewinternet.org/2015/04/09/teens-social-media-technology-2015/

Lenz, E. R. (1984). Information seeking: A component of client decisions and health behavior. *Advances in Nursing Science, 13*(6), 59–72.

Magura, S. (2012). Failure of intervention or failure of evaluation: A meta-evaluation of the National Youth Anti-Drug Media Campaign evaluation. *Substance Use & Misuse, 47*(13–14), 1414–1420.

McNaughton, E. C., Coplan, P. M., Black, R. A., Weber, S. E., Chilcoat, H. D., & Butler, S. F. (2014). Monitoring of internet forums to evaluate reactions to the introduction of reformulated OxyContin to deter abuse. *Journal of Medical Internet Research, 16*(5), e119.

McQueen, A., Kreuter, M. W., Kalesan, B., & Alcaraz, K. I. (2011). Understanding narrative effects: The impact of breast cancer survivor stories on message processing, attitudes, and beliefs among African American women. *Health Psychology, 30*(6), 674–682.

Miller, W. R., Toscova, R. T., Miller, J. H., & Sanchez, V. (2000). A theory-based motivational approach for reducing alcohol/drug problems in college. *Health Education & Behavior, 27*(6), 744–759.

Moreno, M. A., Kota, R., Schoohs, S., & Whitehill, J. M. (2013). The Facebook influence model: A concept mapping approach. *Cyberpsychology, Behavior, and Social Networking, 16*(7), 504–511.

Moreno, M. A., & Whitehill, J. M. (2014). Influence of social media on alcohol use in adolescents and young adults. *Alcohol Research: Current Reviews, 36*(1), 91–100.

Mundt, M. P. (2011). The impact of peer social networks on adolescent alcohol use initiation. *Academic Pediatrics, 11*(5), 414–421.

Nash, C. M., Vickerman, K. A., Kellogg, E. S., & Zbikowski, S. M. (2015). Utilization of a Web-based vs integrated phone/Web cessation program among 140,000 tobacco users: An evaluation across 10 free state quitlines. *Journal of Medical Internet Research, 17*(2), e36.

Newton, R. L., Jr., Han, H., Stewart, T. M., Ryan, D. H., & Williamson, D. A. (2011). Efficacy of a pilot Internet-based weight management program (H.E.A.L.T.H.) and longitudinal physical fitness data in Army Reserve soldiers. *Journal of Diabetes Science and Technology, 5*(5), 1255–1262.

Nicholls, J. (2012). Everyday, everywhere: Alcohol marketing and social media—Current trends. *Alcohol and Alcoholism, 47*(4), 486–493.

Pagoto, S., Waring, M. E., May, C. N., Ding, E. Y., Kunz, W. H., Hayes, R., & Oleski, J. L. (2016). Adapting behavioral interventions for social media delivery. *Journal of Medical Internet Research, 18*(1), e24.

Palmgreen, P., Donohew, L., Lorch, E. P., Hoyle, R. H., & Stephenson, M. T. (2001). Television campaigns and adolescent marijuana use: Tests of sensation seeking targeting. *American Journal of Public Health, 91*(2), 292–296.

Palmgreen, P., Lorch, E. P., Stephenson, M. T., Hoyle, R. H., & Donohew, L. (2007). Effects of the Office of National Drug Control Policy's Marijuana Initiative Campaign on high-sensation-seeking adolescents. *American Journal of Public Health, 97*(9), 1644–1649.

Perrin, A. (2015, October 8). *Social media usage 2005–2015*. Retrieved from http://www.pewinternet.org/2015/10/08/social-networking-usage-2005-2015

Pescosolido, B. (1992). Beyond rational choice: The social dynamics of how people seek help. *American Journal of Sociology, 97*(4), 1096–1138.

Petraglia, J. (2007). Narrative intervention in behavior and public health. *Journal of Health Communication, 12*(5), 493–505.

Portnoy, D. B., Scott-Sheldon, L. A. J., Johnson, B. T., & Carey, M. P. (2008). Computer-delivered interventions for health promotion and behavioral risk reduction: A meta-analysis of 75 randomized controlled trials, 1988–2007. *Preventive Medicine, 47*(1), 3–16.

Ragsdale, K., Difranceisco, W., & Pinkerton, S. D. (2006). Where the boys are: Sexual expectations and behaviour among young women on holiday. *Culture, Health & Sexuality, 8*(2), 85–98.

Reach of leading social media and networking sites used by teenagers and young adults in the United States as of February 2016. 2016. Retrieved from https://www.statista.com/statistics/199242/social-media-and-networking-sites-used-by-us-teenagers/

Reagan, J., & Collins, J. (1987). Sources of health care information in two small communities. *The Journalism Quarterly, 64*(3), 560–563.

Reinhart, A. M., & Feeley, T. H. (2007). Comparing the persuasive effects of narrative versus statistical messages: A meta-analytic review. Paper presented at the 2007 NCA Annual Convention Communicating Worldviews: Faith-Intellect-Ethics, Chicago, IL. Retrieved from http://www.allacademic.com/meta/p194682_index.html

Rideout, V. (2013). *Zero to eight: children's media use in America 2013*. San Francisco, CA: Common Sense Media Retrieved from https://www.commonsensemedia.org/research/zero-to-eight-childrens-media-use-in-america-2013

Rogers, E. M. (2003). *Diffusion of innovations* (5th ed.). New York, NY: Free Press.

Rooke, S., Copeland, J., Norberg, M., Hine, D., & McCambridge, J. (2013). Effectiveness of a self-guided web-based cannabis treatment program: Randomized controlled trial. *Journal of Medical Internet Research, 15*(2), e26.

Rudie, M. (2016). Results from the FY 2015 NAQC Annual Survey of Quitlines. Retrieved from http://c.ymcdn.com/sites/www.naquitline.org/resource/resmgr/2015_Survey/finalweb2242016NAQCFY2015.pdf

Rus, H. M., & Cameron, L. D. (2016). Health communication in social media: Message features predicting user engagement on diabetes-related Facebook pages. *Annals of Behavioral Medicine, 50*(5), 678–689.

Schaub, M. P., Haug, S., Wenger, A., Berg, O., Sullivan, R., Beck, T., & Stark, L. (2013). Can reduce-the effects of chat-counseling and web-based self-help, web-based self-help alone and a waiting list control program on cannabis use in problematic cannabis users: A randomized controlled trial. *BMC Psychiatry, 13*(1), 305.

Scheier, L. M., Grenard, J. L., & Holtz, K. D. (2011). An empirical assessment of the Above the Influence advertising campaign. *Journal of Drug Education, 41*(4), 431–461.

Siebel, T. M., & Mange, S. A. (2009). The Montana meth project: Unselling a dangerous drug. *Stanford Law and Policy Review, 20*(2), 405–416.

Slater, M. D., Buller, D. B., Waters, E., Archibeque, M., & LeBlanc, M. (2003). A test of conversational and testimonial messages versus didactic presentations of nutrition information. *Journal of Nutrition Education and Behavior, 35*(5), 255–259.

Slater, M. D., Kelly, K. J., Edwards, R. W., Thurman, P. J., Plested, B. A., Keefe, T. J., ... Henry, K. L. (2006). Combining in-school and community-based media efforts: Reducing marijuana and alcohol uptake among younger adolescents. *Health Education Research, 21*(1), 157–167.

Slater, M. D., Kelly, K. J., Lawrence, F. R., Stanley, L. R., & Comello, M. L. G. (2011). Assessing media campaigns linking marijuana non-use with autonomy and aspirations: "Be Under Your Own Influence" and ONDCP's "Above the Influence". *Prevention Science, 12*(1), 12–22.

Stephenson, M. T. (2003). Mass media strategies targeting high sensation seekers: What works and why. *American Journal of Health Behavior, 27*(3), S233–S238.

Suls, J. M., & Miller, R. L. (1977). *Social comparison processes*. New York, NY: Hemisphere.

Tait, R. J., McKetin, R., Kay-Lambkin, F., Carron-Arthur, B., Bennett, A., Bennett, K., ... Griffiths, K. M. (2015). Six-month outcomes of a web-based intervention for users of amphetamine-type stimulants: Randomized controlled trial. *Journal of Medical Internet Research, 17*(4), e105.

Tait, R. J., Spijkerman, R., & Riper, H. (2013). Internet and computer based interventions for cannabis use: A meta-analysis. *Drug and Alcohol Dependence, 133*(2), 295–304.

Three technology revolutions. (2012). Retrieved from http://pewinternet.org/Trend-Data-(Adults)/Whos-Online.aspx

The Total Audience Report: Q1 2016. (2016). Retrieved from http://www.nielsen.com/us/en/insights/reports/2016/the-total-audience-report-q1-2016.html

Turner, J. (1982). Towards a cognitive redefinition of the social group. In H. Tajfel (Ed.), *Social identity and intergroup relations* (pp. 15–40). New York, NY: Academic Press.

Turner, R. H., & Killian, L. M. (1992). *Collective behavior* (3rd ed.). Englewood Cliffs, NJ: Prentice-Hall.

Tutenges, S., & Hesse, M. (2008). Patterns of binge drinking at an international nightlife resort. *Alcohol and Alcoholism, 43*(5), 595–599.

The U.S. Digital Consumer Report. (2014). Retrieved from http://www.nielsen.com/us/en/insights/reports/2014/the-us-digital-consumer-report.html

Walther, J. B., Pingree, S., Hawkins, R. P., & Buller, D. B. (2005). Attributes of interactive online health information systems. *Journal of Medical Internet Research, 7*(3), e33.

Walther, J. B., Tong, S. T., DeAndrea, D. C., Carr, C., & Van Der Heide, B. (2011). A juxtaposition of social influences: Web 2.0 and the interaction of mass, interpersonal, and peer sources online. In Z. Birchmeier, B. Dietz-Uhler, & G. Strasser (Eds.), *Strategic uses of social technology: An interactive perspective of social psychology. Cambridge.* Cambridge: Cambridge University Press.

Wang, Z., Walther, J. B., Pingree, S., & Hawkins, R. P. (2008). Health information, credibility, homophily, and influence via the internet: Web sites versus discussion groups. *Health Communication, 23*(4), 358–368.

Werb, D., Mills, E. J., DeBeck, K., Kerr, T., Montaner, J. S., & Wood, E. (2011). The effectiveness of anti-illicit-drug public-service announcements: A systematic review and meta-analysis. *Journal of Epidemiology and Community Health, 65*(10), 834–840.

White, A., Kavanagh, D., Stallman, H., Klein, B., Kay-Lambkin, F., Proudfoot, J., ... Hines, E. (2010). Online alcohol interventions: A systematic review. *Journal of Medical Internet Research, 12*(5), e62.

Woodall, W. G. (1986). Information-processing theory and television news. In J. P. Robinson & M. R. Levy (Eds.)., *The main source: Learning from television news* (pp. 133–158). Beverly Hills, CA: Sage.

Woodall, W. G., Buller, D. B., Saba, L., Zimmerman, D., Waters, E., Hines, J. M., ... Starling, R. (2007). Effect of emailed messages on return use of a nutrition education website and subsequent changes in dietary behavior. *Journal of Medical Internet Research, 9*(3), e27.

Zillman, D., & Bryant, J. (1985). *Select exposure to communication.* Hillsdale, NJ: Lawrence Erlbaum Associates.

Zillman, D., Chen, L., Knobloch, S., & Callison, C. (2004). Effects of lead framing on selective exposure to internet news reports. *Communication Research, 31*(1), 58–81.

A Role for Mindfulness and Mindfulness Training in Substance Use Prevention

Nathaniel R. Riggs, Mark T. Greenberg, and Kamila Dvorakova

Mindfulness and Mindfulness Practice

Mindfulness has been defined as the quality or process of human consciousness characterized by attentive and accepting awareness of the constant stream of lived experience (Brown & Ryan, 2003; Kabat-Zinn, 2003). Mindfully experiencing a thought or emotion involves observing and reflecting on the present experience in a nonjudgmental way, rather than reacting automatically or impulsively (Bishop et al., 2004; Shapiro, Carlson, Astin, & Freedman, 2006), in turn enhancing one's capacity for healthy decision-making (Alfonso, Caracuel, Delgado-Pastor, & Verdejo-Garcia, 2011). Similar to other psychological constructs (e.g., anxiety, self-control), individual differences in mindfulness may reflect both a person's enduring trait or disposition and momentary fluctuations in mindful awareness across time. Considered as a dispositional trait, individual differences in self-reported mindfulness have been associated with several aspects of physical and psychological health and well-being, including substance use, across the lifespan (e.g., Black, Sussman, Johnson, & Milam, 2012; Chambers et al., 2015; Pivarunas et al., 2015). Conceptualized as a state, or mode, conscious attention and awareness to present experience can be cultivated through contemplative, or mindfulness practice. Traditionally, the cultivation of mindfulness has been conducted as part of ancient Eastern spiritual traditions such as meditation, yoga, and other mind-body practices. However, such practices have been active in most major religions and world cultures. More recently, Western clinical, cognitive, and developmental scientists have implemented secular version of mindfulness practices to treat and prevent behavioral and psychological dysfunction, including substance use disorder (SUD) (Wetherill & Tapert, 2013).

Theoretical and empirical support from neuroscience research suggests two interacting neural circuits may be central to mindfulness (Zelazo & Lyons, 2012). The first neural circuit is comprised of prefrontal cortical pathways associated with self-regulation of thought, affect, and behavior. Here, dispositional mindfulness has been associated with "top-down" self-regulated decision-making and executive function processes governed by the prefrontal cortex (PFC)

N. R. Riggs (✉)
Human Development and Family Studies,
Colorado State University, Fort Collins, CO, USA
e-mail: nathaniel.riggs@colostate.edu

M. T. Greenberg
Human Development and Family Studies,
The Pennsylvania State University,
University Park, PA, USA
e-mail: mxg47@psu.edu; kud167@psu.edu

K. Dvorakova
National Institute of Mental Health,
Prague, Czech Republic

including inhibitory control and working memory (Modinos, Ormel, & Aleman, 2010; Riggs, Black, & Ritt-Olson, 2015). The second neural circuit includes "bottom-up" pathways directly responsible for the generation of arousal and affect, where dispositional mindfulness and mindfulness practice have been associated with decreased reactivity in areas of the brain responsible for the generation of affective and motivational impulses (e.g., amygdala and posterior putamen) (e.g., Taylor et al., 2011; Way, Cresewell, Eisenberger, & Lieberman, 2010). Furthermore, recent evidence documents the effect of mindful breathing practices for stimulating integrated functional connectivity between the PFC and the amygdala when responding to emotional stimuli (Doll et al., 2016). This finding suggests that certain mindfulness practices may engage multi-network neural processing.

Cognitive Neuroscience Theories of Substance Use and Abuse

Top-down and bottom-up neuro-cognitive processes are also central to several theories regarding the progression to and treatment of SUD. For example, progression to addiction has been described as a neurobehavioral process of maladaptive habit-based learning whereby substance use shifts from being directed by top-down goal-directed decision-making driven by positively reinforcing properties of the substance, to habitual or automatic behavior, induced by craving (McKim & Boettiger, 2015). Imaging studies in adults have supported habit-based models of substance use demonstrating that when compared to healthy controls, alcohol-dependent adults show decreased activity in the ventral medial PFC and increased activity in areas of the brain related to habitual responding (e.g., posterior putamen) (Sjoerds et al., 2013). Negative affect, including stress, appears to potentiate habit-based learning as experimental research in adults demonstrates that exposure to stressful social and physical situations contributes to preference for stimulus-response over goal-oriented learning (Schwabe et al., 2007; Schwabe & Wolf, 2010).

Complimentary models of substance use have focused on deficits or disruption in top-down executive function processes (Garavan et al., 2015; Nichols & Wilson, 2015). Inhibitory control deficits have been associated with increased likelihood of substance use initiation, suggesting that pre-existing inability to resist impulses functions as a risk factor for initiating substance use during late childhood and adolescence (Riggs, Anthenien, & Leventhal, 2016). Inhibitory control deficits have also demonstrated positive associations with escalation to binge consumption, use in response to cue-induced behavioral scripts, rumination over substance use, and cravings (Garavan, Potter, Brennan, & Foxe, 2015). Individuals with working memory deficits are hypothesized to be less able to maintain goals related to substance nonuse, keep short- and long-term healthy goals in present moment attention, and keep in mind alternative strategies to substance use (Nichols & Wilson, 2015). Additionally, the neuro-toxic effects of substances on working memory have been replicated in several studies strongly suggesting that working memory deficits are both a contributor to and result of substance use (Nichols & Wilson, 2015).

Mindfulness and SUD Treatment

Research on underlying mechanisms of mindfulness is quite preliminary. However, mindfulness practice's potential to alter neural functioning in areas of the brain compromised by SUD suggests these neural processes as potential mechanisms and has provided a rationale for the application of mindfulness-based SUD treatments. Both top-down and bottom-up neural processes are among the hypothesized, but rarely tested, mediators to mindfulness practice's effects on SUD. With respect to top-down processes, mindfulness practice is hypothesized to provide opportunities for individuals to strengthen prefrontal circuits related to self-control, attention regulation, and emotion regulation—all of which are considered by some models as mechanisms through which mindfulness produces its various benefits (Hölzel et al., 2011)—that have either been compromised through repeated exposure to substances and/or ceded executive control to strengthened bottom-up habit-based processes (i.e., craving) (Bechara et al., 2006). For example, 8 weeks of mindfulness-based stress reduction have been shown to directly promote attention subsystems among medical and nursing students and working memory among pre-deployed military personnel (Jha, Krompinger, & Baime, 2007; Jha et al., 2010), and decreased negative mood states (Jha, Stanley, Kiyonaga, Wong, & Gelfand, 2010). However, mindfulness training effects on the underlying neuro-circuitry of these mediating mechanisms and substance use were beyond the scope of these studies (Farb, Anderson, & Segal, 2012).

Mindfulness practice may also directly decrease participants' reactivity to bottom-up affective and craving networks, strengthened through repeated exposure to addictive substances, by training participants to respond nonjudgmentally to uncomfortable emotions and substance use cues. Supporting this hypothesis, Westbrook et al. (2013) used fMRI to demonstrate mindfulness practice effects on decreased activity in the subgenual anterior cingulate cortex (saACC), a neural region associated with substance use craving, more so than effects on neural regions associated with top-down executive control. However, not tested was whether direct effects of mindfulness practice on saACC function and self-reported craving mediated actual nicotine use.

Although the exact neuro-cognitive mediating mechanisms have yet to be confirmed, a review of 24 studies across several substances provides preliminary support that mindfulness practice is associated with reduced substance use and craving in those with SUD (Chiesa & Serretti, 2014). More specifically, mindfulness-based interventions have been associated with reduced substance use and emotional distress in adolescents (Britton et al., 2010), greater tobacco use reductions (Brewer et al., 2011), fewer alcohol-related problems (Bowen et al., 2006), less frequent cannabis use (de Dios et al., 2011), and less opiate use (Hayes et al., 2004). However, it should be noted that several limitations to the generalizability of findings exist including small sample sizes and a lack of randomized controlled trials (Pearson et al., 2015).

The Promise of Mindfulness Practice for Substance Use Prevention

With few exceptions (Galla, Kaiser-Greenland, & Black, 2016), mindfulness-based approaches to youth substance use prevention have not been tested, despite multiple, converging rationales for their potential efficacy. Figure 21.1 illustrates one testable theoretical model, based on existing theory and research, through which mindfulness practice may prevent youth substance use. This model emphasizes hypothesized mediated effects through previously discussed top-down and bottom-up neuro-cognitive processes. Of course, this limited model is considered as a first step in developing more comprehensive prevention models that would include intermediate interpersonal and social-contextual (e.g., family, schools, culture, policy) factors associated with both self-regulation and youth substance use, but which are beyond the current scope of this chapter.

Overlap among the neural circuits associated with substance use and mindfulness, promising mindfulness-based SUD treatment approaches, and research linking mindfulness to top-down and bottom-up neuro-cognitive processes during adolescence (e.g., Ciesla, Reilly, Dickson, Emanuel, and Updegraff, 2012; Riggs et al., 2015) all provide rationale for testing mindfulness practice as an approach to preventing substance use prior to the emergence of problematic use patterns. That is, if mindfulness practice can be implemented to "rewire the brain" after one becomes dependent upon substances, can it also be implemented as a protective factor prior to the progression to dependence? If so, mindfulness practice may function as a strategy for decreasing the high rates of adolescent substance use and associated costs related to the progression to dependence (Johnston et al., 2014). However, mindfulness practice has yet to be systematically tested as an approach to preventing youth substance use.

Neuro-developmental theory supports the premise that implementing mindfulness practice during childhood and adolescence may reduce substance use. Childhood and adolescence represent periods of substantial structural and

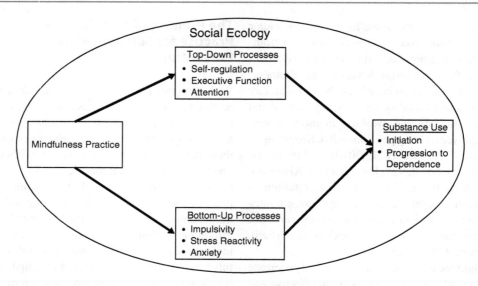

Fig. 21.1 Proposed theoretical model of mindfulness practice's influence on substance use

functional development in areas of the brain responsible for self-regulation. This development occurs asynchronously in that bottom-up mesolimbic dopaminergic structures related to reward sensitivity, sensation seeking, and motivation mature earlier than do top-down PFC systems associated with executive control (Geier, 2013). During adolescence, reward- and affect-related centers of the brain interact with hormonal changes catalyzed by puberty, and developmental changes in the social environment, to influence behavioral regulation and decision-making (Brown et al., 2008). The result is heightened bottom-up reward sensitivity and drive for exploration and novelty that, in combination with relatively late top-down PFC development, contribute to vulnerability to risk-taking behaviors, including substance use, during adolescence (Steinberg, 2014).

This developmental window of risk provides a rationale for implementing neuro-developmentally inspired preventive interventions during childhood and adolescence that can decrease bottom-up emotional and motivational reactivity and promote top-down executive control over affect and behavior. Mindfulness practice may be one approach for modifying these neural circuits among youth (Diamond & Lee, 2011). However, little is known with respect to whether mindfulness practice's effects on neural functioning mediate substance use outcomes. Zelazo and Lyons (2012) note that training youth to mindfully focus attention on their present moment experience, inhibit competing thoughts, emotions, and behaviors from dividing attention, and remember to sustain or bring their attention back to experience hones still developing top-down processes known to be associated with youth substance use (Riggs & Pentz, 2016; Riggs et al., 2012). In fact, several studies have demonstrated cognitive benefits resulting from mindfulness practice including improved attention, self-regulation, and executive function (e.g., Broderick & Metz, 2009; Metz et al., 2013; Napoli, Krech, & Holley, 2005; Schonert-Reichl et al., 2015).

Mindfulness practice may also provide youth with opportunities to decrease reactivity to strong impulses and emotions associated with substance use. Whereas craving-induced cues to the maintenance of substance use may be powerful bottom-up processes once dependent, behavioral impulses, stress, and anxiety may be particularly salient bottom-up risk factors for developing unhealthy coping mechanisms and decision-making skills (i.e., substance use) for young people who have not yet progressed to SUD (Parker & Kupersmidt, 2016). For example, stress can potentiate impulses triggered by the presence of substances in the environment contributing to use among adolescents (Black et al., 2012; Schwabe & Wolf, 2010). Training young people to observe and reflect on their experience, and respond nonjudgmentally to behavioral impulses and stress, may reduce the powerful influence of arousal on behavioral decision-making during developmental periods typified by less efficient prefrontal cortical function. In fact, mindfulness practice has been shown to decrease self-reported emotional reactivity to stress including rumination, intrusive thoughts, and emotional arousal in preadolescents (Mendelson et al., 2010), all of which have been associated with adolescent substance use in other studies (e.g., Kassel, Stroud, & Paronis, 2003; Skitch & Abela, 2008; Steinberg, 2007).

Mindful Awareness Programs for Children and Adolescents

The limited number of mindfulness-based interventions for young people raises questions regarding the feasibility and acceptability of implementing mindfulness-based substance use prevention programs. In this section we briefly review the evidence for mindfulness-based interventions for youth highlighting those programs demonstrating effects on top-down and/or bottom-up processes putatively associated with substance use during childhood and adolescence.

Mindfulness programs have shown the promise to impact both the top-down and bottom-up processes by augmenting self-regulatory functions of coping, cognitive flexibility, and psychological resiliency (Perry-Parrish, Copeland-Linder, Webb, & Sibinga, 2016). Furthermore there is some evidence that mindfulness-based programs with children and youth can be integrated into education or as a part of family prevention programs (Burke, 2009; Greenberg & Harris, 2012). A series of recent reviews and meta-analyses of mindfulness-based interventions for youth conclude that despite methodological limitations, such programs showed the potential to improve psychological symptoms (anxiety, depression) and increase a variety of students' psychosocial characteristics, such as emotion regulation, social-emotional competence, executive functions, or coping skills (Felver, Hoyos, Tezanos, & Singh, 2015; Greenberg & Harris, 2012; (Meiklejohn et al., 2012; Zenner, Herrnleben-Kurz, & Walach, 2014). A substantial limitation to the existing literature is the lack of clear logic models of change and lack of longitudinal follow-up to examine if there are lasting effects. Given the limitations in existing literature, we will turn to a few exemplar studies that represent reasonable evidence.

In a randomized active-control study of 198 middle school students, 8 sessions over 4 weeks of mindfulness instruction using the MBSR program was compared to a hatha yoga program of the same length and a waitlist control. Since both the MBSR and hatha yoga program included similar physical practices aimed to promote present moment awareness, the comparative effectiveness design was able to reveal the distinct benefits of mindfulness meditation. The study found that the intervention group showed significant improvements in a computerized measure of working memory in comparison with both hatha yoga and waitlist control groups (Quach, Mano, and Alexander, 2016). Students were predominantly from low-income minority communities, suggesting that mindfulness practices may be effective in vulnerable populations who are at higher risk for substance use (Garland, Pettus-Davis, & Howard, 2013). Another well-designed study with an active control group randomized 300 urban youth (mean age −12) from urban schools to an adapted 12-week mindfulness-based stress reduction program (MBSR) and health curriculum (Sibinga, Webb, Ghazarian, & Ellen, 2015). At post-test, the MBSR students showed improved coping abilities and lower levels of psychological symptoms, somatization, and self-hostility. Thus, urban youth who are at risk for substance use and/or disorder may benefit from mindfulness skills to prevent its occurrence. Unfortunately, to date there are not randomized trials of mindfulness interventions with youth that have examined changes in brain architecture or functioning.

One randomized trial with youth has reported sustained effects of a mindfulness intervention effects some months after the end of intervention.

A study with high school students in Belgium showed effects of reduced depressive symptoms at 6 months (Raes, Griffith, van der Geuth, & Williams, 2014). Although more longitudinal prevention studies are needed to evaluate if mindfulness programs have lasting preventive effects on substance use per se, the potential of mindfulness programs to improve young people's cognitive, psychological, and neurological processes could be considered promising.

In young adulthood, the multifaceted aspects of mindful awareness become more evident in its relation to substance use. In correlational studies, self-reported dispositional mindfulness has sometimes shown relations to substance use, and different aspects of mindfulness have been associated with both higher and lower substance use. In studies by Leigh and colleagues, greater mind and body awareness was associated with increased alcohol and tobacco use (Leigh, Bowen, & Marlatt, 2005; Leigh & Neighbors, 2009). However, the drinking motives to enhance the positive effects of drinking (rather than drinking to cope) mediated this relationship, suggesting that these students may have been more aware of and craving the positive consequences of drinking (Leigh & Neighbors, 2009).

Other evidence indicates that the mindful capacity to act with awareness is consistently associated with lower alcohol use in terms of quantity, duration, and problematic behaviors (Fernandez, Wood, Stein, & Rossi, 2010; Karyadi & Cyders, 2015). Here, the aspect of mindful acting may serve as a protective factor stimulating the ability to be aware and consequently regulate one's behavior. Stress has also been found to fully mediate the relationship between alcohol use and mindfulness (Bodenlos, Noonan, & Wells, 2013), further suggesting that if young people can actively manage their stress with mindfulness skills, they may be less likely to engage in substance use. Therefore, drinking motives should be investigated when examining the relationship between mindfulness and substance use.

Most recently, a randomized controlled study with college freshmen showed that 8 sessions of a mindfulness program led to a significant decrease in mental health symptoms, and increase in life satisfaction, and marginally significant decrease in alcohol-related consequences (Dvořáková et al., 2017). Furthermore, the effect sizes for alcohol outcomes were larger than the average weighted mean effects found in other alcohol interventions for freshmen (Scott-Sheldon, Carey, Elliott, Garey, & Carey, 2014). By enhancing well-being and providing self-regulation skills to college students, especially during the transition to college, mindfulness interventions may be a promising tool in alcohol prevention efforts.

The effects of mindfulness on young people' drinking uptake and particularly their motivations to drink require more evaluation. In the college population, since there can be resistance to substance use treatment, universal prevention programs that target a variety of protective factors—Stress management, self and emotion regulation, and prosocial behaviors—Might lead to a decrease in stress levels and substance use as well as increases in Well-being. More research is needed to evaluate whether mindfulness strategies could impact the different motivations for drinking by bringing more awareness of one's own personal values (e.g., promoting a healthy peer network and social community). Social influences have been shown to motivate higher levels of drinking (e.g., Gilles, Turk, & Fresco, 2006; Turrisi, Mallett, Mastroleo, & Larimer, 2006) and mindfulness interventions should include a greater focus on offering a way to create alternative healthy communities (Greenberg & Mitra, 2015).

Considerations for the Application of Mindfulness-Based Substance Use Prevention

Mindfulness trials establishing feasibility, acceptability, and preliminary empirical support for decreasing stress and promoting affective and behavioral self-regulation add to the rationale for testing mindfulness-based approaches to youth substance use prevention. However, several conceptual and methodological considerations need to be considered when developing, implementing, and evaluating mindfulness-based preventive intervention for youth. This section describes some of these considerations and the reader is referred to more comprehensive reviews (e.g., Davidson & Kaszniak, 2015; Witkiewitz & Black, 2014).

Prevention Timing and Developmentally Tailored Content

A major consideration when implementing mindfulness practice with youth is ensuring that the content is developmentally appropriate. Mindfulness requires meta-cognitive abilities to reflect on experience, practice introspection, and sit silently for extended periods of time. Although late childhood and adolescence are periods characterized by consolidation of many of these skills, even adolescents lack complete adult capacity to exercise self-regulated abstract and meta-cognitive thought. Consequently, mindfulness practice for adolescents will require developmentally appropriate modifications. Examples will likely include reducing the duration of practices including silent meditations, more time for open discussion and reflection, and integrating more frequent opportunities for interactive and physically active mindfulness activities, such as mindful walking and yoga (Galla et al., 2016).

Contextual Considerations

Whereas treatment for SUD is usually implemented within the clinical context, substance use prevention often takes place in the context of universal prevention (i.e., schools). A number of challenges exist to implementing universal school-based mindfulness programs. Of primary consideration is that teachers, due in part to existing relationships with youth, training in curriculum delivery, and capacity to facilitate diffusion, have traditionally implemented substance use prevention programs. However, teachers will likely vary in their exposure to, buy-in, and expertise with respect to practicing mindfulness. A key issue is whether teachers, who do not have pre-existing knowledge of mindfulness or do not have a consistent mindfulness practice, can effectively teach mindfulness. This variation in experience and commitment is likely to affect the quality of program implementation. Potential strategies for improving teachers' mindfulness practice implementation quality include practitioner-led mindfulness teacher trainings and/or the use of brief and highly scripted mindfulness activities which leave little room for variation in program adherence, both of which have limitations (Galla et al., 2016; Parker & Kupersmidt, 2016).

Integration with Complimentary Strategies for Preventing Substance Use

Most, but not all, mindfulness-based cessation and relapse prevention strategies couple mindfulness practice with other evidence-based approaches to treating SUD including cognitive-behavioral therapy, relapse prevention, acceptance and commitment therapy, among others (e.g., Bowen & Marlatt, 2009). In fact, mindfulness practice combined with other SUD treatments has demonstrated significantly larger effects than several "treatment as usual" comparison groups, supporting the presumed strength that combined treatments produce additive or synergistic effects (Chiesa & Serretti, 2014). A parallel approach to substance use prevention may be to couple mindfulness practice with existing evidence-based preventive interventions for youth, especially those with a shared focus on promoting self-regulation and nonreactivity as mediators to prevention effects.

There are a number of ways that mindfulness might be integrated with existing substance use or social-emotional learning (SEL) curricula. First, there are a number of curricula that already combine some aspects of social and emotional learning with mindfulness. These include Mindup (Schonert-Reichl et al., 2015; Kuyken et al., 2013), and Learning To Breathe (Broderick et al., 2009), but at present these models do not directly apply these skills to substance use contexts/examples. While each has been shown to affect cognitive/affective processes, none have reported effects on substance initiation or progression.

A second example is to add mindfulness to SEL programs that have a primary focus on promoting affect regulation and healthy decision-making. For example, the Promoting Alternative THinking Strategies (PATHS) curriculum is a pre-K through 6th grade evidence-based SEL curriculum, developed upon neuro-developmental theories of brain organization, that promotes self-regulation of affect, executive function, and effective problem-solving strategies as mediators to behavior problems associated with substance use (Greenberg & Kuschè, 1998; Riggs, Greenberg, Kuschè, & Pentz, 2006). Strategies for combining mindfulness practice with PATHS might include the addition of stand-alone mindfulness activities or, when appropriate, integrating mindfulness practices into existing PATHS lessons.

As an example, throughout the PATHs curriculum students are taught to use a Control Signals Poster (CSP) to promote self-regulated decisions-making. The CSP is modeled after a traffic signal with red, yellow, and green lights. At the red light youth are instructed to "stop and take a deep breath." Then at the yellow and green lights youth are instructed to think of potential plans of action, execute the best plan, and ultimately evaluate the effectiveness of the chosen plan. Mindfulness practice can be inserted into the CSP in several ways. For example, at the red light, students could be instructed to take multiple mindful breaths prior to thinking of potential plans of action. Once regulated, youth can be trained to mindfully attend to several individual plans in order to enhance the probability of selecting and executing optimal behavioral responses. Finally, mindfulness training could be used to facilitate evaluation of the plan's effectiveness. Future research should compare the relative effectiveness of a combined approach to substance use prevention relative to mindfulness practice and SEL alone.

A third approach is to integrate mindfulness with existing programs specifically focused on substance use prevention. This would include adding mindfulness practices to evidence-based school models (e.g., Life Skills Training; Botvin, Griffin, & Nichols, 2006) or family-focused models with a strong youth component (e.g., Strengthening Families Iowa—10-14; Coatsworth et al., 2015). Once again, we would recommend examining the added value of the mindfulness component compared to the established programs.

Challenges to the Assessment of Mindfulness in Youth

A potential limitation of the current mindfulness literature is the overreliance on self-report measures of dispositional mindfulness. Self-report assessments, in general, contain several threats to internal validity, including those related to recall and social desirability. Furthermore, those low on ratings of dispositional mindfulness may be particularly poor reporters of their own mental states and processes (Davidson & Kaszniak, 2015). Finally, measures of dispositional mindfulness are less able to detect moment-to-moment fluctuations in mindfulness due to natural within-person variation and/or practice. Some have argued for experience sampling or ecological momentary assessments (EMA) of mindfulness, which may be more precise assessments of within-person variation in mindfulness (Davidson & Kaszniak, 2015). However, few validated objective measures of either state or trait mindfulness exist, particularly for young children.

The context of universal school-based prevention research also presents challenges to the large-scale measurement of mindfulness in youth. For example, experience sampling and EMA may become cost prohibitive in large-scale prevention trials, consisting of hundreds or thousands of study participants. Alternatively, survey-based mindfulness assessments are relatively cheap and can be administered to several students in a group setting. Thus, at present, no single approach to measuring mindfulness is without limitation. One option is to employ multi-method approaches to measuring mindfulness that combine self-report survey assessments for all participants and measures of present moment mindfulness (e.g., EMA) with a randomly selected subpopulation of youth. Multi-method approaches could also be used establishing several forms of measurement validity, including predictive validity vis-à-vis youth substance use.

Conclusion

Substance use during adolescence remains a significant public health issue and there continues to be significant room for the improvement of substance use preventive interventions. Neurodevelopmental theory, empirically supported mindfulness-based SUD treatments, and the feasibility and acceptability of youth mindfulness-based preventive interventions in fields related to substance use suggest the potential value of mindfulness practices as an approach to youth substance use prevention. This approach has yet to be systematically tested and a comprehensive understanding of potential mediating mechanisms to ultimate prevention effects remains unclear. Consequently, this chapter can be viewed as a promissory note to the field of prevention science, attached to which are several conceptual and methodological considerations for future mindfulness-based youth substance use prevention research programs.

References

Alfonso, J. P., Caracuel, A., Delgado-Pastor, L. C., & Verdejo-Garcia, A. (2011). Combined goal management training and mindfulness meditation improve executive functions and decision-making performance in abstinent polysubstance abusers. *Drug and Alcohol Dependence, 117*, 78–81.

Bechara, A., Noel, X., & Crone, E. A. (2006). Loss of willpower: Abnormal neural mechanisms of impulse control and decision-making in addiction. In R. W. Wiers & A. W. Stacy (Eds.), *Handbook of implicit cognition of addiction* (pp. 215–232). Thousand Oaks, CA: Sage.

Bishop, S. R., Lau, M., Shapiro, S., Carlson, L., Anderson, N. D., Carmody, J., ... Devins, G. (2004). Mindfulness: A proposed operational definition. *Clinical Psychology: Science and Practice, 11*, 230–241.

Black, D. S., Sussman, S., Johnson, C. A., & Milam, J. (2012). Testing the indirect effect of trait mindfulness on adolescent cigarette smoking through negative affect and perceived stress mediators. *Journal of Substance Use, 17*, 417–429.

Bodenlos, J. S. J., Noonan, M., & Wells, S. Y. S. (2013). Mindfulness and alcohol problems in college students: The mediating effects of stress. *Journal of American College Health, 61*, 371–378.

Botvin, G. J., Griffin, K. W., & Nichols, T. D. (2006). Preventing youth violence and delinquency through a universal school-based prevention approach. *Prevention Science, 7*, 403–408.

Bowen, S., & Marlatt, A. (2009). Surfing the urge: Brief mindfulness-based intervention for college student smokers. *Psychology of Addictive Behaviors, 23*, 666–671.

Bowen, S., Witkiewitz, K., Dillworth, T. M., Chawla, N., Simpson, T. L., Ostafin, B. D., ... Marlatt, G. A. (2006). Mindfulness meditation and substance use in an incarcerated population. *Psychology of Addictive Behaviours, 20*, 343–347.

Brewer, J. A., Mallik, S., Babuscio, T. A., Nich, C., Johnson, H. E., Deleone, C. M., ... Rounsaville. (2011). Mindfulness training for smoking cessation: Results from a randomized controlled trial. *Drug and Alcohol Dependence, 119*, 72–80.

Britton, W. B., Bootzin, R. R., Cousins, J. C., Hasler, B. P., Peck, T., & Shapiro, S. L. (2010). The contribution of mindfulness practice to a multicomponent behavioral sleep intervention following substance abuse treatment in adolescents: A treatment-development study. *Substance Abuse, 31*, 86–97.

Broderick, P. C., & Metz, S. (2009). Learning to BREATE: A pilot trial of a mindfulness curriculum for adolescents. *Advances in School Mental Health Promotion, 2*, 35–46.

Brown, S. A., McGue, M., Maggs, J., Schulenberg, J., Hingson, R., Swartzwelder, S., ... Murphy, S. (2008). A developmental perspective on alcohol and youths 16 to 20 years of age. *Pediatrics, 121*, S290–S310.

Brown, K. W., & Ryan, R. M. (2003). The benefits of being present: Mindfulness and its role in psychological well-being. *Journal of Personality and Social Psychology, 84*, 822–848.

Burke, C. (2009). Mindfulness-based approaches with children and adolescents: A preliminary review of current research in an emerging field. *Journal of Child and Family Studies, 2*, 133–144.

Chambers, R., Gullone, E., Hassed, C., Knight, W., Garvin, T., & Allen, N. (2015). Mindful emotion regulation predicts recovery in depressed youth. *Mindfulness, 6*, 523–534.

Chiesa, A., & Serretti, A. (2014). Are mindfulness-based interventions effective for substance use disorders? A systematic review of the evidence. *Substance Use Misuse, 49*, 492–512.

Ciesla, J. A., Reilly, L. C., Dickson, K. S., Emanuel, A. S., & Updegraff, J. A. (2012). Dispositional mindfulness moderates the effects of stress among adolescents: Rumination as a mediator. *Journal of Clinical Child & Adolescent Psychology, 41*, 760–770.

Coatsworth, J. D., Duncan, L. D., Nix, R. L., Greenberg, M. T., Gayles, J. G., Bamberger, K. T., ... Demi, M. A. (2015). Integrating mindfulness with parent training: Effects of the mindfulness-enhanced strengthening families program. *Developmental Psychology, 51*, 26–35.

Davidson, R. J., & Kaszniak, A. W. (2015). Conceptual and methodological issues in research on mindfulness and meditation. *American Psychologist, 70*, 581–592.

Diamond, A., & Lee, K. (2011). Interventions shown to aid executive function development in children 4 to 12 years old. *Science, 333*, 959–964.

Doll, A., Hölzel, B. K., Bratec, S. M., Boucard, C. C., Xiyao, X., Wohlschläger, M., & Sorg, C. (2016). Mindful attention to breath regulates emotions via increased amygdala–prefrontal cortex connectivity. *NeuroImage, 134*, 305–313.

de Dios, M. A., Herman, D. S., Britton, W. B., Hagerty, C. E., Anderson, B. J., & Stein, M. D. (2011). Motivational and mindfulness intervention for young adult female marijuana users. *Journal of Substance Abuse Treatment, 42*, 17–33.

Dvořáková, K., Kishida, M., Li, J., Elavsky, S., Broderick, P. C., Agrusti, M. R. & Greenberg, M. T. (2017). Promoting healthy transition to college through mindfulness training with first-year college students: Pilot randomized controlled trial. *Journal of American College Health, 65*, 259–267.

Farb, N. A. S., Anderson, A. K., & Segal, Z. V. (2012). The mindful brain and emotion regulation in mood disorders. *The Canadian Journal of Psychiatry, 57*, 70–77.

Felver, J. C., Hoyos, C. E. C., Tezanos, K., & Singh, N. N. (2015). A systematic review of mindfulness-based interventions for youth in school settings. *Mindfulness*, 34–45.

Fernandez, A. C., Wood, M. D., Stein, L. A. R., & Rossi, J. S. (2010). Measuring mindfulness and examining its relationship with alcohol use and negative consequences. *Psychology of Addictive Behaviors, 24*, 608–616.

Galla, B. M., Kaiser-Greenland, S., & Black, D. S. (2016). Mindfulness training to promote self-regulation in youth: Effects of the Inner Kids program. In K. A. Schonert-Reichl & R. W. Roeser (Eds.), *Handbook of mindfulness in education* (pp. 295–311). New York: Springer.

Garavan, H., Potter, A. S., Brennan, K. L., & Foxe, J. J. (2015). Neural bases of addiction-related impairments in response inhibition. In S. J. Wilson (Ed.), *The Wiley handbook on the cognitive neuroscience of addiction* (pp. 29–54). West Sussex: John Wiley & Sons.

Garland, E. L., Pettus-Davis, C., & Howard, M. O. (2013). Self-medication among traumatized youth: Structural equation modeling of pathways between trauma history, substance misuse, and psychological distress. *Journal of Behavioral Medicine, 36*, 175–185.

Geier, C. F. (2013). Adolescent cognitive control and reward processing: Implications for risk taking and substance use. *Hormones and Behavior, 64*, 333–342.

Gilles, D. M., Turk, C. L., & Fresco, D. M. (2006). Social anxiety, alcohol expectancies, and self-efficacy as predictors of heavy drinking in college students. *Addictive Behaviors, 31*, 388–398.

Greenberg, M. T., & Kuschè, C. A. (1998). Promoting alternative thinking strategies. In *Blueprints for violence prevention: Book 10* (pp. 1–169). Boulder, CO: Institute of Behavioral Science, Regents of the University of Colorado, Center for the Study and Prevention of Violence.

Greenberg, M. T., & Harris, A. R. (2012). Nurturing mindfulness in children and youth: Current state of research. *Child Development Perspectives, 6*, 161–166.

Greenberg, M. T., & Mitra, J. L. (2015). From mindfulness to right mindfulness: The intersection of awareness and ethics. *Mindfulness, 6*, 74–78.

Hayes, S. C., Wilson, K. G., Gifford, E. V., Bisset, R., Piasecki, M., Batten, S., et al. (2004). A preliminary trial of twelve-step facilitation and acceptance and commitment therapy with polysubstance-abusing methadone-maintained opiate addicts. *Behaviour Therapy, 35*, 677–688.

Hölzel, B. K., Lazar, S. W., Gard, T., Schuman-Olivier, Z., Vago, D. R., & Ott, U. (2011). How does mindfulness meditation work? Proposing mechanisms of action from a conceptual and neural perspective. *Perspectives on Psychological Science, 6*, 537–559.

Jha, A. P., Krompinger, J., & Baime, M. J. (2007). Mindfulness training modifies subsystems of attention. *Cognitive, Affective, & Behavioral Sciences, 7*, 109–119.

Jha, A. P., Stanley, E. A., Kiyonaga, A., Wong, L., & Gelfand, L. (2010). Examining the protective effects of mindfulness training on working memory capacity and affective experience. *Emotion, 10*, 54–64.

Johnston, L. D., O'Malley, P. M., Bachman, J. G., et al. (2014). *Monitoring the future national survey results on drug use, 1975–2013: Volume I, secondary school students*. Ann Arbor: Institute for Social Research, The University of Michigan.

Kabat-Zinn, J. (2003). Mindfulness-based interventions in context: Past, present, and future. *Clinical Psychology: Science & Practice, 10*, 144–156.

Karyadi, K. A., & Cyders, M. A. (2015). Elucidating the association between trait mindfulness and alcohol use behaviors among college students. *Mindfulness, 6*, 1242–1249.

Kassel, J. D., Stroud, L. R., & Paronis, C. A. (2003). Smoking, stress, and negative affect: Correlation, causation, and context across stages of smoking. *Psychological Bulletin, 129*, 270–304.

Kuyken, W., et al. (2013). Effectiveness of the mindfulness in schools programme: Non-randomised controlled feasibility study. *The British Journal of Psychiatry, 203*, 126–131.

Leigh, J., Bowen, S., & Marlatt, G. A. (2005). Spirituality, mindfulness and substance abuse. *Addictive Behaviors, 30*, 1335–1341.

Leigh, J., & Neighbors, C. (2009). Enhancement motives mediate the positive association between mind/body awareness and college student drinking. *Journal of Social and Clinical Psychology, 28*, 650–669.

McKim, T. H., & Boettiger, C. A. (2015). Addiction as maladaptive learning, with a focus on habit learning. In S. J. Wilson (Ed.), *The Wiley handbook on the cognitive neuroscience of addiction* (pp. 3–28). West Sussex: John Wiley & Sons.

Mendelson, T., Greenberg, M. T., Dariotis, J. K., Gould, L. F., Rhoades, B. L., & Leaf, P. J. (2010). Feasibility and preliminary outcomes of a school-based mindfulness intervention for urban youth. *Journal of Abnormal Child Psychology, 38*, 985–994.

Metz, S. M., Frank, J. L., Reibel, D., Cantrell, T., Sanders, R., & Broderick, P. C. (2013). The effectiveness of the learning to BREATHE program on adolescent emotion regulation. *Research in Human Development, 10*, 252–272.

Meiklejohn, J., Phillips, C., Freedman, M. L., Griffin, M. L., Biegel, G., Roach, A. T., … Saltzman, A. (2012). Integrating mindfulness training into K-12 education: Fostering the resilience of teachers and student. *Mindfulness, 3*, 291–307.

Modinos, G., Ormel, J., & Aleman, A. (2010). Individual differences in dispositional mindfulness and brain activity involved in reappraisal of emotion. *Social Cognitive and Affective Neuroscience, 5*, 369–377.

Napoli, M., Krech, P. R., & Holley, L. C. (2005). Mindfulness training for elementary school students: The Attention Academy. *Journal of Applied School Psychology, 21*, 99–125.

Nichols, T. T., & Wilson, S. J. (2015). Working memory functioning and addictive behavior. In S. J. Wilson (Ed.), *The Wiley handbook on the cognitive neuroscience of addiction* (pp. 55–75). West Sussex: John Wiley & Sons.

Parker, A. E., & Kupersmidt, J. B. (2016). Two universal mindfulness education programs for elementary and middle-school students: Master Mind and Moment. In K. A. Schonert-Reichl & R. W. Roeser (Eds.), *Handbook of mindfulness in education* (pp. 335–354). New York: Springer.

Pearson, M. R., Roos, C. R., Brown, D. B., & Witkiewitz, K. (2015). Neuroscience and mindfulness-based interventions: Translating neural mechanisms to addiction treatment. In S. W. Feldstein Ewing, K. Witkiewitz, F. M. Filbey, & M. Francesca (Eds.), *Neuroimaging and psychosocial addiction treatment: An integrative guide for researchers and clinicians* (pp. 85–96). New York, NY: Palgrave Macmillan.

Perry-Parrish, C., Copeland-Linder, N., Webb, L., & Sibinga, E. M. S. (2016). Mindfulness-based approaches for children and youth. *Current Problems in Pediatric and Adolescent Health Care, 1–7*.

Pivarunas, B., Kelly, N. R., Pickworth, C. K., Cassidy, O., Radin, R. M., Shank, L. M., … Shomaker, L. B. (2015). Mindfulness and eating behavior in adolescent girls at risk for type 2 diabetes. *Eating Disorders, 6*, 563–569.

Quach, D., Mano, K. E. J., & Alexander, K. (2016). A randomized controlled trial examining the effect of mindfulness meditation on working memory capacity in adolescents. *Journal of Adolescent Health, 58*(5), 489–496.

Raes, P., Griffith, J. W., van der Geuth, K., & Williams, J. M. G. (2014). School-based prevention and reduction of depression in adolescence. A cluster-randomized controlled trial of a mindfulness group program. *Mindfulness, 5*, 477–486.

Riggs, N. R., Anthenien, A., & Leventhal, A. M. (2016). Separating the association between inhibitory control and substance use prevalence versus quantity during adolescence: A hurdle mixed-effects model approach. *Substance Use Misuse, 51*, 565–573.

Riggs, N. R., Black, D. S., & Ritt-Olson, A. (2015). Associations between dispositional mindfulness and executive function in early adolescence. *Journal of Child and Family Studies, 24*, 2745–2751.

Riggs, N. R., Spruijt-Metz, D., Chou, C. P., & Pentz, M. A. (2012). Relationships between executive cognitive function and lifetime substance use and obesity-related behaviors in fourth grade youth. *Child Neuropsychology, 18*, 1–11.

Riggs, N. R., Greenberg, M. T., Kusché, C. A., & Pentz, M. A. (2006). The meditational role of neurocognition in the behavioral outcomes of a social-emotional prevention program in elementary school students: Effects of the PATHS Curriculum. *Prevention Science, 7*, 91–102.

Riggs, N. R., & Pentz, M. A. (2016). Inhibitory control and the onset of combustible cigarette, e-cigarette, and hookah use in early adolescence: The moderating role of socioeconomic status. *Child Neuropsychology, 6*, 613–691.

Schonert-Reichl, K. A., Oberle, E., Lawlor, M., Abbott, D., Thomson, K., Oberlander, T. F., & Diamond, A. (2015). Enhancing cognitive and social-emotional development through a simple-to-administer mindfulness-based school program: A randomized controlled trial. *Developmental Psychology, 51*, 52–66.

Schwabe, L., Oitzl, M. S., Philippsen, C., Richter, S., Bohringer, A., Wippich, W., & Schachinger, H. (2007). Stress modulates the use of spatial versus stimulus-response learning strategies in humans. *Learning & Memory, 14*, 109–116.

Schwabe, L., & Wolf, O. T. (2010). Socially evaluated cold pressor stress after instrumental learning favors habits over goal-directed action. *Psychoneuroendocrinology, 35*, 977–986.

Scott-Sheldon, L. A. J., Carey, K. B., Elliott, J. C., Garey, L., & Carey, M. P. (2014). Efficacy of alcohol interventions for first-year college students: A meta-analytic review of randomized controlled trials. *Journal of Consulting and Clinical Psychology, 82*, 177–188.

Shapiro, S. L., Carlson, L. E., Astin, J. A., & Freedman, B. (2006). Mechanisms of mindfulness. *Journal of Clinical Psychology, 62*, 373–386.

Sibinga, E. M. S., Webb, L., Ghazarian, S. R., & Ellen, J. M. (2015). School-based mindfulness instruction: An RCT. *Pediatrics, 137*, 1–8.

Sjoerds, Z., de Wit, S., van den Brink, W., Robbins, T. W., Beekman, A. T., Penninx, B. W., & Veltman, D. J. (2013). Behavioral and neuroimaging evidence for overreliance on habit learning in alcohol-dependent patients. *Translational Psychiatry, 3*, e337.

Skitch, S. A., & Abela, J. R. Z. (2008). Rumination in response to stress as a common vulnerability factor to depression and substance use in adolescence. *Journal of Abnormal Child Psychology, 36*, 1029–1045.

Steinberg, L. (2007). Risk taking in adolescence: New perspective from brain and behavioral science. *Current Directions in Psychological Science, 16*, 55–59.

Steinberg, L. (2014). *Age of opportunity: Lessons from the new science of adolescence*. New York: Houghton Mifflin Harcourt.

Taylor, V. A., Grant, J., Daneault, V., Scavone, G., Breton, E., Roffe-Vidal, S., ... Beauregard, M. (2011). Impact of mindfulness on the neural response to emotional pictures in experienced and beginner meditators. *NeuroImage, 57*, 1524–1533.

Turrisi, R., Mallett, K. a, Mastroleo, N. R., & Larimer, M. E. (2006). Heavy drinking in college students: who is at risk and what is being done about it? The Journal of General Psychology, 133, 401–420.

Way, B. M., Cresewell, J. D., Eisenberger, N. I., & Lieberman, M. D. (2010). Dispositional mindfulness and depressive symptomatology: Correlations with limbic and self-referential neural activity during rest. *Emotion, 10*, 12–24.

Westbrook, C., Creswell, J. D., Tabibnia, G., Julson, E., Kober, E., Kober, H., & Tindle, H. A. (2013). Mindful attention reduces neural and self-reported cue-induced craving in smokers. *SCAN, 8*, 73–84.

Wetherill, R., & Tapert, S. F. (2013). Adolescent brain development, substance use, and psychotherapeutic change. *Psychology of Addictive Behaviors, 27*, 393–402.

Witkiewitz, K., & Black, D. S. (2014). Unresolved issues in the application of mindfulness-based interventions for substance use disorders. *Substance Use Misuse, 49*, 601–604.

Zelazo, P. D., & Lyons, K. E. (2012). The potential benefits of mindfulness training in early childhood: A developmental social cognitive neuroscience perspective. *Child Developmental Perspectives, 6*, 154–160.

Zenner, C., Herrnleben-Kurz, S., & Walach, H. (2014). Mindfulness-based interventions in schools—A systematic review and meta-analysis. *Frontiers in Psychology, 5*, 603.

Part V
Future Challenges

Bridging the Gap: Microtrials and Idiographic Designs for Translating Basic Science into Effective Prevention of Substance Use

George W. Howe and Ty A. Ridenour

Introduction

Prevention scientists have long advocated using basic research on risk and protective mechanisms in designing effective prevention programs. Coie et al. (1993) articulated a developmental framework for advancing prevention, and Sandler, Braver, Wolchik, Pillow, and Gersten (1991) discussed the use of *small theories*, or delimited models of risk and protection built from research on basic social, psychological, or developmental processes. More recent advocates have focused on basic neuroscience and genetics research as a means of identifying important risk or protective mechanisms (Simons et al., 2013) that could be targeted for prevention of substance use.

The relevant basic science of substance use subsumes all research into behavioral, psychological, social, or biological mechanisms that increase future risk for substance use or protect against substance use in the presence of such risk mechanisms. Such work has accelerated over the past decade. In a quick search of electronic databases using the keywords "risk factor" and "substance abuse," we found over 5800 research reports, over 2200 published in the past 5 years. This has included risk mechanisms such as beliefs or expectancies about the safety of using substances (Simons et al., 2013), involvement with deviant peer groups (Yanovitzky, 2005), and teen-parent conflict (Van Ryzin, Stormshak, & Dishion, 2012). Protective mechanisms have included expectancies about the dangers of substance use (Simons et al., 2013), interpersonal skill in resisting peer influence (Fishbein et al., 2006), and open teen-parent communication or parent monitoring of teen behavior (Perrino et al., 2014). How exactly can prevention scientists best make use of this growing knowledge base? How can they use it to build next-generation prevention programs, and how can it inform recent efforts towards personalized prevention, or the understanding of what works best for whom, and under what conditions (Thibodeau, August, Cicchetti, & Symons, 2016)?

Prevention science is inherently pragmatic. While many mechanisms may contribute to risk for substance use and abuse, we are most concerned with those that are malleable through practical means. Basic research is most often focused on whether some mechanism increases risk or protection, with little attention to whether and how that mechanism can be changed. MacKinnon, Taborga, and Morgan-Lopez (2002) advocated for developing action theories, or models of those processes that change risk or protective mechanisms relevant for substance use. Such theories emphasize *pragmatic mallea-*

G. W. Howe (✉)
Department of Psychology, George Washington University, Washington, DC, USA
e-mail: ghowe@gwu.edu

T. A. Ridenour
Developmental Behavioral Epidemiologist, RTI, International, Research Triangle Park, NC, USA
e-mail: TRidenour@rti.org

bility; as such, they focus on the nexus between theories of change (such as social learning or family systems theories) and theories of etiology (models of risk and protective mechanisms). Some change mechanisms may be very general, while others may be very specific to the risk or protective mechanism in question. Program developers have used these theories to design a range of environmental conditions that make up the specific content and activities of each program component. These include educational messages about the dangers of substance use (Stephens et al., 2009), training exercises to enhance specific interpersonal skills (Fishbein et al., 2006), training teachers in classroom management techniques that shape group behavior (Bowman-Perrott, Burke, Zaini, Zhang, & Vannest, 2016), and family systems interventions designed to reduce conflict and facilitate better communication (Perrino et al., 2014). In this chapter we introduce two research designs that hold promise for developing and testing pragmatic malleability relevant for the prevention of substance use and abuse: microtrials and idiographic designs.

Studying Pragmatic Malleability

Specific risk or protective mechanisms can be useful targets for preventive interventions if they can be changed through practical means. Pragmatic malleability is a function of both the nature of the etiologic mechanism and the mechanisms of action needed to change it. Basic research has been instrumental in identifying promising risk and protective mechanisms that shape the development of substance use, and in describing which of those mechanisms change or remain stable over developmental history. However, research on action mechanisms is necessary to establish how and when these mechanisms can be altered through intervention. Studies of pragmatic malleability attend not only to praxis (what we can do to bring about change) but also to practicality (what effective practices are also practical, given constraints on available resources or time).

As an example, consider recent research on neurobehavioral disinhibition (Tarter, Kirisci, Habeych, Reynolds, & Vanyukov, 2004), or deficiencies in self-regulatory capacities such as attentional control, strategic problem-solving, and goal-directed self-monitoring. Developmental studies using longitudinal designs find that boys with more neurobehavioral disinhibition at age 16 are at increased risk for substance-use disorder at age 19, and disinhibition mediates the association of mother and father substance-use disorder when the child is aged 10–12 with later disorder (Tarter et al., 2004). Ridenour et al. (2009) replicated this finding for cannabis use disorder, and in addition found that neurobehavioral disinhibition mediated the association of early neighborhood disadvantage and residential instability on later disorder. These findings suggest that neurobehavioral disinhibition could prove to be a key target for preventive interventions with youth, particularly if it is malleable. Tarter et al. (2004) found modest stability in this factor across early adolescence, but also substantial variability, suggesting this is the case.

However, developmental studies need to be supplemented with experimental designs to provide formal tests of malleability, and to explore the change mechanisms responsible. Such tests are possible using randomized controlled trials of preventive interventions. For example, Brody, Yu, and Beach (2015) found that African-American youth participating in a family-centered prevention program designed to enhance parent-youth interaction and self-regulation reported fewer positive images of drug-using peers than control participants, and that these changes mediated the impact of the intervention on later substance use. Research on early childhood interventions provides evidence that a variety of enhancement programs can increase executive functioning skills in normative populations, with a few recent studies finding effects in high-risk samples of children who had experienced early adversity (Fisher et al., 2016). Gains in these skills may remediate risk for substance use related to neurobehavioral disinhibition, although we have been unable to locate trials testing this hypothesis.

Randomized prevention trials can be a powerful means of testing both malleability and mediation, but they are limited in several ways. Full-scale prevention trials are expensive, and can take several years to implement. Prevention programs usually combine a range of component intervention activities and target a number of risk and protective factors. This can make it difficult to determine which specific components are influencing each mediator, and tests of mediation can be challenged by mediational collinearity or confounding, especially given the large gaps of time between waves of data collection, usually 6 months or more (Howe, Reiss, & Yuh, 2002). Prevention trials with long-term follow-up can also provide evidence as to whether target mechanisms change permanently or only temporarily, but they may be less useful for determining how and why such change stabilizes or dissipates. Such designs can also provide evidence as to whether targets are more malleable for some people or in specific contexts. For example, Brody et al. (2015) found that their intervention had the strongest impact on youth cognitions for those youth who carried a specific allele of the DRD4 gene and who were in families having the highest levels of conflict and chaos and the lowest levels of support at study onset. However, testing for variation in malleability, particularly in the earlier stages of research when less is known about the sources of that variation, may be more efficient through less resource-intensive designs.

Given that full-scale prevention trials face these limitations, we suggest that testing pragmatic malleability of promising etiologic targets will benefit from brief, focused studies designed specifically for that purpose. With these designs it is possible to study specific intervention components, informed by more detailed action theories, and to assess their impact on very specific etiologic mechanisms. These designs bridge the gap between etiologic studies, which do not study action or intervention, and full-scale prevention trials, which are often unable to disentangle the impact of specific action mechanisms on specific etiologic targets. We next describe two such methods, microtrials and idiographic designs, and consider their utility and limits in furthering our understanding of how to build prevention programs that more effectively target etiologic mechanisms in order to prevent substance use.

Microtrial Designs

Howe, Beach, and Brody (2010) defined microtrials as "randomized experiments testing the effects of relatively brief and focused environmental manipulations designed to suppress specific risk mechanisms or enhance specific protective mechanisms, but not to bring about full treatment or prevention effects in distal outcomes." Such designs have also been referred to as proximal change experiments (Gottman, Ryan, Swanson, & Swanson, 2005). Howe et al. (2010) provide a detailed account of how microtrial designs differ from laboratory or longitudinal studies of etiology on the one hand, and full-scale prevention trials on the other. Unlike longitudinal designs, microtrials are randomized experiments. They assign participants to specific conditions, and study immediate impact. Unlike laboratory studies of etiologic mechanisms, these conditions are designed to bring about meaningful change in those mechanisms that can last after the condition has ended. Microtrials often use components from existing preventive interventions, which can be useful in translating findings back into prevention programming. However, microtrials can also use action theory to design and study specific variations in those components, testing whether theoretically informed modifications increase impact, or whether various modifications can be more effective for specific subgroups of participants.

Unlike full-scale prevention trials, which usually involve multiple sessions over many days, weeks, or months, microtrials employ experimental conditions that are brief, usually involving single sessions. Microtrials allow for more rigorous control of experimental conditions than full-scale prevention trials, because experimental conditions can be designed to focus on very specific targets. Measurement of those targets can also be more extensive and rigorous, because measurement resources are applied to just those targets, rather than being spread out across a range of putative mediators. In addition, microtrials are not designed to bring about lasting preventive effect on more distal outcomes such as substance use, but rather to study pragmatic malleability of specific etiologic mechanisms, given specific intervention actions.

It is important to note that microtrials lie on a continuum between basic laboratory studies and full-scale randomized trials. Investigators have studied experimental manipulations that range from minutes (Fox, Zougkou, Ridgewell, & Garner, 2011) to hours (Fishbein et al., 2006) to a few sessions over a few weeks (Teisl, Wyman, Cross, West, & Sworts, 2012), depending on the nature of the etiologic mechanism being targeted, and the action theory predictions concerning how extensive the manipulation needs to be in order to effect change. These studies all have in common that they are designed to test pragmatic malleability of etiologic mechanisms, and they are not designed to bring about preventive effect in distal targets. This flexibility allows investigators to fit the microtrial design to different etiologic mechanisms which operate across different time scales. We see microtrials not as substitutes for basic etiologic research or full-scale prevention trials; rather they provide a means of refining current prevention programs, and a way of exploring how we can use the burgeoning research on etiology of substance use to inform development of the next generation of prevention programs to be tested in new full-scale trials.

As a prototype example, consider a study by Fishbein et al. (2006), who focused on specific social competencies for resisting peer pressure as a key protective target for preventive interventions. They randomly assigned male teens to either an experimental or a control group. Those in the experimental group participated in a single session emphasizing skills for defusing confrontations without aggression. Session materials were taken from the Positive Adolescent Choices Training (PACT) Program, a prevention program for high-risk adolescents designed to reduce involvement in violence. The study also employed sophisticated measures of putative protective factors, assessing socially competent responses to several vignettes presented by computer in a virtual reality format. These responses were found to be malleable; however, only adolescents who scored higher on pretest measures of executive functioning and emotion perception demonstrated gains in social competence immediately after the intervention.

This study illustrates several elements of microtrials. The experimental manipulation was limited to a very specific and more highly controlled intervention component, explicitly designed to change a specific protective mechanism. Unlike many basic science experiments, the manipulation had elements in common with practical intervention formats used in prevention programming, increasing the likelihood that it could be translated and incorporated more easily into a useful intervention. Such a design was much easier to implement with limited resources. It also allowed the investigators to use more precise and sophisticated methods for assessing proximal changes in the target mechanism without the influence of other intervention components that may be seeking to achieve other outcomes. Leijten et al. (2015) provide a more detailed discussion of the strengths of microtrials, with particular emphasis on using them to test elements of preventive parenting interventions.

More Complex Microtrial Designs

Not only are microtrials useful for assessing the outcomes of specific intervention components but they can also be particularly useful for determining differential impact of these components for subgroups of individuals or when delivered in different contexts. A growing body of basic research indicates that risk and protective mechanisms may themselves operate in different ways for different people in different places. For example, risk for the development of substance-use disorders may vary by genetic characteristics (Lee et al., 2010), personality style (Kotov, Gamez, Schmidt, & Watson, 2010), or neighborhood context (Ridenour et al., 2013). There is much less research as yet on whether action mechanisms influence risk factors in different ways across different populations or contexts. We currently have much more data on what might moderate etiology than we have on what might moderate the impact of preventive interventions on those etiologic mechanisms. As a result, people may differ in how responsive they are to preventive interventions if those interventions have more or less impact on etiologic targets for different participants.

Recent microtrials have provided early evidence for such moderation. The study conducted by Fishbein et al. (2006) presents a cogent example. They assessed early symptoms of conduct disorder at pretest. The brief intervention increased communication skills and resolution of aggressive conflict in teens low on conduct disorder, but significantly decreased use of such skills in those who were initially higher on conduct disorder. These findings suggest that change mechanisms informing the PACT intervention may vary depending on developmental history of aggressive behavior, and prevention programs for higher risk youth may need to be adapted to take this into account. For example, etiologic research suggests that teens who engage in problematic conduct are also more likely to socialize with deviant peers and communication within deviant peer groups involves more direct reinforcement of deviant behavior including substance use (Yanovitzky, 2005). The specific mechanisms of action targeted in the PACT component on defusing conflict may be irrelevant or even counterproductive when conduct-disordered teens are in such contexts. Further microtrials that test mechanisms for changing peer reinforcement of deviant behavior will be useful in identifying more effective methods for targeting this etiologic pathway for teens who are engaging in deviant behavior, as a prelude to developing next-generation prevention programs.

Any design, including randomized prevention trials, can include tests of moderation. Microtrials have two distinct advantages as a means of testing whether change mechanisms vary in their impact across population or context. Many relevant moderators may not be evenly distributed in the population of interest, and so are more difficult to detect in community samples. This is particularly important when relatively rare conditions have substantial impact on change mechanisms. As an example, a microtrial study of attention bias modification by Fox et al. (2011) found the strongest intervention effects for people having low-efficiency polymorphisms of the serotonin transporter gene. Rates of these polymorphisms vary across populations, and can occur at frequencies as low as 15% (Noskova et al., 2008), requiring large samples in order to have enough people with this set of alleles for analysis of moderator effects. Microtrials allow for prescreening and oversampling of lower frequency conditions, greatly increasing power to detect moderation in smaller samples. If a microtrial using this design provides evidence for differential impact on etiologic mechanisms, these findings can inform the development of selective prevention programs designed to target etiologic mechanisms relevant for specific subgroups of individuals.

Microtrials using experimental designs are also inherently more powerful in detecting moderator effects, compared to observational designs employed in studying etiology. McClelland and Judd (1993) demonstrated that residual variance in the product terms of interacting variables greatly reduced power to detect interaction effects in nonexperimental research, compared to experimental designs. Their analyses found that correlational designs had less than 20% of the efficiency of experimental tests, using similar measures in detecting interactions. They attributed these differences to several factors. Measurement is usually more reliable in experimental studies that are conducted under highly controlled conditions, and such studies can also create stronger manipulations than are commonly observed in field studies. In addition, measurement of outcomes immediately after exposure to the manipulation allows for detection of effects that may become harder to detect as other influences add noise over time. This suggests that microtrials using experimental designs can substantially increase statistical power to detect moderator effects, thus requiring smaller samples than field studies or even randomized prevention trials.

Microtrials may also be usefully enhanced by studying how baseline targets moderate impact. Howe, Beach, Brody, and Wyman (2016) suggested that baseline levels of targeted mechanisms are likely to be important moderators of preventive intervention effects. For example, the Familias Unidas program for preventing substance use employed family-based interventions designed to increase positive communication between parents and teens in Hispanic families. Positive communication was the targeted protective mechanism. In a report that combined data from three randomized trials of the Familias Unidas program, Perrino et al. (2014) found that communication measured at baseline (prior to the intervention) moderated the impact of the intervention on this protective factor. Families in the intervention group who began with poorer communication showed greater increases in positive communication compared to those who began with better communication, while the control group showed no changes in communication regardless of baseline level. Such baseline target moderation is likely to occur because those who are deficient on the targeted protective factor are more likely to improve than those who are not, and who have less need for that particular resource.

Microtrials can easily be integrated with baseline target moderator designs through inclusion of pretests measuring the targeted risk or protective mechanism. And if there is reason to believe that proximal change in the target mechanism will have some initial effect on the targeted outcome, this design can be extended to a baseline target moderated mediation (BTMM) design, which allows for a complete test of both moderation and mediation in the same study (see Howe et al., 2016, for a detailed discussion).

Limitations of Microtrials

Interventions employed in microtrials are by definition brief and highly targeted. Some target mechanisms will be more malleable than others, and require either stronger "doses" or some minimal combination of intervention components for change to take place. At the moment questions of preventive intervention dosage are commonly decided through intuition or based on available resources. Microtrials may be particularly useful at this stage in determining whether existing intervention components are up to the task of changing key targets. Full-scale prevention trials can provide some limited evidence concerning dosage if people vary in how much they participate, but variation in dosage is not randomly assigned, and so open to threats of confounding. Microtrials can randomly assign participants to increasing dosages, greatly increasing confidence in causal inference concerning impact on specific targets. Such studies would also contribute to further refinement of action theories concerning specific change mechanisms, which would in the future provide a stronger basis for designing new intervention components.

Preventive intervention programs may also require staging in order to be effective. That is, later components may need to build on foundations laid by earlier components, in order to bring about change in less malleable risk or protective mechanisms. As an example, consider psychoeducational programs for highly stressed populations, such as recently divorced families (Wolchik et al., 2000) or bereaved children who have recently lost a parent (Sandler et al., 2003). Such programs often emphasize skill building, such as helping children develop better methods of coping with stress. However, they also include early components that help children and families develop a sense of trust and safety before moving to more emotionally challenging topics. Microtrials may be less useful for testing malleability when change requires more complex staging of this sort, although microtrials using dismantling designs involving components in isolation and in combination are possible, and have been used to study the impact of such staging on interventions for couples (Babcock, Gottman, Ryan, & Gottman, 2013).

When dosage or staging needs are likely to limit the utility of microtrials, other designs for testing malleability will be called for. We now turn to a discussion of idiographic methods, which hold promise for testing more complex change mechanisms, particularly when combined with microtrial methods.

Idiographic Designs

The term "idiographic" originally referred to single case studies that focused on processes occurring within a single individual. Some of the earliest work emerged in economics, and involved studies of factors that shaped economic changes in single regions or countries. This commonly involved quantitative methods for characterizing a time series, defined as a set of repeated measurements of some economic indicator, such as unemployment rate, made over a number of months or years. Time series could include hundreds of data points, allowing for modeling of change across a range of timescales (such as week to week, month to month, or even year to year). Economists also collected data on the occurrence and timing of "shocks," or changes in the economic environment that were thought to influence that indicator, and developed quantitative methods to test causal hypotheses about these influences.

In its early years, time series measurement and analysis had limited application in other areas of social and behavioral research (but see Gottman, 1981, for an early treatment), whose dominant paradigms involved studying samples of individuals with measurement occurring at one to a few points in time, and employing random assignment to condition and between-group comparisons as a means of testing causal hypotheses concerning intervention impact. Behaviorists proved a notable exception. Behaviorist theories assumed that behavior was under the control of environmental events that were unique to each individual, requiring that researchers study the effects of stimuli and reinforcers on a case-by-case basis. Building on within-subject single-case experimental designs that varied conditions over time in single individuals (Hersen & Barlow, 1976), behaviorists integrated time series analysis with systematic ways of varying stimulus conditions to study the impact on behavior change. Similar to economists' models, these methods assumed that behavior changed quickly when stimulus conditions were altered, a basic assumption of the behaviorist theory of behavior change. A more recent analytic development among behaviorists applies meta-analysis to $N = 1$ time series data using similar techniques as are described later (Owens & Ferron, 2012).

In recent years idiographic methods have expanded to include studies that collect data repeatedly over many days or weeks for a sample of individuals, employ both within-subject and between-subject assignment to intervention conditions, and employ complex multilevel modeling techniques to analyze data and test hypotheses about intervention impact. We provide a brief introduction to these methods, and then discuss how they can be employed by prevention scientists to translate more basic science findings about substance-use risk into next-generation prevention programs.

Intensive Longitudinal Data

Etiologic researchers have turned increasingly to studies that collect many repeated measurements over hours, days, or weeks, as a means of studying how etiologic factors change or stabilize over time. Hamaker and Wichers (2017) documented an eightfold increase in annual publication rates in social and psychological journals from 2000 to 2015, when over 800 papers appeared. Measurement methods have included repeated measurement of physiological variables using wearable sensors (see Fig. 22.1 for an example of a single time series from such measurement), as well as daily diaries or experience sampling using personal digital assistants or smartphones that prompt for responses during the day (also referred to as ecological momentary assessment). As an example, Ferguson, Shiffman, Dunbar, and Schüz (2016) describe two studies of smoking behavior that involved collecting data four to five times a day across 10 days to assess daily fluctuations in smoking rate. They found that smoking rates during the day varied by context, suggesting that smoking behavior was under stimulus control and not just driven by internal cravings.

Shiffman (2009) provided a comprehensive summary of methods for collecting time series data on etiologic factors in studies of substance use, emphasizing the use of ecological momentary assessment.

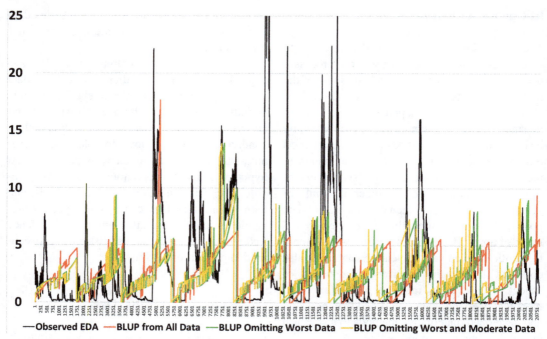

Note: EDA = electrodermal activity. BLUP = Best Linear Unbiased Prediction, also known as Y' or the expected outcomes based on a statistical model (Littell et al., 2006).

Fig. 22.1 Observed vs. modeled electrodermal activity with models based on varying data qualities

This review notes the critical importance for any idiographic study of collecting measures of etiologic mechanisms daily if not more frequently, in order to parse the sequential ordering of risk mechanisms and emerging problem behavior. In addition, such methods can track mechanisms within the participant's "real-life" settings, increasing their ecological validity. In addition, new methods for quantifying dynamic changes over various timescales allow us to make maximal use of such idiographic data, a topic we take up in more detail below.

Intensive Longitudinal Data and Experimental Designs

Although intensive longitudinal data has most often been collected in observational studies of etiologic mechanism, they can also be integrated with experimental designs to test intervention impact. Idiographic methods were originally developed to study treatment impact on single individuals, and to test the causal impact of intervention components by varying when that intervention was active or not. Recent advances in these designs combine intensive repeated measurement within individuals with variation of intervention timing across individuals. Designs combining within-subject data across a set of participants (within/between designs) is common in experimental psychology, but has only recently been applied to intervention research, supported by the development of more complex multilevel statistical modeling, as we discuss in more detail later. When used to study malleability of risk and protective mechanisms, they constitute a form of microtrial, where causal inference is based on variation of intervention and control conditions both within and across participants.

Intensive longitudinal data can be used in a standard between-subject design, where participants are assigned to either intervention or control conditions and intensive follow-up data are used to characterize group differences in change patterns within individuals. We have been unable to find examples of such studies that test the impact on risk mechanisms for substance use. Wichers et al. (2009) provide an example in a randomized trial of antidepressant medication; using experience sampling at 60 time points over 10 days at both baseline and 6-week follow-up, they found that medication reduced stress sensitivity and increased reward experience rates. Medication responders had increased reward experiences compared to nonresponders, but contrary to hypothesis they also had more stress sensitivity.

The utility of within/between designs depends on whether intervention effects generalize to everyone in the sample. Within-person changes can be aggregated at the group level to the degree that they follow some common pattern of change. Intensive longitudinal data allows for a direct test of this assumption, since variation in within-person change can be directly modeled. For example, Madhyastha, Hamaker, and Gottman (2011) found that change and influence patterns based on analysis of repeated behavioral observations during couple interactions often varied across different couples.

In addition, these designs allow us to systematically vary experimental and control conditions within each individual. Perhaps the most common design of this sort uses *staggered baseline phases* (Kazdin, 2011). In place of randomization to groups, a staggered baseline design controls for extraneous influences (such as variation in natural history of an illness, developmental factors, or participant practice) by collecting time series data from each participant during both baseline (or control) phases and intervention phases, and randomly varying phase length among participants. This method of controlling for extraneous influences can be further strengthened by enrolling different participants on different dates (to control for historical events) and using statistical controls as described later. If an intervention has preventive impact, risk mechanisms should abate during intervention phases, but only after onset of the intervention phase, as reflected in changes in time series data for each participant. The strength of intervention impact is then estimated by differences between intercepts, phase means, and/or slopes-over-time among study phases (within individuals as well as in the aggregate).

An alternative set of idiographic designs are the *reversal or ABAB* designs (Kazdin, 2011). Although these were originally developed to test whether the effects of stimulus control can be reversed when it is stopped, these designs can also be useful when theory or prior findings suggest that ongoing conditions are necessary to maintain change in some risk or protective mechanism. A participant begins by providing time series data on the mechanism of interest prior to intervention (condition A). The intervention is then instituted (condition B), in order to assess changes in that mechanism during the next period. The intervention is then stopped (condition A), to determine whether the targeted mechanism returns to baseline, and then instituted again (condition B) to test whether the effects of the intervention replicate. This design can be combined with the staggered phase design by randomly varying the length of time in conditions A and B across participants. An important limitation of reversal designs is that they can only be used with outcomes that could return to baseline levels when withdrawn. For example, many education and psychotherapeutic interventions presume that knowledge, intrapersonal insight, and coping skills will be retained even years later.

Reversal methods were originally designed for treatment rather than prevention, and were based on action theories such as operant conditioning that assumed behaviors were maintained only when specific contextual factors were present. Such treatment targets existing symptoms, while prevention emphasizes bringing about more permanent change in risk or protective factors that precede the onset of symptoms. In studying preventive impact, reversal methods may hold promise for studying more complex mechanisms that stabilize preventive effects. For example, preventive interventions to change parenting behavior have been employed in efforts to reduce risk for adolescent substance use (Prado et al., 2007). However, there is evidence that changes in parenting behavior may be difficult to maintain when parents are depressed or isolated (Dempsey, McQuillin, Butler, & Axelrad, 2016).

More complex reversal designs that vary intervention components targeting both parenting and parent mood or social support can provide initial evidence concerning the set of factors needed to maintain protective mechanisms once they have been established. These include ABCBC designs (Kazdin, 2011), where B and C refer to intervention components targeting the etiologic factor (such as parenting) and the maintaining factor (such as parent depressed mood).

Statistical Methods for Modeling Change and Intervention Impact

Intervention effects can operate at many different timescales, and shape change that follows many different forms. Intensive longitudinal data collection has been employed mostly across periods encompassing hours, days, or weeks, although there have been occasional applications that collect intensive daily data in bouts that are repeated over longer periods of time (Wichers et al., 2009).

Several quantitative methods have been used to characterize patterns of change in intensive longitudinal data, and to test whether those patterns differ by intervention condition. Investigators may be interested in characterizing change that occurs across the entire assessment period. In this case latent growth curve methods are commonly employed to study variation in linear or curvilinear slopes. These methods can be employed with both continuous and categorical outcomes, and latent class or growth mixture models may be employed if patterns of change differ qualitatively (Petras, Masyn, & Ialongo, 2011). For example, McCarthy, Ebssa, Witkiewitz, and Shiffman (2015) used latent class analyses of intensive longitudinal data collected over 27 days following an attempt to quit smoking, finding evidence for five different change patterns that in turn predicted abstinence rates 6 months later.

Two other quantitative methods, building on traditions of time series analysis, hierarchical linear modeling, and Cattell's (1952) q- and p-techniques, have provided a means of assessing patterns of change at shorter timescales, and as it varies across intervention condition within individual participant. These include mixed models trajectory analysis (MMTA) and unified structural equation modeling (USEM).

Similar to growth curve analysis, MMTA uses hierarchical linear modeling, but includes adaptations needed for small samples, described later. MMTA focuses on testing hypotheses regarding change in a single outcome. Each individual provides data in a series of observations collected at regular intervals across some time period. Parameters that index rate of change per unit of time are estimated for each individual, and these individual-level parameters are combined across all participants in the study, allowing for statistical tests of individual differences (Ridenour, Pineo, Maldonado Molina, & Hassmiller Lich, 2013). In large samples, growth mixture models can be used to explore trajectory types for potential identification of subgroups (Petras & Masyn, 2010). Although the applicability of these techniques to small samples and for within-person experiments with varying phase lengths remains largely unexplored, innovative software (described below) and methodologies are evolving to fill this gap (Asparouhov, Hamaker, & Muthén, 2017). Another evolving area is treatment designs for constructing individualized, dynamic interventions that may be altered adaptively, depending on an individual's response to an ongoing intervention (Lei, Nahum-Shani, Lynch, Oslin, & Murphy, 2012).

MMTA models can easily incorporate information about intervention status and can be generally represented using a single regression equation:

$$Y_{it} = \beta_0 + u_{0i} + \beta_1(\text{Time}) + u_{1i}(\text{Time}) \\ + \beta_2(\text{Intx}_{it}) + \beta_3(\text{Intx} \times \text{Time}_{it}) + e_{it} \quad (1)$$

where Y_{it} is an outcome for individual i at time t. The trajectory intercept for individual i is a function of the average sample intercept (β_0) plus individual i's deviation from this average (u_{0i}) which is assumed to have a normal distribution at each time point. Change in the outcome over time is a function of the sample average trend ($\beta_1(\text{Time})$) plus individual i's deviation from that trend ($u_{1i}(\text{Time})$, assumed to be normally distributed). Similar to other regression-based models, additional predictors may be added, such as the intervention intercept, $\beta_2(\text{Intx}_{it})$, and slope, $\beta_3(\text{Intx} \times \text{Time}_{it})$, as presented in (Eq. 1) and described in more detail momentarily. e_{it} denotes random error (an aggregate term that can be parsed into multiple sources of error).

Estimates of individual deviations can be biased by autocorrelation (error of measurements correlated over time). To eliminate this bias, the model usually needs to allow for autocorrelated errors during estimation. It is usually necessary to test a range of error covariance structures and to select the best fitting structure to control for autocorrelation within persons across time. Because the specific sources of correlated error are unknown and cannot be explicitly modeled, fit statistics can be used to identify the best fitting error covariance structure for a sample as well as each participant's time series. This is a critical step as mis-specifying error covariance structures in MMTA can result in biased estimates of effects and of parameter confidence intervals (Ferron, Bell, Hess, Rendina-Gobioff, & Hibbard, 2009).

Unlike basic growth curve models, the MMTA model can also include information concerning intervention status when that status varies over time, and when that pattern of variation differs for different participants. For example, in the staggered baseline phase design, the duration of the baseline phase is randomly varied across participants, to eliminate potential confounds associated with timing of intervention onset.

Intervention effects involve differences between baseline and intervention phases; these are modeled as differences between phase intercepts ($\beta_2\text{Intx}_{it}$) and trends ($\beta_3(\text{Intx} \times \text{Time})_{it}$). When analyzing a single individual's data, the group average terms β_0 and β_1 are dropped, and β_2 and β_3 provide the intervention effects for that individual. When analyzing data for a sample of individuals, that difference reflects the average effect of treatment for the entire sample.

MMTA must be adapted for small samples. This requires switching from full maximum likelihood to restricted maximum likelihood estimation for obtaining model parameters and testing models. Full maximum likelihood under- estimates parameter variance components and this is particularly problematic for small samples (Patterson & Thompson, 1971). Importantly, maximum likelihood estimation is still needed for testing the fit of models to observed data because the restricted maximum likelihood adjustment for number of covariates precludes comparisons between models with different covariates. A second adaptation, the Kenward-Roger adjusted F-test, reduces the potential for type I error that often occurs from poorly estimated covariance structures due to small sample size (Ferron et al., 2009).

A second general analytic method used with idiographic data involves unified structural equation modeling (USEM), also referred to as dynamic structural equation modeling (DSEM). This method resembles standard SEM in many ways, but models day-to-day changes (or more generally changes from time_t to time_{t+1}) across multiple variables. Chow, Ho, Hamaker, and Dolan (2010) review similarities and differences between these approaches, concluding that USEM is best used to model more complex intraindividual dynamics, and can be particularly useful when the number of time points per individual exceeds the sample size.

USEM is particularly useful for studying short-term change in intensive longitudinal data when that change involves multiple outcomes. In USEM, each outcome in a set of outcomes is regressed on contemporaneous and lagged values of all outcomes. The emphasis is usually on day-to-day effects, so models involve lags of only 1 day. As with MMTA, across-time within-person correlated errors may bias estimation, so it is necessary to search for the best fitting model of autocorrelation at longer lags, and to include those autocorrelations in the model to control for their effects.

To test intervention as a moderator of the dynamic processes in a USEM, the full USEM model can be estimated from baseline phase data and contrasted to a full USEM model that is estimated from intervention phase data. This approach to USEM can vary across time points and in different ways for different individuals, as in MMTA (Ridenour, Wittenborn, Raiff, Benedict,

& Kane-Gill, 2016). Because USEM can incorporate more than one outcome and test for lagged associations among outcomes, it is particularly useful for testing hypotheses concerning mediated effects at a day-to-day level, and can be used to model mediation within individuals.

USEM can also be used with multiple time series of a single outcome to control for individual differences in cyclical patterns. Recently, Ridenour and Pineo et al. (2013) measured blood glucose at four times per day in part to account for the circadian rhythm of glucose, which peaks at different times during the day for different individuals. In that study, USEM more accurately modeled observed values as compared to MMTA and time series analysis (ARIMA) with $N = 4$ and a staggered baseline design, based on time series of 400 observations per participant that involved large intraindividual variability. However, compared to MMTA, USEM required such a large number of parameters that for single-person analyses it was unable to converge on a solution. Zheng, Wiebe, Cleveland, Molenaar, and Harris (2013) provided examples of USEM for $N = 1$ in a recent study of substance-use craving and tobacco use.

Although standard software packages such as SAS, SPSS, or STATA include modules for analyzing single time series, MMTA and USEM analyses may require more specialized software. Newer analytic packages simplify the process, allow for a greater range of models to be used, and offer features that are useful specifically for controlled idiographic designs including microtrials. This includes a recently developed set of programs, group iterative multiple model estimation (GIMME) (Beltz & Molenaar, 2016). Unlike other linear algebraic packages, within a single analysis GIMME-MS provides across-person common effects, and individual-specific effects. It can also be used to detect subgroups of participants with similar individual-specific effects. In addition, MPLUS Version 8 has added a full suite of programs for analyzing intensive longitudinal data involving both individual time series and multilevel analyses combining time series across individuals (Muthén & Muthén, 1998–2017).

Using Idiographic Methods to Study Impact on Risk and Protective Mechanisms

To date, idiographic methods using intensive longitudinal assessment have been employed mostly in studies of etiologic mechanisms. Employed within experimental studies that vary intervention conditions both within and across participants, they provide a fertile space for studying whether and how such conditions can influence specific risk and protective mechanisms. As such they represent a new way of conducting microtrials, one that allows for more precise evaluation of proximal change. And because these methods allow for assessment of intervention impact both within and across individuals, they are natural candidates for exploring effect heterogeneity, and identifying characteristics of individuals or contexts that index or account for that heterogeneity. Put another way, predictors of individual variation in intervention effect act as moderators, providing more information concerning which intervention activities influence which people, and under what general conditions.

The second author recently completed a microtrial employing idiographic methods (Ridenour et al., 2017). This study was based on etiologic research indicating that chronic pain can be an important risk factor for the abuse of pain relief medications including opiates (Boscarino et al., 2011). Paraplegic patients who require the use of wheelchairs are at particular risk. Chronic wheelchair use by those with paraplegia can lead to medical complications including pressure sores, muscle spasms, altered blood pressure and flow, joint problems, muscle contractures, and painful discomfort due to sitting in the same position for extended periods. Such patients are likely to be prescribed more powerful pain relief medications, including those that lead to addiction.

Technological advances in the form of powered mobility units hold promise in reducing chronic pain and associated substance use in these patients. Ridenour and colleagues focused on the utilization of one such unit, the Power Seat (PS), developed by the Human Engineering Research Laboratories. The PS was designed to relieve painful discomfort and other complications by allowing users to adjust wheelchair positioning (Dicianno, Mahajan, Guirand, & Cooper, 2012). PS positions range from traditional 90° angles to a nearly supine position using adjustments to the footrest, seat bottom, and seatback. However, during pilot testing of the PS, users failed to follow prescribed methods, instead relying on infrequent and small angle adjustments to their seating position. Pilot study participants continued to experience pain and discomfort (Ding et al., 2008).

Two specific mechanisms of poor adherence were hypothesized: (1) confusion regarding PS usage and (2) neglecting to adjust the PS by more than 15° angles or with enough frequency due to forgetting, failing to self-monitor discomfort levels, or low "buy in." Two interventions were developed to address each of these mechanisms. First, an extended instruction/assistance program was devised to improve comprehension of PS functioning (termed Instruction). Second, the PS computer "Virtual Coach" intervention provided reminders to monitor physical discomfort at the proscribed intervals and to alter PS angles for relief (Ding et al., 2010).

An idiographic microtrial was devised in which all participants first completed baseline phases (staggered in length) and were then randomized to receive either Instruction or Instruction + Virtual Coach. Compared to baseline, both interventions were hypothesized to be associated with decreases in risk factors (physical discomfort) and increases in protective factors (greater compliance with proscribed PS usage, increased frequency of PS usage, and longer duration of large-angle (>15°) positions).

Intensive longitudinal data were collected on PS usage (adjustment frequency, angle sizes); these variables were recorded each minute by the PS computer, resulting in several hundred observations per day. At the end of each study day, participants reported their discomfort levels using a validated assessment measure. The study used a staggered baseline design (randomly assigning patients to 14- or 18-day baseline phases). At the start of baseline phases, an introduction and demonstration of PS use were provided to participants. At the onset of intervention, participants were randomized to receive either Instruction ($n = 11$) or Intervention and Virtual Coach ($n = 6$). Intervention phases lasted 50 days.

Analyses indicated that an autoregressive lag (1) model provided the best fitting error covariance structure for all participants, using SAS Proc Mixed. MMTA tested differences in compliance with PS usage among the study phases. The best fitting MMTA model suggested that after controlling for time (e.g., due to practice) and how long an individual sat in a wheelchair, Virtual Coach + Instruction more than doubled compliance rates on average compared to baseline. In contrast, compared to baseline, compliance lessened slightly for each day of Instruction alone. Results of moderation analyses using USEM found that compared to baseline the Virtual Coach intervention was associated with increased frequency of PS use and large-angle use. In terms of efficacy, general discomfort was equivalent among phases whereas discomfort intensity was less during Virtual Coach—by more than a standard deviation. These findings suggest that interventions to reduce physical discomfort may be important in reducing risk for substance use in people experiencing chronic pain, and provide evidence for one specific method appropriate for a particular population of patients.

Strengths and Challenges of Idiographic Methods

Idiographic methods bring several advantages to the study of pragmatic malleability. Within-subject designs employing intensive repeated measurement with a relatively modest number of individuals are often more highly powered to detect change, as compared to between-subject designs with similar or even much larger sample sizes. Multiple repeated measurements provide more precise estimates of change rates compared to designs measuring outcomes at only two or three time points. Intensive repeated measurement also allows for characterizing more complex patterns of change over a stream of time (rather than using a few waves of essentially cross-sectional data). This can include short-term curvilinear change, sudden discontinuous change, patterns of decay in impact, and even changes in within-subject variability. If two or more outcome variables are repeatedly measured, we can also study coupling or decoupling of outcomes. For example, family interventions are often designed not only to reduce the frequency of some behavior (such as conflict or aggression), but also to reduce reciprocal exchanges of such behavior, decoupling the responses of family members to each other. However, Madhyastha et al. (2011), in a study that repeatedly measured sequential behavior during the interactions of 254 couples, found that individual emotional inertia during the interaction was much more important than coupling of conflict responses in determining the outcome of the discussion.

Idiographic designs are suited to studying immediate impact, detecting influences that operate across hours, days, weeks, or sometimes months. They can also be used to study stabilization or decay of impact, and to test whether combinations of intervention components may be necessary to stabilize or enhance intervention effects.

These designs are also useful when risk or protective mechanisms are unique to small, select subgroups. For example, many barriers preclude using RCTs to research interventions for wheelchair users. The population is small and heterogeneous aside from the characteristic for which participants are recruited. Moreover, clinicians in rehabilitation and assistive technology (like addiction and genetic counselors) are trained to care and value individual's needs and outcomes. Compared to RCTs, idiographic microtrials are more compatible with clinical milieu, interfere less with patient "flow," and offer evidence with more direct clinical interpretation and application (Graham, Karmarkar, & Ottenbacher, 2012). Results from MMTA and USEM also provide more sophisticated information about interactions among study variables, their sequencing, and greater rigor than traditional data analysis methods.

However, as with any research methods, idiographic designs also have challenges and limits (see Hamaker & Wichers, 2017, for a detailed assessment of these issues). They require intensive longitudinal measurement, and this can be challenging to achieve. The recent development of affordable electronic methods for collecting data on multiple occasions has led to burgeoning interest in these approaches. Smartphone apps and Web-based systems provide a means of collecting repeated self-report data, and are increasingly used for momentary ecological assessment or experience sampling (Dempsey, Liao, Klasnja, Nahum-Shani, & Murphy, 2015). Personalized wearable electronic sensors are also becoming affordable and widely available, allowing for collection of physical indicators including heart rate, movement, and skin conductance. However, these new approaches also need critical evaluation to ensure that measures are valid, and may present new threats to validity that need to be assessed and eliminated.

For example, there is evidence for increased risk of substance use in police officers (Ballenger et al., 2011). Although its association with the stress of police activity is unclear, it has been argued that occupational stress is an important contributor to that risk. Furberg (2016) recently used biometric methods to sample electrodermal activity in police personnel as they engaged in stressful episodes of policing. Analyses indicated that, over the course of the officer's shifts, readings of electrodermal activity became more sensitive, probably because conductance increased as perspiration accumulated on the sensors (Gilchrist, personal communication, Sept, 2016). Thus, in MMTA, time had to be "centered," or recalibrated to zero, at the beginning of each shift to account for the expected subsequent change in biosensor functioning during that episode, in order to reduce bias in assessment. Figure 22.1 presents time series data for a single participant, along with estimates that adjust for this and other potential sources of bias that required statistical control before ongoing analyses of what contributes to officer stress could be conducted. One source of bias was the biosensor equipment; the quality of each observation was rated and the effect of poor-quality biosensor readings on predicted outcomes is presented in Fig. 22.1.

Idiographic methods are also limited to the study of short-term change. When employed in experimental designs that combine within-subject and between-subject comparisons, they are an important tool for testing pragmatic malleability of mechanisms amenable to short-term effects. However, they are not useful for studying change that occurs more slowly, over months or years, unless they are integrated into longitudinal designs that repeat measurement at these longer timescales. Wichers et al. (2009) provide an example of such an approach.

Summary and Future Directions

Prevention science follows a rough progression, beginning with etiologic research, translating those findings into promising intervention practices that are then tested for preventive efficacy through full-scale randomized trials. Efficacious interventions can then be moved into practice through research studying dissemination and implementation. But programs are not necessarily effective for everyone, and new etiologic findings may suggest avenues for further refinement of new prevention methods.

In this chapter we have suggested that microtrial and idiographic methods represent two powerful tools for advancing translation of basic research into the development of next-generation programs for effective substance-use prevention. They are relevant for two goals: incorporating new research on etiology into the design of substance-use prevention programs and refining existing programs through testing specific action mechanisms and whether their impact varies across populations or contexts. We have also suggested that these methods require greater attention to the theories of change that should provide the foundation for developing preventive interventions. A number of authors have noted how prevention trials may test theories of etiology (Howe et al., 2002); we would also suggest that microtrials can provide an important means of testing action theories concerning how risk and protective factors can be shaped.

These methods do however require that both basic and prevention scientists step outside their respective silos. Laboratory researchers need to consider more extensive manipulations that can have some practical impact, and use designs that track change in risk or protective mechanisms over longer time periods. Field researchers employing longitudinal observational studies need to think more about the potential malleability of the mechanisms they study. Prevention trial researchers need to think more about the areas where their interventions need improvement (attending more carefully to those instances where candidate mediators of intervention impact don't actually demonstrate such mediation). Researchers who study change mechanisms need to consider how those change processes might differ for different people or in different contexts.

Finally, we suggest that microtrial and idiographic designs may be particularly useful in pursuing questions of moderation, providing us with important initial evidence concerning which interventions for preventing substance use work for whom, and under what conditions. Identifying subgroups for whom our interventions do not lead to change in targets will require that we work to understand why, and look for targets more relevant for those subgroups, ultimately leading to more targeted interventions effective for a greater range of populations and contexts.

References

Asparouhov, T., Hamaker, E. L., & Muthén, B. (2017). Dynamic latent class analysis. *Structural Equation Modeling, 24*(2), 257–269. https://doi.org/10.1080/10705511.2016.1253479

Babcock, J. C., Gottman, J. M., Ryan, K. D., & Gottman, J. S. (2013). A component analysis of a brief psychoeducational couples' workshop: One-year follow-up results. *Journal of Family Therapy, 35*(3), 252–280.

Ballenger, J. F., Best, S. R., Metzler, T. J., Wasserman, D. A., Mohr, D. C., Liberman, A., … Marmar, C. R. (2011). Patterns and predictors of alcohol use in male and female urban police officers. *The American Journal on Addictions, 20*(1), 21–29. https://doi.org/10.1111/j.1521-0391.2010.00092.x

Beltz, A. M., & Molenaar, P. C. M. (2016). Dealing with multiple solutions in structural vector autoregressive models. *Multivariate Behavioral Research, 51*(2–3), 357–373. https://doi.org/10.1080/00273171.2016.1151333

Boscarino, J. A., Rukstalis, M. R., Hoffman, S. N., Han, J. J., Erlich, P. M., Ross, S., … Stewart, W. F. (2011). Prevalence of prescription opioid-use disorder among chronic pain patients: Comparison of the DSM-5 vs. DSM-4 diagnostic criteria. *Journal of Addictive Diseases, 30*(3), 185–194. https://doi.org/10.1080/10550887.2011.581961

Bowman-Perrott, L., Burke, M. D., Zaini, S., Zhang, N., & Vannest, K. (2016). Promoting positive behavior using the good behavior game: A meta-analysis of single-case research. *Journal of Positive Behavior Interventions, 18*(3), 180–190. https://doi.org/10.1177/1098300715592355

Brody, G. H., Yu, T., & Beach, S. R. H. (2015). A differential susceptibility analysis reveals the "who and how" about adolescents' responses to preventive interventions: Tests of first- and second-generation Gene × Intervention hypotheses. *Development and Psychopathology, 27*(1), 37–49. https://doi.org/10.1017/S095457941400128X

Cattell, R. B. (1952). Three basic factor-analytic research designs—their interrelations and derivatives. *Psychological Bulletin, 49*, 499–520. https://doi.org/10.1037/h0054245

Chow, S.-M., Ho, M.-h. R., Hamaker, E. L., & Dolan, C. V. (2010). Equivalence and differences between structural equation modeling and state-space modeling techniques. *Structural Equation Modeling: A Multidisciplinary Journal, 17*(2), 303–332.

Coie, J. D., Watt, N. F., West, S. G., Hawkins, J. D., Asarnow, J. R., Markman, H. J., ... Long, B. (1993). The science of prevention: A conceptual framework and some directions for a national research program. *American Psychologist, 48*(10), 1013–1022. https://doi.org/10.1037/0003-066X.48.10.1013

Dempsey, J., McQuillin, S., Butler, A., & Axelrad, M. (2016). Maternal depression and parent management training outcomes. *Journal of Clinical Psychology in Medical Settings, 23*(3), 240–246. https://doi.org/10.1007/s10880-016-9461-z

Dempsey, W., Liao, P., Klasnja, P., Nahum-Shani, I., & Murphy, S. A. (2015). Randomised trials for the Fitbit generation. *Significance, 12*(6), 20–23. https://doi.org/10.1111/j.1740-9713.2015.00863.x

Dicianno, B. E., Mahajan, H., Guirand, A. S., & Cooper, R. A. (2012). Virtual electric power wheelchair driving performance of individuals with spastic cerebral palsy. *American Journal of Physical Medicine & Rehabilitation, 91*(10), 823–830.

Ding, D., Leister, E., Cooper, R. A., Cooper, R., Kelleher, A., Fitzgerald, S. G., & Boninger, M. L. (2008). Usage of tilt-in-space, recline, and elevation seating functions in natural environment of wheelchair users. *Journal of Rehabilitation Research and Development, 45*(7), 973–983.

Ding, D., Liu, H.-Y., Cooper, R., Cooper, R. A., Smailagic, A., & Siewiorek, D. (2010). Virtual coach technology for supporting self-care. *Physical Medicine and Rehabilitation Clinics of North America, 21*(1), 179–194.

Ferguson, S. G., Shiffman, S., Dunbar, M., & Schüz, N. (2016). Higher stimulus control is associated with less cigarette intake in daily smokers. *Psychology Of Addictive Behaviors: Journal Of The Society Of Psychologists In Addictive Behaviors, 30*(2), 229–237. https://doi.org/10.1037/adb0000149

Ferron, J. M., Bell, B. A., Hess, M. R., Rendina-Gobioff, G., & Hibbard, S. T. (2009). Making treatment effect inferences from multiple-baseline data: The utility of multilevel modeling approaches. *Behavior Research Methods, 41*(2), 372–384. https://doi.org/10.3758/BRM.41.2.372

Fishbein, D. H., Hyde, C., Eldreth, D., Paschall, M. J., Hubal, R., Das, A., ... Yung, B. (2006). Neurocognitive skills moderate urban male adolescents' responses to preventive intervention materials. *Drug and Alcohol Dependence, 82*(1), 47–60.

Fisher, P. A., Beauchamp, K. G., Roos, L. E., Noll, L. K., Flannery, J., & Delker, B. C. (2016). The neurobiology of intervention and prevention in early adversity. *Annual Review of Clinical Psychology, 12*, 331–357. https://doi.org/10.1146/annurev-clinpsy-032814-112855

Fox, E., Zougkou, K., Ridgewell, A., & Garner, K. (2011). The serotonin transporter gene alters sensitivity to attention bias modification: Evidence for a plasticity gene. *Biological Psychiatry, 70*(11), 1049–1054. https://doi.org/10.1016/j.biopsych.2011.07.004

Furberg, R. D. (2016). *Biometrics & policing: Exploring psychophysiology in law enforcement officers*. Paper presented at the 2016 Annual SAPOR Conference, Raleigh, NC.

Gottman, J., Ryan, K., Swanson, C., & Swanson, K. (2005). Proximal change experiments with couples: A methodology for empirically building a science of effective interventions for changing couples' interaction. *Journal of Family Communication, 5*(3), 163–189. 127p.

Gottman, J. M. (1981). *Time-series analysis. A comprehensive introduction for social scientists*. Cambridge: Cambridge University Press.

Graham, J. E., Karmarkar, A. M., & Ottenbacher, K. J. (2012). Small sample research designs for evidence-based rehabilitation: Issues and methods. *Archives of Physical Medicine and Rehabilitation, 93*(12), 2384–2384.

Hamaker, E. L., & Wichers, M. (2017). No time like the present: Discovering the hidden dynamics in intensive longitudinal data. *Current Directions in Psychological Science, 26*(1), 10–15. https://doi.org/10.1177/0963721416666518

Hersen, M., & Barlow, D. H. (1976). *Single case experimental designs. Strategies for studying behavior change*. New York, NY: Pergamon Press.

Howe, G. W., Beach, S., & Brody, G. (2010). Microtrial methods for translating gene-environment dynamics into preventive interventions. *Prevention Science, 11*(4), 343–354. https://doi.org/10.1007/s11121-010-0177-2

Howe, G. W., Beach, S. R. H., Brody, G. H., & Wyman, P. A. (2016). Translating genetic research into preventive intervention: The baseline target moderated mediator design. *Frontiers in Psychology*, 1–9. https://doi.org/10.3389/fpsyg.2015.01911

Howe, G. W., Reiss, D., & Yuh, J. (2002). Can prevention trials test theories of etiology? *Development and Psychopathology, 14*(4), 673–694. https://doi.org/10.1017/S0954579402004029

Kazdin, A. E. (2011). *Single-case research designs: Methods for clinical and applied settings*. Oxford: Oxford University Press.

Kotov, R., Gamez, W., Schmidt, F., & Watson, D. (2010). Linking "big" personality traits to anxiety, depressive, and substance use disorders: A meta-analysis. *Psychological Bulletin, 136*(5), 768–821.

Lee, S.-Y., Hahn, C.-Y., Lee, J.-F., Huang, S.-Y., Chen, S.-L., Kuo, P.-H., ... Lu, R.-B. (2010). MAOA interacts with the ALDH2 gene in anxiety depression alcohol dependence. *Alcoholism: Clinical and Experimental Research, 34*(7), 1212–1218.

Lei, H., Nahum-Shani, I., Lynch, K., Oslin, D., & Murphy, S. A. (2012). A "SMART" design for building individualized treatment sequences. *Annual Review of Clinical Psychology, 8*, 21–48. https://doi.org/10.1146/annurev-clinpsy-032511-143152

Leijten, P., Dishion, T. J., Thomaes, S., Raaijmakers, M. A. J., Orobio de Castro, B., & Matthys, W. (2015). Bringing parenting interventions back to the future: How randomized microtrials may benefit parenting intervention efficacy. *Clinical Psychology: Science & Practice, 22*(1), 47–57. https://doi.org/10.1111/cpsp.12087

Littell, R. C., Milliken, G. A., Stroup, W. W., Wolfinger, R. D., & Schabenberger, O. (2006). *SAS for mixed models* (2nd ed.). Cary, NC: SAS Press.

MacKinnon, D. P., Taborga, M. P., & Morgan-Lopez, A. A. (2002). Mediation designs for tobacco prevention research. *Drug and Alcohol Dependence, 68*(Suppl1), S69–S83. https://doi.org/10.1016/S0376-8716(02)00216-8

Madhyastha, T. M., Hamaker, E. L., & Gottman, J. M. (2011). Investigating spousal influence using moment-to-moment affect data from marital conflict. *Journal of Family Psychology, 25*(2), 292–300. https://doi.org/10.1037/a0023028

McCarthy, D. E., Ebssa, L., Witkiewitz, K., & Shiffman, S. (2015). Paths to tobacco abstinence: A repeated-measures latent class analysis. *Journal of Consulting & Clinical Psychology, 83*(4), 696–708. https://doi.org/10.1037/ccp0000017

McClelland, G. H., & Judd, C. M. (1993). Statistical difficulties of detecting interactions and moderator effects. *Psychological Bulletin, 114*(2), 376–390. https://doi.org/10.1037/0033-2909.114.2.376

Muthén, L. K., & Muthén, B. O. (1998–2017). *Mplus user's guide. Eighth edition* (6th ed.). Los Angeles, CA: Muthén & Muthén.

Noskova, T., Pivac, N., Nedic, G., Kazantseva, A., Gaysina, D., Faskhutdinova, G., ... Seler, D. M. (2008). Ethnic differences in the serotonin transporter polymorphism (5-HTTLPR) in several European populations. *Progress in Neuro-Psychopharmacology & Biological Psychiatry, 32*(7), 1735–1739. https://doi.org/10.1016/j.pnpbp.2008.07.012

Owens, C., & Ferron, J. (2012). Synthesizing single-case studies: A Monte Carlo examination of a three-level meta-analytic model. *Behavior Research Methods, 44*(3), 795–805. https://doi.org/10.3758/s13428-011-0180-y

Patterson, H. D., & Thompson, R. (1971). Recovery of inter-block information when block sizes are unequal. *Biometrika, 58*, 545.

Perrino, T., Pantin, H., Prado, G., Huang, S., Brincks, A., Howe, G., ... Brown, C. H. (2014). Preventing internalizing symptoms among Hispanic adolescents: A synthesis across Familias Unidas trials. *Prevention Science, 15*(6), 917–928. https://doi.org/10.1007/s11121-013-0448-9

Petras, H., & Masyn, K. (2010). General growth mixture analysis with antecedents and consequences of change. In A. Piquero & G. Weisburd (Eds.), *Handbook of quantitative criminology* (pp. 69–100). New York: Springer.

Petras, H., Masyn, K., & Ialongo, N. (2011). The developmental impact of two first grade preventive interventions on aggressive/disruptive behavior in childhood and adolescence: An application of latent transition growth mixture modeling. *Prevention Science, 12*(3), 300–313. https://doi.org/10.1007/s11121-011-0216-7

Prado, G., Lopez, B., Szapocznik, J., Pantin, H., Briones, E., Schwartz, S. J., ... Sabillon, E. (2007). A randomized controlled trial of a parent-centered intervention in preventing substance use and HIV risk behaviors in Hispanic adolescents. *Journal of Consulting and Clinical Psychology, 75*(6), 914–926. https://doi.org/10.1037/0022-006X.75.6.914

Ridenour, T. A., Chen, S. H. K., Liu, H. Y., Hill, K., Bobashev, G., & Cooper, R. (2017). The clinical trials mosaic: Toward a range of clinical trials designs to optimize evidence-based treatment. *Journal of Person Oriented Research, 3*, 28–48.

Ridenour, T. A., Pineo, T., Maldonado Molina, M., & Hassmiller Lich, K. (2013). Toward rigorous idiographic research in prevention science: Comparison between three analytic strategies for testing preventive intervention in very small samples. *Prevention Science, 14*(3), 267–278. https://doi.org/10.1007/s11121-012-0311-4

Ridenour, T. A., Reynolds, M., Ahlqvist, O., Zhai, Z. W., Kirisci, L., Vanyukov, M. M., & Tarter, R. E. (2013). High and low neurobehavior disinhibition clusters within locales: Implications for community efforts to prevent substance use disorder. *American Journal of Drug & Alcohol Abuse, 39*(3), 194–203. https://doi.org/10.3109/00952990.2013.764884

Ridenour, T. A., Tarter, R. E., Reynolds, M., Mezzich, A., Kirisci, L., & Vanyukov, M. (2009). Neurobehavior disinhibition, parental substance use disorder, neighborhood quality and development of cannabis use disorder in boys. *Drug and Alcohol Dependence, 102*(1–3), 71–77. https://doi.org/10.1016/j.drugalcdep.2009.01.009

Ridenour, T. A., Wittenborn, A. K., Raiff, B. R., Benedict, N., & Kane-Gill, S. (2016). Illustrating idiographic methods for translation research: Moderation effects, natural clinical experiments, and complex treatment-by-subgroup interactions. *Translational Behavioral Medicine, 6*(1), 125–134. https://doi.org/10.1007/s13142-015-0357-5

Sandler, I. N., Ayers, T. S., Wolchik, S. A., Tein, J.-Y., Kwok, O.-M., Haine, R. A., ... Griffin, W. A. (2003). The Family Bereavement Program: Efficacy evaluation of a theory-based prevention program for parentally bereaved children and adolescents. *Journal of Consulting and Clinical Psychology, 71*(3), 587–600. https://doi.org/10.1037/0022-006X.71.3.587

Sandler, I. N., Braver, S. L., Wolchik, S. A., Pillow, D. R., & Gersten, J. C. (1991). Small theory and the strategic choices of prevention research. *American Journal of Community Psychology, 19*(6), 873–880. https://doi.org/10.1007/BF00937889

Shiffman, S. (2009). Ecological momentary assessment (EMA) in studies of substance use. *Psychological Assessment, 21*(4), 486–497. https://doi.org/10.1037/a0017074

Simons, R. L., Lei, M. K., Beach, S. R. H., Brody, G. H., Philibert, R. A., Gibbons, F. X., & Gerrard, M. (2013). Differential sensitivity to context: GABRG1 enhances the acquisition of prototypes that serve as intermediate phenotypes for substance use. In J. MacKillop, M. R. Munafò, J. MacKillop, & M. R. Munafò (Eds.), *Genetic influences on addiction: An intermediate phenotype approach* (pp. 303–325). Cambridge, MA: MIT Press.

Stephens, P. C., Sloboda, Z., Stephens, R. C., Teasdale, B., Grey, S. F., Hawthorne, R. D., & Williams, J. (2009). Universal school-based substance abuse prevention programs: Modeling targeted mediators and outcomes for adolescent cigarette, alcohol and marijuana use. *Drug and Alcohol Dependence, 102*(1–3), 19–29. https://doi.org/10.1016/j.drugalcdep.2008.12.016

Tarter, R. E., Kirisci, L., Habeych, M., Reynolds, M., & Vanyukov, M. (2004). Neurobehavior disinhibition in childhood predisposes boys to substance use disorder by young adulthood: Direct and mediated etiologic pathways. *Drug and Alcohol Dependence, 73*(2), 121–132. https://doi.org/10.1016/j.drugalcdep.2003.07.004

Teisl, M., Wyman, P. A., Cross, W., West, J., & Sworts, L. (2012). *Adaptive intervention to address the needs of children with language delays and behavior problems: Proximal impact on emotion-regulation skill knowledge.* Paper presented at the annual meeting of the Society for Prevention Research, Washington, DC.

Thibodeau, E. L., August, G. J., Cicchetti, D., & Symons, F. J. (2016). Application of environmental sensitivity theories in personalized prevention for youth substance abuse: A transdisciplinary translational perspective. *Translational Behavioral Medicine, 6*(1), 81–89. https://doi.org/10.1007/s13142-015-0374-4

Van Ryzin, M. J., Stormshak, E. A., & Dishion, T. J. (2012). Engaging parents in the family check-up in middle school: Longitudinal effects on family conflict and problem behavior through the high school transition. *The Journal of Adolescent Health, 50*(6), 627–633. https://doi.org/10.1016/j.jadohealth.2011.10.255

Wichers, M. C., Barge-Schaapveld, D. Q. C. M., Nicolson, N. A., Peeters, F., de Vries, M., Mengelers, R., & van Os, J. (2009). Reduced stress-sensitivity or increased reward experience: The psychological mechanism of response to antidepressant medication. *Neuropsychopharmacology, 34*(4), 923–931. https://doi.org/10.1038/npp.2008.66

Wolchik, S. A., Griffin, W. A., West, S. G., Sandler, I. N., Tein, J.-Y., Coatsworth, D., ... Greene, S. M. (2000). An experimental evaluation of theory-based mother and mother-child programs for children of divorce. *Journal of Consulting and Clinical Psychology, 68*, 843–856.

Yanovitzky, I. (2005). Sensation seeking and adolescent drug use: The mediating role of association with deviant peers and pro-drug discussions. *Health Communication, 17*(1), 67–89. https://doi.org/10.1207/s15327027hc1701_5

Zheng, Y., Wiebe, R. P., Cleveland, H. H., Molenaar, P. C., & Harris, K. S. (2013). An idiographic examination of day-to-day patterns of substance use craving, negative affect, and tobacco use among young adults in recovery. *Multivariate Behavioral Research, 48*, 241–266.

Dissemination of Evidence-Based Prevention Interventions and Policies

Matthew Chinman, Joie Acosta, Patricia Ebener, Sarah Hunter, Pamela Imm, and Abraham Wandersman

Introduction

In the USA rates of alcohol, marijuana, and other psychoactive drug use among youth remain problematic. In 2015, over half of high school seniors had used alcohol in the past year; over a third had used alcohol in the past month and been drunk in the past year. While some drugs have had declining use, marijuana use has remained steady over the past 5 years, with over 20% of high school seniors using monthly and over a third using in the past year (Johnston, O'Malley, Miech, Bachman, & Schulenberg, 2016). Longitudinal research shows that adolescent substance users are at higher risk for poor physical and mental health and violent behavior in young adulthood (D'Amico, Edelen, Miles, & Morral, 2008; Ford, 2005; Tucker,

M. Chinman (✉)
RAND Corporation, Pittsburgh, PA, USA
e-mail: chinman@rand.org

J. Acosta
RAND Corporation, Arlington, VA, USA
e-mail: jacosta@rand.org

P. Ebener · S. Hunter
RAND Corporation, Santa Monica, CA, USA
e-mail: pateb@rand.org; shunter@rand.org

P. Imm
Private Practice, Lexington, SC, USA

A. Wandersman
Barnwell College, University of South Carolina, Columbia, SC, USA
e-mail: wandersman@sc.edu

Ellickson, Orlando, Martino, & Klein, 2005). They are also more likely to engage in unprotected sex while under the influence of substances (Levy, Sherritt, Gabrielli, Shrier, & Knight, 2009). Early heavy drinking and drug use can also lead to increased alcohol and drug problems in early and late young adulthood (D'Amico, Ellickson, Collins, Martino, & Klein, 2005). In the recent report Facing Addiction, published by the US Surgeon General (U.S. Department of Health and Human Services, 2016), the estimated costs of alcohol misuse, illicit drug use, and substance-use disorders are more than $400 billion which includes costs of premature deaths, lost work productivity, and healthcare spending. These costs often fall disproportionately on minorities and disadvantaged communities (U.S. Department of Health and Human Services, 1985). In addition to these trends, new threats have emerged. The use of opioids has reached epidemic proportions and electronic cigarette use has skyrocketed in just a few years, outpacing the use of regular cigarettes among youth (Johnston et al., 2016). Marijuana continues to be the most frequently used illicit drug with the rate for past month use among those 12 and older in 2014 being significantly higher than any year from 2002 to 2013 (U.S. Department of Health and Human Services, 2016). In a very short time (2013–2014), the prevalence of 30-day marijuana use among those 12 and older increased from 7.5% in 2013 to 8.4% in 2014 (Center for Behavioral Health Statistics and Quality, 2015). In the most recent Monitoring the Future Study, less than a third of high school seniors reported that regular use of marijuana is harmful, which continues a downward trend from 1991, when over three-quarters reported that regular use was harmful (Johnston et al., 2016). While treatment and enforcement are key components of a comprehensive strategy to combat alcohol, tobacco, and other drug use, clearly there is a need to intervene with youth early as delaying use can reduce future problems.

Although substance-use prevention receives much less funding than its cousins, treatment and enforcement (approximately 5% of federal spending), it remains a vital part of the US effort to combat the use of psychoactive substances. After several years of failed approaches using scare tactics, the "just say no" campaign, and education-only programs in the 1970s–1980s, substance-use prevention has made tremendous progress. Rigorous research trials have yielded evidence-based substance-use prevention programs (EBPs) shown to prevent or reduce use by emphasizing active skill building, addressing social norms, and involving families. However, few of these EBPs directly targeted populations in disadvantaged communities including populations of color.

Despite the successes, it remains unclear how much substance-use prevention programs have impacted use rates among youth for the USA as a whole. While studies provided communities with several effective prevention options, and some communities have been successful in adopting these, the adoption of EBPs more broadly across the nation's schools and other youth-serving organizations remains low. Further, even when EBPs are adopted, they are often not implemented well enough to achieve their potential impact. It should be noted that by themselves, these programs are not panaceas. Impacts of the best programs (as measured by effect size) are often small. However, when implemented well across a large group, these impacts can save more dollars than they cost to operate. The phrase "implemented well" is key. In addition to the actual service delivery, these programs need to be part of an overall effort that involves implementation best practices such as setting realistic goals, thoughtfully planning multiple aspects of a program, and carrying out ongoing evaluation, quality improvement, and program sustainability. Thus, a goal shared by many in the prevention field is to support youth-serving organizations (particularly in disadvantaged communities) to not only adopt EBPs, but then also to assist them in implementing these best practices.

Status of the Dissemination of Evidence-Based Substance-Use Prevention Programs

Over the last two decades, several researchers have carried out studies designed to document the extent to which EBPs are being implemented, primarily in schools. Overall, the picture has been disappointing. One of the earliest efforts was conducted by Silvia and Thorne (1997). Starting in 1991, they followed annually for 4 years about 10,000 5th and 6th graders from 19 districts across the country and gathered program implementation data from those districts. They found a classic bell curve distribution on a measure of "program strength" that included program comprehensiveness and stability, community support, and teacher training. The variability in program strength was due to the varying amounts of funding, time, type of content, delivery methods, training, and clear leadership support available for effective substance-use prevention. For example, districts were found to have implemented programming shown not to work—in particular D.A.R.E. and "special events" such as school assemblies—at equal or greater rates than effective classroom-based programs. As shown below, several studies conducted since that time have found similar results.

Hallfors and Godette (2002) surveyed Safe and Drug Free Coordinators from 81 districts (primarily large and urban) about their prevention practices in the late 1990s. Fifty-nine percent reported using one of the six most commonly used EBPs at the time. However, 53% reported using locally developed curricula, and the three most commonly cited programs were not evidence based: D.A.R.E. (82%), Here's Looking at You (63%), and McGruff Drug Prevention (52%). When asked about how their programs were implemented, only 19% responded that they followed basic best practices (i.e., adequately trained teachers, adhered to program delivery guidelines, implemented to all students at the appropriate age). In 1999, Ennett et al. (2003) assessed substance-use prevention practices in a representative sample of 1795 public and private high and middle schools. About 14% reported using content known to be effective and implementing that content with evidence-based delivery methods. Using the same sample, Ringwalt et al. (2002) reported that while about 82% of schools were implementing some kind of program, only about a quarter of the schools were using an EBP. Again, D.A.R.E. (53%), Here's Looking at You (16%), and McGruff Drug Prevention (16%) were the most commonly used curricula. In 2005, Ringwalt et al. (2008) surveyed a representative sample of 1392 high schools and found that while over half (57%) were implementing some kind of substance-use prevention program, only about 10% were using an EBP. Over a third (36%) were using locally developed programs. The same year, Ringwalt et al. (2009) collected similar data on public middle schools and found that 43% used some kind of EBP, which was up from 35% of public middle schools in 1999. However, most schools (77%) reported not using an EBP and 40% reported using locally developed programs. An even larger survey of schools sponsored by the Department of Education found far less penetration of EBPs. In a survey of over 6000 schools (K-12), Crosse et al. (U.S. Department of Education, 2011) found that, while 85% of schools implemented at least one substance-use prevention program of any type during the 2004–2005 school year, only a small proportion (about 8%) reported implementing EBPs. Further, less than one-half of those implementing EBPs (about 44%) met minimal standards for fidelity of implementation. Finally, using annual samples of schools from the Monitoring the Future initiative from 2001 to 2007 (totaling 1206), administrators responded to questions about prevention practices with their eight, tenth, and 12th graders (Kumar, O'Malley, Johnston, & Laetz, 2013). While only 8% of the schools reported that they did not implement any type of substance-use prevention program, the four most common types that were being used were locally developed (47%), D.A.R.E. (30%), state developed (9%), and health education curricula (3%), which were not evidence based.

A common assumption about the low level of EBP implementation is that schools do not have time to spend on substance-use prevention as they are under increasing pressure to deliver positive educational outcomes. However, while that factor may play a role, several of the studies above show that schools are in fact delivering prevention programming of some kind; it is just that the programming tends not to be evidence based. In fact, using the data collected by Ringwalt and colleagues, Cho et al. investigated (Cho, Dion Hallfors, Iritani, & Hartman, 2009) the impact of the No Child Left Behind policy and found that it had little impact on schools' prevention practices and that program funding was the key factor related to implementation. This may be a particular hardship in disadvantaged communities where schools' resources are particularly strained. In the following section, we discuss additional factors related to successful implementation of EBPs.

Factors that Facilitate and Hinder the Adoption and Successful Implementation of EBP Based on the Consolidated Framework for Implementation Research

The Consolidated Framework of Implementation Research (Damschroder et al., 2009) is an organizational framework of theory-based constructs related to evidence-based practice implementation. More specifically, the CFIR outlines five major domains (with 39 subdomains, see Table 23.1) that may impact program implementation: the outer setting, inner setting, intervention characteristics, individual characteristics, and implementation process. *Outer setting* refers to factors outside of the organizational setting in which the evidence-based practice is being

Table 23.1 Domains and subdomains of the consolidated framework for implementation research

Intervention characteristics	Outer setting	Inner setting	Characteristics of individuals	Process

A. Intervention source
B. Evidence strength and quality
C. Relative advantage
D. Adaptability
E. Trialability
F. Complexity
G. Design quality and packaging
H. Cost
	A. Patient needs and resources
	B. Cosmopolitanism
	C. Peer pressure
	D. External policy and incentives
		A. Structural characteristics
		B. Networks and communications
		C. Culture
		D. Implementation climate
		  1. Tension for change
		  2. Compatibility
		  3. Relative priority
		  4. Organizational incentives and rewards
		  5. Goals and feedback
		  6. Learning climate
		E. Readiness for implementation
		  1. Leadership engagement
		  2. Available resources
		  3. Access to knowledge and information
			A. Knowledge and beliefs about the intervention
			B. Self-efficacy
			C. Individual stage of change
			D. Individual identification with organization
			E. Other personal attributes
				A. Planning
				B. Engaging
				  1. Opinion leaders
				  2. Formally appointed internal implementation leaders
				  3. Champions
				  4. External change agents
				C. Executing
				D. Reflecting and evaluating

implemented (e.g., external policy and incentives, patient needs and resources in the community). Outer setting factors may be particularly important to program dissemination policy and strategies while the remaining domains relate more to quality and effectiveness of actual implementation. The *inner setting* refers to factors within the organizational context (e.g., culture, climate, organizational incentives, and structural characteristics of the organization). *Intervention characteristics* refer to the aspects of the EBP itself, such as its complexity, adaptability, cost, and source. *Individual characteristics* refer to aspects of the people charged with implementation, such as their knowledge and attitudes about the EBP, and self-efficacy to deliver it. Finally, the *process* domain refers to the methods by which the intervention is designed to be implemented, including planning, use of opinion leaders, reflection, and evaluation of its execution. We use the CFIR as our organizing framework to discuss the factors related to the successful implementation of substance-use prevention EBPs because it is based on a systematic review of the literature that synthesizes information from several theories and approaches. Moreover, the CFIR is one of the most widely used and cited frameworks in implementation science to date.

The CFIR can systematically characterize how EBPs have been studied and help identify elements that are essential for explaining adoption, implementation, and sustainment. The CFIR, first introduced in 2009 (Damschroder et al., 2009), is consistent with previous observations of implementation challenges in prevention science. For example, over a decade ago, leaders from the Center of Substance Abuse Prevention's Centers for the Application of Prevention Technologies (CAPTs) documented several lessons learned from their experiences supporting the adoption, implementation, and sustainability of EBPs across the USA (Hogan et al., 2003). First, they emphasized that the perception of the innovation as being superior to current practices (i.e., relative advantage) is critical to EBP adoption. This is consistent with CFIR's *intervention characteristics* domain. Second, they argued the importance of the EBP to be consistent with the system (i.e., community, operating organization) it is to be delivered in, demonstrating alignment with the CFIR *inner setting* domain. Finally, they recommended that successful EBP implementation required support from the community (*outer setting*), operating organization (*inner setting*), and resources to address implementation barriers as they arise (*implementation process*), thereby highlighting many of the elements in the CFIR.

Around the time that the CFIR was developed Forman, Olin, Hoagwood, Crowe, and Saka (2009) outlined seven critical elements needed to support school-based prevention program implementation and sustainment based on qualitative interviews with 25 developers of evidence-based programs. The seven elements align with four of the CFIR domains: inner setting—(1) administrative support, (2) program alignment with school goals and mission, (3) fiscal stability, and (4) a strategy to address staff turnover; *individual characteristics*—(5) teacher support; *intervention characteristics*—(6) result demonstrability; and *implementation process*—(7) high-quality training and technical assistance. Holder (2009) identified six important elements to institutionalization of community/environmental prevention efforts rather than school-based prevention programs: (1) community leadership support; (2) media advocacy efforts; (3) local alliance building; (4) local and national resources; (5) political support; and (6) local cultural "fit" or alignment. These elements primarily map onto the *outer setting* factors represented in CFIR, that is, the importance of the environmental context in which an EBP operates.

Despite the explosive growth in the development of effective strategies to prevent substance use from the 1980s to 2000s (Barrera & Sandler, 2006), there have been relatively fewer empirical studies examining how developers and government and other sponsors disseminate EBPs and how communities and organizations effectively adopt, implement, and sustain such approaches. Adoption is considered the first step in implementation, i.e., the decision to implement a new program or strategy. For example, Little, Pokhrel, Sussman, and Rohrbach (2015) assessed various factors associated with the adoption of an evidence-based tobacco-use prevention program. Factors associated with the *inner setting* (school district size, receipt of funding), *outer setting* (presence of a mandate to use a program), *implementation process* (use of a program champion), and *intervention characteristics* (perceived effectiveness of the program by administrators) were all found relevant to tobacco-use EBP adoption. These findings suggest that multiple factors related to the CFIR model have been shown to be critical for the adoption of EBPs.

Predictors of implementation and implementation quality have also been investigated for several different EBPs. For example, Beets et al. (2008) examined the implementation of an EBP (i.e., positive action) after a school adopted it. The investigators found that the *inner setting* factors, such as administrator support for prevention programming and positive school climate whereby teachers felt a high level of school connectedness, along with *individual characteristics*, such as positive teacher perceptions about the program, influenced the quality of implementation of this school-based prevention program. Another example is the work by Cho and colleagues (Cho et al., 2009) that examined certain *inner setting* characteristics—specifically, the variability in funding sources and the district size—among a representative sample of school districts containing middle schools across the USA. This study indicated that diverse funding sources in larger school districts were more likely to implement evidence-based prevention curricula as compared to school districts that had less varied funding sources and were smaller in size.

EBP sustainability has been even less well studied than adoption and implementation. In exception, Tibbitts, Bumbarger, Kyler, and Perkins (2010) examined the sustainment of crime and delinquency prevention programming in school settings 1–3 years post-initial funding. The investigators found that *inner setting* and *process* factors such as leadership support, school support, adequate staffing, and planning were related to self-reported program sustainment albeit with a small self-selected sample of programs ($n = 15$). More recently, Cooper, Bumbarger, and Moore (2015) examined 2-year sustainment among 77 grantees who received seed money for youth delinquency and substance-use prevention programs. Predictors of programs operating 2 years after receiving the initial seed funding included *outer setting* characteristics, like the patient need and community engagement; *inner setting* factors, such as administrator support; *process* factors, such as staff training and sustainability planning; and *individual characteristics*, such as knowledgeable staff. These findings again show that factors from multiple domains influence the support for EBPs.

In sum, researchers have found that many factors across multiple domains of CFIR are relevant to EBP adoption, implementation, and sustainment. One notable challenge to this research is that it can be difficult to assess the full range of possible factors in one study. One study that did evaluate a wide range of CFIR domains, Payne and Eckert (2010), suggests that *implementation process* and *intervention characteristics* may be more influential than other domains. Payne and Eckert (2010) reported that when all program-level factors were considered, program structural characteristics, such as the use of standardized materials, supervision over the program, integration into normal school operations, high-quality training, and use of the intervention during normal school hours, were related to the implementation quality of the program. In fact, these indicators of the structure of the intervention were the most consistent predictors of implementation quality throughout all analyses. However, much more research is needed that considers the relative impact of all the CFIR domains.

Efforts to Improve Dissemination and Use of EBPs

Over the last three decades, researchers, and federal and state agencies, have attempted to improve the uptake of EBPs, with some success. Much of this research utilizes an implementation science perspective (Eccles & Mittman, 2006). Implementation science is defined as a scientific study of methods to promote the systematic uptake of research findings and other EBPs into routine practice to improve the quality and effectiveness of health services and care. The Interactive Systems Framework for Dissemination and Implementation (Wandersman et al., 2008) conceptualizes the processes by which EBPs can be introduced into communities. There are three systems in the ISF. The Delivery System is the organization(s) or community setting (e.g., mental health centers, schools, community coalitions) and its policies and resources that actually implement a new EBP. The Synthesis and Translation System synthesizes the products of research and translates them into user-friendly formats that can be easily accessed and understood by practitioners in the Support System (Rapkin et al., 2012), which in turn uses various implementation strategies like training and technical assistance to strengthen the Delivery System's ability to implement EBPs with quality (Wandersman, Chien, & Katz, 2012). The efforts below tap into many of the elements of the ISF but systematic research on the interactions among the systems is needed to identify important connections and how to strengthen them to produce wider dissemination and implementation.

Research-Developed Support and Delivery Systems

There are many researcher-developed systems to support the work of those delivering EBPs. This section reviews the evidence for several of the most prominent prevention support systems—Getting To Outcomes, Communities that Care, Blueprints, and PROSPER. For each example, we first describe a bit about the prevention support system itself and then provide a brief review of the evidence supporting its effectiveness and sustainability.

Getting To Outcomes. Developed by RAND, Getting To Outcomes® (GTO) builds capacity for implementing EBPs by strengthening the knowledge, attitudes, and skills needed to plan, implement, evaluate, improve, and sustain EBPs. GTO does this in ten "steps," by posing questions that program staff should address in order to obtain positive results. Each step represents an activity critical to running any program successfully (Chinman et al., 2008). The first six steps involve planning; the next two are process and outcome evaluation. The last two steps involve using data to improve and sustain programs. These steps are facilitated by the support system which provides (1) the GTO manual of text and tools published by the RAND Corporation in a variety of content domains including drug prevention (Chinman, Imm, & Wandersman, 2004) and underage drinking prevention (Imm et al., 2007); (2) face-to-face training; and (3) ongoing, technical assistance (TA). GTO has worked with a variety of delivery systems, in particular low-resource community-based settings where program staff have limited professional expertise in program implementation (e.g., Boys and Girls Clubs, community coalitions). In addition, the Centers for Disease Prevention and Control (CDC) used GTO to organize its teen pregnancy initiative from 2005 to 2010 and currently the Office of Adolescent Health has required its current grantees to use it in their teen pregnancy efforts. The Substance Abuse and Mental Health Services Administration has provided GTO guidance to those conducting town halls supporting underage drinking prevention. Several states have used it in contracting or to support evidence-based child welfare services (see descriptions at http://www.rand.org/health/projects/getting-to-outcomes/news.html).

GTOs effectiveness has been examined in several randomized trials. During the first randomized trial, researchers examined the impact of GTO on program staff responsible for running 30 existing prevention programs of varying types as part of a larger community-based coalition. This study found that higher exposure to GTO significantly improved knowledge and behaviors program staff needed to run a high-quality program. Programs that received the highest number of technical assistance hours showed the most program improvement (Acosta et al., 2013; Chinman et al., 2013). Multiple quasi-experimental trials have found similar results (Chinman et al., 2014; Hunter et al., 2009). A randomized control trial examined the impact of GTO on 16 Boys and Girls Clubs carrying out a teen pregnancy prevention EBP compared to 16 Boys and Girls Clubs implementing the same program without GTO (although the EBP was not substance-use prevention, the implementation process was very similar). After 2 years, those Clubs with GTO were rated by outside observers to run their programs better and with greater fidelity (Chinman, Acosta, Ebener, Malone, & Slaughter, 2015; Chinman, Acosta, Ebener, Malone, & Slaughter, 2016). Also, after 2 years, Clubs with GTO had greater improvement on several outcomes that mediate sex behavior than Clubs that did not use GTO (Chinman, Acosta, Ebener, Malone, & Slaughter, 2018). In these GTO studies, participating communities are typically provided only a small amount of funding as an award for participating, but not significant enough resources to hire new staff. GTO has not been evaluated for sustainability, but an ongoing RCT is assessing the cost and cost-effectiveness of GTO.

Communities that Care (CTC) (Hawkins, Catalano, & Arthur, 2002) is a prevention system created to provide drug prevention and delinquency prevention training and materials to community-based coalitions. Similar to GTO, the CTC approach prescribed that coalitions walk through several steps, including using the CTC Youth Survey to assess risk and protective factors in the community, selecting and implementing evidence-based drug and delinquency prevention programs targeted at the identified community risk factors, and evaluating outcomes (Arthur et al., 2007; Arthur, Hawkins, Pollard, Catalano, & Baglioni, 2002; Fagan, Hawkins, & Catalano, 2008; Glaser, Van Horn, Arthur, Hawkins, & Catalano, 2005). Participating coalitions receive funding to cover the staff and resources to run selected EBPs. The CTC prevention support system is intended to encourage adoption of EBPs to reduce community risk factors and build protective factors, and in turn reduce substance use and delinquent behaviors in youth in the community. Similar to GTO, CTC does not prescribe specific programs, but encourages the community-based coalition to choose EBPs that best address the community's risk factors.

Research has shown that the CTC system has been implemented with fidelity in communities (Quinby et al., 2008) and that CTC communities use more EBPs than non-CTC communities (Brown, Hawkins, Arthur, Briney, & Abbott, 2007). In addition, targeted risk factors have improved and the incidence of delinquent behavior has decreased 3 years after implementation of CTC in communities (Fagan, Hanson, Hawkins, & Arthur, 2008). A randomized trial of CTC coalitions in 24 small towns in 7 states (12 receiving CTC and 12 control matched within state) followed a panel of 4407 fifth-grade students annually through eighth grade and found that incidences of alcohol, cigarette and smokeless tobacco initiation, and delinquent behavior were significantly lower in CTC than in control communities for students in grades five through eight (Hawkins et al., 2009). A 2012 study also examined whether these gains could be sustained after study funding to coalitions ended. Twenty months after CTC funding to coalitions ended, 11 out of 12 coalitions had maintained a relatively high level of implementation fidelity; however, there was a downward trend in some of the benchmarks. Ability to sustain funding was the strongest predictor of sustainability. The one coalition that was not able to maintain funding dissolved (Gloppen, Arthur, Hawkins, & Shapiro, 2012). Additionally, research has shown that CTC is cost beneficial with a return of $5.30 (in the form of lower criminal justice, crime victim, and healthcare costs, and increased earnings and tax revenues) for every dollar invested in CTC (Kuklinski, Briney, Hawkins, & Catalano, 2012).

PROSPER: Similar to CTC, the PROmoting School–community–university Partnerships to Enhance Resilience (PROSPER) was designed as a prevention support system for substance use EBPs implemented in schools. PROSPER is built on the existing infrastructure of land grant universities' Cooperative Extension Systems (CES) and consists of a prevention coordinator from CES, teams of school-based stakeholders led by local CES staff, and a team of state-level university researchers and CES faculty. Prevention Coordinators act as an intermediary between the community and university teams, and provide ongoing, proactive technical assistance to school-based teams to support program delivery (Spoth, Clair, Greenberg, Redmond, & Shin, 2007; Spoth, Greenberg, Bierman, & Redmond, 2004).

Research has shown that PROSPER has improved participant recruitment (Spoth, Guyll, Lillehoj, Redmond, & Greenberg, 2007), maintenance of implementation quality (Spoth et al., 2007), and sustainability of intervention delivery (Greenberg et al., 2015), and has had positive effects on intervention-targeted youth and parent skills likely to reduce substance misuse (Redmond et al., 2009). After four and a half years, PROSPER has also been shown to significantly reduce students' substance misuse (Spoth et al., 2011). A recent randomized trial of PROSPER used a cohort sequential design with 28 public school districts (14 randomly assigned to PROSPER and 14 control) to follow 11,960 students from 6th to 12th grades to examine PROSPERs effects on student outcomes. The study found significantly lower substance misuse and significantly slower growth in misuse in the intervention group, as well as significantly greater intervention benefits for higher versus lower risk youth (Spoth et al., 2013). Research has also suggested that PROSPER is sustainable, with community teams generating funding and resources to sustain team operations and EBP implementation for 11 years (average of $23,000 per year) (Greenberg et al., 2015; Perkins et al., 2011). Another study (Guyll, Spoth, Crowley, & Jones, 2011) found that communities that make use of the PROSPER implementation support are able to implement family programs at lower costs at 59–67% less than comparable communities not using PROPSER (albeit not counting the cost of the implementation support itself).

Blueprints for Violence Prevention Initiative

The Blueprints for Violence Prevention Initiative ("Blueprints") is one of the largest EBP dissemination and replication efforts. The Center for the Study and Prevention of Violence at the University of Colorado first identified model violence and drug prevention programs using stringent criteria (improvement 1 year beyond treatment and replicated at more than one site (Mihalic, Irwin, Elliott, Fagan, & Hansen, 2001)). Then, using funds from the Office of Juvenile Justice and Delinquency Prevention, Blueprints provided funds and implementation support (ongoing technical assistance) to 42 communities across the USA to replicate the identified EBPs with a high degree of quality (Mihalic et al., 2002).

One of the most striking findings across the Blueprints replications was that most communities were initially unprepared to implement and sustain programs with fidelity (Elliott & Mihalic, 2004). Thus, building community capacity has become a critical component of supporting Blueprints model program replications. In particular, research on Blueprints programs has found that a well-connected and respected local champion, strong administrative support, formal organizational commitments and organizational staffing/stability, up-front commitment of necessary resources, program credibility within the community, and some potential for program routinization are the capacities that predict successful implementation (Elliott & Mihalic, 2004). A 2003 study of common implementation obstacles across 42 sites implementing eight of the Blueprints programs also found that the quality and, to a lesser extent, quantity of technical assistance were the most consistent and direct influences on implementation success (defined as program adherence, sustainability, dosage, and percent of core program components achieved (Mihalic & Irwin, 2003)).

Looking at these programs via the ISF multisystem framework and a CFIR lens suggests why these support models have generally been successful. The primary domain influenced by these prevention support systems is the CFIR *implementation process*. These models used external change agents to intensively improve communities' capacity to use a systematic implementation process—i.e., carry out key programming practices such as diagnosing needs, setting goals, and then choosing, planning, implementing, and evaluating EBPs. The capacity building used ongoing technical assistance and training to increase program implementers' knowledge, efficacy, and skills to implement EBPs (i.e., *individual characteristics*). These models also addressed various factors within the *inner setting*. For example, these approaches not only provided concrete resources (this varied with CTC covering the full costs of program implementation to GTO providing a small stipend), but they also attempted to increase program implementers' access to information, and change the norms, culture, implementation climate, and level of readiness among the community organizations. Another similarity across models is their use of collaborative groups (e.g., CTC coalitions, PROSPER community teams) comprised of stakeholders that are knowledgeable about the *outer setting* (e.g., community needs and resources, policies) and that can influence the *inner settings* responsible for program implementation (e.g., organizational culture and relationships). Finally, all of these approaches addressed the *intervention characteristics* domain by having participating communities choose an EBP from a small list or choose one program, collaboratively, with the research team. This arrangement favored implementation according to CFIR because the available programs had low costs (because the cost of the programs was covered by the research studies) and were likely perceived as having strong evidence (i.e., high evidence quality). Complexity, another *intervention characteristic* subdomain, may have also been favorably influenced because the communities received intensive technical assistance (compared to running other programs in which they would not have received any assistance). Our GTO research has shown that practitioners receiving implementation support perceive programs they are implementing as less complex (Hunter, Ober, Paddock, Hunt, & Levan, 2014). While these approaches did help communities understand their target population's needs more, for the most part, these approaches did not address the *outer setting*. For example these support systems were not in the position to establish requirements that the communities implement EBPs.

Government-Developed Synthesis and Translation and Support Systems

In addition to researchers and practitioners working to help disseminate effective programs, the federal government also works to support the dissemination of effective prevention programs and practices. Specifically, agencies such as SAMHSA, the Office of National Drug Control Policy, and the Department of Education have created opportunities (and sometimes requirements) for funding to states and communities. Consistent with the ISF's Prevention Support System, SAMHSA facilitates the adoption and utilization of effective programs among the states and Native American tribes through training and technical assistance (TA) centers. Specifically, SAMHSA's Center for the Application of Prevention Technologies (CAPT) is a national substance-use prevention training and TA system dedicated to strengthening prevention systems and improving the nation's behavioral health workforce. CAPT offers training and technical assistance to states and communities supported under SAMHSA's Substance Abuse Prevention and Treatment Block Grant program, and to SAMHSA's discretionary grant programs of regional and national significance (e.g., Partnership for Success grantees). The CAPT has regional centers to help promote capacities at different locations (e.g., states, tribes) and disseminate effective prevention strategies and programs.

State-level efforts include block grant funding from SAMHSA that has 20% funding set aside for effective prevention initiatives that are based on research evidence. This might be a specific program for certain populations, but also includes evidence-based strategies for community organization and environmental change (e.g., community coalitions, enforcing underage drinking laws). While many states benefitted from Safe and Drug Free Schools money through the 2000s, this funding consistently produced few outcomes and was reorganized to include shared funding from several agencies to offer grant support through programs such as Safe Schools Healthy Students and Drug Free Communities and Support Program. This latter initiative, funded through the Office of National Drug Control Policy (ONDCP), requires the development of a community coalition to facilitate the planning, implementation, and evaluation of these efforts. There is a priority to create lasting community changes in the community by addressing the underlying needs and conditions of substance use (e.g., availability, accessibility, social norms).

Other government grant-making efforts (e.g., ONDCP) and other agencies frequently require the use of evidence-based programming. Frequently, this is facilitated by requiring potential grantees to select specific programs from a predetermined list of evidence-based programs. Recognizing the challenge for prevention practitioners to identify and select effective programs/strategies that match identified needs (e.g., risk factors), these initiatives sometimes provide technical assistance to communities to select the best programs. Similarly, states frequently require that local communities implement evidence-based programs that they have identified to be effective. In some states, tribes, and jurisdictions (STJ), evidence-based workgroups (EBW) are convened to help promote the use of evidence-based programs across these settings. For example, Iowa's EBW was established in 2008 to provide guidance for its infrastructure grants (e.g., State SPF, Partnership for Success). The group, co-chaired by the Iowa Department of Public Health and the Iowa Department of Education, reviews and selects programs, policies, and practices relevant to the factors that underlie underage alcohol use and binge drinking. The EBW provides guidance on fidelity and requested EBP adaptations by funded counties. This group also developed a guide on the selection of EBPs which has been a helpful resource for the prevention field in Iowa.

While many states utilize their EBW for a grant program (e.g., state infrastructure grants), the initial intent was that the EBWs would be integrated into a state's block grant funding to ensure that all communities have knowledge about effective programs. Because implementing EBPs with fidelity remains a challenge, many states (e.g., South Carolina, Vermont) develop technical assistance systems in their states where staff are trained as coaches and provide in-person technical assistance on implementation.

To facilitate the dissemination of evidence-based programs in the areas of substance-use prevention and mental health promotion, a variety of evidence-based registries have been developed including those from the federal government. Specifically, SAMHSA sponsors the National Registry for Effective Programs and Practices (http://nrepp.samhsa.gov/landing.aspx, NREPP), the CDC sponsors the Community Guide (https://www.thecommunityguide.org/), and various other agencies and organizations maintain registries/clearinghouses in other content areas (e.g., education, criminal justice). The registries are primarily developed to ensure that practitioners have access to programs that have been shown to be effective. Thus, these registries are a good example of the ISF's synthesis and translation system, because they are designed to take information in journal articles and make them more easily accessible and understandable by community practitioners.

The most popular of all the registries is NREPP, which was initially developed in 1997 as a centralized repository where practitioners could access information about the effectiveness of substance-use prevention programs in a database searchable by program type, target population, desired outcome, and setting. The programs were originally categorized as Model, Effective, or Promising. These labels were discontinued in 2004 when a new type of "consumer reports" registry was developed that included a 4-point rating system in two major categories of information: the quality of the research and the readiness for dissemination. Programs accepted into NREPP received a summary score of 0 (low rating) to 4 (highest rating) on these two major categories. Consumers were able to review each program's findings and related scores to decide what level of evidence/dissemination they were willing to accept. This approach, which lasted about 10 years, caused significant confusion among communities. Many developers continued to present their programs as being "in NREPP" to mean being evidence based, even when their scores were very low. SAMHSA relaunched NREPP in late 2015, returning it to the old model of reviewing programs and assigning labels that very quickly reflect the amount and quality of the research evidence for each program (effective, promising, ineffective, or inconclusive). NREPP is also adding information about high-quality implementation, evaluation, cultural and behavioral health, and information from program developers and is actively looking for programs in addition to receiving nominations.

While NREPP has a strong focus on making available information about evidence-based programs and broad-level practices (e.g., Assisted Outpatient Treatment), the Community Preventive Services Task Force, established in 1996 by the US Department of Health and Human Services, publishes recommendations in the Community Guide to identify population health interventions that are scientifically proven to save lives, increase life spans, and improve quality of life. Many of these interventions include programs, services, and policies. Topics are varied and include alcohol and tobacco prevention/treatment as well as other areas such as policies/interventions that address obesity, diabetes, cancer, oral health, cancer, etc. The Task Force bases its recommendations on rigorous, replicable systematic reviews of scientific literature. These reviews are conducted, with Task Force oversight, by scientists and subject matter experts from the CDC in collaboration with a wide range of government, academic, policy, and practice-based partners. There are no voluntary submissions of programs/policies for the Community Guide as the recommendations/results published are entirely based on reviews and analyses of existing research literature.

Reviewing the government-developed efforts to support EBPs using CFIR reveals the challenges faced by community practitioners. The primary support the government provides is funding, which is one of the subdomains within the *inner setting*. However, compared to the vast number of schools and community-based organizations in the USA, only a small fraction receives funding. While organizations such as the CAPT and NREPP provide information about available EBPs to increase practitioner knowledge (a subdomain of *characteristics of individuals*), these efforts do not impact many of the other key domains and subdomains identified in CFIR and shown above to be critical for successfully implementing an EBP.

Promising Approaches: Social Bonds

Given the challenges in the provision of resources necessary to implement effective prevention programming, innovative funding approaches such as "Pay for Success" financing models (PFS, also known as "Social Innovation Bonds") are starting to be used (e.g., see https://obamawhitehouse.archives.gov/administration/eop/sicp/initiatives/pay-for-success). These initiatives engage nontraditional funding sources, such as the private sector (e.g., investment banks), to provide initial resources for program implementation. A set of performance metrics is negotiated between the investors, an intermediary that oversees program implementation, and the traditional funding source, usually the government. Following initial program implementation (typically 3–5 years), an independent evaluator determines whether the performance targets are met. If targets are met, then the traditional funding source pays back the private sector funders through the intermediary plus interest. The payments are typically based on an estimate of the program costs and benefits. For example, the costs of operating the program (e.g., training, staffing, program materials) and the program benefits (e.g., the reduction in juvenile justice costs, such as number of youth diverted from the juvenile justice system) are estimated as part of the payment structure.

Estimated benefits of PFS models include the emphasis on the use of effective prevention models using an influx of new funding sources (Roman, 2015). Challenges to the use of PFS models include a complex arrangement between multiple entities, identification and negotiation of performance targets, a program payment structure, and a guaranteed source of payment plus interest at the end of the initial program period (Lantz, Rosenbaum, Ku, & Iovan, 2016). While there are over 40 PFS initiatives currently under way across the USA, the success of these approaches in building the capacity of local communities to provide effective prevention programming is not well known (Callanan, Law, & Mendonca, 2012). That is, the impact of these initiatives to lead to long-lasting improvements in the delivery of effective substance-use prevention programming is currently based more on theory than data. Only time will tell whether PFS initiatives facilitate the institutionalization of EBPs.

Implications and Future Directions

Implementation science theory, in particular CFIR, can be used to understand the successes and challenges of previous efforts to improve EBP implementation. Different risk and protective factors can influence any individual youth to use substances. Analogously, as shown above, many factors can influence an organization's ability to adopt and run an EBP successfully. If one were to consider how prevention EBPs could have a much larger impact in the nation than they have had to date, what would the above review suggest about how to accomplish that? Studies of research-developed support and delivery systems discussed above have shown that with investment of some funds, personnel, translation, and support, individual communities can implement EBPs well. Looking at CFIR shows why: several subdomains of the *inner setting*, *individual characteristics*, and *implementation process* domains were addressed by such projects. They provided resources (some more than others) and built capacity at the group level (*inner setting*—could be a coalition or school) and at the individual level (*individual characteristics*) to engage in all the key steps of prevention (including setting goals, planning, using data to improve) and follow a certain *implementation process* that included working with key stakeholders. Further, most of these initiatives did not make communities choose from all the available programs, but instead presented communities with a short list of EBPs in such a way that addressed many of the *intervention characteristics* subdomains (e.g., evidence strength, complexity). However, what is notable about the implementation research described above is the finding that results were achieved without really addressing the *outer setting* domain (overall, policies to promote and provide incentives for high-quality prevention across public schools are minimal). Instead, what is consistent in these projects is that the participating coalitions/schools/community groups demonstrated some level of readiness to engage in these projects (i.e., agreed to participate in a study). Their innate willingness appeared to obviate the need for outside mandates.

Compare the impact of these research-developed efforts to the government-developed efforts, which have had modest impact. First, most communities do not receive government funding for EBPs, even communities that do typically receive much less outside support to engage in a genuine implementation process. Thus, domains like the *inner setting*, *individual characteristics*, and *implementation process* are not as impacted by these grants. Structural and program-type support systems like the CAPT, NREPP, The Community Guides are helpful, but are not of sufficient intensity to improve the use of prevention EBPs across the nation as a whole. These efforts tend to build some knowledge and can be a useful component of an overall strategy, but by themselves do not address most of the CFIR domains.

Using CFIR, certain changes to how EBPs are organized and funded could improve implementation. To increase the successful implementation of prevention EBPs overall, a first step could be to strengthen and, in some cases to introduce, a mandate to use EBPs. Given that most coalitions/schools/community groups are not inherently able and willing to conduct EBPs (as shown in studies reviewed in the "Status of the Dissemination" section above), concrete incentives and rewards for participation and consequences for not participating could strengthen adoption. Over time, if all schools for example are supposed to run EBPs, a peer pressure (another *outer setting* subdomain) could build up, which would further reinforce implementation. Along with such a mandate, communities would need better *access to EBPs* and *implementation support*.

Access mostly means funding. Currently, many of the federal and state resources mentioned above award grant funding to a relatively small number of communities, relative to the nationwide need. However, many EBPs are not expensive. Thus, as an alternative, smaller amounts of funding could be dispersed to a much wider number of communities for greater impact.

Research shows that community organizations, including schools, clearly need support to implement EBPs well. However, like funding for the EBPs themselves, there are not large amounts of funds available to deliver intensive support. Yet, research has found that even a modest amount of support could go a long way. In our study of using GTO to support the implementation of an EBP in Boys and Girls Clubs, only 32 h of TA time a year was needed to help the Clubs adopt and implement programming that achieved outcomes. Research on CTC has shown that even factoring in the cost of the assistance, the money saved due to better outcomes outweighed the costs. Further, EBP developers and implementation support system developers could collaborate on developing streamlined tools to help users set goals, assess their fit and capacity to run the program, make detailed plans, and conduct simple evaluation of implementation and outcomes. Such tools could be appended to EBPs when they are distributed. Federal and state funds could be used to deploy a set of TA providers to support communities for the EBPs most widely adopted. Given the GTO, CTC, and PROSPER results, even a small number of these providers in each state could make a big impact on EBP implementation.

In disadvantaged or minority communities, more attention is needed to develop EBPs that work for those communities. EBPs vary in terms of how difficult and how costly they are to implement *(intervention characteristics)*. In particular, it can be difficult to find universal programs designed for high-risk youth in disadvantaged and minority communities. While EBP registries like NREPP offer search functions to find EBPs that have included minority populations in samples from the original research studies, they often do not have information about whether these programs are beneficial specifically for various minority or disadvantaged populations (i.e., via subgroup analyses). That is because those studies have typically not been conducted. More research is needed to not only develop programs that work in these communities, but also test whether existing programs (already deemed EBPs) work in these communities. In addition, NREPP could invest in this important area by more proactively identifying programs and practices for review that show promising outcomes in culturally diverse and underserved populations. Further, supporting the development of practice-based evidence, especially for programs developed for those in disadvantaged communities and underserved populations through NREPP's revised Learning Center (https://nrepp-learning.samhsa.gov/), has the potential to significantly address issues related to the development and use of culturally appropriate programs across all settings.

Disadvantaged and minority communities may especially benefit from resources and support to achieve strong implementation of EBPs. Tools and TA could be of most assistance in disadvantaged and minority communities, which tend to receive less funding for these types of support. The Surgeon General's report (U.S. Department of Health and Human Services, 2016) addresses this area as a priority of focus to ensure that evidence-based programs (and even program components) address sociocultural factors that exist for various populations. If one goal is to ensure population-level exposure (and outcomes) including various subgroups, there is a need to assess the needs and conditions of local participants and then provide adequate support so they can make the necessary adaptations while preserving the integrity of the program (Burlew, Copeland, Ahuama-Jonas, & Calsyn, 2013; Chinman et al., 2004). The report highlights some key areas for this including the utilization of diverse coalitions to promote cultural responsiveness in programming, clear understanding of population needs and fit, and enhancing of capacities of those who implement programs (U.S. Department of Health and Human Services, 2016).

Conclusion

When implemented well across a population, EBPs can have impacts that save more dollars than they cost to operate. While most communities and schools are not using EBPs, studies of implementation support efforts demonstrate that community practitioners can adopt EBPs and run them well when provided adequate support. Use of implementation science theories reveals why some efforts at improving community-based implementation are stronger than others. These theories also offer guidance about what changes could be made to better support community-based organizations in their EBP implementation. Disadvantaged and minority communities would benefit from additional research identifying which EBPs work for their own communities and from receiving implementation support on how to adapt EBPs to their own communities. These changes could vastly improve the level of EBP implementation.

References

Acosta, J., Chinman, M., Ebener, P., Malone, P. S., Paddock, S., Phillips, A., ... Slaughter, M. E. (2013). An intervention to improve program implementation: Findings from a two-year cluster randomized trial of Assets-Getting To Outcomes. *Implementation Science, 8*, 87. https://doi.org/10.1186/1748-5908-8-87

Arthur, M. W., Briney, J. S., Hawkins, J. D., Abbott, R. D., Brooke-Weiss, B. L., & Catalano, R. F. (2007). Measuring risk and protection in communities using the Communities That Care Youth Survey. *Evaluation and Program Planning, 30*(2), 197–211. https://doi.org/10.1016/j.evalprogplan.2007.01.009

Arthur, M. W., Hawkins, J. D., Pollard, J. A., Catalano, R. F., & Baglioni, A. J., Jr. (2002). Measuring risk and protective factors for substance use, delinquency, and other adolescent problem behaviors. The Communities That Care Youth Survey. *Evaluation Review, 26*(6), 575–601.

Barrera, M., Jr., & Sandler, I. N. (2006). Prevention: A report of progress and momentum into the future. *Clinical Psychology Science and Practice, 13*(3), 221–226.

Beets, M. W., Flay, B. R., Vuchinich, S., Acock, A. C., Li, K. K., & Allred, C. (2008). School climate and teachers' beliefs and attitudes associated with implementation of the positive action program: A diffusion of innovations model. *Prevention Science, 9*(4), 264–275. https://doi.org/10.1007/s11121-008-0100-2

Brown, E. C., Hawkins, J. D., Arthur, M. W., Briney, J. S., & Abbott, R. D. (2007). Effects of Communities That Care on prevention services systems: Findings from the community youth development study at 1.5 years. *Prevention Science, 8*(3), 180–191. https://doi.org/10.1007/s11121-007-0068-3

Burlew, A. K., Copeland, V. C., Ahuama-Jonas, C., & Calsyn, D. A. (2013). Does cultural adaptation have a role in substance abuse treatment? *Social Work in Public Health, 28*(3–4), 440–460. https://doi.org/10.1080/19371918.2013.774811

Callanan, L., Law, J., & Mendonca, L. (2012). *From potential to action: Bringing social impact bonds to the US*. New York, NY: McKinsey&Company.

Center for Behavioral Health Statistics and Quality. (2015). *Results from the 2015 National Survey on Drug Use and Health: Detailed tables*. Rockville, MD: Author.

Chinman, M., Acosta, J., Ebener, P., Burkhart, Q., Malone, P. S., Paddock, S. M., ... Tellett-Royce, N. (2013). Intervening with practitioners to improve the quality of prevention: One-year findings from a randomized trial of assets-getting to outcomes. *The Journal of Primary Prevention, 34*(3), 173–191. https://doi.org/10.1007/s10935-013-0302-7

Chinman, M., Acosta, J., Ebener, P., Malone, P. S., & Slaughter, M. (2015). A novel test of the GTO implementation support intervention in low resource settings: Year 1 findings and challenges. *Implementation Science, 10*(suppl 1), A34.

Chinman, M., Acosta, J., Ebener, P., Malone, P. S., & Slaughter, M. (2018). A cluster-randomized trial of Getting To Outcomes' impact on sexual health outcomes in community-based settings. *Prevention Science, 19*, 437–448.

Chinman, M., Acosta, J., Ebener, P., Malone, P. S., & Slaughter, M. E. (2016). Can implementation support help community-based settings better deliver evidence-based sexual health promotion programs? A randomized trial of Getting To Outcomes(R). *Implementation Science, 11*(1), 78. https://doi.org/10.1186/s13012-016-0446-y

Chinman, M., Ebener, P., Burkhart, Q., Osilla, K. C., Imm, P., Paddock, S. M., & Wright, P. A. (2014). Evaluating the impact of getting to outcomes-underage drinking on prevention capacity and alcohol merchant attitudes and selling behaviors. *Prevention Science, 15*(4), 485–496. https://doi.org/10.1007/s11121-013-0389-3

Chinman, M., Hunter, S. B., Ebener, P., Paddock, S. M., Stillman, L., Imm, P., & Wandersman, A. (2008). The getting to outcomes demonstration and evaluation: An illustration of the prevention support system. *American Journal of Community Psychology, 41*(3–4), 206–224. https://doi.org/10.1007/s10464-008-9163-2

Chinman, M., Imm, P., & Wandersman, A. (2004). *Getting To Outcomes™ 2004: Promoting accountability through methods and tools for planning, implementation, and evaluation*. Retrieved from http://www.rand.org/pubs/technical_reports/TR101.html

Cho, H., Dion Hallfors, D., Iritani, B. J., & Hartman, S. (2009). The influence of "No Child Left Behind" legislation on drug prevention in US schools. *Evaluation Review, 33*(5), 446–463. https://doi.org/10.1177/0193841X09335050

Cooper, B. R., Bumbarger, B. K., & Moore, J. E. (2015). Sustaining evidence-based prevention programs: Correlates in a large-scale dissemination initiative. *Prevention Science, 16*(1), 145–157. https://doi.org/10.1007/s11121-013-0427-1

D'Amico, E. J., Edelen, M. O., Miles, J. N., & Morral, A. R. (2008). The longitudinal association between substance use and delinquency among high-risk youth. *Drug and Alcohol Dependence, 93*(1–2), 85–92. https://doi.org/10.1016/j.drugalcdep.2007.09.006

D'Amico, E. J., Ellickson, P. L., Collins, R. L., Martino, S., & Klein, D. J. (2005). Processes linking adolescent problems to substance-use problems in late young adulthood. *Journal of Studies on Alcohol, 66*(6), 766–775.

Damschroder, L. J., Aron, D. C., Keith, R. E., Kirsh, S. R., Alexander, J. A., & Lowery, J. C. (2009). Fostering implementation of health services research findings into practice: A consolidated framework for advancing implementation science. *Implementation Science, 4*, 50. https://doi.org/10.1186/1748-5908-4-50

Eccles, M. P., & Mittman, B. S. (2006). Welcome to implementation science. *Implementation Science, 1*(1), 1. https://doi.org/10.1186/1748-5908-1-1

Elliott, D. S., & Mihalic, S. (2004). Issues in disseminating and replicating effective prevention programs. *Prevention Science, 5*(1), 47–53.

Ennett, S. T., Ringwalt, C. L., Thorne, J., Rohrbach, L. A., Vincus, A., Simons-Rudolph, A., & Jones, S. (2003). A comparison of current practice in school-based substance use prevention programs with meta-analysis findings. *Prevention Science, 4*(1), 1–14.

Fagan, A., Hawkins, J., & Catalano, R. (2008). Using community epidemiologic data to improve social settings: The Communities That Care prevention system. In M. Shinn & H. Yoshikawa (Eds.), *Toward positive youth development transforming schools and community programs* (pp. 292–312). New York, NY: Oxford University Press.

Fagan, A. A., Hanson, K., Hawkins, J. D., & Arthur, M. W. (2008). Bridging science to practice: Achieving prevention program implementation fidelity in the community youth development study. *American Journal of Community Psychology, 41*(3–4), 235–249. https://doi.org/10.1007/s10464-008-9176-x

Ford, J. (2005). Substance use, the social bond, and delinquency. *Sociological Inquiry, 75*, 109–128.

Forman, S. G., Olin, S. S., Hoagwood, K. E., Crowe, M., & Saka, N. (2009). Evidence-based interventions in schools: Developers' views of implementation barriers and facilitators. *School Mental Health, 1*, 26–36.

Glaser, R., Van Horn, M., Arthur, M., Hawkins, J., & Catalano, R. (2005). Measurement properties of the Communities That Care Youth Survey across demographic groups. *Journal of Quantitative Criminology, 21*(1), 73–102.

Gloppen, K. M., Arthur, M. W., Hawkins, J. D., & Shapiro, V. B. (2012). Sustainability of the Communities That Care prevention system by coalitions participating in the Community Youth Development Study. *The Journal of Adolescent Health, 51*(3), 259–264. https://doi.org/10.1016/j.jadohealth.2011.12.018

Greenberg, M. T., Feinberg, M. E., Johnson, L. E., Perkins, D. F., Welsh, J. A., & Spoth, R. L. (2015). Factors that predict financial sustainability of community coalitions: Five years of findings from the PROSPER partnership project. *Prevention Science, 16*(1), 158–167. https://doi.org/10.1007/s11121-014-0483-1

Guyll, M., Spoth, R., Crowley, D. M., & Jones, D. (2011). *Economic analysis of the PROSPER partnership trial: Direct costs and substance use outcomes 18 months past baseline*. Paper presented at the Society for Prevention Research 19th Annual Meeting, Washington, DC.

Hallfors, D., & Godette, D. (2002). Will the 'principles of effectiveness' improve prevention practice? Early findings from a diffusion study. *Health Education Research, 17*(4), 461–470.

Hawkins, J. D., Catalano, R. F., & Arthur, M. W. (2002). Promoting science-based prevention in communities. *Addictive Behaviors, 27*(6), 951–976.

Hawkins, J. D., Oesterle, S., Brown, E. C., Arthur, M. W., Abbott, R. D., Fagan, A. A., & Catalano, R. F. (2009). Results of a type 2 translational research trial to prevent adolescent drug use and delinquency: A test of

Communities That Care. *Archives of Pediatrics & Adolescent Medicine, 163*(9), 789–798. https://doi.org/10.1001/archpediatrics.2009.141

Hogan, J. A., Baca, I., Daley, C., Garcia, T., Jaker, J., Lowther, M., & Klitzner, M. (2003). Disseminating science-based prevention: Lessons learned from CSAP's CAPTs. *Journal of Drug Education, 33*(3), 233–243.

Holder, H. D. (2009). Current challenges faced by efforts to prevent alcohol and other drug problems: Lessons from science-to-practice. *Drug and Alcohol Review, 28*(2), 99–102. https://doi.org/10.1111/j.1465-3362.2008.00037.x

Hunter, S. B., Chinman, M., Ebener, P., Imm, P., Wandersman, A., & Ryan, G. W. (2009). Technical assistance as a prevention capacity-building tool: A demonstration using the getting to outcomes framework. *Health Education & Behavior, 36*(5), 810–828. https://doi.org/10.1177/1090198108329999

Hunter, S. B., Ober, A. J., Paddock, S. M., Hunt, P. E., & Levan, D. (2014). Continuous quality improvement (CQI) in addiction treatment settings: Design and intervention protocol of a group randomized pilot study. *Addiction Science & Clinical Practice, 9*, 4. https://doi.org/10.1186/1940-0640-9-4

Imm, P., Chinman, M., Wandersman, A., Rosenbloom, D., Guckenburg, S., & Leis, R. (2007). *Preventing underage drinking: Using getting to outcomes with the SAMHSA strategic prevention framework to achieve results* (TR-403-SAMHSA). Santa Monica, CA: RAND. Retrieved from http://www.rand.org/pubs/technical_reports/TR403/

Johnston, L. D., O'Malley, P. M., Miech, R. A., Bachman, J. G., & Schulenberg, J. E. (2016). *Monitoring the future national survey results on drug use, 1975–2015: Overview, key findings on adolescent drug use.* Ann Arbor, MI: Institute for Social Research, The University of Michigan.

Kuklinski, M. R., Briney, J. S., Hawkins, J. D., & Catalano, R. F. (2012). Cost-benefit analysis of communities that care outcomes at eighth grade. *Prevention Science, 13*(2), 150–161. https://doi.org/10.1007/s11121-011-0259-9

Kumar, R., O'Malley, P. M., Johnston, L. D., & Laetz, V. B. (2013). Alcohol, tobacco, and other drug use prevention programs in U.S. schools: A descriptive summary. *Prevention Science, 14*(6), 581–592. https://doi.org/10.1007/s11121-012-0340-z

Lantz, P. M., Rosenbaum, S., Ku, L., & Iovan, S. (2016). Pay for success and population health: Early results from eleven projects reveal challenges and promise. *Health Affairs, 35*(11), 2053–2061. https://doi.org/10.1377/hlthaff.2016.0713

Levy, S., Sherritt, L., Gabrielli, J., Shrier, L. A., & Knight, J. R. (2009). Screening adolescents for substance use-related high-risk sexual behaviors. *Journal of Adolescent Health, 45*(5), 473–477. https://doi.org/10.1016/j.jadohealth.2009.03.028

Little, M. A., Pokhrel, P., Sussman, S., & Rohrbach, L. A. (2015). The process of adoption of evidence-based tobacco use prevention programs in California schools. *Prevention Science, 16*(1), 80–89. https://doi.org/10.1007/s11121-013-0457-8

Mihalic, S., Ballard, D., Michalski, A., Tortorice, J., Cunningham, L., & Argamaso, S. (2002). *Blueprints for violence prevention, violence initiative: Final process evaluation report.* Boulder, CO: Center for the Study and Prevention of Violence, Institute of Behavioral Science, University of Colorado.

Mihalic, S., Irwin, K., Elliott, D., Fagan, A., & Hansen, D. (2001). *Blueprints for violence prevention.* Washington, DC: US Department of Justice, Office of Justice Programs.

Mihalic, S. F., & Irwin, K. (2003). Blueprints for violence prevention from research to real-world settings—Factors influencing the successful replication of model programs. *Youth Violence and Juvenile Justice, 1*(4), 307–329.

Payne, A. A., & Eckert, R. (2010). The relative importance of provider, program, school, and community predictors of the implementation quality of school-based prevention programs. *Prevention Science, 11*(2), 126–141. https://doi.org/10.1007/s11121-009-0157-6

Perkins, D. F., Feinberg, M. E., Greenberg, M. T., Johnson, L. E., Chilenski, S. M., Mincemoyer, C. C., & Spoth, R. L. (2011). Team factors that predict to sustainability indicators for community-based prevention teams. *Evaluation and Program Planning, 34*(3), 283–291. https://doi.org/10.1016/j.evalprogplan.2010.10.003

Quinby, R., Fagan, A., Hanson, K., Brooke-Weiss, B., Arthur, M., & Hawkins, J. (2008). Installing the communities that care prevention system: Implementation progress and fidelity in a randomized controlled trial. *Journal of Community Psychology, 36*(3), 313–332.

Rapkin, B. D., Weiss, E. S., Lounsbury, D. W., Thompson, H. S., Goodman, R. M., Schechter, C. B., … Padgett, D. K. (2012). Using the interactive systems framework to support a quality improvement approach to dissemination of evidence-based strategies to promote early detection of breast cancer: Planning a comprehensive dynamic trial. *American Journal of Community Psychology, 50*(3–4), 497–517. https://doi.org/10.1007/s10464-012-9518-6

Redmond, C., Spoth, R. L., Shin, C., Schainker, L. M., Greenberg, M. T., & Feinberg, M. (2009). Long-term protective factor outcomes of evidence-based interventions implemented by community teams through a community-university partnership. *Journal of Primary Prevention, 30*(5), 513–530. https://doi.org/10.1007/s10935-009-0189-5

Ringwalt, C., Hanley, S., Vincus, A. A., Ennett, S. T., Rohrbach, L. A., & Bowling, J. M. (2008). The prevalence of effective substance use prevention curricula in the nation's high schools. *Journal of Primary Prevention, 29*(6), 479–488. https://doi.org/10.1007/s10935-008-0158-4

Ringwalt, C., Vincus, A. A., Hanley, S., Ennett, S. T., Bowling, J. M., & Rohrbach, L. A. (2009). The prevalence of evidence-based drug use prevention curricula in U.S. middle schools in 2005. *Prevention*

Science, 10(1), 33–40. https://doi.org/10.1007/s11121-008-0112-y

Ringwalt, C. L., Ennett, S., Vincus, A., Thorne, J., Rohrbach, L. A., & Simons-Rudolph, A. (2002). The prevalence of effective substance use prevention curricula in U.S. middle schools. *Prevention Science, 3*(4), 257–265.

Roman, J. (2015). *Solving the wrong pockets problem: How pay for success promotes investment in evidence-based best practices*. Washington, DC: Urban Institute.

Silvia, E. S., & Thorne, J. (1997). *School-based drug prevention programs: A longitudinal study in selected school districts*. Research Triangle Park, NC: Research Triangle Institute.

Spoth, R., Clair, S., Greenberg, M., Redmond, C., & Shin, C. (2007). Toward dissemination of evidence-based family interventions: Maintenance of community-based partnership recruitment results and associated factors. *Journal of Family Psychology, 21*(2), 137–146. https://doi.org/10.1037/0893-3200.21.2.137

Spoth, R., Greenberg, M., Bierman, K., & Redmond, C. (2004). PROSPER community-university partnership model for public education systems: Capacity-building for evidence-based, competence-building prevention. *Prevention Science, 5*(1), 31–39.

Spoth, R., Guyll, M., Lillehoj, C. J., Redmond, C., & Greenberg, M. (2007). Prosper study of evidence-based intervention implementation quality by community-university partnerships. *Journal of Community Psychology, 35*(8), 981–999. https://doi.org/10.1002/jcop.20207

Spoth, R., Redmond, C., Clair, S., Shin, C., Greenberg, M., & Feinberg, M. (2011). Preventing substance misuse through community-university partnerships: randomized controlled trial outcomes 4½ years past baseline. *American Journal of Preventive Medicine, 40*(4), 440–447. https://doi.org/10.1016/j.amepre.2010.12.012

Spoth, R., Redmond, C., Shin, C., Greenberg, M., Clair, S., & Feinberg, M. (2007). Substance-use outcomes at 18 months past baseline: The PROSPER Community-University Partnership Trial. *American Journal of Preventive Medicine, 32*(5), 395–402. https://doi.org/10.1016/j.amepre.2007.01.014

Spoth, R., Redmond, C., Shin, C., Greenberg, M., Feinberg, M., & Schainker, L. (2013). PROSPER community-university partnership delivery system effects on substance misuse through 6 1/2 years past baseline from a cluster randomized controlled intervention trial. *Preventive Medicine, 56*(3–4), 190–196. https://doi.org/10.1016/j.ypmed.2012.12.013

Tibbits, M. K., Bumbarger, B. K., Kyler, S. J., & Perkins, D. F. (2010). Sustaining evidence-based interventions under real-world conditions: Results from a large-scale diffusion project. *Prevention Science, 11*(3), 252–262. https://doi.org/10.1007/s11121-010-0170-9

Tucker, J. S., Ellickson, P. L., Orlando, M., Martino, S. C., & Klein, D. J. (2005). Substance use trajectories from early adolescence to emerging adulthood: A comparison of smoking, binge drinking, and marijuana use. *Journal of Drug Issues, 35*, 307–332.

U.S. Department of Education, Office of Planning, Evaluation and Policy Development, Policy and Program Studies Service. (2011). *Prevalence and implementation Fidelity of research-based prevention programs in public schools: Final report*. Washington, DC: Author.

U.S. Department of Health and Human Services. (1985). *Report of the Secretary's Task Force on Black and Minority Health: Volume I: The executive summary*. Includes bibliographical references and appendices. (Document) MH10D9924. Washington, DC: Author. xii, 239 p. Retrieved from https://minorityhealth.hhs.gov/assets/pdf/checked/1/ANDERSON.pdf

U.S. Department of Health and Human Services. (2016). *Facing addiction in America. The surgeon general's report on alcohol, drugs, and health*. Washington, DC: Author.

Wandersman, A., Chien, V. H., & Katz, J. (2012). Toward an evidence-based system for innovation support for implementing innovations with quality: Tools, training, technical assistance, and quality assurance/quality improvement. *American Journal of Community Psychology, 50*(3–4), 445–459. https://doi.org/10.1007/s10464-012-9509-7

Wandersman, A., Duffy, J., Flaspohler, P., Noonan, R., Lubell, K., Stillman, L., … Saul, J. (2008). Bridging the gap between prevention research and practice: The interactive systems framework for dissemination and implementation. *American Journal of Community Psychology, 41*(3–4), 171–181. https://doi.org/10.1007/s10464-008-9174-z

24. Supporting Prevention Science and Prevention Research Internationally

Jeremy Segrott

Prevention Science

Substance misuse is a global phenomenon and represents a major public health issue worldwide. Though the exact nature and patterning of the problem varies across countries there are also striking similarities which provide a starting point for thinking about substance misuse internationally. Similar risk and protective factors are seen in contrasting national contexts. For example, parenting practices and family relationships have been identified as key influences on young people's substance-related behaviours in a wide range of settings, including the United States of America, European countries, and Asia (Kumpfer and Alvarado, 2003; McArdle, et al. 2002; Yen, et al. 2007). Similarly, the short and longterm health effects of substance misuse by young people manifest themselves across contrasting cultural and socio-economic settings. There is growing recognition by national governments and local health systems that primary prevention of substance misuse is key to addressing this public health issue. Whilst the development and effectiveness of prevention efforts vary widely, many countries have introduced prevention initiatives aimed at young people that address known risk and protective factors. School- and family-based interventions are common in many parts of the world for instance. At their best such efforts comprise well-theorised interventions with clear mechanisms of action, and they operate within broader prevention systems which support intervention development, evaluation and long-term implementation. But there is considerable variation in the development of prevention systems, particularly when comparing high and low/middle income nations.

Whilst prevention science has always had international connections and networks, it could be argued that its early development sat primarily within national systems and organisations. In recent years there has been increasing interest in the development of international collaborations and networks within the field. We might think of two related, though distinct, ways in which this has occurred. First, there have been various attempts to develop prevention systems and prevention science in countries where they had not hitherto been established or extensive. So for instance, countries which have previously not supported prevention activities have now begun to develop, evaluate and implement evidence-based interventions. Another indicator of the growth of prevention science internationally has been the formation of academic societies in Australia, Europe and South America, which are built on the earlier formation of the SPR in the United States. This could be thought of as a form of globalisation of prevention science and the

J. Segrott (✉)
Centre for Trials Research, DECIPHer Centre,
Cardiff University, Cardiff, Wales, UK
e-mail: segrottj@cardiff.ac.uk

creation of prevention systems, which whilst interconnected exist primarily to address the public health needs of a nation or region. Traditionally prevention science and systems have been distributed unevenly with a concentration of resources and prevention systems in high-income countries. The lack of resources and capacity within lower and middle-income countries has been noted as a key challenge (Romano and Israelashvili, 2017; Catalano et al., 2012), and efforts to build networks in these settings have increased, the formation of the Brazilian Association for Research on Prevention and Health Promotion (BRAPEP) for instance being an example of this.

Alongside the development of prevention systems that address the needs of national and regional population health needs, there have also been important efforts to develop various forms of international connections and networks which link these systems, and the researchers and practitioners working within them. Whilst differing in their structure and specific aims, what unites these efforts is the goal of building capacity through the sharing of knowledge, skills and resources (financial, cognitive and technical). For example, collaboration between researchers working in different national contexts brings together previously separate bodies of knowledge on the factors shaping young people's use of substances, enables the transfer of interventions developed and implemented in one country to new settings and permits studies which evaluate programmes delivered simultaneously in multiple countries. The activities needed for these networks and collaborations are multifaceted but include linking national prevention systems, enabling the sharing of knowledge (e.g. research findings) across national boundaries and building of collaborative partnerships. These activities form part of building an international prevention system, which whilst still uneven and fragmented has and continues to make an important contribution to the development of the field. International prevention science is characterised by a commitment to collaborate with others, and to share knowledge. It values difference and diversity and recognises that we can learn from different experiences and cultures and appreciate the situatedness of our perspectives and assumptions.

The Importance of International Prevention Science

International Networks as Advocates for Building National Prevention Systems

Following Hosman and Clayton (2000) we might think of three interconnected rationales for the building of international prevention science. The first concerns the role of international networks in helping to promote the development of prevention activities in countries where they are poorly resourced, and where government support for prevention may be lacking. Especially in contexts where prevention scientists may be limited in number, international networks can help generate the critical mass needed to advocate for government resources and health policies to promote prevention activities. Such advocacy is also important for the provision of adequate funding for prevention infrastructure which enables new interventions to be designed in line with existing evidence, and to be evaluated prior to decisions being made about wide-scale implementation. International networks can also provide a way of sharing knowledge and expertise on how to build prevention science systems, and effective strategies for building research capacity within a country.

Developing the Evidence Base Within Prevention Science Through International Networks and Collaboration

Secondly, as Hosman and Clayton rightly note, the field of prevention science is a broad and complex one, taking in as it does the aetiology of substance misuse, theorisation of mechanisms through which interventions can modify behaviours, implementation of these interventions in a range of settings and the science of how to evaluate these interventions. No one country—however well resourced—possesses all the resources, knowledge or experience needed to address these questions. Collaboration across countries can increase intellectual capacity and financial resources to address some of the key questions which prevention science is currently grappling with. Bringing together researchers, policymakers and practitioners from different geographical and cultural contexts also offers other potential benefits. There are opportunities to be exposed to different sets of knowledge, experience and perspectives, and to reflect on the cultural assumptions and specificity of our knowledge and practices. We can develop our understanding of how key risk and protective factors function by learning about how they may operate differently in contrasting cultural and political contexts. As Freshwater, Sherwood, and Drury (2006) argue, "International research collaboration presents health researchers with opportunities to share experiences, data and methods that can provide the basis for new and important perspectives on existing practices" (p. 296). These benefits accrue both to the teams involved in collaboration and to the individual researchers who form part of them.

A key basis on which all research collaborations are enabled is the sharing of knowledge. Academic journals, institutional websites and social media enable individuals to discover others working on similar issues, read the findings of their work and identify potential collaborators or interventions which they might implement. Face-to-face events (conferences, seminars) perform a similar role, both through formal presentations and informal conversations and chance encounters which take place at such events. Sometimes when researchers access such information it does not lead to collaboration but provides a source of information (on how to build capacity, theoretical frameworks which might be applied within a new intervention or approaches to methodological designs) which researchers then apply within their own research teams. However, these exchanges are also often an essential stepping stone to the development of collaborations across national borders and the identification of international colleagues whom it might be fruitful to work with.

These flows of information and encounters between researchers therefore provide the basis on which collaborations across national borders can develop. They sometimes begin with informal discussions or more formal collaboration in conference symposia, visits to respective research teams or use of online meetings (teleconferences, Skype, etc.) to explore avenues for collaboration in more depth. Where they lead to the formation of international research teams these may take various forms. A researcher, or group of researchers, may wish to conduct a study within their own local setting, and engage researchers from other countries to provide input—perhaps on specific aspects of the project. For instance, project teams may involve international colleagues to provide leadership on the process evaluation or health economic evaluation component of a randomised controlled trial (RCT). Involvement of international colleagues in this way may reflect the fact that the particular form of expertise or skills does not exist (or is limited) in the country where the research is taking place, and that prevention science draws on interdisciplinary and specialised knowledge which may only be held by a few individuals. Such international collaboration is also about identifying individuals who can work well within a team, have an appreciation of the value of international work and understand its challenges and how they can be overcome. As with all collaboration, international research depends on the formation of effective relationships. Another form of international collaboration comprises studies that take place simultaneously across multiple countries. For example, the EUDAP study tested the Unplugged substance-misuse prevention intervention in schools in seven European countries (Giannotta, et al., 2014).

In Hosman and Clayton's description of international work, a third key rationale is that collaboration and knowledge exchange allow interventions which have been implemented and found to be effective in one national setting to be replicated in new contexts. Such sharing of interventions avoids wasteful duplication of resources, and enables knowledge and expertise developed in one location to be harnessed to inform the implementation of the intervention in its new context. The replication of interventions in new settings also builds knowledge at a broader level about the extent to which the risk and protective factors affecting substance misuse might vary in different contexts, and therefore the degree to which intervention theories and hypothesised causal mechanisms may apply. We can learn too about the best ways to implement interventions in different kinds of systems, where organisational structures, resources and social norms may differ. This should push us to think of international research on substance-misuse prevention as less about the linear dissemination of interventions from 'place to place' and more about a collaborative exchange of knowledge which builds understanding of intervention theories and implementation.

Challenges in Developing International Prevention Science

Given the importance of developing international capacity and activity within prevention science it is perhaps surprising that relatively little has been written on the topic within the academic literature. Hosman and Clayton (2000) provide one of the few detailed explorations of the subject and examine some of the key challenges to the development of international collaboration in prevention science. Written at a time when the Society for Prevention Research was in its infancy it is interesting to note that a number of these challenges persist. However, whilst these challenges are complex and may require long-term action, much has been done in recent years within the field of prevention science to promote international collaboration and capacity building and a great deal of progress has been achieved. Of course, much of these efforts have been driven at a national level and the efforts of researchers, policymakers and practitioners to build prevention systems. My focus here is on the work of international organisations and networks to support these efforts and connect them at a more global level.

Building Capacity for Prevention Science

A key barrier to international prevention science is the limited levels of capacity within many countries. North America and Europe—overall—now have well-developed public health systems. These provide financial resources for intervention development and research infrastructure. Prevention activities gain legitimacy and recognition through their inclusion in government policy, and the building of a cadre of policymakers who value and promote the development of theoretically informed interventions and their rigorous evaluation. However, there are wide geographical variations in the extent to which such systems and infrastructure exist (Catalano et al., 2012). Many lower and middle-income countries lack research capacity, and prevention is often poorly supported by policymakers and government health agendas. Where funding and support for prevention science within university and other education systems are limited this creates several barriers to the development and evaluation of interventions, partly because the number of prevention scientists may be limited. Where present, prevention scientists can play a key role in the development of new interventions by ensuring that they are based on well-evidenced theories of change, that implementation processes and systems are considered from an early stage and that new interventions are rigorously tested before decisions are made concerning large-scale utilisation. Training of future researchers (e.g. through Masters-level and PhD courses) builds long-term skills and capacity to provide such expertise. Awareness raising and support for policymakers who are tasked with setting broad public health policy and commissioning or developing specific interventions are also important. The absence of funding and other support for these activities limits the development of cohesive prevention systems and the building of skills which will sustain it over the long term. Thus, some countries with the highest levels of substance use have the least resources and capacity to do so.

To address these challenges several organisations have developed international guidance and standards for prevention activities. For example, the UNODC's (2015) International Standards on Drug Prevention aim to provide guidance on effective interventions and policies, and the characteristics of successful prevention systems. Such work aims not only to provide practical guidance on key strategies which can be adopted, but also to increase the legitimacy and value placed on prevention systems by governments and other organisations working in the health and related sectors. Another example of efforts to build capacity at an international level is the development of the Universal Prevention Curriculum which seeks to strengthen and expand the education of practitioners who deliver interventions and who train others to do so. Drawing on the UNODC's International Standards, the curriculum seeks to ensure that training of practitioners working in the field of prevention is of good quality and informed by scientific and ethical principles (ISSUP, n.d.).

Developing International Collaboration

International collaboration depends on the operation of networks that allow researchers to discover the work of others in their field and to identify potential collaborators. As Hosman and Clayton (2000) argue, such networks are often poorly developed, and researchers in one country may be unaware of similar efforts to address substance misuse and develop interventions in other contexts. Equally they note that international networks sometimes overlap and duplicate each other. International networks are also uneven in their coverage, with some countries much better connected than others. Limited research infrastructure in some low- and middle-income countries acts as a barrier to greater integration of these nations within international networks.

Promoting and enabling international collaboration has been an important focus of the work of the Society for Prevention Research (SPR), the European Society for Prevention Research and related organisations. For example, the SPR's International Committee promotes international work at two interconnected levels. First it is concerned with encouraging and supporting international research collaboration by raising awareness of funding opportunities and creating opportunities for researchers to identify and meet others working in their specific area of work. Face-to-face events such as dedicated sessions and an International Networking Forum at the annual SPR conference are a key part of this work, but the Committee is also concerned with developing online networks and resources to connect prevention scientists. Secondly the Committee develops links with organisations (including professional societies, funders, NGOs) around the world to facilitate the sharing of information and identify systems and activities through which these organisations can collaborate (e.g. on the development of international positional statements or other advocacy activities). As Hosman and Clayton note, it is important for efforts to promote international collaboration to assess their effectiveness. The International Committee has built such assessment into its work through the development of a long-term strategy (with regular review of key goals), and the engagement of external stakeholders who can provide advice and guidance on its progress. Organisations such as the SPR and EUSPR aim to coordinate and reduce duplication of networks, pool together a critical mass of researchers and other stakeholders and identify efficient systems for maintaining international links. This is important, as Hosman and Clayton note that it is often difficult to sustain the activities and initial enthusiasm generated by international networks.

Working as Part of an International Team

Whilst working as part of any research team raises potential challenges (as well as opportunities) there are several aspects of international teams which make them distinctive. As Stokols, Misra, Moser, Hall, and Taylor (2008) argue, building effective relationships and trust (key ingredients of effective partnerships) may be more difficult to achieve when researchers are geographically distant and are not able to meet face to face. Physical co-location helps build trust because it allows collaborators to interact with (and monitor the behaviour of) others in various ways. The authors note that such 'virtual teams' have to negotiate differences in social and cultural norms, and the potentially limited extent of their shared experiences. There may also be challenges in the use of 'tacit' knowledge, which whilst part and parcel of face-to-face interactions may hinder understanding and communication in teams that must interact mainly online.

Working across different languages is another challenge which many international research teams must address. Few research teams will have the necessary resources to provide simultaneous translation of meetings, and/or to translate documents. Given the dominance of English in many academic spaces (conferences, journals, etc.) researchers from non-English-speaking countries often find themselves having to communicate complex ideas and terms through a second (or even third) language. Concepts and words may be understood in different ways across cultural contexts, whilst expressions and idioms may have culturally specific sets of meanings. Even the name given to the field in which we collaborate (e.g. prevention science) does not hold constant across different countries, with a range of terms used to cover work in this area, including Public Health, Health Improvement and Health Promotion. Likewise, some of the ways in which we categorise and therefore describe prevention activities may be specific to particular places. The notion of 'universal' prevention for example is not necessarily universal (Hosman & Clayton, 2000).

There are many practical challenges of collaborating across space and time zones (Hosman & Clayton, 2000; Stokols et al., 2008). Organising meetings which coincide with working (or even waking) hours across multiple regions of the world may be challenging and some participants may have to take part at night or very early in the morning. Whilst telephone conferencing and Web-based/videoconference meeting systems have made virtual meetings easy to organise, the lack of face-to-face contact can make interaction and the building of relationships more difficult, and technical difficulties and poor sound quality are not uncommon.

As well as the internal dynamics of research teams, international collaboration must also negotiate broader differences in social and cultural norms and prevention systems which exist across the contexts which team members come from. Though global in nature, the ways in which substance-misuse problems occur may differ across countries, and cultural context will likely shape the functioning of risk and protective factors. There will also often be differences in the ways in which health systems operate. More broadly, all researchers work within national, organisational and disciplinary norms and there may be challenges in translating these norms, such as those concerning appropriate methods, values and conceptual approaches across different cultures. International teams frequently must translate and negotiate differences between their respective members' research systems (Freshwater et al., 2006; Hosman & Clayton, 2000). For instance, governance arrangements, financial procedures, ethical review requirements and everyday practices within institutions may differ in important ways, reflecting varying norms and assumptions of how research 'gets done'.

Despite these multiple challenges, many international research teams operate successfully, and there are a number of strategies which can be put in place to facilitate the functioning of 'virtual teams' (Stokols et al., 2008) which stretch across national borders. Perhaps the most important advice provided by researchers with experience of international collaboration is the importance of promoting clear communication between members of the team on all aspects of the project (e.g. Stokols et al., 2008). de Grijs (2015) stresses the value of being clear from the start as to the reason for the international collaboration being engaged in (e.g. to share knowledge, to access resources). Articulation and consensus on clear roles and responsibilities should proceed from this. Clear written agreements on how data and resources will be managed and shared, and policies on authorship and dissemination strategies, are also helpful (de Grijs, 2015).

Whilst many international collaborations will by necessity have to conduct most of their communication online or teleconference, where resources exist it can be extremely helpful for geographically distant researchers to travel to team member countries—especially at the outset of a project—such visits can promote trust and group norms and identify and facilitate greater understanding of the national and local contexts in which colleagues are working (Stokols et al., 2008). Bagshaw, Lepp and Zorn (2007) stress the importance of individual researchers being willing to learn from others, and to reflect on the specificity and assumptions of their cultural context and existing knowledge. International research collaboration can be conceptualised as a process of capacity building whereby team members from different places develop the skills and systems necessary to overcome the challenges identified above when working across borders.

Transporting and Adapting Interventions in New National Contexts

An important aspect of international work in prevention science concerns the transfer of interventions found to be effective in one country to new settings. For example, many US-based parenting and family interventions have been adapted for, and implemented within, European countries. The transportation of interventions in this way aims to avoid duplication of effort that might occur if developers in multiple countries were to work in silos and create similar programmes. It enables researchers in different countries to bring together their separate sets of knowledge, and to focus these on some of the most promising interventions which have the potential to prevent substance misuse.

A key challenge in the international transportation of interventions is that we cannot presume that an intervention found to be effective in one setting will necessarily replicate these effects in the new setting into which it is introduced (Bonell, Oakley, Hargreaves, Strange, & Rees, 2006; Evans, Craig, Hoddinott, et al., 2018). Whilst some interventions have equalled or even strengthened their effectiveness in new settings (Gardner, Montgomery, & Knerr, 2016) there are also many examples where programmes have failed to replicate impacts. The evidence base for interventions on a range of health behaviours has tended to be dominated by work in high-income countries, and there is a need to assess the extent to which it can be applied to low/middle-income countries to which such interventions are often transported (e.g. Mejia, Ulph, & Calam, 2016; Sweetland et al., 2014).

Work in the field of prevention science over a number of decades has increased our understanding of the factors which may affect the replication of intervention effectiveness from one setting to another. A key dilemma facing implementers in new countries is the extent to which implementation of the intervention should be a faithful replication of the original version (with no or few changes made) or adapted for the new social and cultural context into which it is introduced (Castro, Barrera, & Martinez, 2004). Interventions comprise a set of components or activities that are theorised to achieve their impacts through particular sets of mechanisms. Implementation fidelity (e.g. including the key components *and* delivering them as intended) is therefore important to ensure that the intervention's hypothesised casual mechanisms are enacted.

Though methodological guidance on cultural adaptation and evaluation of adapted interventions is still limited (Evans et al., 2018), a number of authors have described ways in which the task might be approached to balance intervention integrity on the one hand and fit with local context on the other. Castro et al. (2004) suggest that there are two levels at which an intervention's content may be adapted for new settings. First, surface-level changes involve changing the appearance or ethnicity of role models used in the programme, or other modifications to everyday cultural references and expressions. Second, deeper or structural level changes involve making changes to the content and underlying messages to fit cultural norms, world views and other aspects of the new social and cultural context.

A key point is that such adaptation needs to consider the extent to which the mechanisms (or risk and protective factors) which shape the behaviours being addressed by the intervention may vary across contexts (Bonell et al., 2006; Evans et al., 2018). For instance, Colby et al. (2013) describe how the operation of family relationships and networks (which function as important risk/protective factors for substance use) may differ across urban and rural settings, and such differences are likely to occur at the scale of national settings also. Intervention theory (which informs the design and content of activities) may need to be modified to take account of variation in the operation of the mechanisms which shape substance use across settings. The extent to which interventions need to be adapted in this way will vary—but may be greater where there are more extensive differences between relevant aspects of the cultural and social factors in the original and the new setting (Evans et al., 2018).

Recent work in this area has been helpful in highlighting the need to think about contexts (i.e. the setting into which an intervention is introduced) as complex systems which interact with interventions. For Hawe, Shiell, and Riley (2009) interventions can be conceptualised as 'events in systems'. Many prevention interventions seek to change aspects of the system into which they are introduced, and so contextual variations in outcomes might be expected (Evans et al., 2018; Moore et al., 2015). Interventions which take a whole-school approach are a good example of such interventions, seeking to change not only individual behaviours and attitudes, but also aspects of the broader physical and social environment of the institution and its connections with families and the wider community. Existing aspects of local contexts (including social and cultural norms) may facilitate or act as barriers to the changes an intervention seeks to bring about (Evans et al., 2018). An intervention with poor cultural fit may have less relevance to the intended population and levels of participation (Castro et al., 2004).

Another important aspect of adaptation outlined by Castro and colleagues concerns the form of programme delivery (see also Stirman, Miller, Toder, & Calloway, 2013). Changes may be made to the delivery channel (e.g. replacing online components with face-to-face activities), the individual or organisation who delivers the intervention and the location of implementation. We need to consider the feasibility of implementation and whether there are differences in resources and systems which may require changes to how the intervention is delivered. Issues around resources may be particularly pertinent when an intervention is transferred from high- to middle/low-income settings. It is also important—as for the intervention mechanisms themselves—to think about how the new intervention interacts with the system into which it is introduced, and the factors which may help support and embed it or frustrate implementation (May, 2013). For instance, which organisations might need to support and integrate a new intervention for it to be funded and sustained in the long term?

These different aspects of intervention transportation, implementation and adaptation are clearly complex. Addressing them will often benefit from or indeed require collaboration between researchers in the country where the intervention was originally developed, and the new context into which it is being introduced. Such collaboration brings together knowledge of how the intervention was designed (its intended mechanisms and how the components are intended to enact these) with an understanding of how it may need to be adapted to achieve cultural fit in the new setting without undermining the intervention's intended change processes. Within these collaborations there is learning for researchers in both countries and opportunities to increase the understanding of how interventions interact with the contexts into which they are introduced, insights which can strengthen our approaches to their design and evaluation.

Conclusion

International research has a key role to play in the field of prevention science and the development and evaluation of interventions to prevent substance misuse. The key goals of international research revolve around the desire to improve the evidence base on the ways in which risk and protective factors function in different contexts, and how best to design, implement and evaluate interventions. These actions are driven by a desire to improve equity in the development of prevention systems and provision of resources across countries which have often been unevenly distributed. These goals—and the commitment and to work collaboratively and share knowledge and resources—are closely aligned with the values and mission of prevention science as a whole. International collaboration is critical for increasing the capacity in countries where it is less developed, for answering some of the key questions in prevention science which are too large or complex to be fully answered by research teams working in national silos, and for promoting the transportation of effective interventions to new contexts.

This chapter has identified a number of challenges in achieving these aims and developing international networks and research collaborations. They include the limited capacity for prevention science—particularly in low/middle-income countries, the difficulties of identifying potential overseas collaborators and the complexities of working as part of international teams where relationships must be developed across geographical and cultural contexts, but often without the benefit of regular face-to-face communication. A number of challenges arise when transporting interventions to new contexts, including the need to consider what adaptations may be needed to their content or delivery whilst ensuring that causal mechanisms still function as intended.

Whilst these challenges may be complex, this chapter has also demonstrated that they are not insurmountable. For instance, progress has been made in developing international networks that help connect researchers across countries, and we are seeing the emergence of more coherent systems which can sustain these activities over the long term, and which avoid duplication of effort. We now have a greater understanding of some of the key principles which need to be considered when interventions are transported to new settings, in terms of both the importance of considering how intervention theories operate across contexts and how contexts themselves are dynamic and interact with interventions, rather than merely acting as a passive space within which interventions operate.

As has been seen, collaborating as part of international teams, with the challenges of limited face-to-face communication, working across contrasting cultural norms and prevention systems, and practical issues of language and time zones, is not without its difficulties. But here also, there are ways of overcoming the challenges if there is a willingness to do so. This is perhaps one of the defining characteristics of international collaboration when done well. For as much as a set of procedures or functional steps, international collaboration is defined by a set of values. They include valuing difference and diversity, of being willing to reflect on the specificity of our knowledge and to acknowledge the assumptions which underlie it. Perhaps more than anything else it is about being willing to listen and to learn from others. Of course, these values are far from exclusive to international research. But they are sometimes brought into sharper view when we collaborate across national borders. Working internationally may have its challenges, but it also offers important opportunities – both for prevention science and the populations it seeks to benefit, and the networks of individual researchers and practitioners working around the world to fulfil the potential of international research for the field.

References

Bagshaw, D., Lepp, M., Zorn., C. (2007) International research collaboration: Building teams and managing conflicts. *Conflict Resolution Quarterly 24*(4), 433–446

Bonell, C., Oakley, A., Hargreaves, J., Strange, V., & Rees, R. (2006). Assessment of generalisability in trials of health interventions: Suggested framework and systematic review. *BMJ: British Medical Journal, 333*(7563), 346.

Castro, F., Barrera, M., Jr., & Martinez, C., Jr. (2004). The cultural adaptation of prevention interventions: Resolving tensions between fidelity and fit. *Prevention Science, 5*(1), 41–45.

Catalano, R., Fagan, A., Gavin, L., Greenberg, M., Irwin, C., Jr., Ross, D., & Shek, D. (2012). Worldwide application of prevention science in adolescent health. *The Lancet, 379*(9826), 1653–1664.

Colby, M., Hecht, M., Miller-Day, M., Krieger, J., Syvertsen, K., Graham, J., & Pettigrew, J. (2013). Adapting school-based substance use prevention curriculum through cultural grounding: A review and exemplar of adaptation processes for rural schools. *American Journal of Community Psychology, 51*(1-2), 190–205.

de Grijs, R. (2015). Ten simple rules for establishing international research collaborations. *PLoS Computational Biology, 11*(10), e1004311.

Evans, E., Craig, P., Hoddinott, P., Littlecot, H., Moore, L., Murphy, S., O'Cathain, A., Pfadenhauer, L., Rehfuess, E., Segrott, J., Moore, G. (2018). Adaptation of population health interventions for new contexts: The need for guidance. Under review by *Journal of Epidemiology and Community Health*.

Freshwater, D., Sherwood, G., & Drury, V. (2006). International research collaboration: Issues, benefits and challenges of the global networks. *Journal of Research in Nursing, 11*(4), 295–303.

Gardner, F., Montgomery, P., & Knerr, W. (2016). Transporting evidence-based parenting programs for child problem behavior (age 3–10) between countries: Systematic review and meta-analysis. *Journal of Clinical Child and Adolescent Psychology, 45*(6), 749–762.

Giannotta, F., Vigna-Taglianti, F., Galanti, R., Scatigna, M., & Faggiano, F. (2014). Short-term mediating factors of a school-based intervention to prevent youth substance use in Europe. *Journal of Adolescent Health, 54*(5), 565–573.

Hawe, P., Shiell, A., & Riley, T. (2009). Theorising interventions as events in systems. *American Journal of Community Psychology, 43*(3-4), 267–276.

Hosman, C., & Clayton, R. (2000). Prevention and health promotion on the international scene: The need for a more effective and comprehensive approach. *Addictive Behaviors, 25*(6), 943–954.

International Society of Substance Use Professionals (ISSUP). (n.d.) *Universal prevention curriculum*. Retrieved June 6, 2018, from https://www.issup.net/training/universal-prevention-curriculum.

Kumpfer, K., & Alvarado, R. (2003). Family-strengthening approaches for the prevention of youth problem behaviors. *American Psychologist, 58*(6–7), 457–465.

May, C. (2013). Towards a general theory of implementation. *Implementation Science, 8*(1), 18.

McArdle, P., Wiegersma, A., Gilvarry, E., Kolte, B., McCarthy, S., Fitzgerald, M., ..., & Quensel, S.. (2002). European adolescent substance use: The roles of family structure, function and gender. *Addiction, 97*(3), 329–336.

Mejia, A., Ulph, F., & Calam, R. (2016). Preventing interpersonal violence in Panama: Is a parenting intervention developed in Australia culturally appropriate? *International Journal of Public Health, 61*(8), 915–922.

Moore, G., Audrey, S., Barker, M., Bond L., Bonell C., Hardeman W., ..., Baird J. (2015). Process evaluation of complex interventions: Medical Research Council guidance. *British Medical Journal, 350*: h1258.

Romano, J., & Israelashvili, M. (2017). Prevention science: A call for global action. Chapter 43. In M. Israelashvili & J. Romano (Eds.), *The Cambridge handbook of international prevention science* (pp. 1021–1036). New York: Cambridge University Press.

Stirman, S., Miller, C., Toder, K., & Calloway, A. (2013). Development of a framework and coding system for modifications and adaptations of evidence-based interventions. *Implementation Science, 8*, 65.

Stokols, D., Misra, S., Moser, R., Hall, K., & Taylor, B. (2008). The ecology of team science: understanding contextual influences on transdisciplinary collaboration. *American Journal of Preventive Medicine, 35*(2 suppl), S96–S115.

Sweetland, A., Oquendo, M., Sidat, M., Santos PF, Vermund SH, Duarte CS, ..., Wainberg ML (2014). Closing the mental health gap in low-income settings by building research capacity: Perspectives from Mozambique. *Annals of Mental Health, 80* (2), 126–133.

United Nations Office on Drugs and Crime. (2015). *International standards on drug use prevention*. Retrieved June 6 2018, from https://www.unodc.org/documents/prevention/UNODC_2013_2015_international_standards_on_drug_use_prevention_E.pdf

Yen, J., Yen, C., Chen, C., Chen, S., & Ko, C. (2007). Family factors of internet addiction and substance use experience in Taiwanese adolescents. *Cyber Psychology & Behavior, 10*(3), 323–329.

The Substance-Use Prevention Workforce: An International Perspective

Harry R. Sumnall

Professional Cultures in Prevention

Professionalisation of an occupation signifies special knowledge or skill in the performance of a service or commitment that distinguishes it from others, and which may be certified by accredited organisations as a condition of practice (Mattingly, 1977). Although there is no normative definition, professional culture can be understood as *'an emergent property of underlying social structures, intrinsically infused with differences, shifting allegiances and variable attitudes, values and predispositions'* (Allen, Braithwaite, Sandall, & Waring, 2016, p. 190). This suggests that there is an interaction between individual behaviour (not just related to occupational duties) with shared meanings and cognition at organisational and societal (including policy) level, which serves to guide collective and individual action. However, although there is a relationship between individual behaviour and professional culture, dominant professional culture and other external forces (e.g. funding decisions) may exert the greatest influence (Mattingly, 1977). For example, substance-use prevention professionals may have an orientation towards, and shared understanding of, evidence-based practice, which would be reflected in their working activities, but this perspective would have been shaped by funding and policy that supported the stability and expansion of organisations that attracted them into the field in the first place. There has been no contemporary work exploring the psychoactive substance-use prevention professional culture, but in keeping with discussions in the wider health sector, it may be understood with respect to those shared values which determine the motivations, standards, actions, and goals of prevention to which members attribute intrinsic worth (Allen et al., 2016). Although it is not possible, nor is it useful, to try and define a unitary prevention culture with which all professionals might identify, there are some key values that are shared, and these might include an orientation towards evidence-based programmes; the relative prioritisation of utilitarian perspectives on health and well-being over harms caused by restricting individual rights and behavioural freedoms; or the professional status of preventive activities compared to other clinical and treatment approaches to substance use. In one prevention training needs analysis conducted in California, USA, the most frequently cited reasons for entering the field were a 'desire to help others and make an impact', 'opportunities to work with youth', and an 'interest in developing a specialism' (Center for Applied Research Solutions, 2013). Professional prevention culture may also reflect broader perspectives on behaviour and how those individuals and groups that engage in such behaviours are viewed and managed by society. Here the changes in legal regulation of cannabis in

H. R. Sumnall (✉)
Public Health Institute, Liverpool John Moores University, Liverpool, UK
e-mail: h.sumnall@ljmu.ac.uk

some US states and other countries provide a good example, whereby the ambitions of primary prevention work designed to reduce the health and social harms of substance use may be at odds with a policy environment that expands and normalises access to potentially harmful substance (Werb, 2018). Professional cultures may also represent a social power which influences individual and collective choices, and prioritises certain ways of working over others (Bloor & Dawson, 1994). So with respect to substance-use prevention, this may be reflected, for example, in culturally influenced debates about the relative value of neuroscientific understandings of substance use (e.g. Heim, 2014; Volkow, Koob, & McLellan, 2016), or whether a focus on delivery of programmed approaches to prevention ignores the political and social determinants of health (Marmot, 2005; Roumeliotis, 2015; Viner et al., 2012). Comparison can also be drawn to broader debates in the evidence-based medicine model which dominates clinical practice and to which prevention advocates aspire, but which has been criticised for its inflexibility and adherence to a flawed 'brand' (Greenhalgh, Howick, & Maskrey, 2014).

The prevention workforce, as defined in this chapter, typically includes practitioners, policymakers, coordinators, and programme designers, although as discussed below the range of relevant roles is much greater than this. Prevention researchers should not be considered independently from the workforce, as there is likely to be reciprocal influence due to how prevention is defined, assessed, and delivered, and how prevention policy and practice are typically co-produced.

Quality Standards and Promotion of High-Quality Prevention Practice

The European Drug Prevention Quality Standards (EDPQS) were published by the European Monitoring Centre for Drugs and Drug Addiction (EMCDDA), and aimed to provide a European framework to support the planning, implementing, and evaluation of high-quality substance-use prevention activities (Brotherhood & Sumnall, 2011). The work emerged from identification of gaps in EU prevention activity concerning the lack of concordance between policy ambitions and low level of implementation of effective evidence-based prevention programmes in practice (Faggiano et al., 2014; Ferri, Ballotta, Carra, & Dias, 2015). During the development of EDPQS the project team presented a researcher-informed definition of 'high-quality' prevention work to communicate the aims of the quality standards. This was defined by factors such as being relevant to target populations (assessed through exercises such as needs assessment and screening using validated tools); made reference to relevant policy; was in line with principles of ethical conduct; made use of the best available scientific evidence (including evidence of effectiveness); generated evidence through delivery; achieved specified objectives; was practically feasible; and was sustained for as long as the target population required it (in accordance with life-course perspectives on health and well-being). Interestingly, whilst the members of the prevention workforce who were consulted shared many of these aims, they highlighted additional considerations aligned with practice-based definitions of quality, including prioritisation of acutely presented needs (e.g. prevention of homelessness, responding to emergent mental health crisis); importance of secondary outcomes such as developing positive relationships with target groups; adaption of programmes in response to public, political, funding, and commissioning priorities rather than developments in the scientific evidence base; utilisation of a range of sources of evidence, not just traditional scientific evidence (cf. Oliver and de Vocht (2015)); and sustaining actions only for as long as funding was available.

Although the research phase of the EDPQS has ended, project outputs continue to contribute to several current EU initiatives supporting improvements in (substance-use prevention) policy and practice (Ferri et al., 2016). The standards included in EDPQS were developed through a consensus-building process across the EU member states and were produced in consultation with the prevention workforce. Professional culture was considered as an interacting *input* (e.g. acceptance of quality standards would depend on initial acceptance of and orientation towards evidence-based prevention) and *impact* (e.g. implementation of the standards would lead to greater acceptance of high-quality evidence-based prevention) in the hypothesised EDPQS theory of change (Brotherhood & European Prevention Standards Partnership, 2015).

Development of the standards and subsequent use in several EU member states (including endorsement in national policy, e.g. H.M. Government (2017)) was hypothesised to meet the conditions for supporting (positive) professional cultural change through responding to a 'felt need' (resulting from a 'crisis' in the quality of prevention provision in the EU where professional culture was not orientated towards evidence-based approaches (Burkhart, 2015; Faggiano et al., 2014)); promoting shared ownership of expertise (Allen et al., 2016); being compatible with existing systems and structures (Roche & Nicholas, 2017); and mobilisation of effective and influential stakeholder networks to support change (e.g. national and regional professional bodies; funding agencies, (inter)national policymakers, the EMCDDA) (Ferri et al., 2016).

Minimum quality standards (termed 'basic standards' in the EDPQS) are applied at the organisational level but include items such as ensuring the recruitment and development of appropriately skilled team members. This approach is based upon the development of a training needs analyses and staff development plans that support the training of relevant staff in the general knowledge and skills relating to effective substance-use prevention (based on the prevention science cycle; Gottfredson et al. (2015); Institute of Medicine Committee on Prevention of Mental Disorders (1994)). Although the EDPQS include competencies relevant to the delivery of prevention interventions, many can also be applied to general health and social care work (e.g. respectful, participant-focused working; accessing and understanding prevention research). Prevention meta-competencies are specified to support responses to individual participant needs (Le Deist & Winterton, 2005). These include, but are not limited to, cultural sensitivity, ethical substance-use prevention, and respecting the multiple needs and identities of target groups (i.e. a participant is not just a 'substance user'). Of relevance to the substance use field, the EDPQS present prevention workers as role models to target groups, and whilst assuming that workers abstain from substance use themselves staff are encouraged to reflect and consider personal attitudes and experiences of substance use and substance users to ensure that these characteristics do not affect the quality of support provided. This position was developed in accordance with the preferences of consultees, but it was acknowledged that for some high-risk groups, where primary prevention or abstention from substance use is not a realistic aim, a shared substance-use history may increase engagement with professionals and improve acceptability of interventions designed to prevent escalation of use (Fletcher, Calafat, Pirona, & Olszewski, 2010). Where it is in accordance with national legislation, and where appropriate skills and qualifications are evident, the EDPQS support the involvement of people with a history of substance use, or who are currently in receipt of treatment, in the delivery of prevention programmes. In some countries, where diagnosed substance-use disorders are recognised as a disability (e.g. the US Americans with Disabilities Act of 1990-ADA-42 U.S. Code Chapter 126), legislation aims to prohibit employment discrimination against a history of, but not current, substance use (but see Westreich (2002) for a critique). Partly as a result of national differences in how disability is viewed and approached, disability discrimination employment laws are less common in the EU, although some associated co-morbidities are protected (e.g. mental ill health; HIV resulting from injecting drug use) (Brotherhood & Sumnall, 2012). In contrast, the EDPQS do not support the use of ex-substance users as prevention staff where their personal history and testimonial are used as the basis of intervention (Israelashvili, 2011; UNODC, 2013).

These considerations are important because stigmatisation of some types of substance users, or of populations who have a greater propensity towards substance use, is evident in the general population, from which social and healthcare professionals are drawn (van Boekel, Brouwers, van Weeghel, & Garretsen, 2013). Negative views may also be held towards users of some types of substances and not others, particularly where substance use intersects with other demographic characteristics such as ethnicity, religion, deprivation, and social class (Farrugia, 2014; Järvinen & Demant, 2011; Pennay & Measham, 2016;

UNODC, 2004). Stigmatising attitudes towards substance use and substance users can also be culturally endorsed and reinforced by policy, laws, and practices (Santos da Silveira, Andrade de Tostes, Wan, Ronzani, & Corrigan, 2018). Whilst holding stigmatising views can be protective against individual substance use (Adlaf, Hamilton, Wu, & Noh, 2009), this can also lead to prejudice and discriminatory practice and behaviour towards people who use substances and associated groups (e.g. siblings, children of substance users). Although no research has been undertaken with prevention professionals, and it is less commonly observed than in the broader health and social care workforce, negative attitudes and practices have also been reported in some groups of specialist drug and alcohol treatment professionals (Russell, Davies, & Hunter, 2011; Skinner, Feather, Freeman, & Roche, 2007; van Boekel et al., 2013; von Hippel, Brener, & von Hippel, 2008). Professional stigmatisation can result from factors such as perceptions of lower professional status in working with affected groups compared to non-substance users (e.g. similar groups such as young people with mental ill health); structural barriers that make working with these groups more challenging (e.g. within criminal justice and under-resourced settings); perceived lack of effective treatment/intervention approaches; personally held causal attributions towards patients and clients using substances; and beliefs that (problematic) substance use is caused by poor individual choices (Gilchrist et al., 2011; van Boekel et al., 2013). Overall, this can lead to negative professional (self-) labelling, prejudice, exclusion, and discrimination, which can undermine the provision, access, and quality of treatment, and which serves to reproduce and reinforce broader health and social inequity (Smith, Earnshaw, Copenhaver, & Cunningham, 2016). A systematic review of interventions to reduce stigma related to substance-use disorders concluded that despite limited evidence, effective strategies to reduce stigma in professional groups included the incorporation of regular reflective practices, and providing early opportunities for recipients to meet relevant target groups as part of their professional training (Livingston, Milne, Fang, & Amari, 2012). Exposure to such programmes led to positive outcomes such as increased self-reported comfort in working with target groups and a reduction in negative attitudes.

Whilst there are clearer parallels between substance-use treatment and selective and indicated preventive actions, stigmatising and negative attitudes may also affect the delivery of universal approaches. Despite these types of programme being delivered without an assumption of target group substance use or elevated risk of use (UNODC, 2013), societal views on substance use and its potential consequences might be reflected in working practices, and in the content of programmes (Edman, 2012). Farrugia (2017), for example, argued in a review of Australian school substance-use education programmes that these activities served to problematise young women's substance-related behaviour to a greater extent than men's, and by presenting a normative view of femininity (by defining 'acceptable' feminine behaviour) may inadvertently reinforce unhelpful gender stereotypes and prioritise some types of harms or behaviours over others (e.g. female responsibility in relation to alcohol-related sexual assault rather than male perpetrator behaviour). The continued popularity in many EU countries of ineffective prevention approaches based on fear arousal techniques (EMCDDA, 2017; Esrick et al., 2018) suggests not only an implementation and training gap, but also the potential for marginalisation of young people (at risk of) using substance (Thompson, Barnett, & Pearce, 2009).

Who Is the Prevention Workforce?

During the development of the EDPQS, a consultation exercise was undertaken with prevention professionals in six EU countries using a Delphi survey methodology. Although the purpose of this exercise was to help prioritise the final selection of standards, as part of construction of a sampling frame, information was also collected on the types of professional roles involved in delivering prevention work (Brotherhood & Sumnall, 2010). General occupational/sector categories were firstly pre-specified, based upon knowledge of the types of general and specialist roles, and settings involved the delivery of prevention actions in project partner countries. Specialist workers were those whose central role objective was the development and delivery of prevention programmes, and who would typically be employed by dedicated substance use- or adolescent health- and social care-focused organisations or provide specialist support in non-specialist organisations across government, non-government, public, and private sectors. These professions would be expected to develop and deliver structured prevention programmes or undertake individual-level interventions. General workers were those who would have non-prevention-related core roles, but worked in organisations or sectors that would likely encounter target populations using or at risk of use. Policy- and other decision makers (including funders, co-ordinators, and commissioners) were considered as both generalists and non-specialists as these groups would include those who had expertise in substance-use policy and those whose remit included areas broadly related to substance use such as mental health and education.

Specified roles included central government representatives such as policymakers; prevention planning/co-ordinators; prevention providers; education; health; mental health; social services; children, young people, and family services; criminal justice; the wider voluntary and community sector; and media. Participants in the Delphi exercise were then asked to self-identify their specific role, and this data was synthesised (Table 25.1). Although not intending to be representative, similar findings have been found in other surveys (e.g. Canadian Centre on Substance Abuse (2015); Center for Applied Research Solutions (2013)). This exercise was important as it illustrated the diverse multisectoral nature of the EU prevention field, and highlighted the difficulties in identifying *who* comprises the prevention workforce, and whether the specialist 'prevention professional' was even a role that was consistently understood across countries. Different roles predominated across participating countries and so for example, in Italy, prevention work was frequently delivered by qualified psychologists, whilst in the UK there was no requirement for specialisation, and prevention was typically delivered by school teachers who had not received any formal training, or by substance-use treatment workers who would not be considered prevention specialists. These findings also suggested that the workforce comprised individuals with diverse skills and qualifications, ranging from those with little or no formal training to those with significant specialist educational and professional experience, although not always related to prevention (e.g. medical training in the EU is highly specialised, but few medical students received education on substance use (Ayu, Schellekens, Iskandar, Pinxten, & De Jong, 2015; Klimas, 2015)).

Whilst a multisectoral approach, overseen by a co-ordinating body, is promoted in substance-use prevention/treatment system frameworks, in reality there may only be loose policy and infrastructural harmonisation (Armstrong, Doyle, Lamb, & Waters, 2006; Babor, Stenius, & Romelsjo, 2008; UNODC, 2013). As suggested by the EDPQS sample, overall, only a small proportion of professionals delivering prevention in Europe could be considered specialists, but effective workforce development requires role clarity, a shared culture, and clear boundaries in relation to other sectors (Nelson, 2017). Greater professionalisation and coordination might support the ambitions of improved delivery of evidence-based prevention (Ferri et al., 2016), but considering the diversity of the prevention field there will be challenges, and there is also the attendant risk of minimising the unique contributions that diverse informal roles can make to supporting prevention work (e.g. through local advocacy, or infusion of evidence-based prevention principles into general youth programmes).

Scientific Advances in Understanding Effective Preventive Responses to Substance Use Pose Challenges to the Workforce and to Researchers

Popular definitions of substance-use prevention have focused on intervention outcomes such as abstention from substance use, delay in initiation age, and avoidance of substance-use disorders. However, as prevention science has developed as a discipline, this classic definition, and the range of relevant actions, has also become more complex. With an improved understanding of substance-use aetiology and epidemiology, the

Table 25.1 The diversity of professional roles delivering substance-use prevention activities in the EU

Regional prevention planning
Regional substance-use prevention—e.g. prevention action co-ordinating teams, area manager (responsible for planning and implementation of drug policy)
(Local) Drug monitoring network, observatory on drugs and alcohol, databank on prevention programmes
Local government, municipal district, association of municipalities—e.g. representative, specialist for young people or social policies, local politician
Local management/coordination of social programmes—e.g. representative responsible for young people's policies
Education
Ministry of Education—e.g. representative, school counsellor
Health education—e.g. lead teacher with responsibility for health and social education in schools
National agency implementing prevention programmes in educational system—e.g. substance-use prevention specialist
Regional educational bureau—e.g. director, school counsellor, 'healthy schools' policy advisor
School lead in substance-use policy—e.g. head teacher/principal
Substance-use education/prevention/addiction specialist teacher
Teacher with pastoral role, teacher responsible for pupil's health and well-being
Alternative education programme/schools—e.g. facility manager
University lecturer
School nurse, health worker
School counsellor, education welfare officer/educational psychologist
Students' university associations—e.g. president, student union welfare officer
Health
(NGO) Drug treatment units—e.g. manager, staff, young person specialist
Health service/department, national treatment agency, public health districts—e.g. regional substance misuse lead, regional officer, director
GP (general practitioner/family doctor) representative
Paediatrician/family doctor
Accident and emergency service—e.g. emergency physician, children's manager, substance-use specialist
Drug counselling centre—physician
Workplace physician
Trade union representative responsible for health and safety in the workplace
Community pharmacy representative
Mental health
Addiction psychiatrist
Psychologist with specialisms in substance use
Young people mental health prevention/treatment services—e.g. manager, substance-use specialist, specialists in dual diagnoses, and co-morbidities
Social services/children, young people, and families
Social work—e.g. social worker working with looked-after children, young persons, families with substance-use problems
Family/adolescent support centre—e.g. practitioner, psychologist with substance-use specialisms, manager
National authority for child protection—e.g. specialist regarding young substance users/child protection
Local team/board for safeguarding children
Young people substance-use services—e.g. practitioner, manager
Young persons' counselling services
Housing officer
Minority and underserved groups—e.g. representative for young people
Criminal justice
Ministry of the Interior

(continued)

Table 25.1 (continued)

Police—e.g. general representative, local officers; specialised police (e.g. officer responsible for prevention programmes, young people, school drug education)
Ministry of Justice
Child courts, youth justice legal sector
Youth offending teams (preventing children from offending, supporting young offenders)
Probation workers
Voluntary and community sector
Specialist NGO substance-use prevention centres and programmes—e.g. practitioner, manager, social worker specialising in substances
General NGOs working with populations likely to be affected by substance use (e.g. homeless youth)
Representative from voluntary organisations and networks
Substance user representatives
Youth groups, community-based prevention initiatives and coalitions, parent and family groups, therapeutic/recovery communities
Religious organisations
Government representatives
National department/agency with responsibility for substances—e.g. representative, specialist in drug education
Department for families/children—representative
Department/Ministry of Health—representative
Ministry of Labour—representative
Ministry of Social Affairs—representative
Prevention consultants
Academic—e.g. researchers with expertise in substance use, health promotion, programme development, and evaluation
Consultants in planning prevention policies
Media
(Local) Journalists—drug-specific publications (drug magazines); popular press used as partners in prevention campaigns
Governmental media or press departments, e.g. public prevention campaigns, informing the public on government's substance-use prevention work and policy priorities

interaction of multiple risk behaviours, associated comorbidities, and identification of substance use as a broader indicator of health and well-being (Cordova et al., 2014; Hale & Viner, 2016; Vanyukov et al., 2012), these developments suggest that 'real-world' prevention work should not be limited to a focus on substance-related outcomes. Indeed, examining prevention service configurations in EU countries as part of the EDPQS development, most non-universal actions were supported by a range of other professionals such as those working in social services, youth justice, housing, mental health, and education. However, in contrast to this, domain-specific prevention programmes still dominate the substance use research field (e.g. Allara, Ferri, Bo, Gasparrini, & Faggiano, 2015; Faggiano et al., 2008; Foxcroft & Tsertsvadze, 2011a, 2011b), although there is an emerging evidence base on actions that take a multiple risk behaviour perspective (Hale, Fitzgerald-Yau, & Viner, 2014; Hale & Viner, 2012; Hickman et al., 2014; Meader et al., 2017). In part, this is a product of the research process, whereby funding for research and decisions on the effectiveness of programmes and inclusion in evidence-based registries are incentivised by criteria that focus on a relatively small number of pre-specified indicators in single-outcome domains (Becona et al., 2013; Flay et al., 2005; Gottfredson et al., 2015). Furthermore, only a relatively small number of prevention programmes with demonstrated effectiveness are delivered in European settings (ACMD, 2015; EMCDDA, 2013, 2017; Faggiano et al., 2014), and as most substance-use interventions with young people tend to be on an individual needs-led basis (analogous to treatment approaches) rather than through structured prevention programmes it is unclear whether much of the existing body of prevention evidence provides great practical value and relevance to those working in the field.

Socioecological models of health (Bambra et al., 2010; Brofenbrenner, 1979; Hawkins, Catalano, & Miller, 1992; McLeroy, Bibeau, Steckler, & Glanz, 1988) describe how health-related behaviours, including substance use, emerge as a result of complex associations and interactions between public policy, social and structural factors, physical environment, and individual practices (Connell, Gilreath, Aklin, & Brex, 2010). Such framing is becoming more influential in prevention-related policy, as it is helpful in understanding not only the determinants of individual-level behaviour, but also how extra-individual factors may lead to inequalities, and how actions that focus only on individual-level behaviour change may also generate inequality (Adams, Mytton, White, & Monsivais, 2016; Lorenc, Petticrew, Welch, & Tugwell, 2013; Saunders, Barr, McHale, & Hamelmann, 2017). In the broader public health field, health behaviour has been conceptualised as emerging from a complex system of influence whereby focus on individual inputs, such as the effects of the delivery of a single intervention, is unlikely to provide sufficient explanation for any observed changes (Rutter et al., 2017). Taking a similar systems-based approach towards substance-use behaviour moves emphasis away from the impact of individual prevention actions towards understanding how those actions may influence system properties. Similarly, policy approaches towards prevention, such as restrictions on availability, marketing, and accessibility of health-harming goods (Foxcroft, 2014), have been shown to have greater impact on reducing population-level substance-related harms (tobacco and alcohol) than prevention programmes (Babor et al., 2010; Burton et al., 2017; World Health Organization, 2008). This presents challenges to the workforce, as these approaches do not require the same level of specialist input, which may reduce the visibility of prevention programmes, and the influence of prevention professionals in leading responses (Sussman et al., 2013). However, considering international variability in the quality and timing of implementation of such polices (Anderson, Moller, & Galea, 2012), prevention programmes fill important intervention gaps, and are especially useful in addressing community, societal, and intra- and interpersonal determinants of health in higher risk targets that are not necessarily influenced by policy. Alternatively, taking a systems perspective may even improve advocacy for prevention work. For example, one of the moderating factors that have historically meant that most evaluated alcohol prevention initiatives have shown to be ineffective (Foxcroft, 2014; Foxcroft & Tsertsvadze, 2012) is the absence of 'boundary conditions' on pricing and marketing set by government (Rehm, Babor, & Room, 2006). Without the presence of social and policy conditions that set 'healthier' social norms, prevention programme effects may be suboptimal. Presenting preventive responses to alcohol use as part of an overall system approach may not only counter simplistic arguments that prevention 'doesn't work' but also help to persuade decision makers that judgements on prevention effectiveness should be made alongside evaluation of the dynamics of other systems-modifying actions (Hawe, Shiell, & Riley, 2009; McKay, Sumnall, Harvey, & Cole, 2018).

Strategies Designed to Improve the Professional Competency and the Use of Evidence-Based Prevention Programmes

Most EU member states offer formal training and professional development activities for the prevention workforce (Ferri et al., 2016; Pavlovská, Miovský, Babor, & Gabrhelík, 2017). These range from specialist university programmes offered in countries such as Austria, Croatia, Germany, and the Czech Republic to continued professional development courses on prevention-related topics in other countries. In the UK, where the author is based, the National Institute for Health and Care Excellence (NICE), a non-departmental public body of the Department of Health, provides learning tools for its national prevention-related guidance (e.g. targeted interventions; National Institute for Health and Care

Excellence (2017)) such as interactive online presentations of guidelines and quality standards; implementation guides; audit tools and progress trackers; resource impact assessment tools to help assess the costs of implementing guidelines; and funding of implementation consultants who are tasked with supporting local organisations in delivery of recommended actions. The UK Government-funded Alcohol and Drug Education and Prevention Information Service (ADEPIS) provides guidance to inform schools on good practice for effective education and prevention, but in the absence of other forms of support its user group also extends to more specialist roles (Thurman & Boughelaf, 2015). However, there is a lack of evidence on whether these two UK systems improve implementation of recommended activities in practice (cf. Durlak and DuPre (2008).

The Czech Republic has attempted to address diversity in the school-system workforce through the development of a tiered approach to prevention competencies (Miovsky, 2013). Whilst school-based work only represents a small proportion of the total prevention activities delivered in the country, a four-level system has been constructed that describes basic to advanced competencies, and these are targeted at relevant roles depending on the level of specialism required. A teacher delivering a simple education programme or substance-use awareness session would only be required to achieve the basic level of competency, whilst an education specialist responsible for screening and delivering of an indicated prevention programme would be expected to demonstrate advanced competencies (Charvat, Jurystova, & Miovsky, 2012; Miovsky, 2013).

Internationally, the Canadian Centre on Substance Abuse (2015) has developed 11 professional prevention competencies across four levels of proficiency (introductory, developing, intermediate, and advanced) that reflect consensual principles for working effectively with young people. These cover (1) child and youth development; (2) health promotion and prevention knowledge; (3) substances and substance use; (4) advocacy; (5) building and sustaining relationships; (6) community engagement and partnership building; (7) comprehensive planning, implementation and evaluation; (8) early and brief intervention, harm minimisation, and referral; (9) media savvy; (10) personal and professional development; and (11) teamwork and leadership. The competencies were based on nine key principles which are intended to guide all types of prevention work. With respect to professional activities, achievement of the competencies demonstrates that regardless of background and specialism, those delivering prevention activities have the 'appropriate aptitude, commitment, flexibility, knowledge, training, skills and support to do so effectively, and thus build and sustain relationships and serve as role-models for youth' (Canadian Centre on Substance Abuse, 2015, p. 3). The US Department of State-funded International Centre for Credentialing and Education of Addiction Professionals (ICCE) has introduced credentialing in lower and middle-income countries (LMIC) (*International Centre for Credentialing and Education of Addiction Professionals*, 2016). There is a requirement for all candidates to have received approved prevention training (the Universal Prevention Curriculum (UPC) see below) and to sit for an examination. The International Certified Prevention Specialist I (ICPS I) is a basic-level certification option for professionals who already possess an undergraduate degree and have at least 2 years of supervised working in the prevention field (or 5 years if only in possession of a high school diploma). The advanced certification (ICPS II) increases the working requirement to 5 and 7 years, respectively. In keeping with other professions (e.g. medical practitioners), accredited status must be renewed every 2 years and evidence provided of an additional 40 h of continuing education. This system of accreditation represents one of the first (international) attempts to define a prevention specialist, but there may be greater acceptance and more opportunities for implementation in LMIC countries with (presumed) less well-developed prevention systems. In countries with more mature health and social support systems, there may be resistance towards harmonisation of professional standards, and a greater focus on domestic accreditation processes for existing occupations that have been formulated in line with policy priorities and historical occupational development (Miovský et al., 2015). In many countries, this process is further complicated by national drug policy being situated in Interior and Justice Ministries, but often delivery is primarily through the health and education sector (Ysa et al., 2014). This can lead to the prioritisation of one sector (e.g. police) to the detriment of other contributors, or difficulties in ensuring that all groups deliver prevention work in a consistent, high-quality, and ethically coordinated manner.

Training for delivery of manualised prevention programmes is usually embedded in the early phases of delivery, and ongoing support is associated with improved programme effectiveness (Sloboda, Dusenbury, & Petras, 2014). Core components of such training include presentation of theoretical background and evidence supporting the programme; discussion and prioritisation of target group needs; programme features and skills required for delivery; and reflection and evaluation of learning goals (Sloboda et al., 2014; van der Kreeft, Jongbloet, & Van Havare, 2014a). Typically, where non-specialists (e.g. teachers) are responsible for delivery as part of routine working (outside a research trial), attention is also paid to the identification of those core and variable programme concepts and delivery mechanisms that should be retained so that programme integrity is preserved in the face of the informal adaptations that are often introduced in different delivery settings and contexts (Cohen et al., 2008; Ennett et al., 2011).

However, prevention is an 'umbrella discipline' (Cates, 1995), and for the specialist worker or programme developer the evolution of prevention science necessitates knowledge and skills across a diverse range of disciplines, including basic pharmacology (e.g. understanding substance effects and toxicity), developmental psychology, programme design, epidemiology, mental health, criminology, and relevant health systems. Reflecting on the challenges of developing European 'addiction education' more generally, Pavlovska and colleagues (2017) have concluded that previous attempts to promote a multidisciplinary perspective in the treatment field, as part of actions to develop a specialist profession, have not been successful. Instead, training is usually incorporated into existing professional roles (e.g. social worker, psychologist, psychiatrist), and is considered supplementary to the core skills of those occupations. Training was predominately provided post-qualification (or as part of postgraduate education); a practical response to lack of undergraduate opportunities, and national workforce requirements. This has subsequently led to the prioritisation of discipline-specific perspectives on treatment in accordance with prevailing pedagogy and praxis. Therefore, conceptualisation and responses to substance use were secondary to the identity and practices of these professional groups, and not considered a specialism. This suggests that incorporating a new approach to prevention into practice, such as through the delivery of a new intervention, would only be successful where that intervention was designed, delivered, and understood in relation to the language and routine practice of that occupation.

No equivalent analysis has been undertaken with respect to specialised training of the prevention workforce, but over-specialisation and segmentation are evident in the prevention research field, particularly in early career phases. Although academic specialism in the university system is essential in developing individual careers, expertise, and contributions to multidisciplinary research teams, Eddy, Smith, Brown, and Reid (2005) noted with concern that whilst senior researchers in the USA had high levels of knowledge in traditional domains across the prevention science cycle (e.g. problem analysis, innovation design, field trials, and innovation diffusion), this was largely gained through a process of self-directed learning and years of professional experience. Early career prevention researchers lacked confidence in their knowledge and competence in these areas, possibly as a result of the lack of specialist provision at both undergraduate and postgraduate levels, and potentially leading to disconnection with workforce demands. In Europe, a number of dedicated Master's and doctoral training courses in prevention have been developed. The EU-funded Science for Prevention Academic Network (SPAN) mapped prevention science training provision across 90 courses in 21 countries (van der Kreeft et al., 2015). Common components of these courses included basic skills in programme development and evaluation, epidemiology, implementation, and project management. However, despite this provision for early career colleagues, senior European researchers have identified significant gaps in all areas of prevention work amongst their peers, including programme development (Ostaszewski et al., 2017), suggesting that it will take time before early recipients progress to senior positions, and that in contrast to the USA (Eddy et al., 2005) advancement of basic skills through self-development activities has not matched career development stage. An earlier mapping exercise in the prevention workforce (including practitioners and decision makers) conducted as part of the same research project suggested prioritisation of knowledge and skills relating to the theoretical background of prevention actions and associated evidence base (van der Kreeft et al., 2014b). Promotion of the skills required for programme implementation quality, funding, and embedding ethics in preventive activities was also endorsed by a majority of respondents.

The EDPQS formed the basis of the prevention component of the European Council's conclusions on the implementation of the EU Action Plan on Drugs 2013–2016 regarding minimum quality standards in drug demand reduction (Council of the European Union, 2015). Standard b (there was a total of four prevention standards) specified that *'Those developing prevention interventions have competencies and expertise on prevention principles, theories and practice, and are trained and/or specialised professionals who have the support of public institutions (education, health and social services) or work for accredited or recognised institutions or NGOs'*. At the time of writing one European-co-funded action is underway to support this recommendation. The Universal Prevention Curriculum in Europe (UPC-ADAPT) project (http://upc-adapt.eu/) aims to adapt the international Universal Prevention Curriculum (UPC) for European contexts, and is currently piloting implementation in nine EU member states (Belgium, the Czech Republic, Croatia, Estonia, Germany, Italy, Poland, Slovenia, and Spain). The original UPC was based on UNODC's International Standards on Drug Use Prevention and the EDPQS (European Drug Prevention Quality Standards), and currently exists in two forms that target prevention co-ordinators (e.g. professionals with responsibilities for co-ordination and supervision of the implementation of prevention interventions and/or policies) and implementers (currently under development) (International Society of Substance Use Professionals, 2017). The UPC aims to develop core skills and competencies in prevention and includes modules on physiology and pharmacology, monitoring and evaluation, and prevention programmes in the areas of family, school, workplace, media, and community. However, it is a resource-intensive curriculum (288 h of training), and so the European adaption aims to pilot a short module (e.g. 1 week and a follow-up session), an extended academic module (e.g. a series of courses in one semester at a faculty), and an online e-learning module.

Although training courses such as the UPC (ADAPT) offer opportunities for workforce development, considering the diversity of the prevention workforce (as outlined above and in Table 25.1) it is uncertain what demand there might be for specialised international prevention qualification in those countries that already have standardised qualification requirements for relevant roles. Systems such as the European Credit and Transfer System[1] (for university students transferring across institutions in different countries) and the European Qualifications Framework[2] (for comparing formal and non-formal learning outcomes across countries) can be used to standardise qualifications, but most European countries set their own occupational competencies, and these national standards may take preference. In the UK, for example, professional registration (e.g. social worker), chartered status (e.g. practicing psychologist), and certifi-

---

[1] https://ec.europa.eu/education/resources/european-credit-transfer-accumulation-system_en
[2] https://ec.europa.eu/ploteus/

cation of specialist roles (e.g. counsellor) are governed by recognised national bodies. Professionals in non-protected roles, such as those working in substance-use treatment and prevention services, demonstrate specialist competence and skills to employers through work-based vocational qualifications, approved apprentices, and occupational standards.

Knowledge transfer frameworks have been developed to improve the use of research-based innovations and guidelines in practice and to inform professional behavioural change (Boaz, Baeza, & Fraser, 2011; Bywood, Lunnay, & Roche, 2008a, 2008b, 2008c; Grimshaw et al., 2001; Grimshaw, Thomas, MacLennan, Fraser, & Ramsay, 2004; Ward, House, & Hamer, 2009). These share five main components: problem identification and communication; knowledge/research development and selection; analysis of context; knowledge transfer activities or interventions; and knowledge/research utilisation (Ward et al., 2009). Accordingly, passive approaches such as publishing research evidence or guidelines can raise awareness of the desired professional behaviour change but rarely change practice.

In a comprehensive review, Bywood et al. (2008a) identified four general strategies to change individual professional practice in the substance use field. These were: practice audits, reminders, and feedback about practice innovations; educational meetings, including interactive learning technologies (e.g. online resources); educational outreach (the use of trained persons who meet with users of guidelines in their practice settings to give information with the intent of changing behaviour); and support of influential local opinion leaders. It was concluded that individual actions were less likely to be successful than the sustained delivery of a coherent package of activities. Knowledge transfer and innovation is also a social activity that depends upon the interaction of different communities and actors, and so professional culture may encourage or inhibit innovation (Greenhalgh, Robert, MacFarlane, Bate, & Kyriakidou, 2004) and so Bywood et al. (2008a) also described core features of professional development strategies that were sensitive to professional culture:

- The strategy begins with an assessment of, and focus on, barriers to change.
- The strategy provides clear and succinct messages, with simple, focused objectives that require small practical changes and are easy to comply with.
- The strategy highlights the relevance of information to the professional and their client needs.
- The strategy identifies organisational changes that require professionals to respond or take action (e.g. automatic prompts and obligatory responses).
- There is clear identification of roles and activities, and who is responsible for taking action.
- The strategy refers to reliable and credible sources such as national guidelines from trusted organisations, and provides accurate, evidence-based information.
- Information can be tailored so that it is personalised and can be modified to the local setting without disrupting the overall aims of the strategy.
- The strategy reinforces key messages with additional materials and support.
- The strategy provides for the sustainability of itself over a prolonged period.

Comprehensive workforce development should not just attend to improving individual-level skills and competencies. Staff may recognise the need to change and may want to change, but organisational and systemic barriers beyond individual worker's control often prevent them from doing so. Roche and colleagues (Roche & Nicholas, 2017; Roche, Pidd, & Freeman, 2009) have presented a structured systems-based model of workforce development that incorporates facilitators of individual (drug treatment) workers' training and career development, and that incorporates consideration of professional culture, including the workforce's position within the systems in which they are employed, and the broader physical, social, and policy environments in which they operate. Detailed discussion is beyond the scope of this chapter, but these authors highlight the importance for individual and collective development of organisational orientation towards evidence-based practice; clearly defined staff roles and functions (professionalisation); opportunities for practice development and experimentation; and workforce well-being. Noting the difficulties in attracting and retaining high-quality workers, they identified key measures to enhance the workforce, including reducing stigma associated with working with substance users; promoting the substance use sector as a career of choice; developing appropriate qualifications; enhancing early career exposure to substance-use issues; and increasing relevant teaching in non-specialist undergraduate higher education courses.

The Interactive Systems Framework (ISF) (Wandersman et al., 2008) is one popular example of an integrated tool that incorporates these types of strategies, and has been used to help prevention researchers understand ways to bridge the research-to-practice gap in order to improve implementation of evidence-based programmes (e.g. implementation of the Good Behavior Game in after-school settings; Halgunseth et al., 2012). The framework consists of three interactive systems: the prevention synthesis and translation system, the prevention support system, and the prevention delivery system. Briefly, the prevention synthesis and translation system focuses on how to make prevention research accessible for practitioners by synthesising and disseminating knowledge in ways that are most appropriate for target groups. The prevention support system centres on how to facilitate and support implementation through programme-specific support and general capacity building. Programme-specific support includes information about an intervention before delivery, including pre-implementation training, coaching, and ongoing support once delivery begins. Capacity building is not intervention specific, but focuses on the infrastructure, skills of a delivery organisation that will enable it to successfully deliver an intervention or to promote stability of funding and operation. Finally, the prevention delivery system addresses how prevention interventions are delivered in practice and what organisation and system barriers and facilitators might affect implementation. These include both individual and organisational factors such as fit with the organisation's goals and ethos, size and structure, and education, experience, and attitudes to evidence-based prevention of the practitioner.

Summary and Concluding Remarks

The diversity of the prevention workforce and organisation and delivery of multisectoral services means that it is uncertain that there will be great demand for further professional specialism, at least in the EU. Implementation of structured prevention programmes is already low in the EU, and an increasing focus on multiple vulnerabilities and interdisciplinary working may lead to further de-emphasis unless new programmes reflecting policy and practice priorities are developed. In some respects, and in contrast to the substance-use treatment field, the occupation of 'prevention specialist' in the EU is one that has been largely externally defined, and preventive activities are often secondary to the core duties and responsibilities of those tasked with responding to drug use. Workforce skill development may be best served by development of core prevention competencies in these occupational groups in accordance with the approaches adopted by countries such as Canada and the Czech Republic. Actions to develop frameworks for interprofessional education to support collaborative practice may provide opportunities to infuse prevention skills across the general workforce that is delivering most of the prevention activity in the EU (EMCDDA, 2017; Reeves, Perrier, Goldman, Freeth, & Zwarenstein, 2013).

Transferring experiences from the treatment field suggests that existing knowledge and skills that are critical for performance of the primary professional duty (e.g. social work) are prioritised and perceived as exceeding those gained through dedicated prevention training, and this is reinforced by national systems governing occupational competency. Although accreditation systems would help define standards of competence for prevention workers and support professionalisation, these would have to be developed nationally and may work best as sub-components of broader occupational competencies.

The development of resources such as quality standards and evidence-based guidelines has been justified as a means to improve the quality and impact of substance-use prevention activities in the EU. Inclusion in European and member state national drug policy is one indicator of success, but there is currently no data on how frequently these have been implemented in practice and if programmes developed in accordance with the included principles are more likely to lead to positive outcomes for target groups. Although much is known about strategies to improve professional awareness and utilisation of evidence, individual knowledge and skills are only one component of an overall systems approach to workforce development. Strategies that fail to take into account professional culture and the organisational, structural, and systemic factors that determine practice are unlikely to lead to sustained change.

Acknowledgments This chapter is based upon materials published to support implementation of the EDPQS (Brotherhood, Sumnall, & Partnership, 2015). An early draft of this chapter was presented at the European Society for Prevention Research Conference, Vienna, Austria, September 2017. I am extremely grateful to Angelina Brotherhood for her expert insights which informed the content of this chapter, and to the EU Prevention Standards Partnership for their collaboration on the EDPQS project.

References

ACMD. (2015). *Prevention of drug and alcohol dependence*. London: Home Office.
Adams, J., Mytton, O., White, M., & Monsivais, P. (2016). Why are some population interventions for diet and obesity more equitable and effective than others? The role of individual agency. *PLoS Medicine, 13*(4), e1001990.
Adlaf, E. M., Hamilton, H. A., Wu, F., & Noh, S. (2009). Adolescent stigma towards drug addiction: Effects of age and drug use behaviour. *Addictive Behaviors, 34*(4), 360–364.
Allara, E., Ferri, M., Bo, A., Gasparrini, A., & Faggiano, F. (2015). Are mass-media campaigns effective in preventing drug use? A Cochrane systematic review and meta-analysis. *British Medical Journal Open, 5*(9), e007449.
Allen, D., Braithwaite, J., Sandall, J., & Waring, J. (2016). Towards a sociology of healthcare safety and quality. *Sociology of Health and Illness, 38*(2), 181–197.
Anderson, P., Moller, L., & Galea, G. (2012). *Alcohol in the European Union Consumption, harm and policy approaches*. Copenhagen: World Health Organization.
Armstrong, R., Doyle, J., Lamb, C., & Waters, E. (2006). Multi-sectoral health promotion and public health: The role of evidence. *Journal of Public Health, 28*(2), 168–172.
Ayu, A. P., Schellekens, A. F., Iskandar, S., Pinxten, L., & De Jong, C. A. (2015). Effectiveness and organization of addiction medicine training across the globe. *European Addiction Research, 21*(5), 223–239.
Babor, T. F., Caetano, R., Casswell, S., Edwards, G., Giesbrecht, N., Graham, K., ... Rossow, I. (2010). *Alcohol: No ordinary commodity. Research and public policy*. New York: Oxford University Press.
Babor, T. F., Stenius, K., & Romelsjo, A. (2008). Alcohol and drug treatment systems in public health perspective: Mediators and moderators of population effects. *International Journal of Methods in Psychiatric Research, 17*(Suppl 1), S50–S59.
Bambra, C., Gibson, M., Sowden, A., Wright, K., Whitehead, M., & Petticrew, M. (2010). Tackling the wider social determinants of health and health inequalities: Evidence from systematic reviews. *Journal of Epidemiology and Community Health, 64*(4), 284–291.
Becona, E., Martinez, U., Calafat, A., Fernandez-Hermida, J. R., Juan, M., Sumnall, H. R., ... Gabrhelik, R. (2013). Parental permissiveness, control, and affect and drug use among adolescents. *Psicothema, 25*(3), 292–298.
Bloor, G., & Dawson, P. (1994). Understanding professional culture in organizational context. *Organization Studies, 15*(2), 275–295.
Boaz, A., Baeza, J., & Fraser, A. (2011). Effective implementation of research into practice: An overview of systematic reviews of the health literature. *BMC Research Notes, 4*, 212.
Brofenbrenner, U. (1979). *The ecology of human development: Experiments by nature and design*. Cambridge, MA: Harvard University Press.
Brotherhood, A., & European Prevention Standards Partnership. (2015). *EDPQS theory of change: How can the introduction of quality standards help improve prevention practice and lead to better outcomes for target populations?* Liverpool: Centre for Public Health.
Brotherhood, A., Sumnall, H., & European Prevention Standards Partnership. (2015). *EDPQS Toolkit 4: Promoting quality standards in different contexts (Adaptation & Dissemination Toolkit)*. Liverpool: Centre for Public Health, Liverpool John Moores University.
Brotherhood, A., & Sumnall, H. R. (2010). *European drug prevention quality standards. Final report to the Executive Agency for Health and Consumers*. Liverpool: Centre for Public Health.
Brotherhood, A., & Sumnall, H. R. (2011). *Drug prevention quality standards*. Luxembourg: Publications Office of the European Union.

Brotherhood, A., & Sumnall, H. R. (2012). *Social reintegration and employment: evidence and interventions for drug users in treatment*. Luxembourg: Publications Office of the European Union.

Burkhart, G. (2015). International standards in prevention: How to influence prevention systems by policy interventions? *International Journal of Prevention and Treatment of Substance Use Disorders, 1*(3–4), 18–37.

Burton, R., Henn, C., Lavoie, D., O'Connor, R., Perkins, C., Sweeney, K., ... Sheron, N. (2017). A rapid evidence review of the effectiveness and cost-effectiveness of alcohol control policies: An English perspective. *The Lancet, 389*(10078), 1558–1580.

Bywood, P. T., Lunnay, B., & Roche, A. M. (2008a). *Effective dissemination: A systematic review of implementation strategies for the AOD field*. Adelaide: National Centre for Education and Training on Addiction.

Bywood, P. T., Lunnay, B., & Roche, A. M. (2008b). *Effective dissemination: An examination of the costs of implementation strategies for the AOD field*. Adelaide: National Centre for Education and Training on Addiction.

Bywood, P. T., Lunnay, B., & Roche, A. M. (2008c). *An examination of theory and models of change for research dissemination in the AOD field*. Adelaide: National Centre for Education and Training on Addiction.

Canadian Centre on Substance Abuse. (2015). Competencies for the youth substance use prevention workforce: Prevention workforce competencies report. In *Canadian Centre on substance abuse*. Ontario: Ottawa.

Cates, W. (1995). Prevention science: The umbrella discipline. *American Journal of Preventive Medicine, 11*(4), 211.

Center for Applied Research Solutions. (2013). *CA prevention workforce development survey report*. Santa Rosa, CA: Community Prevention Initiative.

Charvat, M., Jurystova, L., & Miovsky, M. (2012). Four-level model of qualifications for the practitioners of the primary prevention of risk behaviour in the school system. *Adiktologie, 12*(3), 190–211.

Cohen, D. J., Crabtree, B. F., Etz, R. S., Balasubramanian, B. A., Donahue, K. E., Leviton, L. C., ... Green, L. W. (2008). Fidelity versus flexibility: Translating evidence-based research into practice. *American Journal of Preventive Medicine, 35*, S381–S389.

Connell, C. M., Gilreath, T. D., Aklin, W. M., & Brex, R. A. (2010). Social-ecological influences on patterns of substance use among non-metropolitan high school students. *American Journal of Community Psychology, 45*(0), 36–48.

Cordova, D., Estrada, Y., Malcolm, S., Huang, S., Hendricks Brown, C., Pantin, H., & Prado, G. (2014). Prevention science: An epidemiological approach. In Z. Sloboda & H. Petras (Eds.), *Defining prevention science*. New York: Springer.

Council of the European Union. (2015). *Council conclusions on the implementation of the EU action plan on drugs 2013–2016 regarding minimum quality standards in drug demand reduction in the European Union*. General Secretariat of the Council (Ed.). Brussels, Belgium.

Durlak, J. A., & DuPre, E. P. (2008). Implementation matters: A review of research on the influence of implementation on program outcomes and the factors affecting implementation. *American Journal of Community Psychology, 41*(3–4), 327–350.

Eddy, J. M., Smith, P., Brown, C. H., & Reid, J. B. (2005). A survey of prevention science training: Implications for educating the next generation. *Prevention Science, 6*(1), 59–71.

Edman, J. (2012). Swedish drug treatment and the political use of conceptual innovation 1882–1982. *Contemporary Drug Problems, 39*(3), 429–460.

EMCDDA. (2013). *North American drug prevention programmes: are they feasible in European cultures and contexts?* Luxembourg: Publications Office of the European Union.

EMCDDA. (2017). *European drug report 2017: Trends and developments*. Luxembourg: Publishing Office of the European Union.

Ennett, S. T., Haws, S., Ringwalt, C. L., Vincus, A. A., Hanley, S., Bowling, J. M., & Rohrbach, L. A. (2011). Evidence-based practice in school substance use prevention: Fidelity of implementation under real-world conditions. *Health Education Research, 26*(2), 361–371.

Esrick, J., Kagan, R. G., Carnevale, J. T., Valenti, M., Rots, G., & Dash, K. (2018). Can scare tactics and fear-based messages help deter substance misuse: A systematic review of recent (2005–2017) research. *Drugs: Education, Prevention and Policy, 25*, 1–10. https://doi.org/10.1080/09687637.2018.1424115

Faggiano, F., Allara, E., Giannotta, F., Molinar, R., Sumnall, H. R., Wiers, R., ... Conrod, P. (2014). Europe needs a central, transparent, and evidence-based approval process for behavioural prevention interventions. *PLoS Medicine, 11*(10), e1001740.

Faggiano, F., Vigna-Taglianti, F. D., Versino, E., Zambon, A., Borraccino, A., & Lemma, P. (2008). School-based prevention for illicit drugs use: A systematic review. *Preventive Medicine, 46*(5), 385–396.

Farrugia, A. (2014). Assembling the dominant accounts of youth drug use in Australian harm reduction drug education. *International Journal of Drug Policy, 25*(4), 663–672.

Farrugia, A. (2017). Gender, reputation and regret: the ontological politics of Australian drug education. *Gender and Education, 29*, 281–298.

Ferri, M., Ballotta, D., Carra, G., & Dias, S. (2015). A review of regional drug strategies across the world: How is prevention perceived and addressed? *Drugs: Education, Prevention and Policy, 22*(5), 444–448.

Ferri, M., Dias, S., Bo, A., Ballotta, D., Simon, R., & Carrá, G. (2016). Quality assurance in drug demand reduction in European countries: An overview. *Drugs: Education, Prevention and Policy, 25*(2), 1–7.

Flay, B. R., Biglan, A., Boruch, R. F., Gonzalez Castro, F., Gottfredson, D., Kellam, S., ... Ji, P. (2005). Standards of evidence: Criteria for efficacy, effectiveness and dissemination. *Prevention Science, 6*(3), 151–175.

Fletcher, A., Calafat, A., Pirona, A., & Olszewski, D. (2010). Young people, recreational drug use and harm reduction. In T. Rhodes & D. Hedrich (Eds.), *Harm reduction: Evidence, impacts and challenges* (pp. 357–379). Lisbon: EMCDDA.

Foxcroft, D. R. (2014). Can prevention classification be improved by considering the function of prevention? *Prevention Science, 15*(6), 818–822.

Foxcroft, D. R., & Tsertsvadze, A. (2011a). Universal family-based prevention programs for alcohol misuse in young people. *Cochrane Database of Systematic Reviews*, (9), CD009308.

Foxcroft, D. R., & Tsertsvadze, A. (2011b). Universal multi-component prevention programs for alcohol misuse in young people. *Cochrane Database of Systematic Reviews*, (9), CD009307.

Foxcroft, D. R., & Tsertsvadze, A. (2012). Universal alcohol misuse prevention programmes for children and adolescents: Cochrane database of systematic reviews. *Perspectives in Public Health, 132*(3), 128–134.

Gilchrist, G., Moskalewicz, J., Slezakova, S., Okruhlica, L., Torrens, M., Vajd, R., & Baldacchino, A. (2011). Staff regard towards working with substance users: A European multi-centre study. *Addiction, 106*(6), 1114–1125.

Gottfredson, D. C., Cook, T. D., Gardner, F. E. M., Gorman-Smith, D., Howe, G. W., Sandler, I. N., & Zafft, K. M. (2015). Standards of evidence for efficacy, effectiveness, and scale-up research in prevention science: Next generation. *Prevention Science, 16*(7), 893–926.

Greenhalgh, T., Howick, J., & Maskrey, N. (2014). Evidence based medicine: A movement in crisis? *British Medical Journal, 348*, g3725.

Greenhalgh, T., Robert, G., MacFarlane, F., Bate, P., & Kyriakidou, O. (2004). Diffusion of innovations in service organizations: Systematic review and recommendations. *The Milbank Quarterly, 82*(4), 581–629.

Grimshaw, J., Thomas, R., MacLennan, G., Fraser, C., & Ramsay, C. (2004). Effectiveness and efficiency of guideline dissemination and implementation strategies. *Health Technology Assessment, 8*(6), 84.

Grimshaw, J. M., Shirran, L., Thomas, R., Mowatt, G., Fraser, C., Bero, L., ... O'Brien, M. A. (2001). Changing provider behavior: An overview of systematic reviews of interventions. *Medical Care, 39*(8 Suppl 2), Ii2–I45.

H.M. Government. (2017). *2017 Drug strategy*. London: H.M. Government.

Hale, D. R., Fitzgerald-Yau, N., & Viner, R. M. (2014). A systematic review of effective interventions for reducing multiple health risk behaviors in adolescence. *American Journal of Public Health, 104*(5), e19–e41.

Hale, D. R., & Viner, R. M. (2012). Policy responses to multiple risk behaviours in adolescents. *Journal of Public Health (Oxford, England), 34*(Suppl 1), i11–i19.

Hale, D. R., & Viner, R. M. (2016). The correlates and course of multiple health risk behaviour in adolescence. *BMC Public Health, 16*(1), 458.

Halgunseth, L. C., Carmack, C., Childs, S. S., Caldwell, L., Craig, A., & Smith, E. P. (2012). Using the interactive systems framework in understanding the relation between program capacity and implementation in afterschool settings. *American Journal Community Psychology, 50*, 311–320.

Hawe, P., Shiell, A., & Riley, T. (2009). Theorising interventions as events in systems. *American Journal of Community Psychology, 43*(3–4), 267–276.

Hawkins, J. D., Catalano, R. F., & Miller, J. Y. (1992). Risk and protective factors for alcohol and other drug problems in adolescence and early adulthood: Implications for substance abuse prevention. *Psychological Bulletin, 112*(1), 64–105.

Heim, D. (2014). Addiction: Not just brain malfunction. *Nature, 507*(7490), 40.

Hickman, M., Caldwell, D. M., Busse, H., MacArthur, G., Faggiano, F., Foxcroft, D. R., ... Campbell, R. (2014). Individual-, family-, and school-level interventions for preventing multiple risk behaviours relating to alcohol, tobacco and drug use in individuals aged 8 to 25 years (Protocol). *Cochrane Database of Systematic Reviews*, (11). Art. No.: CD011374. https://doi.org/10.1002/14651858.CD011374

Institute of Medicine Committee on Prevention of Mental Disorders. (1994). *Reducing risks for mental disorders: Frontiers for preventive intervention research*. Washington, DC: National Academies Press.

International Centre for Credentialing and Education of Addiction Professionals. (2016). White Paper. Colombo Plan.

International Society of Substance Use Professionals. (2017). *Universal prevention curriculum*. Retrieved from https://www.issup.net/training/universal-prevention-curriculum

Israelashvili, M. (2011). *The paradox of realism in exposing students to ex-addicts*. Lisbon: European Society for Prevention Research.

Järvinen, M., & Demant, J. (2011). The normalisation of cannabis use among young people: Symbolic boundary work in focus groups. *Health, Risk & Society, 13*(2), 165–182.

Klimas, J. (2015). Training in addiction medicine should be standardised and scaled up. *British Medical Journal, 351*, h4027.

Le Deist, F. D., & Winterton, J. (2005). What is competence? *Human Resource Development International, 8*(1), 27–46.

Livingston, J. D., Milne, T., Fang, M. L., & Amari, E. (2012). The effectiveness of interventions for reducing stigma related to substance use disorders: A systematic review. *Addiction (Abingdon, England), 107*(1), 39–50.

Lorenc, T., Petticrew, M., Welch, V., & Tugwell, P. (2013). What types of interventions generate inequalities? Evidence from systematic reviews. *Journal* of *Epidemiology and Community Health, 67*(2), 190–193.

Marmot, M. (2005). Social determinants of health inequalities. *Lancet, 365*(9464), 1099–1104.

Mattingly, P. (1977). The meaning of professional culture. *The Review of Education, 3*(6), 435–445.

McKay, M. T., Sumnall, H. R., Harvey, S. A., & Cole, J. C. (2018). Perceptions of school-based alcohol education by educational and health stakeholders: "Education as usual" compared to a randomised controlled trial. *Drugs: Education, Prevention and Policy, 25*(1), 77–87.

McLeroy, K. R., Bibeau, D., Steckler, A., & Glanz, K. (1988). An ecological perspective on health promotion programs. *Health Education Quarterly, 15*(4), 351–377.

Meader, N., King, K., Wright, K., Graham, H. M., Petticrew, M., Power, C., ... Sowden, A. J. (2017). Multiple risk behavior interventions: Meta-analyses of RCTs. *American Journal of Preventive Medicine, 53*(1), e19–e30.

Miovský, M., Miller, P., Grund, J. P., Belackova, V., Gabrhelik, R., & Libra, J. (2015). Academic education in addictology (addiction science) in the Czech Republic: Analysis of the (pre-1989) historical origins. *Nordic Studies on Alcohol and Drugs, 32*, 527–538.

Miovsky, M. (2013). An evidence-based approach in school prevention means an everyday fight: A case study of the Czech Republic's experience with national quality standards and a national certification system. *Adicciones, 25*(3), 203–207.

National Institute for Health and Care Excellence. (2017). *Drug misuse prevention: Targeted interventions. NICE guideline [NG64]*. London: NICE.

Nelson, A. (2017). Addiction workforce development in Aotearoa New Zealand. *Drugs: Education, Prevention and Policy, 24*(6), 461–468.

Oliver, K. A., & de Vocht, F. (2015). Defining 'evidence' in public health: A survey of policymakers' uses and preferences. *European Journal of Public Health, 27*(suppl_2), 112–117.

Ostaszewski, K., Feric, M., Foxcroft, D. R., Kosir, M., Kranzelic, V., Mihic, J., ... Talic, S. (2017). European prevention workforce competencies and training needs: An exploratory study. *Adiktologie, 1*, 7–15.

Pavlovská, A., Miovský, M., Babor, T. F., & Gabrhelík, R. (2017). Overview of the European university-based study programmes in the addictions field. *Drugs: Education, Prevention and Policy, 24*(6), 485–491.

Pennay, A. M., & Measham, F. C. (2016). The normalisation thesis—20 years later. *Drugs: Education, Prevention and Policy, 23*(3), 187–189.

Reeves, S., Perrier, L., Goldman, J., Freeth, D., & Zwarenstein, M. (2013). Interprofessional education: effects on professional practice and healthcare outcomes (update). *Cochrane Database of Systematic Reviews*, (3), Cd002213.

Rehm, J., Babor, T., & Room, R. (2006). Education, persuasion and the reduction of alcohol-related harm: A reply to Craplet. *Addiction, 101*(3), 452–453.

Roche, A., & Nicholas, R. (2017). Workforce development: An important paradigm shift for the alcohol and other drugs sector. *Drugs: Education, Prevention and Policy, 24*(6), 443–454.

Roche, A. M., Pidd, K., & Freeman, T. (2009). Achieving professional practice change: From training to workforce development. *Drug and Alcohol Review, 28*(5), 550–557.

Roumeliotis, F. (2015). Politics of prevention: The emergence of prevention science. *International Journal of Drug Policy, 26*(8), 746–754.

Russell, C., Davies, J. B., & Hunter, S. C. (2011). Predictors of addiction treatment providers' beliefs in the disease and choice models of addiction. *Journal of Substance Abuse Treatment, 40*(2), 150–164.

Rutter, H., Savona, N., Glonti, K., Bibby, J., Cummins, S., Finegood, D. T., ... White, M. (2017). The need for a complex systems model of evidence for public health. *Lancet, 390*(10112), 2602–2604.

Santos da Silveira, P., Andrade de Tostes, J. C., Wan, H. T., Ronzani, T. M., & Corrigan, P. W. (2018). The stigmatization of drug use as mechanism of legitimation of exclusion. In T. M. Ronzani (Ed.), *Drugs and social context: Social perspectives on the use of alcohol and other drugs* (pp. 15–25). Cham: Springer International Publishing.

Saunders, M., Barr, B., McHale, P., & Hamelmann, C. (2017). *Key policies for addressing the social determinants of health and health inequities*. Copenhagen: World Health Organization.

Skinner, N., Feather, N., Freeman, T., & Roche, A. M. (2007). Stigma and discrimination in health-care provision to drug users: The role of values, affect, and deservingness judgements. *Journal of Applied Social Psychology, 37*, 163–186.

Sloboda, Z., Dusenbury, L., & Petras, H. (2014). Implementation of science and the effective delivery of evidence-based prevention. In Z. Sloboda & H. Petras (Eds.), *Defining prevention science*. New York: Springer.

Smith, L. R., Earnshaw, V. A., Copenhaver, M. M., & Cunningham, C. O. (2016). Substance use stigma: Reliability and validity of a theory-based scale for substance-using populations. *Drug and Alcohol Dependence, 162*(Supplement C), 34–43.

Sussman, S., Levy, D., Lich, K. H., Cene, C. W., Kim, M. M., Rohrbach, L. A., & Chaloupka, F. J. (2013). Comparing effects of tobacco use prevention modalities: Need for complex system models. *Tobacco Induced Diseases, 11*(1), 2.

Thompson, L. E., Barnett, J. R., & Pearce, J. R. (2009). Scared straight? Fear-appeal anti-smoking campaigns, risk, self-efficacy and addiction. *Health, Risk & Society, 11*(2), 181–196.

Thurman, B., & Boughelaf, J. (2015). "We don't get taught enough": An assessment of drug education provision in schools in England. *Drugs and Alcohol Today, 15*(3), 127–140.

UNODC. (2004). *Drug abuse prevention among youth from ethnic and indigenous minorities*. New York: United Nations.

UNODC. (2013). *International standards on drug use prevention*. Vienna: UNODC.

van Boekel, L. C., Brouwers, E. P., van Weeghel, J., & Garretsen, H. F. (2013). Stigma among health professionals towards patients with substance use disorders and its consequences for healthcare delivery: Systematic review. *Drug Alcohol Dependence, 131*(1–2), 23–35.

van der Kreeft, P., Jongbloet, J., Schamp, J., Becona, E., Foxcroft, D. R., Gabrhelik, R., ... Mulligan, K. (2015). *Mapping prevention science education courses across Europe*. Ghent: University College Ghent.

van der Kreeft, P., Jongbloet, J., & Van Havare, T. (2014a). Factors affecting implementation: Cultural adaptation and training. In Z. Sloboda & H. Petras (Eds.), *Defining prevention science*. New York: Springer.

van der Kreeft, P., Jongbloet, J., Schamp, J., Becona, E., Foxcroft, D. R., Gabrhelik, R., ... Feric, M. (2014b). *Mapping prevention science workforce education and training needs in Europe*. Oxford: Oxford Brookes University.

Vanyukov, M. M., Tarter, R. E., Kirillova, G. P., Kirisci, L., Reynolds, M. D., Kreek, M. J., ... Ridenour, T. A. (2012). Common liability to addiction and "gateway hypothesis": Theoretical, empirical and evolutionary perspective. *Drug Alcohol Dependence, 123*(Suppl 1), S3–S17.

Viner, R. M., Ozer, E. M., Denny, S., Marmot, M., Resnick, M., Fatusi, A., & Currie, C. (2012). Adolescence and the social determinants of health. *The Lancet, 379*(9826), 1641–1652.

Volkow, N. D., Koob, G. F., & McLellan, A. T. (2016). Neurobiologic advances from the brain disease model of addiction. *New England Journal of Medicine, 374*(4), 363–371.

von Hippel, W., Brener, L., & von Hippel, C. (2008). Implicit prejudice toward injecting drug users predicts intentions to change jobs among drug and alcohol nurses. *Psychological Science, 19*(1), 7–11.

Wandersman, A., Duffy, J., Flaspohler, P., Noonan, R., Lubell, K., Stillman, L., ... Saul, J. (2008). Bridging the gap between prevention research and practice: The interactive systems framework for dissemination and implementation. *American Journal of Community Psychology, 41*(3–4), 171–181.

Ward, V., House, A., & Hamer, S. (2009). Developing a framework for transferring knowledge into action: A thematic analysis of the literature. *Journal of Health Services Research & Policy, 14*(3), 156–164.

Werb, D. (2018). Post-war prevention: Emerging frameworks to prevent drug use after the War on drugs. *International Journal of Drug Policy, 51*, 160–164.

Westreich, L. M. (2002). Addiction and the Americans with disabilities act. *The Journal of the American Academy of Psychiatry and the Law, 30*(3), 355–363.

World Health Organization. (2008). *WHO report on the global tobacco epidemic*. Geneva: World Health Organization.

Ysa, T., Colom, J., Albareda, A., Ramon, A., Carrion, M., & Segura, L. (2014). *Governance of addictions: European public policies*. Oxford: Oxford University Press.

Prevention Systems: Structure and Challenges: Europe as an Example

26

Gregor Burkhart and Stefanie Helmer

Introduction

The primary focus, mostly in North America, has been on developing and implementing "manualised" interventions. These are generally structured in a modular standardised format, which defines the number and sequence of sessions, as well as their content (e.g. social skills, awareness, normative education), their delivery (e.g. by interactive teaching strategies or by means of open discussions, role play, group work), contextual factors such as the composition of the target group, the person who should deliver the intervention, and above all the materials that have to be used. Such interventions allow for accounting for the active ingredients of a program, facilitate knowing how much dosage the target group actually received and therefore properly evaluate the effects of an intervention. Most of the evidence about substance-use prevention comes from such manualised programmes. A plausible and logical strategy is therefore to bring such interventions to scale. It is in this context that research has increasingly been focusing on "systems", since the importance of implementation quality is highlighted by evidence suggesting that even if effective programmes are available, this is not sufficient in itself to produce positive outcomes in target groups (Chan, Oldenburg, & Viswanath, 2015; Grimshaw, Eccles, Lavis, Hill, & Squires, 2012; Hunter, Han, Slaughter, Godley, & Garner, 2015; Ringwalt et al., 2010, 2011). It has often been reported that interventions that were highly effective in efficacy studies were then generally not widely implemented under real-world conditions (Tibbits, Bumbarger, Kyler, & Perkins, 2010) or did not yield results when implemented widely (Dzewaltowski, Estabrooks, Klesges, Bull, & Glasgow, 2004; Institute of Medicine and National Research, 2009). Additionally, many evidence-based interventions are not sustained after initial implementation (Scheirer & Dearing, 2011).

One key question has therefore been whether such effective and well-implemented programmes can actually be scaled up system-wide to such a degree that they can produce detectable impacts at the community or population level. For this purpose, the understanding and development of implementation factors such as policy, structure, organisation, workforce and its prevention ethos and culture may be as important (Aarons et al., 2014) as identifying effective interventions (Grol, 1997; Ritter & McDonald, 2008) since scaling up continues to be the main

G. Burkhart (✉)
European Monitoring Centre for Drugs and Drug Addiction, Lisbon, Portugal
e-mail: Gregor.Burkhart@emcdda.europa.eu

S. Helmer
Institute of Social Medicine, Epidemiology and Health Economics, Charité - Universitätsmedizin Berlin, Berlin, Germany
e-mail: stefanie.helmer@charite.de

challenge. Hence, there is a need for comprehensive system-level processes that facilitate and accelerate the cycle of implementing findings of evidence-based research in a sustainable manner to practice and policy (Fishbein, Ridenour, Stahl, & Sussman, 2016; Wang, Moss, & Hiller, 2006).

What Does a Systems Approach Offer?

General systems theory (Von Bertalanffy, 1968) is a way of describing all kinds of systems with interacting components. The aim is to discover patterns and to find principles that can be distilled from and applied to all types of systems, be it in biology, social sciences, administration or mathematics. Within this framework, the prevention field could be conceived as a complex system, since there are many components (some of them unknown or undetermined) that interact with each other in almost unpredictable, complex ways, similar to an organism or the climate. Complex systems typically have feedback loops, a certain degree of spontaneous order or self-organisation (which is stable) and an emergent hierarchical organisation (Simon, 1991). Such a complex system is adaptive to changes in its local environment, is composed of other complex systems (for example, the human body) and behaves in a non-linear fashion so that change in outcome is not proportional to change in input (Shiell, Hawe, & Gold, 2008). Common to all system thinking is a comparison of an environment (or situation) as it is, and some models of the environment as it might or could be. This comparison can lead to a better understanding of the environment (the research and analytic part), and to proposals about how to improve it, and hence the rationale of this analysis.

Systems theory and the concept of a "prevention system" per se are relatively recent. It has been used predominantly to describe prevention delivery systems, such as the Community That Cares[1] system, which motivates and brings together community stakeholders assisting them in making science-based choices about the most adequate evidence-based prevention interventions to be implemented in their community (Arthur et al., 2010; Fagan, Arthur, Hanson, Briney, & Hawkins, 2011; Van Horn, Fagan, Hawkins, & Oesterle, 2014). This is in line with the main focus of implementation science, which is concerned with improving the scaling up, fidelity, acceptance and sustainability of manualised prevention programmes (Palinkas et al., 2015; Spoth, Guyll, Redmond, Greenberg, & Feinberg, 2011). During the collaborative work that took place across Europe while developing the European Drug Prevention Quality Standards—EDPQS—(Brotherhood & Sumnall, 2011), the concept of a "prevention system" achieved a broader meaning that includes different kinds of prevention activities, services and policies, including manualised, behavioural interventions. The essential feature of this prevention systems approach is to recognise the dynamic interactions of interventions within the broader context into which they are introduced. Such complex ecological systems can be schools, municipalities or entire societies. Hawe, Shiell, and Riley (2009) posit that three dimensions are particularly important: (1) the activity settings (e.g. clubs, assemblies, classrooms); (2) the social networks that connect the people and the settings; and (3) time. An intervention, for example a local policy or an evidence-based intervention, may then be seen as a critical and innovative event in the history of a system, leading to the evolution of new structures of interaction and new meanings. This can include changing relationships, displacing existing activities, and redistributing and transforming resources.

Prevention systems are directly interwoven with existing substance-use policies which generally aim to develop and deploy infrastructure, interventions and services in order to reduce the incidence of substance-use problems and associated or antecedent problem behaviours, mostly at the population level. In addition, there are higher level factors that are likely to influence the functioning of prevention systems, such as national legislation, social capital and social inequality.

---

[1] http://www.communitiesthatcare.net/

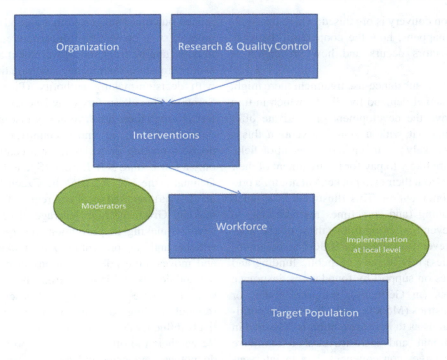

Fig. 26.1 The schematic composition of a prevention system

We propose five putative components of a prevention system, based on the information and data from and the experiences in Europe (Fig. 26.1): (1) *organisation*, i.e. decision-making structures; (2) *research and quality control*; (3) *interventions*; (4) prevention *workforce*; and (5) *target populations* themselves. This is complemented by a set of *moderators* that influence the interaction of these components. Furthermore, the implementation at the local level needs to be taken into account. In this chapter, we discuss the system components and moderators and include examples from available data sources from EU countries and transnational projects in the European Union.

Since this system-focused way of looking at prevention is relatively new, to gather information on these aspects is challenging: some important pieces of information are not readily available: political will or cooperation and professional cultures are difficult to assess and there is few information about the composition of the prevention workforce and its training. Countries do however report about the type of interventions, research and development, quality criteria, funding and organisational aspects. Besides this structural system, it is important to describe contextual mediators (elements, whose modification through policies changes the overall effect) such as administrative organisation, intersectorial cooperation, interaction with academia, implementation and moderators (that affect overall effects without being easily modified) that we hypothesise to influence the overall delivery of prevention. This model is conceptually similar to a recently proposed community systems model for obesity (Allender et al., 2015), or for behavioural change through environmental structures (e.g. MINDSPACE, Institute for Government, 2009), all of which propose interaction of different contextual and behavioural elements.

Organisation

It goes without saying that the term 'organisation' might cover a vast array of aspects, but we use it here only to subsume three aspects of how prevention delivery is organised: where decision-making happens, how the cooperation between policy sectors occurs and how prevention is funded.

While for substance-use treatment there might exist an actual demand by clients, which in turn could drive the development of a private offer responding to it, without state intervention, this is much less likely to happen in the prevention field. Parents are likely to pay for the treatment of their offspring from their own pocket, but not for a prevention intervention. This illustrates how much policymaking (and sometimes research) has to drive prevention. In addition, most of the non-public prevention providers (NGOs, associations, universities) rely heavily on public funding and sometimes on support by foundations, insurance companies (in Germany), religious bodies or even industries (Moodie et al., 2013). The political decisions as to how prevention is delivered in organisational and infrastructural terms have therefore larger consequences than in intervention fields where people themselves (or their insurances) would pay for services, actively look for them, choose the most adequate and create hence a client-driven demand. Whether, how, where and for whom prevention interventions are developed, funded and deployed depend to a far larger degree on political decisions (at least at local level) than on "demand" (as in treatment) or than on bottom-up initiatives of those affected (as in harm reduction). The different political organisation of countries therefore plays a major role in implementing evidence-based prevention. Furthermore, policies can have an impact on the sustainability of prevention at local and national levels (Aarons et al., 2014).

Where Are Decisions Made?

Another factor is the level of strategic decision-making and the cooperation structures between sectors that can be critical when moving from policy decisions to policy implementation. A US evaluation study that assessed state substance-use prevention system infrastructure in order to examine their role in achieving prevention-related outcomes suggested that a good development of state prevention infrastructure is linked to both funding from state government and presence of a state interagency coordinating body with decision-making authority (Piper, Stein-Seroussi, Flewelling, Orwin, & Buchanan, 2012). Even though there are several key institutions on different levels, in most countries strategic decision-making priorities lie at a central level; only a few countries in Europe (Spain, Germany, Denmark, the UK, Austria, the Czech Republic and Latvia) reported local and regional decision-making. Given the high leverage of centralised decision-making in prevention, the question is whether and how prevention policymaking shifts and moves alongside innovations in prevention methodologies and insights from the prevention sciences. There is no theory that describes how research findings and interventions can effectively influence decision makers' use of evidence. Researchers too often assume that policymakers do not use evidence and that the use of more research evidence would benefit policymakers and populations. By focussing on "getting evidence into policy", less attention has been paid to how research and policy actually interact in vivo. "Rather than asking how research evidence can be made more influential, academics should aim to understand what influences and constitutes policy, and produce more critically and theoretically informed studies of decision-making" (Oliver, Lorenc, & Innvær, 2014). A recent analysis (Langer, Tripney, & Gough, 2016) of the factors that influence policymakers' decisions outlines six intervention mechanisms of evidence use: awareness of evidence-based interventions; agreement about what is evidence; communication and access to evidence; facilitation of engagement between researchers and decision-makers; decision-makers' skills to access and use evidence; and influencing decision-making structures and processes. Several of these elements will appear again in the analysis presented in this chapter. Research and research findings should be more attuned to the needs of policymakers and practitioners, thus fundamentally changing the way in which research is produced and consumed. Rather than academics exclusively setting the agenda, in a new approach to knowledge, researchers, and those they are seeking to address, need to work together to define the research questions, agree on the methods and assess the implications of the data analysis and findings for policy and practice (Hunter, 2009).

Factual Cooperation Between Policy Sectors

A recent joint publication by UNESCO, UNODC and WHO (2017) about the role of the education sector in substance-use prevention sheds light on an often-overlooked detail: policy sectors that could reach the most important shares of the target populations for prevention, in many countries, don't cooperate with those sectors or entities that develop prevention policies. Even if interventions have been proven effective and been successfully implemented in an array of countries, many school authorities nevertheless refuse to have them implemented. Ideological perspectives about how prevention should be delivered (Burkhart, 2013, 2015) are not the only reason; often the relevant policy sectors do not see their own interests being served in exchange for yielding resources for prevention and it isn't only the education (school-based prevention) or the social sectors (family-based prevention) that are not enthusiastic. Also ministries for economy and trade are used to having alcohol, gambling and tobacco tax incomes and value the interests of the respective industries, including advertising, publicity, etc. This aspect is often more pronounced in municipalities who depend sometimes heavily on the nightlife industry (Calafat et al., 2011; Hall, 2005; Hobbs, 2005; Winlow & Hall, 2005). There are therefore tensions between addictive goods as revenue raisers and as burdens upon health (Casswell & Thamarangsi, 2009; Moodie et al., 2013). Different ministries may also be looking for different outcomes. Health ministries will be interested in morbidity and mortality, justice in crime and education in educational achievement. In the European example, several countries have inter-ministerial commissions (Lithuania and France) or official institutions that are only responsible for prevention tasks (Hungary) and that are in charge of coordinating prevention among the different ministries. The information from only a third of the countries[2] suggests however that there is any actual cooperation. Albeit in Austria, where there is no national coordinating body for prevention, access to the school system for the implementation of programs is facilitated by the Ministry of Education, whereas in a few other countries evidence-based prevention programmes are not accepted by the school system. Often though, there are instances when cooperation can succeed at the local level. In Denmark, for instance, the BTI model (Danish for *Improved Interdisciplinary Efforts*) for systematic interdisciplinary cooperation targets staff in local services to provide guidance and tools. This model can be adapted to existing work in other municipalities with the aim to assure quality in integrated, coordinated efforts without interrupting follow-up of children, young people and families that need help. Similar systems exist in Norway and in some regions in Northern Italy. This is also why many prevention quality standards[3] highlight the importance of establishing alliances and coalitions with key actors for prevention at local level.

How Is Prevention Funded?

Funding avenues are an essential requirement for the development of effective interventions but also for successful implementation and sustainability (Fixsen, Naoom, Blase, Friedman, & Wallace, 2005). However, data on funding are scarce and there is not enough information available for precise estimates of what is needed and given to finance prevention activities. In Europe, almost all countries report central national

---

[2]The Czech Republic, Denmark, Ireland, Greece, Lithuania, Poland, Romania, Luxembourg, Finland, Sweden and Norway.
[3]http://prevention-standards.eu/toolkit-4/
http://www.emcdda.europa.eu/attachements.cfm/att_218446_EN_TD0113424ENN.pdf
http://www.communitiesthatcarecoalition.org/

funding allocations but some countries such as Spain, Germany, the UK, Austria, the Czech Republic, France and Latvia also mention regional funding resources for prevention. As an exception, in Denmark local funding services are predominant.

Since many European societies consider prevention as pertaining to public health, it does not come as a surprise that European countries have ministries or drug coordinators on federal and local levels that are responsible for prevention and are its key financing sources. Even if public funding continues to play a central role in supporting prevention, funding by insurance companies as direct service is likely to increase, as is the case in Germany and France. In Bulgaria, Austria and Poland, small parts of alcohol and tobacco tax revenues are used as investments for substance-use prevention, whereas in Spain, the confiscated assets of drug traffickers can be channelled into prevention funds. In some countries in the northern Europe, revenues from the gambling industry feed into prevention funding. Such funding sources are primarily at a central level as well.

Research and Quality Control

There are four aspects of the research and quality control component that are important to mention: funding, availability of technical assistance, assessment of local needs identified for prevention programming and prevention standards.

Conditional Funding

In some countries, specific funding programmes only support interventions that are highly rated in evidence-based registries[4] or by commissions. These funding schemes however do not represent the main financing stream for prevention. Currently, only two countries make full use of this mechanism at the national level: Portugal and the Czech Republic. In the latter, institutions can only receive public funding if they are accredited and if their interventions or programs have been certified (Charvát, Jurystová, & Miovsky, 2012). This is the result of an implementation and negotiation process that lasted more than 10 years, but which now communicates to the population that prevention is taken as seriously as treatment. In Portugal the most vulnerable areas in the country are identified in collaboration with local NGOs working in the field. The existing resources (services, NGOs, interventions) in the different intervention areas are mapped as well. Local institutions, NGOs or associations can then propose joint (i.e. they should make use of all locally available resources) intervention proposals to the central drug coordination office, SICAD,[5] which allocates funding and provides technical advice about how to improve interventions. The system seems to respond both to the need of quality assurance and to the importance of involving local stakeholders in the needs assessment and in intervention development.

Obviously, in a number of other countries as well, projects have to comply with the priorities of the existing National Plan. Such priorities are however often open to interpretation, so that interventions of dubious quality might still get funding.

Given the above-described situation, i.e. prevention funding in Europe is mostly public and mostly centralised, it seems that there is an important increase in the motivation to apply evidence and process standards in a more binding and rigorous way, by making funding conditional upon current widely accepted quality criteria, both for internal validity and for the evidence that they are based on. More complexity arises when prevention funding is specifically labelled (such as grants for a prevention program) or when prevention spending is part of more general activities (e.g. an early-years development fund or an educational engagement program).

---

[4]For example http://cayt.mentor-adepis.org/ in the UK

[5]General Directorate for Intervention on Addictive Behaviours and Dependencies: http://www.sicad.pt/EN/Paginas/default.aspx

Technical Assistance

As conditional funding is clearly the exception in Europe, and since local prevention agencies in most countries enjoy quite a high level of independence—only the prevention centres in Greece, Lithuania and Romania seem to be bound to stricter guidelines—technical assistance is the next important strategy that can theoretically improve the quality of prevention, as well as the uptake and sustainability of innovations. Technical assistance aims to enhance the readiness of practitioners to implement evidence-based prevention interventions, but some studies suggest that technical assistance is rarely delivered to professionals who are seeking to sustain innovations subsequent to adoption and implementation (Katz & Wandersman, 2016). This limitation might be a reflection that these studies are more concerned with technical assistance for the implementation of specific manualised interventions as they prevail in the Americas, and less concerned with scientific support for practitioners in general. Scientific support, advice and guidance are particularly important in countries where the delivery of prevention is largely delegated to the local level and where manualisation is rare. If the technical assistance partnerships create a collaborative relationship with local practitioners, science-based innovation can be moulded to local conditions. "Improvement science" has become the term for such approaches in which local practitioners are trained to use evidence to experiment with local pilots and learn and adapt to their experiences. In contrast, models such as the *Early Years Collaborative* in Scotland reverse this emphasis, using scholarship as one of many sources of information and focusing primarily on the assets of practitioners and service users (Cairney, 2015). The abandoned prevention training modules of CICAD[6] in Central America and the Caribbean used such a model, where, after each training module, practitioners had to experiment with evidence-based approaches in their environments and feed these experiences back into the next training module.

The Portuguese system within the above-described PORI (*Plano Operacional de Repostas Integradas*—Operational Plan for Integrated Responses) which provides technical assistance to all the local prevention partnerships, NGOs and associations in vulnerable areas uses such a methodology of improvement science and has produced a number of reasonably evaluated local interventions that are innovative and grounded in local conditions and needs. This program focuses however on prevention, harm reduction and social reintegration regarding drugs, in vulnerable areas, and belongs exclusively to the National Drugs Institute SICAD (*Serviço de Intervenção nos Comportamentos Aditivos e nas Dependências*).

The countries in the north of Europe also seem to have embraced this approach in a broader perspective, but with differing intensity. Public health institutes organise quality trainings for local prevention agencies and NGOs, or regional competence centres advise municipalities on science-based prevention principles. The training measures target county governors as well as key personnel in the municipalities beyond prevention practitioners, such as administrative decision-makers, politicians, relevant sector managers, retail and licensed trades, police, health personnel, local school managers, teachers, parents/guardians and voluntary organisations. Different from most other countries, this testifies to a conceptualisation of prevention beyond the narrow concept of "drug education" towards a stronger focus on socio-environmental determinants of behaviour.

Such strategies are even more important when quality control is delegated, alongside delivery, to the local level, as seems to be the case in the Nordic countries, Germany and the Netherlands. Responsible prevention policymakers would strive to make sure that local prevention professionals, agencies and NGOs implement interventions other than those that are only instinctively appealing approaches (educating, awareness raising, risk communication). Yet many professionals in the field continue to be fond of awareness raising and cognitive or educational interventions. These however may be more effective for

---

[6] http://www.cicad.oas.org/main/default_eng.asp

less vulnerable populations with sufficient cognitive abilities and superior executive functions (e.g. impulse control and knowing on how to translate knowledge into behaviour). They might therefore further enhance the already existing educational inequalities in problem substance use, in analogy to the trends observed in obesity (Adams, Mytton, White, & Monsivais, 2016) and tobacco smoking. One of the few studies addressing this (Legleye et al., 2016) found that in France, the risk of transition from cannabis initiation to daily use has remained consistently higher among less educated cannabis initiators over three generations.

If there are systems in place to assure that local prevention providers are well trained, well coached, open to evidence and innovation and well aware about the otherwise harmful effects of prevention, then high levels of delegation to the local level are safe. Otherwise, manualised approaches might offer an alternative. There seems to be an interaction between the level of science-practice dialogue and the way prevention is delivered: whether by programs or by highly flexible activities or services.

Assessing Local Needs

Different from harm reduction and treatment, a systematic approach to assess the health needs of the population is often missing in prevention. However, to improve the health of the population and to ensure the use of resources in the most efficient way systematic assessment (Wright, Williams, & Wilkinson, 1998) is essential in preventive work. The European country reports do not allow a clear picture as to whether interventions do correspond to the actual health needs or vulnerability profiles. Some countries however do explicitly report that data from municipal levels is used to inform important decisions regarding the overall strategy (Bulgaria) or that officials on the local level are consulted and allowed to participate in establishing strategies and priorities for prevention (i.e. Denmark, Croatia, the Netherlands, Austria, Portugal and Norway). Norway stands out for its "Ungdata" surveys,[7] a standardised system for local questionnaire surveys on various aspects of young people's lives, including the use of drugs, alcohol and tobacco. Also the implementation of Communities That Care[8] approach to planning and sustaining prevention programming at the community level in Lower Saxony in Germany[8,9] and in the Netherlands (Steketee et al., 2013) uses specific youth surveys in order to create local risk profiles that provide information used for deciding if and which kind of program should be implemented in a given neighbourhood or town.

An additional challenge is that the pathway from evidence via policies to practice is predominantly conceived as unidirectional. Rarely does research address the gaps of prevention practice and the needs of practitioners.[10] Drawing from the reports from European countries, only a few[11] mention consultations with the local level in designing and defining prevention strategies. Again, the countries with communitarian traditions (mostly protestant ones, see Burkhart (2013a) for the historical accounts) are overrepresented among them. This might be related to the above-mentioned degree to which local delivery agencies (municipalities or prevention centres) are independent from the central level. Especially in prevention, central governments often delegate delivery to agencies, charities or the private sector with differing degrees of autonomy in service delivery, often based on principles such as "localism" and the need to include service users in the design of public services. For scientists and for the translation of evidence this is a problem because many effective interventions (especially the manualised ones) do not fare

---

[7] http://www.ungdata.no/English

[8] CTC is a coalition-based prevention operating system that uses an evidence-based approach to prevent youth problem behaviours such as violence, delinquency, school dropout and substance abuse.

[9] http://www.ctc-info.de/nano.cms/umsetzung

[10] See for example http://euspr.hypotheses.org/276 and the ensuing discussion

[11] Denmark, Spain, Croatia, the Netherlands, Austria, Portugal, Sweden and Norway

well if they undergo too many modifications to local conditions and ad libitum.

Standards: They Are not Self-Implementing

Standards that include practitioners' and local policymakers' perspectives and experiences would solve part of these tensions. On the European level the European Drug Prevention Quality Standards (EDPQS) were set up to support *the development and evaluation of high-quality drug prevention* (i.e. "how to carry out prevention?"). Those standards have been agreed upon by a wide range of different professional groups, in several waves and often across many countries (Brotherhood & Sumnall, 2011), and can confidently be considered consensual common denominators for establishing "good quality" regarding content, design and implementation of prevention. They have afterwards been complemented with numerous tools[12] to improve adherence and acceptance in the prevention field.

At the international level, UNODC (2013) has published guidelines for the use of the current evidence (i.e. "what works?"), the International Standards on Drug Use Prevention. Both are examples of a variety of standards with different objectives (Burkhart, 2015).

But although standards can be used as a reference point on high-quality prevention, the applicability of the standards to local circumstances also has to be taken into account. The phase II of the EDPQS project[13] has dealt with this point, focusing on this aspect in a considerable number of European countries. Standards in prevention seem to be widely available in Europe: according to the workbooks only a third of the countries report no use of any prevention standard; and the EDPQS are the most predominantly mentioned, while a few countries[14] report using their own standards. The open question remains as to what extent are these standards followed and adhered to in the field at the local level. Since addressing this question through official national sources is not possible, the EDPQS project itself is seeking to monitor the use and application of its standards. Following the Capacity-Opportunity-Motivation model (Michie, van Stralen, & West, 2011), the tools provided by EDPQS have certainly contributed to increasing the opportunities of critical reflection and improving the work of professionals. The evidence mentioned above might have increased the capacity of doing so, but whether professionals and service providers actually are motivated to rigorously follow standards and to work accordingly depends ultimately on their motivation to do so. Self-improvement and professionalisation are relevant but financial incentives are likely to be stronger motivations.

There is consensus among experts and professionals that adherence to such standards will provide an optimal platform for the delivery of evidence-based programmes, which might make the delivery of effective approaches more likely. But there is currently no direct evidence in Europe that fully applying standards like the EDPQS actually leads to demonstrable improvements in prevention and outcomes. The attitudes of practitioners to them might be analogous to those of psychologists towards the NICE guidelines on psychotherapy (Court, Cooke, & Scrivener, 2016): they valued summaries of the latest evidence regarding effective practices but were also very concerned about the implication that the evidence is "neat "and that there is a correct approach across the board. Practitioners tend therefore to feel that their freedom to use their judgment and tailor their approach to individual situations would be curtailed.

Only some studies around the Communities That Care prevention system in the United States (Brown et al., 2013; Kim, Gloppen, Rhew, Oesterle, & Hawkins, 2015; Oesterle et al., 2015) provide evidence that a prevention system which offers only evidence-based interventions targeted for each community's vulnerability profile does not only improve programme delivery,

---

[12] See http://prevention-standards.eu/

[13] http://prevention-standards.eu/the-prevention-standards-partnership-in-phase-ii/

[14] Belgium, the Czech Republic, France, Hungary, Lithuania, the Netherlands and Finland

implementation and adoption but ultimately also youth outcomes such as violence and substance use in the areas using this approach.

Prevention Interventions: Programmes, Policies or Services?

Manualised prevention concepts, interventions and having easy access to them are certainly important to ensure efficient knowledge translation within countries but also beyond national borders. Therefore, much of the prevention literature focuses on their evaluation, effectiveness and readiness for dissemination. But then the most distinctive aspect of European prevention systems is that manualised interventions play a significant role in only a few countries. In Spain some regions (such as *Castilla-la-Mancha*) have catalogues of certified programmes from which local prevention services and schools can make a choice. This allows for registering how much the programmes are adopted, but not how much they are implemented in real life. Also, Germany, the Netherlands, the UK, Poland, Lithuania and Croatia have increased the development or adaptation and implementation of evidence-based programmes in the past years. Accordingly, in these countries registries of programmes (see below) are also available. On the other end of the continuum, Sweden and Norway are deliberately reducing the role and importance of manualised programmes in order to give more space for communities to develop their own interventions. In Denmark, Finland and France manualised interventions have never had an importance and only very recently some programmes such as the Good Behaviour Game and Strengthening Families Program are beginning to raise the interest of policymakers in France. In the remaining countries, manualised interventions might coexist with a majority of interventions that are less complex and don't demand adherence to a given protocol. The scarcity of manualised interventions is often intended, in cultures where such programmes are seen as "American" and behaviourist in their modus operandi, rigid and not suitable to a given European country's reality (Burkhart, 2013). However, even in those countries where manualised interventions play a role and are evaluated, adapted and disseminated, their delivery still covers only a small part of the possible target populations: even in Spain, which offers 100 manualised programmes (*Memoria Plan Nacional sobre Drogas*, 2013), only around 10% (800,000) of the school population participated in any of them. Therefore, only by looking at the content, effects or dissemination readiness of manualised interventions, we can hardly assess the potentials of European prevention systems. This leads to the question: How non-manualised interventions can be monitored? Below we explore prevention services, regulations and policies.

Services

When we discuss prevention services we refer to the whole plethora of counselling, advice, personal help and support to vulnerable youth, vulnerable families and substance-using youth, delivered on the street, in recreational settings, at home visits or in service facilities. They might range from universal to indicated prevention but the contents of such interventions are mostly not known, except for specialised interventions such as crisis intervention in party settings or Brief Interventions with Motivational Interviewing. There are however some data on how these services predominantly operate, i.e. whether they actively reach out to vulnerable youth and families (Go-Strategies) or whether their professionals expect people to come into their facilities (Come-Strategies). In Europe, Come-Strategies prevail for most vulnerable groups.

For indicated prevention, individualised services have particular importance. While universal and selective prevention are manageable by local policies and population-based interventions (even nightlife venues frequented by a subset of high-risk young people can be accordingly managed or regulated), indicated prevention involves work with vulnerable individuals that cannot be defined by demographic or geographic factors. Instead they are coming from all classes and backgrounds and seem personally vulnerable to several kinds of problems, especially psychological disorders or problems brought on by a poor/dysfunctional family situation. Thus, individual- or family-oriented services seem to make most sense. Also, good coordination and involvement of treatment services are important in this context, particularly when it comes to approaching substance-using parents. The challenge lies in the development of appropriate detection and intervention systems at the local level and to ensure for this purpose the cooperation with specialised services from the treatment and mental health areas. Data on the availability of such systems are lacking and there are few reports about their functioning (Espelt et al., 2012; Ramírez de Arellano, 2015) as these services are often not primarily conceived or developed for substance-use prevention purposes. This might be the reason that in European real-life conditions indicated prevention is predominantly implemented in its narrowest form, which exclusively is concerned with detecting and addressing substance use at intensities beneath clinical criteria of dependence or problem use. Even though they do not address individual behavioural, temperamental or psychological difficulties that mostly occur earlier than substance use and are considered precursors for it (Sloboda, Glantz, & Tarter, 2012), mostly such approaches are nevertheless called "early interventions". They probably comprise a vast array of services, ranging from stationary counselling services for young people and/or their parents, telephone helplines and home visits up to youth work on the streets. About the contents of these services not much is known and they are not subject to any monitoring. Drawing on accounts from multiple reports by European countries, counselling, education and street conversations[15] and other cognitive pedagogical approaches seem to be the most common ingredients.

These multiple services to address substance use on an individual basis and in an overlapping grey zone between prevention, harm reduction and minimal treatment are an important and distinctive feature of European prevention systems, while in other continents prevention seems to be more based on manualised interventions.

More is known about Brief Interventions (BI), an evidence-based (Carney & Myers, 2012; Foxcroft et al., 2016; Glass et al., 2015; O'Donnell et al., 2013; Yuma-Guerrero et al., 2012) form of intervention, which is—like the above—delivered at the individual level, but has been quasi-manualised and has clearly defined contents: normative feedback and motivational interviewing. Also in contrast to the above, much has been published about scaling it up and inserting it into routines of primary healthcare (Abidi, Oenema, Nilsen, Anderson, & van de Mheen, 2016; McCormick et al., 2010; Parkes et al., 2011) and emergency rooms (Cherpitel, Moskalewicz, Swiatkiewicz, Ye, & Bond, 2009; Kohler & Hofmann, 2015). Since the evidence for BI (and the majority of the implementations) comes from treatment settings, we have included Brief Interventions only marginally in this description of prevention systems.

Policies

Services and (quasi-)manualised interventions deliver prevention predominantly by means of personal interaction, by skill training, discussions, education or individual counselling. However, much of human behaviour is automatic, driven by impulses and habits, and unconscious (Marteau, Hollands, & Fletcher, 2012; Papies, 2016). This limits somehow the power of education and reflexive motivation when behaviour is supposed to be changed. With the increasing evidence for the potentials of interventions that shape the physical, economic and normative environment of people (Burkhart, 2011; Hollands et al., 2013; Hollands, Marteau, & Fletcher, 2016), local environmental policies are becoming more visible components of prevention systems, because they can complement current approaches in addressing the automatic and non-conscious determinants of behaviours such as substance use, violence and obesity (Adams et al., 2016). Most of them are however at local level and are

---

[15] For example http://www.streetworkinstitute.org/lms/

seldom defined and labelled as "substance-use prevention interventions". Therefore, we propose to focus monitoring and analysis on the following types that are most frequently described in the literature.

Regulations of Nightlife

Nightlife or entertainment venues are a good example of where social and physical environments, prices and serving practices significantly affect substance use and related problems, including violence (Hughes et al., 2011; Miller, Holder, & Voas, 2009). In such settings, the modification of physical spaces, visual cues and affordances[16] (Fleming & Bartholow, 2014; Ostlund, Maidment, & Balleine, 2010; Withagen, de Poel, Araujo, & Pepping, 2012) offer—in theory—multiple intervention opportunities that require low personal agency, which is essential in environments where people don't go in order to control, "be responsible" or moderate their behaviours. Accordingly, the potential (and the existing evidence) for multicomponent local policies regulating nightlife and its corollary (transport, nuisance, drunk driving, etc.) is higher than for the prevailing interventions that provide information and sometimes personalised advice (Bolier et al., 2011; Calafat, Juan, & Duch, 2009).

Municipalities, especially in regions with declining or weak economies, depend on or need to promote nightlife as a source of wealth and well-being (Hobbs, 2005) while trying to minimise the problems associated with the practice of this kind of entertainment. Local governments can play a major role in promoting and supporting environmental approaches (e.g., regulation of opening hours, banning of certain places and/or certain times for alcohol trade, increasing and reorganising police surveillance, ensuring strict compliance of the law, securing perimeters to reduce social nuisances) that can be undertaken by professionals and technical staff of the different municipal areas that they cover (Duch, Calafat, & Juan, 2016).

Since tourism to international nightlife destinations contributes also to the escalation of substance use in other countries (Calafat et al., 2010), especially in regions of Europe where regulations are weak (Greece and Spain), the strength of regulatory policies is important to be included in the assessment of any prevention system. Policies regulating nightlife, such as access by intoxicated patrons, alcohol-serving practices, happy hours or flat-rate offers, crowdedness, chill-out rooms and areas around the premises, are often reported from the North of Europe (Belgium, some German regions, France, Luxembourg, the Netherlands, Sweden and the UK) but barely from the South (only from Catalonia) where however the big international nightlife resorts are located. This might be one of the reasons why nightlife tourism in Europe seems to follow a North-South gradient, where not only the South's favourable climate but also the laxer regulations in its big tourist resorts would attract young tourists from the more regulated North of Europe.

Implementation and Reinforcement of (Alcohol) Policy at the Local Level

National alcohol policies are not always completely implemented at local level, particularly in smaller municipalities, where local decision-makers might be more compromised to the local trade and to cultural drinking traditions. Municipalities have nevertheless possibilities to effectively intervene in their jurisdictions (Giesbrecht & Haydon, 2006) since often they have also quite a decision latitude in defining local regulations to address, for example, density and concentration of outlets, type of selling venues, and selling and serving policies. Legislation in several countries allow for alcohol consumption to be addressed locally at a broader level than the individual premises, for example, through early morning restrictions and late-night levies in the UK (Martineau, Graff, Mitchell, &

---

[16]The possibility of a behaviour or action within an individual–environment transaction. A sofa, for example, provides an obvious affordance for sitting; free water for drinking. It is independent of an individual's ability to recognise it or even take advantage of it.

Lock, 2014). There as well, local authorities can also designate so-called cumulative impact zones (CIZs) to control new alcohol outlets in areas where the cumulative stress caused by existing overprovision of alcohol outlets threatens the licensing objectives. A number of studies have already suggested a clear relationship between outlet density and alcohol-related harm (Holmes et al., 2014; Livingston, 2011; Young, Macdonald, & Ellaway, 2013). For Europe, where for long such local policies have been limited to Sweden (van Poppel, 2008)—with the Trelleborg (Stafström, Ostergren, Larsson, Lindgren, & Lundborg, 2006) and the STAD (Gripenberg Abdon, Wallin, & Andréasson, 2011) projects—there is recently increasing evidence for the impacts of local alcohol policies, also in Spanish, Dutch and UK administrative and legal contexts. A recent study in England (de Vocht, Heron, Angus et al., 2016) rated at national level the intensity of licensing scrutiny aimed at controlling licensing and alcohol availability in local areas and found a relationship with alcohol-related hospital admissions, showing that local government areas in England with more intensive alcohol licensing policies are also the places where measurably larger reductions in alcohol harm have taken place. The analogue effect was also found regarding rates of violent crimes, sexual crimes and public order offences (de Vocht, Heron, Campbell et al., 2016). In the Netherlands, two of three regions in which municipalities adhered to a regional alcohol prevention policy had beneficial outcomes (compared to the non-adhering region) in regard to weekly drinking, increase in adolescents' age at consuming their first alcoholic drink, and changes in heavy weekly drinking (de Goeij et al., 2016). Whether direct causation of the policies themselves or association, this suggests a population health benefit of local government initiatives to restrict alcohol licences. Also regarding opening hours, a recent study (de Goeij, Veldhuizen, Buster, & Kunst, 2015) compared two districts of Amsterdam, one of which established longer opening hours for bars. There was a significant difference between the districts, with an increase in alcohol-related harm and nuisance in the district with longer opening hours. Also the city of Barcelona has successfully reinforced specific regulations (e.g. no sales to minors and late night, no consumption in the public space) and monitored the development over several years with a view to change the social perception that minors have of alcohol consumption. There have been no documented episodes of heavy drinking in masses in public spaces (known as "botellón") in the city in that period (Villalbí et al., 2015). In most other countries, the local implementation of alcohol policies is difficult to assess or to monitor from the central level. A parents' empowerment initiative in Spain is a good example how civil society can monitor and reinforce alcohol legislation at local level: the local parents' associations of FERYA[17] denounce and lobby against alcohol selling, serving and promotion practices that would violate principles of alcohol legislation. Cooperation with civil society initiatives like these could improve the monitoring in prevention systems. The EU-funded multinational Take Care Project has monitored (until 2012) implementations of alcohol legislation in some locations in Belgium, Denmark, Germany, Greece, Ireland, Portugal, Slovakia, Slovenia, Cyprus and Italy (South Tyrol). In some countries local alcohol policies as the above described for England seem to be particularly difficult to implement, e.g. in Germany, where they can be legally challenged with ease (Schmidt, 2014).

Supporting School Policies/Environments

There is emerging evidence that positive school climates that make pupils feel safe, stimulated and accepted may have a protective effect against violence and substance use (Bonell et al., 2013; Jamal et al., 2013; Thapa, Cohen, Guffey, & Higgins-D'Alessandro, 2013). Students' perceptions of whether they are treated fairly and of school safety as well as teacher support are also related to the prevention of substance use. Interventions that increase student participation,

---

[17] http://ferya.es/

improve relationships and promote a positive school ethos (involvement, engagement and positive teacher–pupil relations) therefore appear to contribute to a reduction of substance use. Programmes based on this concept have been shown to be transferable between countries (Markham, Young, Sweeting, West, & Aveyard, 2012). Again, except for such programmes, school climate is difficult to monitor without specific audit instruments (Embry, 1997). Such interventions should not be confounded with health promotion in schools, which has repeatedly failed to show evidence for effects on substance-use behaviour (Langford et al., 2015; Stewart-Brown, 2006). Interestingly, there are only a few published attempts to combine an effective structural (on school climate or norms) intervention with content components of social-emotional and behavioural training in order to create synergistic effects (Domitrovich et al., 2009) and the best known European example (the Healthy Schools and Drugs Program) failed to yield significant effects (Malmberg et al., 2014, 2015).

But also school norms and rules are supporting policies since they reduce the visibility and therefore the illusion of normality and social acceptance of substance use on school premises (and sometimes around) which is associated with substance use (Kuntsche & Jordan, 2006; Kuntsche & Kuendig, 2005). They are easier to monitor as well. In Europe, such environmental prevention approaches in schools have expanded and today almost all countries report total smoking bans in all schools, and a majority of them report high availability of drug policies in schools, i.e. rules on the use and sale of substances on school premises and procedures how to deal with violations. As indicated in the International Standards, key to effective school policies on substance use is to have policies that are clearly specific as what substances are targeted and to what locations and/or occasions they apply, that the infractions are dealt with using positive sanctions such as providing referral to counselling or other support services and not suspensions or expulsions, and that all stakeholders (students, parents and school staff) participate in the development of the policies (Fig. 26.2).

The advantages of manualised interventions are certainly that their ingredients are known, that their evaluations provide trust in their safety and effectiveness and that those who implement them get clear instructions or deepened training and do therefore not have to know everything about prevention. A priori however, they don't provide the feeling of ownership and identity that local self-made interventions or practices can provide. Adaptations to local conditions that create such ownership feelings are demanding.

Locally developed services or interventions are based on an understanding and an involvement of the local situation, resources, actors and mentalities, but tend to be less complex than manualised interventions, in the sense that content-wise they tend to rely more on information and education rather than on skill training, or on regulating, incentivising or limiting behaviour directly. They are generally not theory based. If such approaches are meant to become more evidence based, such local services require above all a very motivated and well-trained prevention workforce who is aware that prevention is something else than just educating about risks, informing about dangers, giving advice, using fear tactics or organising external lectures by police officers and ex-users or drug awareness days; in short they require professionals who can use other than cognitive strategies in changing behaviours.

But after all, both concepts—manualised evidence-based programmes and locally relevant experiences—are not mutually exclusive and could be combined, as the experiences with CTC in some member states show: this system allows communities to first objectively analyse their specific need and problem profile and then to choose the most suitable programme(s) that address their particular situation. Ideally, science-based manualised interventions that train competences and skills should ideally be complemented with local environmental policies.

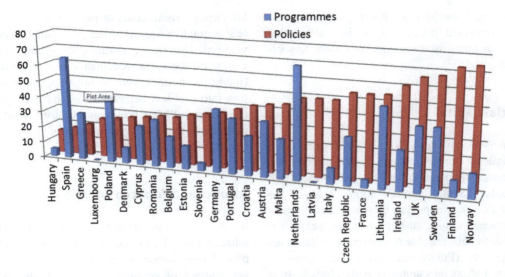

Fig. 26.2 Comparison of the importance given to manualised interventions versus local policies across European countries (high values indicate a high importance)

Moderators

There are accounts from Sweden that evidence-based programmes, such as Unplugged (Faggiano et al., 2008), Strengthening Families Program (Skärstrand, Larsson, & Andréasson, 2008) and MultiSystemic Therapy (Sundell et al., 2008), were not superior to usual Swedish services or interventions. This might however be related to additional factors in societies like Sweden that have low social inequality, high social capital and strong social norms against substance use. These factors might lower the overall vulnerability of the target group so much that additional interventions yield little additional effects to the existing prevention infrastructure.

As moderators within a prevention system we conceive those aspects of social, political and cultural life that influence the functioning, implementation and effects of prevention. They are however difficult to be modified by prevention systems themselves. For the purposes of a comprehensive overview of prevention systems, these possible moderators should be taken into account. This is particularly relevant as moderators are not foreseen to be involved in most conceptualisations of prevention strategies or cannot be considered in research studies in an adequate way, but may have a high practical relevance especially in the field of cross-national exchange of intervention programmes. Due to the lack of data on these moderators in European prevention activities public-use data of cross-national surveys from research fields that are not primarily related to prevention were reviewed, such as the Tobacco Control Scale, the Alcohol Control Score, the World Values Survey and the Gini Score[18] data by OECD.

Social Inequality

It has been argued that a range of social problems, including substance use, teenage pregnancy and violence, are more prevalent in countries with high levels of social and health inequality (Wilkinson & Picket, 2010) because of the increased competition for status and positional goods which affects people's physiological and physical well-being. A WHO (CSDH, 2008)

---

[18]The Gini inequality index measures income inequality between the richest decile of a population and the poorest. It ranges from 0 (everyone has the same income) to 100 (one person has all the income) and is a good proxy for social inequality.

report and the Marmot Review (2010) for the UK confirmed that inequalities in health including substance-use problems are related to social inequality.

Social Capital

Francis Fukuyama (2001, p. 7) defined social capital as "an instantiated informal norm that promotes cooperation between two or more individuals". Social capital norms lead to co-operation in groups and therefore are related to traditional virtues such as honesty, keeping of commitments, reliable performance of duties and reciprocity (Fukuyama, 2011). One important factor for social capital is particularistic trust, which is characterised by three different forms: trust in family, trust in neighbours and trust in people one personally knows. Data of the World Values Survey (years 2010–2014) suggest that in general, the level of trust in family is comparably high among all European countries and trust in neighbourhood or personal acquaintances never approach family trust in any researched country. This in turn has impact on community organisations and the openness towards adopting new social interventions: if societies with low social capital have a "narrow radius of trust" (Fukuyama, 2001), their members do not easily co-operate with outsiders. The result is that, in some societies, social capital resides largely in families and a rather narrow circle of friends. If members of such groups do not co-operate with each other and do not get involved in new activities, the adoption of preventive interventions would be difficult.

Social Norms

We focus here on general social norms at the population level, which cannot be modified by prevention policies or interventions and are therefore considered moderators (in analogy to why we have included alcohol and tobacco policies among the moderators). This is different from in-group social norms which are obviously malleable through some kinds of prevention strategies (e.g. normative education and environmental prevention). Descriptive norms ("Everybody does that") and the social acceptance of a behaviour (injunctive norms) seem to influence the initiation into problem behaviour and substance use (Berkowitz, 2002). They can therefore boost or undermine the reach and impact of prevention interventions.

Alcohol and Tobacco Policies

In an ideal situation, macro-level alcohol and tobacco control policies would be an integral part of a prevention system. In a slowly increasing number of countries, such as France and the Nordic countries, this is indeed the case. However, in many countries alcohol and tobacco policies continue to be policy domains apart from substance-use prevention. Besides, the alcohol industry in some countries has a participatory role in (influencing) policymaking, not necessarily protecting public health (Brown, 2015; Knai, Petticrew, Durand, Eastmure, & Mays, 2015). While at the policy level national drug coordinators sometimes cannot touch the interests of the alcohol industries with regulatory approaches on advertising, prizing or taxation (Burkhart, 2011), professionals strive to compensate for such macro policymaking with local prevention interventions. Therefore, national alcohol and tobacco policies are considered as moderators, since they often continue to be independent from prevention systems, sometimes counteracting their objectives.

Drug-Use Legislation

There is currently no evidence that the harshness of legislation on illicit drugs (consumption or possession for use) has an impact on substance-use behaviour (EMCDDA, 2011, p. 45). There are concerns that harsh drug laws, which increase the stigma (Lloyd, 2010) for drug users in general and punish vulnerable young people for behaviour that is ultimately beyond their control, might hamper the reach and implementation possibilities of selective and indicated prevention interventions if vulnerable substance users cannot openly be enrolled and engaged in them, because they have to conceal their drug use (Booth, Kwiatkowski, Iguchi, Pinto, & John, 1998; Cunningham, Sobell, Sobell, Agrawal, & Toneatto, 1993; Finney & Moos, 1995).

We hypothesise that strong alcohol and tobacco policies, together with low inequality (low Gini score), paired with high social capital (generalised trust, i.e. not only towards the family) and strong social norms against antisocial behaviour, as well as a public health-oriented legal framework (less punitive) would all contribute in supporting prevention systems and boosting their outcomes in terms of substance use-related problems. The limitation for a comprehensive analysis is that (a) complete data—i.e. covering all EU countries—are available only for alcohol and tobacco control, and for income inequality; (b) a score on the harshness of drugs legislation does not yet exist; and (c) the available data on social capital and social norms do not allow for developing a stringent theoretical framework and a clear interaction with prevention systems, similar to, e.g., the alcohol control score. A conceptual limitation is that the premises of this model are based on a "modern" state (Fukuyama, 2011), while in many countries in the South of Europe social life and support continue to be driven by family, thus affecting the relevance of people outside the family. There is often less trust, less "social capital" and hence less public solutions for problems, which are taken care of by the families. These "private solutions" continue to contribute to buffering the impact of a number of social and public health problems, even if the system of "public solutions" might be weaker.

To give nonetheless an overview of moderators at the national level, in the original EMCDDA report a composite score was calculated of only those moderators that are consistently available and interpretable. It includes social inequalities (Gini score), as well as alcohol and tobacco control policies. For all three variables we calculated quartiles and subsequently all variables were summed up. Lower scores of the composite score indicated less supportive moderators on national level (Fig. 26.3). In a direct comparison, the Nordic countries show a high score of supportive moderators whereas Greece, Cyprus, Luxembourg, Portugal, Spain and particularly Germany show less supportive structures. In Luxembourg and Austria, inequality is relatively low but both countries do have weak alcohol and tobacco policies. In Ireland the alcohol and tobacco control regulations are quite stricter but social inequality is one of the highest in Europe, with the second highest Gini score.

The Prevention Workforce

The success and positive outcomes of prevention strategies in general and of a prevention programme in particular depend on a careful selection of the practitioners who implement them: their skills, motivation, dedication and personality. Moreover, the infrastructure (social, legislative, technical and physical) that support them are of vital importance (Burkhart, 2013).

The professional background and training level of professionals do play a crucial role in the delivery of prevention strategies, but for the majority of countries it is difficult to describe and analyse the composition of the prevention workforce and how they have been trained (Fixsen et al., 2005).

This is very distinct from the treatment field, where most professionals (except in non-publicly funded therapeutic communities in some countries), before they are allowed to treat and deal with clients, need to have accreditation and specific training, which is easier to register.

Nevertheless, even in therapy, a non-irrelevant portion of clients gets worse (Crawford et al., 2016) and several findings (Dishion & Dodge, 2005; Hornik, Jacobsohn, Orwin, Piesse, & Kalton, 2008; Moos, 2005) suggest that prevention can be harmful as well. However, there seems to be little concern or awareness among parents and policymakers about potential harms arising from prevention activities that might be well intended, but without evidence or carried out

Moderators

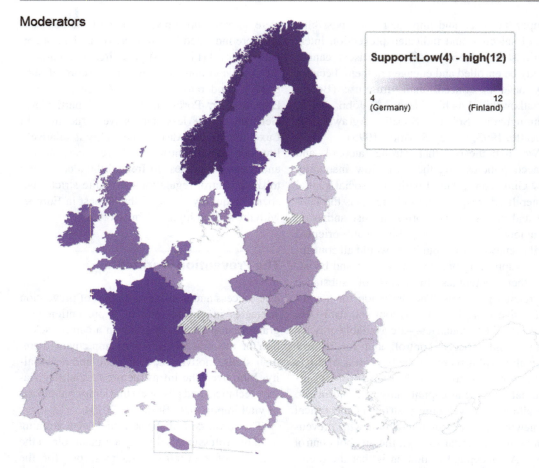

Fig. 26.3 Composite score of moderators that support functioning, implementation and effects of prevention (high scores indicate a composition of highly supportive moderators)

by suboptimally trained staff. Many standards (see also Brotherhood and Sumnall (2011) for the EDPQS) therefore address the issue of staff qualification. According to the country reports only in the Czech Republic a proper accreditation is required for any prevention professional who wants to deliver prevention in the education system.

The prevention workforce can be categorised by prevention services, local prevention decision makers and implementing professionals.

Services

Providers and facilities that deliver prevention are mostly public service settings like schools, prevention centres and health centres or sometimes through law enforcement, but differing from country to country other settings such as NGOs, associations and universities play a crucial role. Most countries report predominantly about their public prevention services, since those—alike those in the treatment field—are accredited and tend to have stable funding. Less seems to be known about the activities of private associations. This might be related to the fact that accreditation is not a prerequisite for entities to deliver prevention and to enter into contact with youth and children. Therefore, it is often the case that some NGOs, charities and mainstream (and fringe) faith groups deliver ineffective activities that are typically based on informational, awareness-raising approaches, sometimes combined with blunt scare tactics. The available information from European countries suggests that most local services are also not obliged to follow existing standards and don't seem to be audited for this.

Monitoring of such services for prevention is almost impossible because of this diversity of different services, which are not necessarily bound to a physical installation; for example, a small NGO operating from a home office can implement several school-based prevention interventions. Several countries report an incalculable plethora of organisations that somehow carry out prevention.

Local Decision Makers

Among regional or local decision makers there is no common understanding of what substance-use prevention (or prevention of problem behaviour) would consist of, and possibly because of the frequent assumption that "prevention is informed decision-making" purely informative approaches are still used in many countries (EMCDDA, 2015). It seems for example that in countries with a preponderance of psycho-analytically trained prevention professionals, all approaches are repudiated that could be marked as "behaviourist" or "normative" (Burkhart, 2013). In one country in Latin America the implementers of the Good Behaviour Game (Kellam et al., 2014) had to change the "packaging information" of the intervention (description of theory base, working mode and objectives) in order to overcome the fierce resistance by the Ministry of Education which considered it behaviourist and manipulative and therefore unacceptable for the country's educational philosophy, according to which the children have to consciously and knowingly adopt the desirable behaviour but should not be nudged towards it. A similar concept seems to be the reason that "drug education" is the prevailing term used for prevention—virtually exclusively—in the UK: the assumption that prevention has to be done via education, i.e. by only applying conscious processes of persuasion, information provision and reflection. Accordingly, comprehensive social influence programmes are repeatedly denounced as "American" and manipulative.[19] Such specific professional cultures among decision makers seem also be the basis as to why in some countries manualised programmes have been seen as too standardised, rigid and not suitable for diversified local conditions (Burkhart, 2013).

Since the publication of the International Standards on Prevention (UNODC, 2013) and the European Drug Prevention Quality Standards—EDPQS (Brotherhood & Sumnall, 2011)—training initiatives and curricula[20] have been developed that aim both to train prevention decision makers and prevention implementers in effective prevention principles and in how to implement them. Once adapted to Europe they might improve the current situation where it seems to be difficult for local decision makers to select the most suitable prevention approaches.

Professionals Who Actually Carry Out the Interventions

Not only should prevention specialists and decision makers be considered in a prevention system, but also above all implementing professionals such as teachers and educators, family counsellors, staff in health, counselling and youth centres, policemen, outreach and social workers, and other professionals enrolled in delivering prevention. Their role is crucial. Horton (2014) postulates that in order to achieve safe, effective, patient-centred, efficient, timely and equitable care, a revolution in the quality of care is needed, which would constitute "a third revolution in global health", but this depends on staff training and less on interventions. Often there is no relation between health outcomes and coverage with key interventions because the missing ingredient is quality of the care provided by the specialised workforce. This applies to prevention as well. A pivotal point here however is

---

[19] http://findings.org.uk/PHP/dl.php?file=drug_ed.hot
[20] https://www.issup.net/training/universal-prevention-curriculum

that there is yet no agreed-upon means to monitor the quality of prevention work. There is not even a common professional profile of a prevention worker and for this reason it is difficult to obtain information about who makes up the prevention workforce in Europe, except for the teachers who deliver interventions in schools. Professional cultures, beliefs and assumptions are influential: for example the situation in which an entire professional group in a country decides that certain intervention types—e.g. indicated prevention—are unacceptable because they'd "medicalise" certain behaviours, or if other professional groups fiercely oppose local regulatory approaches because they sometimes have been developed from the crime prevention or law enforcement sector, or because they see them as limiting "personal freedom".

If there was a unified prevention training syllabus for prevention professionals in Europe, such ideological prejudices or misunderstandings about the nature and scope of prevention might be reduced. The open question remains, why not-so-well-paid prevention workers would invest in such a training curriculum of about 280 h, like the Universal Prevention Curriculum (see Footnote 20), which is currently being adapted to Europe. Based on the UNODC standards of evidence (UNODC, 2013) and the EDPQS (Brotherhood & Sumnall, 2011) it transmits key competences such as Needs and Resource Assessment; Preparation and Implementation of Interventions and/or Policies; Selection of Evidence-Based Interventions and/or Policies; Specifying and Defining Outcomes; Monitoring and Evaluation; and Dissemination and Improvement.

The Target Populations

The characteristics of the target population should be considered as part of the prevention system as well, since the target population is not only the final recipient of prevention, but also have an active role in how prevention measures can (or cannot) be implemented. There is an obvious interaction between the characteristics of the target population and the adequacy and relevance of interventions or policies for them (Brotherhood & Sumnall, 2011).

The most obvious characteristic that comes to mind is the vulnerability profile of the populations in terms of social exclusion, for example how many vulnerable groups are there and how deprived are they. A target population with a high vulnerability is often associated with low education (Legleye et al., 2016; Legleye, Beck, Khlat, Peretti-Watel, & Chau, 2012) or personal resources, such as self-control (Teasdale & Silver, 2009; Vaughn, Beaver, DeLisi, Perron, & Schelbe, 2009; Wills, Ainette, Mendoza, Gibbons, & Brody, 2007). As a consequence, informational strategies to raise awareness about drugs and their risks are even less adequate, relevant and pertinent for them since they require a very high level of "personal agency" (Adams et al., 2016), i.e. the capacity of transforming knowledge and intentions into behavioural change. Such informational strategies require a level of cognitive and executive skills that is often lacking for the most vulnerable. In other words, more effective contents of interventions for vulnerable groups and individuals are either environmental measures or policies (since they require low personal agency) or interventions that address underlying or associated behavioural challenges and obstacles by training social competence, academic performance and motivation (Sussman et al., 2004) or positive family management (Bailey, Hill, Oesterle, & Hawkins, 2009; Hill et al., 2010).

Families and students sometimes have participated in a number of prevention interventions so they are reluctant to engage in new and additional interventions, even if they are perhaps more evidence based (Burkhart, 2013). If however prevention interventions or policies provide added value to their lives and development, their reception might be different. The reception of "Unplugged" and "the Strengthening Families Program" by pupils, teachers and vulnerable families, respectively, was unexpectedly enthusiastic in Brazil for example, because in its deprived public schools and marginalised families these programmes provided for the first time interactive role play, and a focus on social inclusion and competence. When programmes originating from another country are adapted to new contexts and cultures, it is good practice to involve the target group in the adaptation process, by assessing its relevance and adequacy and in making suggestions in order to guarantee that the intervention is meaningful to them (Burkhart, 2013; UNODC, 2009). This principle does not apply only to manualised interventions but could—in a participatory approach—generally improve and perfect more elements of a prevention system. These arguments provide strong support to those prevention systems where the central level and research centres closely work together with local communities in developing interventions at local level. These same principles can be applied also to manualised interventions.

Conclusions

It appears that system thinking can be helpful in overcoming the current major focus only on (evidence-based) manualised interventions or programmes. Many more determinants have to be optimised in order to achieve sustainable and detectable prevention effects at a population level. This chapter therefore aimed at inventorying these different factors and conditions that need to be known in order to describe how "prevention systems" could be conceptualised. These elements characterise how and by whom prevention is conceived, planned, organised, delivered, evaluated, improved and received. We have proposed additional variables and aspects of a society (e.g. its inequality) that can boost (or impede) the implementation and impact of prevention interventions or policies, and have called them "moderators". Even if they are often not seen as pertaining to prevention and difficult to be modified by prevention policies, they certainly are determining aspects of a prevention system and important for understanding the multifaceted cultural and structural reality. We have seen that in the example of Europe, many variables of a prevention system change substantially from each country to another, particularly the training and professional cultures of the workforce. It seems often difficult for people in one country to realise that the conditions of implementing and improving prevention in other countries are fundamentally different, solely because of system conditions, without even going into cultural comparisons. Evidence-based interventions are an innovation for much of the prevention field, which has been dominated by untested approaches. If such innovations in interventions, policies or training have to be rolled out into other countries, it is advisable to first apply some system thinking and to have a look at the variations of the systems components that are essential for the functioning, uptake and sustainment of these interventions or initiatives. For example manualised programmes might be particularly difficult to implement in certain countries while environmental strategies might be hard to implement in others. Under the current trend where effective interventions, evaluation and relevance for the population are demanded at all levels, this chapter might help to draw the attention to the additional aspects that need to be considered in order to achieve this aim.

Since the prevention strategies of many countries are quite compartmentalised into crime prevention, drug prevention, alcohol prevention, etc., a systems approach is even more necessary for instance in clarifying that evidence-based crime and violence prevention share most aetiological factors and almost all principles of effective action with substance-use prevention, and that (illicit) drug prevention cannot be effectively carried out when alcohol policies are not considered.

A weakness of this analysis is that the model is static: for the most part, we are not able to predict how the different components might influence each other over time and have therefore used general systems theory only to a limited extend in presenting the components of a system, which are interlinked. The processes involved have not been discussed since this would require longitudinal information about changes in the countries' prevention systems. In the future, hopefully specific organisational system research methods might also help in detecting how the different components affect individual components and how this synergism affects systems for drug prevention.

Given the low popularity of manualised interventions in Europe, as a particular example, it is unlikely that evidence-based prevention can be taken to scale in the continent by focusing only on the large-scale dissemination of programmes. Manualised evidence-based programmes are an effective way of reaching relatively large populations, but they collide often with professional traditions about how to deliver prevention in many countries.

An important share of prevention practice in Europe continues to be much ingrained in treatment traditions: by providing services that target, approach and counsel people *individually*. This has facilitated developing flexible responses for vulnerable groups (selective prevention) and for vulnerable individuals (indicated prevention) in Europe, but the unique potential of prevention as population-based intervention is underused and sometimes even unpopular. Nevertheless, a good collaboration and integration with the treatment field are essential in order to reach all target groups and to provide a multi-tiered offer of prevention interventions and services.

Institutions at national or regional levels in Europe have often a stronger role than communities and civil society. But siloed institutions and sectors make cooperation for a multi-context, multidisciplinary activity like substance-use prevention particularly difficult, if for example the education sector does not share the interests of the health sector, criminal justice or other essential stakeholders. This integration is easier in countries with communitarian traditions, where most of prevention is delivered at the municipal level, where multi-sector co-operation is straightforward.

The moderators in the prevention system model proposed here should be taken into account carefully when for example an ambitious new prevention strategy or an evidence-based programme is supposed to be implemented or introduced from one country into another. It would be naïve to assume that offering evidence-based interventions, mapping and involving key stakeholders and professionals, forming community coalitions and getting political support would be sufficient to bring evidence-based prevention to scale and to have population-level effects. In a country with weak alcohol policies and indulgent social norms about antisocial behaviour, substance-use and violence prevention interventions are less likely to make an impact, and in countries with low social capital they might be much more difficult to implement. These are not trivial details. International publications for example tend to assume that parenting programmes, which have achieved great progress in effectiveness in the recent past (Foxcroft & Tsertsvadze, 2011; Mihalic & Elliott, 2015), should and could be widely implemented (Leslie et al., 2016), for instance through primary care. Most parenting programmes however require parents to meet and to interact with each other (sharing experiences, challenges, problems and progresses). But contrary to schools, where almost all young people can be found and by default are expected to interact with each other, families interact with others better in societies with high social (bridging) capital. North American societies have much stronger traditions of communitarian self-organisation (de Tocqueville, 1838; Fukuyama, 2011) than many European societies, where social capital is accordingly lower. In Portugal for example, the recruitment of families for the Strengthening Families Program has been difficult for this reason. Often preferred in this country is therefore a locally developed intervention (Melo, 2009) that targets each family individually, i.e. not requiring them to interact with unknown people. For countries with low social capital it is recommended that interventions be developed to respond to this cultural peculiarity. In a similar way, social norms, attitudes and policies about alcohol and tobacco have to be taken into account when prevention systems are to be optimised, especially for Europe, with its worldwide high consumption rates for alcohol (World Health Organisation, 2014).

To sum up, a systems approach can be useful to researchers and practitioners, as well as to policymakers:

- By opening their thinking towards a view of prevention as a system, in which many different components and their interaction need to be considered.
- By considering that for an intervention within a system, the research question should not be "is it effective?" but rather "how and when does it contribute to effectiveness?"
- By going beyond a particular focus, e.g. on evidence-based programmes only and their implementation towards a broader consideration of supporting factors and actors.
- By planning and providing different resources for different aspects of a system that need to be developed.
- By assessing beforehand the "system compatibility" of new approaches and programmes, and for deciding what adaptations are needed in order to increase system readiness.
- By developing multi-modular interventions and policies with modules that allow reducing complexity or intensity according to system characteristics.
- By developing implementation checklists that assess the most relevant system components before implementing programmes or policies. This might help to make multi-site evaluations more meaningful and comparable.
- By informing national prevention action plans at different levels to consider a wider range of policy options and stakeholders.
- By recognising that professionals' behaviour and attitudes might only change if multi-component implementation strategies are employed, particularly for new, more science-based and evidence-based approaches.

Applying some of these examples might help in actually achieving sustained behavioural change by setting up multilevel, multi-tiered, multicomponent prevention systems, where important but non-obvious stakeholders such as the police, commercial outlets and treatment sector have a clearly recognised role, optimising thus their unique contributions to prevention.

References

Aarons, G. A., Green, A. E., Willging, C. E., Ehrhart, M. G., Roesch, S. C., Hecht, D. B., & Chaffin, M. J. (2014). Mixed-method study of a conceptual model of evidence-based intervention sustainment across multiple public-sector service settings. *Implementation Science, 9*(1), 183. https://doi.org/10.1186/s13012-014-0183-z

Abidi, L., Oenema, A., Nilsen, P., Anderson, P., & van de Mheen, D. (2016). Strategies to overcome barriers to implementation of alcohol screening and brief intervention in general practice: A Delphi study among healthcare professionals and addiction prevention experts. *Prevention Science, 17*(6), 689–699. https://doi.org/10.1007/s11121-016-0653-4

Adams, J., Mytton, O., White, M., & Monsivais, P. (2016). Why are some population interventions for diet and obesity more equitable and effective than others? The role of individual agency. *PLoS Medicine, 13*(4), e1001990. https://doi.org/10.1371/journal.pmed.1001990

Allender, S., Owen, B., Kuhlberg, J., Lowe, J., Nagorcka-Smith, P., Whelan, J., ... Hammond, R. (2015). A community based systems diagram of obesity causes. *PLoS One, 10*(7), e0129683. https://doi.org/10.1371/journal.pone.0129683

Arthur, M. W., Hawkins, J. D., Brown, E. C., Briney, J. S., Oesterle, S., & Abbott, R. D. (2010). Implementation of the Communities that Care prevention system by coalitions in the Community Youth Development study. *Journal of Community Psychology, 28*(2), 245–258.

Bailey, J. A., Hill, K. G., Oesterle, S., & Hawkins, J. D. (2009). Parenting practices and problem behavior across three generations: Monitoring, harsh discipline, and drug use in the intergenerational transmission of externalizing behavior. *Developmental Psychology, 45*(5), 1214–1226. https://doi.org/10.1037/a0016129

Berkowitz, A. D. (2002, August). The social norms approach: Theory, research, and annotated bibliography. *Social Norms Theory and Research*, 1–47. Retrieved from www.alanberkowitz.com

Bolier, L., Voorham, L., Monshouwer, K., Van Hasselt, N., Bellis, M., & van Hasselt, N. (2011). Alcohol and drug prevention in nightlife settings: A review of experimental studies. *Substance Use and Misuse, 46*(13), 1569–1591.

Bonell, C., Parry, W., Wells, H., Jamal, F., Fletcher, A., Harden, A., ... Moore, L. (2013). The effects of the school environment on student health: A systematic review of multi-level studies. *Health & Place, 21C*, 180–191. https://doi.org/10.1016/j.healthplace.2012.12.001

Booth, R. E., Kwiatkowski, C., Iguchi, M. Y., Pinto, F., & John, D. (1998). Facilitating treatment entry among out-of-treatment injection drug users. *Public Health Reports, 113*(Suppl 1), 116–128. Retrieved from http://www.ncbi.nlm.nih.gov/pubmed/9722817

Brotherhood, A., & Sumnall, H. R. (2011). *European drug prevention quality standards—A manual for prevention professionals.* Lisbon: EMCDDA. https://doi.org/10.2810/48879

Brown, E. C., Hawkins, J. D., Rhew, I. C., Shapiro, V. B., Abbott, R. D., Oesterle, S., ... Catalano, R. F. (2013). Prevention system mediation of communities that care effects on youth outcomes. *Prevention Science, 15*(5), 623–632. https://doi.org/10.1007/s11121-013-0413-7

Brown, K. (2015). The public health responsibility deal: Why alcohol industry partnerships are bad for health? *Addiction, 110*(8), 1227–1228. https://doi.org/10.1111/add.12974

Burkhart, G. (2011). Environmental drug prevention in the EU. Why is it so unpopular? *Adicciones, 23*(2), 87–100.

Burkhart, G. (2013). *North American drug prevention programmes: are they feasible in European cultures and contexts?* Lisbon: EMCDDA. https://doi.org/10.2810/41791

Burkhart, G. (2015). International standards in prevention: How to influence prevention systems by policy interventions? *International Journal of Prevention and Treatment of Substance Use Disorders, 1*(3–4), 18–37. https://doi.org/10.4038/ijptsud.v1i3-4.7836

Cairney, P. (2015). *Briefing: Using evidence to guide policy decisions.* Edinburgh. Retrieved from http://www.lgiuscotland.org.uk/briefing/using-evidence-to-guide-policy-decisions/

Calafat, A., Blay, N. T., Hughes, K., Bellis, M., Juan, M., Duch, M., & Kokkevi, A. (2010). Nightlife young risk behaviours in Mediterranean versus other European cities: Are stereotypes true? *European Journal of Public Health* (1464–360X (Electronic)). Retrieved from file://v/RES/02 Common outputs/7 Literature/GB/JabRef_pdf_files/gregorbiblio/1121/Calafat - Nightlife young risk behaviours in mediterranean Eur J Public Health-2010.pdf

Calafat, A., Juan, M., & Duch, M. A. (2009). Preventive interventions in nightlife: A review. *Adicciones, 21*(4), 387–413.

Calafat, A., Mantecón, A., Juan, M., Adrover-Roig, D., Blay, N., & Rosal, F. (2011). Violent behaviour, drunkenness, drug use, and social capital in nightlife contexts. *Psychosocial Intervention, 20*(1), 45–51. https://doi.org/10.5093/in2011v20n1a4

Carney, T., & Myers, B. (2012). Effectiveness of early interventions for substance-using adolescents: Findings from a systematic review and meta-analysis. *Substance Abuse Treatment, Prevention, and Policy, 7*, 25. (1747–597X (Electronic)). https://doi.org/10.1186/1747-597X-7-25

Casswell, S., & Thamarangsi, T. (2009). Reducing harm from alcohol: Call to action. *The Lancet, 373*, 2247–2257. https://doi.org/10.1016/S0140-6736(09)60745-5

Chan, C. K. Y., Oldenburg, B., & Viswanath, K. (2015). Advancing the science of dissemination and implementation in behavioral medicine: Evidence and progress. *International Journal of Behavioral Medicine, 22*(3), 277–282. https://doi.org/10.1007/s12529-015-9490-2

Charvát, M., Jurystová, L., & Miovsky, M. (2012). Four-level model of qualifications for the practitioners of the primary prevention of risk behaviour in the school system. *Adiktologie: Časopis pro Prevenci, Léčbu a Výzkum Závislostí, 12*(3), 190–211.

Cherpitel, C. J., Moskalewicz, J., Swiatkiewicz, G., Ye, Y., & Bond, J. (2009). Screening, brief intervention, and referral to treatment (SBIRT) in a Polish emergency department: Three-month outcomes of a randomized, controlled clinical trial. *Journal of Studies on Alcohol and Drugs, 70*(6), 982–990.

Court, A. J., Cooke, A., & Scrivener, A. (2016). They're NICE and neat, but are they useful? A grounded theory of clinical psychologists' beliefs about and use of NICE guidelines. *Clinical Psychology & Psychotherapy, 24*, 899–910. https://doi.org/10.1002/cpp.2054

Crawford, M. J., Thana, L., Farquharson, L., Palmer, L., Hancock, E., Bassett, P., ... Parry, G. D. (2016). Patient experience of negative effects of psychological treatment: Results of a national survey. *The British Journal of Psychiatry, 208*(3), 260–265. https://doi.org/10.1192/bjp.bp.114.162628

CSDH. (2008). Closing the gap in a generation: health equity through action on the social determinants of health. In *Final Report of the Commission on Social Determinants of Health.* Geneva: World Health Organization.

Cunningham, J. A., Sobell, L. C., Sobell, M. B., Agrawal, S., & Toneatto, T. (1993). Barriers to treatment: Why alcohol and drug abusers delay or never seek treatment. *Addictive Behaviors, 18*(3), 347–353. https://doi.org/10.1016/0306-4603(93)90036-9

de Goeij, M. C. M., Jacobs, M. A. M., van Nierop, P., van der Veeken-Vlassak, I. A. G., van de Mheen, D., Schoenmakers, T. M., ... Kunst, A. E. (2016). Impact of cross-sectoral alcohol policy on youth alcohol consumption. *Journal of Studies on Alcohol and Drugs, 77*(4), 596–605. https://doi.org/10.15288/jsad.2016.77.596

de Goeij, M. C. M., Veldhuizen, E. M., Buster, M. C. A., & Kunst, A. E. (2015). The impact of extended closing times of alcohol outlets on alcohol-related injuries in the nightlife areas of Amsterdam: A controlled before-and-after evaluation. *Addiction, 110*(6), 955–964. https://doi.org/10.1111/add.12886

de Melo, A. T. (2009). *Em Busca do Tesouro das Famílias Intervenção familiar em prevenção primária das toxicodependências* (2nd ed.). Viana do Castelo: GAF.

de Tocqueville, A. (1838). Of the use which the Americans make of public associations in civil life. Democracy in America. New York: G. Adlard

de Vocht, F., Heron, J., Angus, C., Brennan, A., Mooney, J., Lock, K., ... Hickman, M. (2016). Measurable effects of local alcohol licensing policies on population health in England. *Journal of Epidemiology* and *Community Health, 70*(3), 231–237. https://doi.org/10.1136/jech-2015-206040

de Vocht, F., Heron, J., Campbell, R., Egan, M., Mooney, J. D., Angus, C., ... Hickman, M. (2016). Testing the impact of local alcohol licencing policies on reported crime rates in England. *Journal of Epidemiology and Community Health, 71*, 137–145. https://doi.org/10.1136/jech-2016-207753

Dishion, T. J., & Dodge, K. a. (2005). Peer contagion in interventions for children and adolescents: Moving towards an understanding of the ecology and dynamics of change. *Journal of Abnormal Child Psychology, 33*(3), 395–400.

Domitrovich, C. E., Bradshaw, C. P., Greenberg, M. T., Embry, D., Poduska, J. M., & Ialongo, N. S. (2009). Integrated models of school-based prevention: Logic and theory. *Psychology in the Schools, 47*(1), 71–88. https://doi.org/10.1002/pits.20452

Duch, M., Calafat, A., & Juan, M. (2016). Preventing and reducing risks of nightlife: The role of local corporations. *Revista Española de Drogodependencias, 41*(2), 120–134.

Dzewaltowski, D. A., Estabrooks, P. A., Klesges, L. M., Bull, S., & Glasgow, R. E. (2004). Behavior change intervention research in community settings: How generalizable are the results? *Health Promotion International, 19*(2), 235–245. https://doi.org/10.1093/heapro/dah211

Embry, D. D. (1997). Does your school have a peaceful environment? Using an audit to create a climate for change and resiliency. *Intervention in School and Clinic, 32*(4), 217–222.

EMCDDA. (2011). *Annual report 2011: The state of the drug problems in Europe*. Luxembourg: Publications Office of the European Union.

EMCDDA. (2015). *European drug report—Trends and developments*. Luxembourg: Publications Office of the European Union. https://doi.org/10.2810/084165

Espelt, A., Villalbí, J. R., Brugal, M. T., Castellano, Y., Guilañá, E., Guitart, A. M., & Bartroli, M. (2012). Prevención indicada del consumo problemático de drogas en adolescentes de Barcelona. *Revista Española de Salud Pública, 86*(2), 189–198. Retrieved from http://www.redalyc.org/resumen.oa?id=17023094007

Fagan, A. A., Arthur, M. W., Hanson, K., Briney, J. S., & Hawkins, J. D. (2011). Effects of Communities that Care on the adoption and implementation fidelity of evidence-based prevention programs in communities: Results from a randomized controlled trial. *Prevention Science, 12*(3), 223–234.

Faggiano, F., Galanti, M. R., Bohrn, K., Burkhart, G., Vigna-Taglianti, F., Cuomo, L., ... Wiborg, G. (2008). The effectiveness of a school-based substance abuse prevention program: EU-Dap cluster randomised controlled trial. *Preventive Medicine, 47*(5), 537–543.

Finney, J. W., & Moos, R. H. (1995). Entering treatment for alcohol abuse: A stress and coping model. *Addiction (Abingdon, England), 90*(9), 1223–1240. Retrieved from http://www.ncbi.nlm.nih.gov/pubmed/7580820

Fishbein, D. H., Ridenour, T. A., Stahl, M., & Sussman, S. (2016). The full translational spectrum of prevention science: Facilitating the transfer of knowledge to practices and policies that prevent behavioral health problems. *Translational Behavioral Medicine, 6*(1), 5–16. https://doi.org/10.1007/s13142-015-0376-2

Fixsen, D. L., Naoom, S. F., Blase, K. a., Friedman, R. M., & Wallace, F. (2005). Implementation research: A synthesis of the literature. *Components, 311712*, 1–119.

Fleming, K. A., & Bartholow, B. D. (2014). Alcohol cues, approach bias, and inhibitory control: Applying a dual process model of addiction to alcohol sensitivity. *Psychology of Addictive Behaviors, 28*(1), 85–96.

Foxcroft, D. R., Coombes, L., Wood, S., Allen, D., Almeida Santimano, N. M., & Moreira, M. T. (2016). Motivational interviewing for the prevention of alcohol misuse in young adults. *Cochrane Database of Systematic Reviews*. https://doi.org/10.1002/14651858.CD007025.pub4

Foxcroft, D. R., & Tsertsvadze, A. (2011). Universal family-based prevention programs for alcohol misuse in young people. *Cochrane Database of Systematic Reviews*, (9), CD009308.

Fukuyama, F. (2001). Social capital, civil society and development. *Third World Quarterly, 22*(1), 7–29.

Fukuyama, F. (2011). *The origins of political order*. New York: Farrar, Straus and Giroux.

Giesbrecht, N., & Haydon, E. (2006). Community-based interventions and alcohol, tobacco and other drugs: Foci, outcomes and implications. *Drug and Alcohol Review, 25*(6), 633–646. https://doi.org/10.1080/09595230600944594

Glass, J. E., Hamilton, A. M., Powell, B. J., Perron, B. E., Brown, R. T., & Ilgen, M. A. (2015). Specialty substance use disorder services following brief alcohol intervention: A meta-analysis of randomized controlled trials. *Addiction, 110*(9), 1404–1415. https://doi.org/10.1111/add.12950

Grimshaw, J. M., Eccles, M. P., Lavis, J. N., Hill, S. J., & Squires, J. E. (2012). Knowledge translation of research findings. *Implementation Science, 7*, 50. https://doi.org/10.1186/1748-5908-7-50

Gripenberg Abdon, J., Wallin, E., & Andréasson, S. (2011). Long-term effects of a community-based intervention: 5-year follow-up of "Clubs against Drugs". *Addiction (Abingdon, England), 106*(11), 1997–2004. https://doi.org/10.1111/j.1360-0443.2011.03573.x

Grol, R. (1997). Personal paper: Beliefs and evidence in changing clinical practice. *British Medical Journal, 315*(7105), 418–421. https://doi.org/10.1136/bmj.315.7105.418

Hall, S. (2005). Night-time leisure and violence in the breakdown of the pseudo-pacification process. *Probation Journal, 52*(4), 376–389. https://doi.org/10.1177/0264550505058943

Hawe, P., Shiell, A., & Riley, T. (2009). Theorising interventions as events in systems. *American Journal of Community Psychology, 43*(3–4), 267–276. https://doi.org/10.1007/s10464-009-9229-9

Hill, K. G., Hawkins, J. D., Bailey, J. A., Catalano, R. F., Abbott, R. D., & Shapiro, V. B. (2010). Person-environment interaction in the prediction of alcohol abuse and alcohol dependence in adulthood. *Drug and Alcohol Dependence, 110*(1–2), 62–69.

Hobbs, D. (2005). Violent hypocrisy: Governance and the night-time economy. *European Journal of Criminology, 2*(2), 161–183.

Hollands, G. J., Marteau, T. M., & Fletcher, P. C. (2016). Non-conscious processes in changing health-related behaviour: A conceptual analysis and framework. *Health Psychology Review*, 1–14. https://doi.org/10.1080/17437199.2015.1138093

Hollands, G. J., Shemilt, I., Marteau, T. M., Jebb, S. A., Kelly, M. P., Nakamura, R., ... Ogilvie, D. (2013). Altering micro-environments to change population health behaviour: Towards an evidence base for choice architecture interventions. *BMC Public Health, 13*(1), 1218. https://doi.org/10.1186/1471-2458-13-1218

Holmes, J., Guo, Y., Maheswaran, R., Nicholls, J., Meier, P. S., & Brennan, A. (2014). The impact of spatial and temporal availability of alcohol on its consumption and related harms: A critical review in the context of UK licensing policies. *Drug and Alcohol Review, 33*(5), 515–525. https://doi.org/10.1111/dar.12191

Hornik, R., Jacobsohn, L., Orwin, R., Piesse, A., & Kalton, G. (2008). Effects of the National Youth Anti-Drug Media Campaign on youths. *The American Journal of Public Health, 98*(12), 2229–2236.

Horton, R. (2014). Offline: The third revolution in global health. *The Lancet, 383*(9929), 1620. https://doi.org/10.1016/S0140-6736(14)60769-8

Hughes, K., Quigg, Z., Eckley, L., Bellis, M., Jones, L., Calafat, A., ... van Hasselt, N. (2011). Environmental factors in drinking venues and alcohol-related harm: The evidence base for European intervention. *Addiction, 106*(Suppl 1), 37–46.

Hunter, D. J. (2009). Relationship between evidence and policy: A case of evidence-based policy or policy-based evidence? *Public Health, 123*(9), 583–586. https://doi.org/10.1016/j.puhe.2009.07.011

Hunter, S. B., Han, B., Slaughter, M. E., Godley, S. H., & Garner, B. R. (2015). Associations between implementation characteristics and evidence-based practice sustainment: A study of the Adolescent Community Reinforcement Approach. *Implementation Science, 10*(1), 173. https://doi.org/10.1186/s13012-015-0364-4

Institute for Government. (2009). *MINDSPACE: Influencing behaviour through public policy.* London: Institute for Government Retrieved from http://www.instituteforgovernment.org.uk/sites/default/files/publications/MINDSPACE.pdf

Institute of Medicine and National Research. (2009). *Preventing mental, emotional, and behavioral disorders among young people.* Washington, DC: National Academies Press. https://doi.org/10.17226/12480

Jamal, F., Fletcher, A., Harden, A., Wells, H., Thomas, J., & Bonell, C. (2013). The school environment and student health: A systematic review and meta-ethnography of qualitative research. *BMC Public Health, 13*, 798. https://doi.org/10.1186/1471-2458-13-798

Katz, J., & Wandersman, A. (2016). Technical assistance to enhance prevention capacity: A research synthesis of the evidence base. *Prevention Science, 17*(4), 417–428. https://doi.org/10.1007/s11121-016-0636-5

Kellam, S. G., Wang, W., Mackenzie, A. C. L., Brown, C. H., Ompad, D. C., Or, F., ... Windham, A. (2014). The impact of the good behavior game, a universal classroom-based preventive intervention in first and second grades, on high-risk sexual behaviors and drug abuse and dependence disorders into young adulthood. *Prevention Science, 15*(Suppl 0 1), S6–S18. https://doi.org/10.1007/s11121-012-0296-z

Kim, B. K. E., Gloppen, K. M., Rhew, I. C., Oesterle, S., & Hawkins, J. D. (2015). Effects of the communities that care prevention system on youth reports of protective factors. *Prevention Science, 16*(5), 652–662. https://doi.org/10.1007/s11121-014-0524-9

Knai, C., Petticrew, M., Durand, M. A., Eastmure, E., & Mays, N. (2015). Are the Public Health Responsibility Deal alcohol pledges likely to improve public health? An evidence synthesis. *Addiction, 110*(8), 1232–1246. https://doi.org/10.1111/add.12855

Kohler, S., & Hofmann, A. (2015). Can motivational interviewing in emergency care reduce alcohol consumption in young people? A systematic review and meta-analysis. *Alcohol and Alcoholism (Oxford, Oxfordshire), 50*(2), 107–117. https://doi.org/10.1093/alcalc/agu098

Kuntsche, E. N., & Jordan, M. D. (2006). Adolescent alcohol and cannabis use in relation to peer and school factors. Results of multilevel analyses. *Drug and Alcohol Dependence, 84*(2), 167–174.

Kuntsche, E. N., & Kuendig, H. (2005). Do school surroundings matter? Alcohol outlet density, perception of adolescent drinking in public, and adolescent alcohol use. *Addictive Behaviors, 30*(1), 151–158.

Langer, L., Tripney, J., & Gough, D. (2016). *The science of using science: Researching the use of research evidence in decision-making.* London: EPPI—Centre, Social Science Research Unit, UCL Institute of Education, University College London.

Langford, R., Bonell, C., Jones, H., Pouliou, T., Murphy, S., Waters, E., ... Campbell, R. (2015). The World Health Organization's health promoting schools framework: A Cochrane systematic review and meta-analysis. *BMC Public Health, 15*(1), 130. https://doi.org/10.1186/s12889-015-1360-y

Legleye, S., Beck, F., Khlat, M., Peretti-Watel, P., & Chau, N. (2012). The influence of socioeconomic status on cannabis use among French adolescents. *The Journal of Adolescent Health, 50*(4), 395–402.

Legleye, S., Khlat, M., Mayet, A., Beck, F., Falissard, B., Chau, N., & Peretti-Watel, P. (2016). From cannabis initiation to daily use: Educational inequalities in consumption behaviours over three generations in France. *Addiction, 111*, 1856–1866. https://doi.org/10.1111/add.13461

Leslie, L. K., Mehus, C. J., Hawkins, J. D., Boat, T., McCabe, M. A., Barkin, S., ... Beardslee, W. (2016). Primary health care: Potential home for family-focused preventive interventions. *American Journal of Preventive Medicine.* https://doi.org/10.1016/j.amepre.2016.05.014

Livingston, M. (2011). Alcohol outlet density and harm: Comparing the impacts on violence and chronic harms. *Drug and Alcohol Review, 30*(5), 515–523. https://doi.org/10.1111/j.1465-3362.2010.00251.x

Lloyd, C. (2010). Sinning and sinned against: The stigmatisation of problem drug users. UK Drug Policy Commission: London. Retrieved from http://www.ukdpc.org.uk/wp-content/uploads/Policy%20report%20%20Sinning%20and%20sinned%20against_%20the%20stigmatisation%20of%20problem%20drug%20users.pdf

Malmberg, M., Kleinjan, M., Overbeek, G., Vermulst, A., Lammers, J., Monshouwer, K., ... Engels, R. C. M. E. (2015). Substance use outcomes in the Healthy School and Drugs program: Results from a latent growth curve approach. *Addictive Behaviors, 42*, 194–202. https://doi.org/10.1016/j.addbeh.2014.11.021

Malmberg, M., Kleinjan, M., Overbeek, G., Vermulst, A., Monshouwer, K., Lammers, J., ... Engels, R. C. M. E. (2014). Effectiveness of the "Healthy School and Drugs" prevention programme on adolescents' substance use: A randomized clustered trial. *Addiction, 109*(6), 1031–1040. https://doi.org/10.1111/add.12526

Markham, W., Young, R., Sweeting, H., West, P., & Aveyard, P. (2012). Does school ethos explain the relationship between value-added education and teenage substance use? A cohort study. *Social Science & Medicine, 75*(1), 69–76.

Marmot, M. (2010). Fair Society Healthy Lives. *Nursing Standard, 25*(6), 30–30.. https://doi.org/10.7748/ns2010.10.25.6.30.p4603

Marteau, T. M., Hollands, G. J., & Fletcher, P. C. (2012). Changing human behavior to prevent disease: The importance of targeting automatic processes. *Science, 337*(6101), 1492–1495. https://doi.org/10.1126/science.1226918

Martineau, F. P., Graff, H., Mitchell, C., & Lock, K. (2014). Responsibility without legal authority? Tackling alcohol-related health harms through licensing and planning policy in local government. *Journal of Public Health (Oxford, England), 36*(3), 435–442. https://doi.org/10.1093/pubmed/fdt079

McCormick, R., Docherty, B., Segura, L., Colom, J., Gual, A., Cassidy, P., ... Heather, N. (2010). The research translation problem: Alcohol screening and brief intervention in primary care – Real world evidence supports theory. *Drugs: Education, Prevention, and Policy, 17*(6), 732–748.

Memoria Plan Nacional Sobre Drogas. (2013). Madrid. Retrieved from http://www.pnsd.msssi.gob.es/profesionales/publicaciones/catalogo/catalogoPNSD/publicaciones/pdf/memo2013.pdf

Michie, S., van Stralen, M. M., & West, R. (2011). The behaviour change wheel: A new method for characterising and designing behaviour change interventions. *Implementation Science, 6*, 42.

Mihalic, S. F., & Elliott, D. S. (2015). Evidence-based programs registry: Blueprints for healthy youth development. *Evaluation and Program Planning, 48*, 124–131. https://doi.org/10.1016/j.evalprogplan.2014.08.004

Miller, B. A., Holder, H. D., & Voas, R. B. (2009). Environmental strategies for prevention of drug use and risks in clubs. *Journal of Substance Use, 14*(1), 19–38.

Moodie, R., Stuckler, D., Monteiro, C., Sheron, N., Neal, B., Thamarangsi, T., ... Casswell, S. (2013). Profits and pandemics: Prevention of harmful effects of tobacco, alcohol, and ultra-processed food and drink industries. *The Lancet, 381*(9867), 670–679.

Moos, R. H. (2005). Iatrogenic effects of psychosocial interventions for substance use disorders: Prevalence, predictors, prevention. *Addiction, 100*(5), 595–604.

O'Donnell, A., Anderson, P., Newbury-Birch, D., Schulte, B., Schmidt, C., Reimer, J., & Kaner, E. (2013). The impact of brief alcohol interventions in primary healthcare: A systematic review of reviews. *Alcohol and Alcoholism (Oxford, Oxfordshire), 49*(1), 66–78. https://doi.org/10.1093/alcalc/agt170

Oesterle, S., Hawkins, D. J., Kuklinski, M. R., Fleming, C., Rhew, I. C., Brown, E. C., ... Catalano, R. F. (2015). Preventing adolescent violence using the communities that care prevention system: Findings from a community-randomised trial. *Injury Prevention, 21*(Suppl 2), A23.2–A2A23. https://doi.org/10.1136/injuryprev-2015-041654.64

Oliver, K., Lorenc, T., & Innvær, S. (2014). New directions in evidence-based policy research: A critical analysis of the literature. *Health Research Policy and Systems/BioMed Central, 12*, 34. https://doi.org/10.1186/1478-4505-12-34

Ostlund, S. B., Maidment, N. T., & Balleine, B. W. (2010). Alcohol-paired contextual cues produce an immediate and selective loss of goal-directed action in rats. *Frontiers in Integrative Neuroscience, 4.* https://doi.org/10.3389/fnint.2010.00019

Palinkas, L. A., Spear, S. E., Mendon, S. J., Villamar, J., Valente, T., Chou, C.-P., ... Brown, C. H. (2015). Measuring sustainment of prevention programs and initiatives: A study protocol. *Implementation Science, 11*(1), 95. https://doi.org/10.1186/s13012-016-0467-6

Papies, E. K. (2016). Goal priming as a situated intervention tool. *Current Opinion in Psychology, 12*, 12–16. https://doi.org/10.1016/j.copsyc.2016.04.008

Parkes, T., Atherton, I., Evans, J., Gloyn, S., McGhee, S., & Stoddart, B. (2011). *An evaluation to assess the implementation of NHS delivered Alcohol Brief Intervention.* Edinburgh: NHS Health Scotland.

Piper, D., Stein-Seroussi, A., Flewelling, R., Orwin, R. G., & Buchanan, R. (2012). Assessing state substance abuse prevention infrastructure through the lens of CSAP's Strategic Prevention Framework. *Evaluation and Program Planning, 35*(1), 66–77. https://doi.org/10.1016/j.evalprogplan.2011.07.003

Ramírez de Arellano, A. (2015). La estrategia de la prevención indicada: un problema de infraestructura. *Consumo de alcohol en jóvenes y adolescentes. Una mirada ecológica.* Bilbao: Publicaciones de la Universidad de Deusto.

Ringwalt, C. L., Clark, H. K., Hanley, S., Shamblen, S. R., & Flewelling, R. L. (2010). The effects of Project ALERT one year past curriculum completion. *Prevention Science, 11*(2), 172–184. https://doi.org/10.1007/s11121-009-0163-8

Ringwalt, C., Vincus, A. A., Hanley, S., Ennett, S. T., Bowling, J. M. M., & Haws, S. (2011). The prevalence of evidence-based drug use prevention curricula in U.S. middle schools in 2008. *Prev Sci, 12*(1), 63–69.. https://doi.org/10.1007/s11121-010-0184-3

Ritter, A., & McDonald, D. (2008). Illicit drug policy: Scoping the interventions and taxonomies. *Drugs: Education, Prevention, and Policy, 15*(1), 15–35. https://doi.org/10.1080/09687630701204344

Scheirer, M. A., & Dearing, J. W. (2011). An agenda for research on the sustainability of Public Health Programs. *American Journal of Public Health, 101*(11), 2059–2067. https://doi.org/10.2105/AJPH.2011.300193

Schmidt, A. (2014). Kommunale Alkoholprävention in Niedersachsen—Formale und rechtliche Grundlagen. In *Professionalisierung kommunaler Alkoholprävention: Was kann eine lokale Alkoholpolitik leisten?* Hannover: Niedersächsische Landesstelle für Suchtfragen.

Shiell, A., Hawe, P., & Gold, L. (2008). Complex interventions or complex systems? Implications for health economic evaluation. *British Medical Journal, 336*(7656), 1281–1283. https://doi.org/10.1136/bmj.39569.510521.AD

Simon, H. A. (1991). The architecture of complexity. In *Facets of systems science* (pp. 457–476). Boston, MA: Springer US. https://doi.org/10.1007/978-1-4899-0718-9_31

Skärstrand, E., Larsson, J., & Andréasson, S. (2008). Cultural adaptation of the strengthening families programme to a Swedish setting. *Health Education, 108*(4), 287–300. https://doi.org/10.1108/09654280810884179

Sloboda, Z., Glantz, M. D., & Tarter, R. E. (2012). Revisiting the concepts of risk and protective factors for understanding the etiology and development of substance use and substance use disorders: Implications for prevention. *Substance Use and Misuse, 47*, 944–962. https://doi.org/10.3109/10826084.2012.663280

Spoth, R., Guyll, M., Redmond, C., Greenberg, M., & Feinberg, M. (2011). Six-year sustainability of evidence-based intervention implementation quality by community-university partnerships: The PROSPER study. *American Journal of Community Psychology, 48*(3–4), 412–425. https://doi.org/10.1007/s10464-011-9430-5

Stafström, M., Ostergren, P. O., Larsson, S., Lindgren, B., & Lundborg, P. (2006). A community action programme for reducing harmful drinking behaviour among adolescents: The Trelleborg Project. *Addiction, 101*(6), 813–823.

Steketee, M., Oesterle, S., Jonkman, H., Hawkins, J. D., Haggerty, K. P., & Aussems, C. (2013). Transforming prevention Systems in the United States and The Netherlands Using Communities that Care. *European Journal on Criminal Policy and Research, 19*(2), 99–116. https://doi.org/10.1007/s10610-012-9194-y

Stewart-Brown, S. (2006). *What is the evidence on school health promotion in improving health or preventing disease and, specifically, what is the effectiveness of the health promoting schools approach?* Copenhagen: WHO Regional Office for Europe Retrieved from http://www.euro.who.int/document/e88185.pdf

Sundell, K., Hansson, K., Löfholm, C. A., Olsson, T., Gustle, L.-H., & Kadesjö, C. (2008). The transportability of multisystemic therapy to Sweden: Short-term results from a randomized trial of conduct-disordered youths. *Journal of Family Psychology, 22*(4), 550–560. https://doi.org/10.1037/a0012790

Sussman, S., Earleywine, M., Wills, T., Cody, C., Biglan, T., Dent, C. W., & Newcomb, M. D. (2004). The motivation, skills, and decision-making model of "drug abuse" prevention. *Substance Use & Misuse, 39*(10–12), 1971–2016.

Teasdale, B., & Silver, E. (2009). Neighborhoods and self-control: Toward an expanded view of socialization. *Social Problems, 56*(1), 205–222. https://doi.org/10.1525/sp.2009.56.1.205

Thapa, A., Cohen, J., Guffey, S., & Higgins-D'Alessandro, A. (2013). A review of school climate research. *Review of Educational Research, 83*(3), 357–385. https://doi.org/10.3102/0034654313483907

Tibbits, M. K., Bumbarger, B. K., Kyler, S. J., & Perkins, D. F. (2010). Sustaining evidence-based interventions under real-world conditions: Results from a large-scale diffusion project. *Prevention Science, 11*(3), 252–262. https://doi.org/10.1007/s11121-010-0170-9

UNESCO, UNODC, & WHO. (2017). *Education sector responses to the use of alcohol, tobacco and drugs.* Paris: United Nations Educational, Scientific and Cultural Organization Retrieved from http://unesdoc.unesco.org/images/0024/002475/247509E.pdf

UNODC. (2009). *Guide to implementing family skills training programmes for drug abuse prevention.* New York: United Nations.

UNODC. (2013). International standards on drug use prevention. Vienna: United Nations.

Van Horn, M. L., Fagan, A. A., Hawkins, J. D., & Oesterle, S. (2014). Effects of the communities that care system on cross-sectional profiles of adolescent substance use and delinquency. *American Journal of Preventive Medicine, 47*, 188–197. https://doi.org/10.1016/j.amepre.2014.04.004

van Poppel, D. G. H. (2008). *Effective municipal and community alcohol prevention strategies across the world.* Utrecht: STAP (Stichting Alcoholpreventie).

Vaughn, M. G., Beaver, K. M., DeLisi, M., Perron, B. E., & Schelbe, L. (2009). Gene-environment interplay and the importance of self-control in predicting polydrug use and substance-related problems. *Addictive Behaviors, 34*(1), 112–116. https://doi.org/10.1016/j.addbeh.2008.08.011

Villalbí, J. R., Bartroli, M., Bosque-Prous, M., Guitart, A. M., Serra-Batiste, E., Casas, C., & Brugal, M. T. (2015). Enforcing regulations on alcohol sales and use as universal environmental prevention. *Adicciones, 27*(4), 288–293. Retrieved from http://www.ncbi.nlm.nih.gov/pubmed/26706811

Von Bertalanffy, L. (1968). *General system theory* (Vol. 1). New York: George Braziller Retrieved from http://books.google.es/books?id=N6k2mILtPYIC

Wang, S., Moss, J. R., & Hiller, J. E. (2006). Applicability and transferability of interventions in evidence-based public health. *Health Promotion International, 21*, 76–83. https://doi.org/10.1093/heapro/dai025

Wilkinson, R., & Picket, K. (2010). *The spirit level: Why equality is better for everyone.* London: Penguin.

Wills, T. A., Ainette, M. G., Mendoza, D., Gibbons, F. X., & Brody, G. H. (2007). Self-control, symptomatology, and substance use precursors: Test of a theoretical model in a community sample of 9-year-old children. *Psychology of Addictive Behaviors, 21*(2), 205–215. https://doi.org/10.1037/0893-164X.21.2.205

Winlow, S., & Hall, S. (2005). *Violent night. Urban leisure and contemporary culture.* Oxford: Berg. Retrieved from file://v/RES/02 Common outputs/7 Literature/GB/JabRef_pdf_files/gregorbiblio/1248/Hall y Winlow - Night-time leisure and violence in the breakdown of the pseudo-pacification process.pdf

Withagen, R., de Poel, H. J., Araujo, D., & Pepping, G. J. (2012). Affordances can invite behavior: Reconsidering the relationship between affordances and agency. *New Ideas in Psychology, 30*(2), 250–258. https://doi.org/10.1016/j.newideapsych.2011.12.003

World Health Organisation. (2014). *Global status report on alcohol and health* (pp. 1–392). Geneva: WHO. Retrieved from http://www.who.int/substance_abuse/publications/global_alcohol_report/msbgsruprofiles.pdf

Wright, J., Williams, R., & Wilkinson, J. R. (1998). Development and importance of health needs assessment. *British Medical Journal, 316*(7140), 1310–1313. https://doi.org/10.1136/bmj.316.7140.1310

Young, R., Macdonald, L., & Ellaway, A. (2013). Associations between proximity and density of local alcohol outlets and alcohol use among Scottish adolescents. *Health & Place, 19*, 124–130.

Yuma-Guerrero, P. J., Lawson, K. A., Velasquez, M. M., von Sternberg, K., Maxson, T., & Garcia, N. (2012). Screening, brief intervention, and referral for alcohol use in adolescents: A systematic review. *Pediatrics, 130*(1), 115–122. https://doi.org/10.1542/peds.2011-1589

Index

A

Adaptation, 391–393
Adapting interventions, 141, 142
Adaptive preventive interventions
   alcohol abuse, 264
   baseline characteristics, 263
   vs. business, 277
   classroom-based universal prevention, 278
   contributions, 264
   development of, 271, 272
   Fast Track study, 277
   indicated, 266–271
   individual and family-based intervention models, 263
   intervention type, 264
   one-size-fits-all, 264
   selective, 266
   SMART, 272–276
   substance abuse, 265
   substance use, 263
   substantive and methodological work, 277
   universal, 266
   USI, 266
   Web-BASICS *vs.* In-Person BASICS, 277
Addiction, 281
   biomarkers, 68
   definition, 59
   disease phenotypes, 60
   epigenetic modifications, 67
   experimental models, 60
   "genes implicated in addiction", 68
   genetics, 60
   human behavioral phenotype, 60
   liability, 60
   opiate, 65
Adolescence
   in cognitive skills, 3
   cultures change, 3
   description, 8
   phenotypic changes, 3
   puberty, 3
Adolescent brain development
   ABCD, 4
   and alcohol (*see* Alcohol and the adolescent brain)
   axon, 5
   corpus callosum and sex differences, 10, 11
   in emotional reactivity and risky behaviors
      (*see* Brain structures, in emotional reactivity and risky behaviors)
   frontal lobes, changes, 6, 7
   glial cells, 5
   gray matter, 4, 5
   human brain, 5
   moodiness and general tumult, 4
   neuron, depiction of, 6
   occipital lobes, 7
   parietal lobes, 7
   prefrontal cortex, 6
   research, 4
   temporal lobes, 7
   white matter, 5
Adolescents, 217
   adult consumption, 123
   alcohol marketing, 120, 121
   binge drinking, 119
   prevalence, adult drinking, 119
Advertising exposure, 122, 124
Aetiology, 224
Affordable Care Act, 103, 105, 107
Age restrictions, 165
   alcohol, 166
   marijuana, 170
   tobacco, 168
Age-prevalence gradient, 78–80
Alcohol, 227
   advertising, 167
   age, 166
   age-standardised DALYs, 30
   alcohol-attributable burden, 30
   bans, 166
   dependence, 25, 28
   epidemiological data, 21
   government control, 167
   health burden, 28
   mortality rates, 28
   prevalence, 22
   price, 167

Alcohol (*cont.*)
　　research, 172
　　restrictions, 167
　　tax, 167
Alcohol and adolescent brain
　　adolescent neuroplasticity, 14
　　age of onset, drinking, 14
　　amygdala and corpus callosum, 12
　　BACs, 12
　　cumulative levels, 12
　　family interventions, 14
　　healthy coping skills, 15
　　high peak levels, drinking, 12
　　inpatient substance abuse treatment
　　　　program, 11
　　ISFP, 15
　　learning and memory, tests of, 11
　　levels, drinking, 12
　　neuropsychological functioning, 12
　　online prevention program, 15
　　PDFY, 15
　　risk factors, 14
　　sensitivity, adolescents *vs.* adults, 13, 14
　　substance use, 11
Alcohol and Drug Education and Prevention Information
　　Service (ADEPIS), 403
Alcohol marketing
　　alcohol advertising, 125
　　branding (*see* Branding)
　　counter-advertising, 127
　　media literacy, 126
　　non-compliant advertising, 126
　　restricting outdoor advertising, 126
　　and young people (*see* Youth)
　　WHO, 125
Alcohol taxes, 120
Alcohol, tobacco and other drugs (ATOD), 194, 195,
　　198, 199
Alcohol use, 119
ALDH2 finding, 69
Amphetamine-type stimulants, 19, 22, 28
Amygdala, 9, 10
Anthropological methods
　　copping, 212
　　cultural, 210
　　ethnographic monographs, 210
　　"exotic" drug, 211
　　formalization (*see* Formalization)
　　getting off, 212
　　the hustle, 212
　　museum artifacts, 210
　　national statistics, 210
　　open-ended interviews, 211
　　theory of addiction, 211
Anthropologists, 210, 211, 213, 214
Attachment theory, 136
Avoid RP32, 305
Axons, 5, 6
Ayahuasca, 209

B
Behavioral Assessment System for Children (BASC), 268
Behavioral parent training
　　in childhood, 140
　　component meta-analysis, 138, 139
　　family-based preventive interventions, 137
　　management skills, 136
　　meta-analyses, 138
　　RCT, 137
　　SPR, 137
　　systemic review, 137, 138
Binge drinking, 76, 119, 121, 125
Biometrics genetic studies
　　ALDH2 gene, 62
　　binary trait definition, 62
　　dizygotic (DZ) twins, 60, 61
　　DNA variation, 61
　　environmental components, 61
　　GLA, 62, 63
　　heritability, 61, 62
　　human genetic program, 61
　　monozygotic (MZ) twins, 60
　　parent-child transmission, SUD risk, 63
　　prevalence, smoking, 63
　　significant heritability, 58
Blood alcohol concentrations (BACs), 12
Body count, 99
Brain structures, in emotional reactivity and risky
　　behaviors
　　adolescence, 8
　　amygdala, 10
　　brain activity, 8
　　changes, in frontal lobes, 7
　　cortisol levels, 9
　　frontalization, 8
　　HPA axis, 9
　　immature cognitive control, 8
　　maturation, frontal lobes, 8
　　nucleus accumbens, 8
　　risk-taking behavior, 8
　　skin-conductance changes, 9
　　stress response, 9
　　VTA, 8
Branding
　　advertising campaigns, 122
　　advertising exposure, 122
　　beer, 122
　　brands of alcohol, 122
　　research, on youth alcohol consumption, 125
　　tequila, 122
　　young people
　　　　adult consumption, 123
　　　　advertising exposure, 124
　　　　alcohol advertising, 125
　　　　brand choice, 124
　　　　cheapest brands, consumption, 123
　　　　magazine advertising behavior, 124
　　　　social sources, 123
　　youth alcohol consumption, 122, 123

Index

Brief Alcohol Screening and Intervention for College
    Students (BASICS), 275, 276
Brief intervention (BIs)
    alcohol, 181
    evidence, 184–186
    expected effects, 187, 188
    illicit drugs, 181
    implementation, 188
    prevention, 181
    researchers and practitioners, 181
    substance use, 182–184
    types of services, 182
Burden of disease, 30

C

Canadian Centre on Substance Use and Addiction, 403
Cannabis use, 19, 22, 25, 28, 34
Card clusters, 212
Center for Behavioral Health Statistics and Quality
    (CBHSQ), 281
Center for the Application of Prevention Technologies
    (CAPT), 376, 377, 379
Center on Alcohol Marketing and Youth (CAMY), 120
Centers for the Application of Prevention Technologies
    (CAPT), 370
Certificate of Confidentiality (CoC), 290
Children and adolescents, mindful awareness programs,
    339, 340
Chutaderos, 214
Cigarette smoking, 99, 100, 103, 107, 110, 114
Cocaine, 19, 22, 28, 34
Cognitive Mediation Model, 323
Cognitive neuroscience theories, 336
Collaboration
    academic journals, 387
    in conference symposia, 387
    institutional websites, 387
    international, 387–391, 393
    and networks, 386
    prevention science, 385, 386
    social media, 387
Communities that Care (CTC), 373–375, 379
Community advisory board (CAB), 201
Community-based participatory research (CBPR), 201
    ATOD prevention, 194–196, 198, 199
    collaborative, 201
    contractual, 201
    consultative, 201
    implementation stage, 202
    social determinants, 200
    US-based prevention research, 201
Comorbid mental disorders, 293
Components, EQUIP model
    inform, 309–311
    interacting requisites, 306–308
    persuade, 311, 312
    question phase, 308, 309
    undermine, 309

Confidentiality, 284, 287, 289, 290, 292
Consolidated Framework for Implementation Research
    (CFIR), 370–372, 375, 377–379
Consolidated Standards of Reporting Trials
    (CONSORT), 257, 258
Content Appealing to Youth (CAY), 125
Control Signals Poster (CSP), 342
Corpus callosum, 10
Cortisol, 9
Counter-advertising, 102, 104, 107, 127
Criminal justice agencies, 226
Crush the Crave (CTC) campaign, 327
Cultural competence, 196, 197
The Centers for Disease and Prevention
    (CDC), 173
Cumulative impact zones (CIZs), 425

D

DARE campaign, 108, 310
Data collection methods
    feedback loops, 225
    geographical area, 225
    interplay and iterative process, 225–226
    overview, 226
    prevention needs, 225
    prevention programs, 224
    risk assessment, 223, 225
    tailoring process, 226
    target outcomes, 224
Data interpretation, 218
Decision-making, 416
Defining problematic substance use
    binge drinking, 76
    clinical SUD diagnosis, 76
    for illicit drugs, 76
    problematic/risky substance involvement, 76
Demographics, 226
Department of Health and Human Services (DHHS),
    102, 103
Dependence, substance, *see* Substance dependence
Desistance
    cohort changes, 84
    historic differences, 84
    maturing out *vs.* natural recovery models,
        88, 90
    mechanisms, 90
    naturally-occurring factors, 84
    older-adult health, 90
    in young adulthood, 88
Deviance proneness pathway, 80, 81
Differential taxation, 111
Diffusion of Innovations Theory (DIT), 327
DNA methylation, 66
DNA methyltransferases (DNMT), 66
Dopamine D2 receptor gene (DRD2), 39
Dopaminergic mesocorticolimbic system, 63
Drug alerts, 223
Dynamic structural equation modeling (DSEM), 359

E

Ecobiodevelopmental theoretical framework, 37, 38
Ecological momentary assessments (EMA), 342
Elaboration likelihood model (ELM), 314
Elements, persuasive communications
    credibility and trustworthiness, 313
    risk or usage status, 313–315
    the source ("Who"), 312, 313
Endophenotype, 65
Environmental influences, 38, 39, 49
Epidemiology, 215
    alcohol, 77
    illicit-drug use, 77
    national studies, 77
    pharmaceuticals, 77
    prevalence rates, 77
    risky/problematic use, 77
    smoking and nicotine use, 77
Epidemiology monitoring information, 223, 224
Epigenetics, substance use
    acetylation-related processes, 67
    addiction-related behaviors, 67
    DNA methylation, 66
    environmental variance, 67
    genetic variation, 68
    mechanisms, 57, 66, 68
    modifications, 67
    phenotypic changes, 66
EQUIP model
    components (*see* Components, EQUIP model)
    judgment of media failures, 304
    persuasive message development, 305, 306
    PSU, 303
    resistance in persuasion, 305
Ethnicity
    ATOD, 194, 195, 198, 199
    in US, 193, 194
Ethnographers
    extensive conversation, 210
    house-to-house survey, 210
    photograph, 210
Ethnographic methods, 228
Ethnography, 210, 211, 217, 219
Ethnoscience, 211
Etiology, SUD
    developmental and integrative framework, 38
    deviance proneness pathway, 80, 81
    heterotypic continuity, 80
    integrative perspective
        competency, levels of, 49
        contextual systems, 48
        and developmental perspective, 50
        EBPs, 49
        ECF's, 49
        neurodevelopment, 50
        prevention practices and interventions, 48
        programs and interventions, 48
        protective factors, 48
        research, 49
        responsiveness, 48
        social and emotional skills, 48
    inter-related biopsychosocial risk pathways, 80
    macro-level influences
        income/resources, 46, 47
        neighborhood and physical environment, 45, 46
        public policy/government influence, 47, 48
    micro-level influences
        parenting and family functioning, 43, 44
        peer influences, 45
        schools and educational opportunities, 44, 45
    personal level
        characteristics, 38
        genetic influences, 40
        genetic susceptibility, 38
        mental and behavioral health, 40
        neurobiological development, 41
        neurological development, 40
        personality traits, 39
        stress exposures (*see* Stress)
    practical implications, 81
Etymology, 210
European Drug Addiction Prevention trial (EU-DAP), 248, 252
European Drug Prevention Quality Standards (EDPQS), 396, 397, 399, 401, 405, 414, 421, 430–432
European Monitoring Centre for Drugs and Drug Addiction (EMCDDA), 223, 228, 230
Evidence-based prevention (EBPs)
    adoption, 368
    alcohol and drug problems, 367
    blueprints, 374, 375
    CFIR, 369–372
    coalitions/schools/community groups, 379
    CTC, 373, 374
    disadvantages and minority communities, 379, 380
    dissemination, 368, 369, 372
    government-developed synthesis, 375–377
    GTO, 372, 373
    implementation science theory, 378, 379
    interventions
        classrooms, 154, 155
        prevention of substance use, 156, 157
        school culture and bonding, 154
    longitudinal research, 367
    marijuana use, 367
    opioids, 367
    PROSPER, 374
    research-developed support and delivery systems, 372
    social bonds, 377, 378
    substance-use, 368
    translation and support systems, 375–377
    the US rates, 367
Evidence-based programs (EBPs), 49
Evidence-based workgroups (EBW), 376
Executive cognitive functions (ECFs), 41, 49
Expectancy violation theory (EVT), 307
Experience-dependence, brain, 37
Ex-substance users, self-esteem, 157, 158
Extra-medical use, 19, 20

Index

F
Facebook, 326–328
Fairness Doctrine, 101, 104, 109
Familias Unidas program, 354
Family Check-Up (FCU) Program, 270
Family functioning, 133, 134, 137, 141, 142
Family processes
 beliefs, attitudes and values, 134
 communication, 135
 human well-being, 133
 organization, 134, 135
 problem solving, 135
 protective processes, 133
Family skill programs, 138, 140
Family Smoking Prevention and Tobacco Control Act of 2009, 102
Family structures, 133, 134, 143
Family systems theory, 136
Family therapy, 216
Fast Track Program, 270
Federal Cigarette Labeling and Advertising Act of 1965, 100
Federal Trade Commission, 100, 120, 126
Formalization
 cannabis consumption, 213
 evaluation studies, 218
 field notes, 212, 213
 injecting behavior, 213
 narrative texts, 213
 population prevention, 215
 prevention messages, 218
 prevention, process, 217
 prodromal signs, 216
 quantitative instruments, 212
 target population, 215, 218
 terrain, 212
 textual descriptions, 212
 word processing software, 213
Framework Convention on Tobacco Control, 109–110
Frontal lobes, 6, 7
Funding, 415–419, 430

G
Gateway drug, 63
Gene mapping, 64
Genetic program, 57, 61
Genetics, substance use
 behavioral variation, 68
 biometric, 57 (*see also* Biometrics genetic studies)
 and environment, 57
 in GWAS, 58
 mechanistic causes, 57
 molecular, 57 (*see also* Molecular genetics)
 trait and phenotypes (*see* Trait and phenotypes)
Genetic susceptibility, 38–40
Geospatial mapping, 290–291
Getting To Outcomes® (GTO), 373, 375, 379
Glial cells, 5
Global Burden of Disease (GBD) study, 20, 22, 25, 28, 30

Good Behavior Game (GBG), 154, 155
Government monopolies, 165, 167, 170, 171
Graphic cigarette package warnings, 108
Graphic warning labels (GWLs), 102
Group Iterative Multiple Model Estimation (GIMME), 360
Growth mixture models (GMM), 247, 251

H
Hallucinogenic plant, 209
Harm reduction, tobacco control, 114
Harms, 282, 284, 285, 294
Health belief model, 321
Health care provider accountability, 175, 176
Hepatitis B and C, 215, 226
Heritability
 addiction, 60
 alcoholism liability, 62
 binary trait definition, 62
 description, 57
 epigenetic modifications, 67
 genetic variation, 58
 GLA heritability, 63
 Mendelian traits, 61
 "missing heritability", 66
Heroin, 19, 22, 211, 212, 214, 227
Heterotypic continuity, 80, 81
Hieracium type of inheritance, 58
Hippocampus, 9, 10, 12, 13
HIV
 contagion, 214
 pandemic, 214
 transmission, 217
Human Genome Project, 68
Hypothalamic-pituitary-adrenal (HPA) axis, 9

I
Illegal drugs, 170, 171
Illicit drugs
 burden attributable, 30
 cannabis and opioid dependence, 25
 epidemiological data, 21
 GBD study, 28
 global prevalence, 22
 health burdens, 25
 mortality rates, 28
 MTF data, 77
 NPS, 24
 in potency and purity, 76
 public policy reactions, 77
Implementation
 CFIR, 375
 CTC, 374
 EBP, 369–372, 380
 GTO, 375
 PROSPER, 374
Implementation program, ATOD, 199, 200
Impulsivity, 81–83, 86–88
Increase taxes, 100, 104, 110
Inculcation process, 216

Indicated prevention interventions, 266–271
Indigenous people, 193, 194
Informed by scientific and ethical principles (ISSUP), 389
Informed consent, 283, 285–291, 293
Injecting drug use (IDU), 22, 32, 214
In-person BASICS, 274, 275
Instagram, 326, 328, 329
Institute for Health Metrics and Evaluation (IHME), 20
Institutional review boards (IRBs), 282, 294
Intensive longitudinal data, 355–362
Interactive Systems Framework (ISF), 372, 375–377, 407
Interactive voice response (IVR), 272
International Centre for Credentialing and Education of Addiction Professionals (ICCE), 403
International Certified Prevention Specialist I (ICPS I), 403
International collaboration, 387–391, 393
International networks, 386, 389, 393
International prevention science
    building capacity, 388
    collaboration, 387
    collaboration and knowledge exchange, 387
    development, international collaboration, 389
    international capacity and activity, 388
    international guidance and standards, 389
    international networks, 386
    substance misuse prevention, 388
    transporting and adapting interventions, 391–392
    working, 389–391
International research collaboration, 387, 389, 391
Internet
    audience activity, 324
    displays of alcohol use, 329
    monitoring, behavior and discourse, 329
    substance use prevention, 324
    web-based interventions, 324
Intervention theory, 388, 392
Intoxication, 209, 217
Iowa Strengthening Families Program (ISFP), 15

K
Kessler, D., 103

L
Latent class analysis (LCA), 247, 250, 251, 257
Latent class growth model (LCGM), 251
Latent transition analysis (LTA), 251
Law of demand, 109
Lecturing, 157
Legislation, 414, 425, 428
Linkage, 64
Local threats, 224
Lock in alcohol effect, 13
Low level of response (LLR) model, 83
Lower and middle-income countries (LMIC), 403

M
Macro-level environments, 215
Marihuana, 211, 216
Marijuana, 11, 227, 321, 327, 329, 330
    advertising, 170
    age restrictions, 170
    bans, 169, 170
    government monopolies, 170
    price, 170
    research, 173
    sale, 170
    tax, 170
Mass media, 319
    opinion followers, 315
    opinion leaders, 315
    prevention campaigns, 303
    prevention failures, 315
    UNODC, 303
Mass media campaigns, 321–323
Master Settlement Agreement, 103
Mature minor, 287
Maturing out
    contextual transitions, 84
    epidemiologic data, 88
    in desistance, 88
    maturing out *vs.* natural recovery models, 90
    in new onsets, 88
    older-adult health and desistance, 90, 91
    personality development, 86
    severe alcohol use disorder, 88
Mechanistic model test, 65
Media
    Internet (*see* Internet)
    mass media, 319 (*see also* Mass media)
    messages, 319
    print media, 319 (*see also* Social media)
    in substance use prevention, 320
    television, 319
Media campaigns, 102, 106, 107, 109
    campaign exposure (*see* Role of campaign exposure)
    nature and effectiveness
        Above the Influence, 321
        Be Under Your Own Influence campaign, 321
        emotional climate, puberty, 322
        marijuana use, 321
        My Anti-Drug, 321, 322
        non-randomized observational designs, 321
Media literacy, 126, 127
Mediation
    analysis, 233
    description, 233
    practical implications, 235, 236
    prevention programs, 242
    programs, substance-use, 233
    substance-use, 236, 237
    theoretical mediation model, 234, 235
Mediators, 186, 236, 237
Meta-analysis, 247, 252, 255, 256, 259
Micro-level environments, 215

Index

Microtrials, 350–354, 360, 362, 363
Middle-range theories
   communication-persuasion model, 305
   optimal model, 305
Mindfulness
   ancient Eastern spiritual traditions, 335
   application, 340–342
   children and adolescents, 339, 340
   field of prevention science, 343
   neuroscience research, 335
   PFC, 336
   practice, 337–339
   psychological constructs, 335
   substance use and abuse, 336
   and SUD treatment, 336, 337
Mindfulness-based stress reduction (MBSR) program, 339
Mixed Models Trajectory Analysis (MMTA), 358–362
Mobile computing, 320
Modeling change, 358–360
Moderators, 186
Molecular genetics
   alcohol dehydrogenases, 65
   association approaches, 64
   AVPR1A gene, 65
   behavioral disorders, 66
   family-based approach, 64
   functional polymorphism, 65
   gene mapping, 64
   GWAS, 64, 65
   linkage disequilibrium (LD) methods, 65
   mediation analysis, 65
   non-SNP genetic variation, 66
   "novel" genes, 65
Monetary incentives, 291–293
Monitoring the Future (MTF), 77–79
Monogenic/Mendelian traits, 58
Mortality and morbidity, 25, 28, 30
Multiple mediator model, 240, 241
My Anti-Drug, 321–324

N

National Institute for Health and Care Excellence (NICE), 402
National Longitudinal Alcohol Epidemiologic Survey (NLAES), 77
National Registry for Effective Programs and Practices (NREPP), 376, 377
National Youth Anti-drug Media Campaign (NYADMC), 321, 323, 330
Neurobiology, 41, 215
Neuroimaging techniques, 4
Neurological development, 40–42
New psychoactive substances (NPS), 20
   description, 24
   monitoring, 25
   morbidity and mortality, 25
   new type, 24
   prevalence, of use, 24

Nicotine replacement therapy (NRT), 111
Nightlife resorts, 417, 422, 424
Nurse Family Partnership program, 139

O

Occipital lobes, 7
Office of National Drug Control Policy (ONDCP), 376
Online alcohol interventions, 325
Online prevention program, 15
Opiates, 227

P

Pan American Health Organization (PAHO), 125
Parenting, 134, 138, 139
   attitudes, 135
   behaviors, 135
   developmental status, 135
   knowledge, 135
   practices, 135
   principles, 140
Parietal lobes, 7
Patient Review and Restriction Programs (PRRPs), 174, 175
Patterns and trends
   hypothesis, 227
   period prevalence, 227
   psychoactive substances, 227
   risk perceptions, 227
   school and general population surveys, 227
   stakeholders, 226
   substance use treatment data, 228
   targeted surveys and modelling, 227
Peer group therapy, 157, 216
Personality traits, 39, 40, 45
Personalized normative feedback (PNF) intervention, 269
Persuasion
   campaigns, 304, 315
   dual process models, 313
   and message-based PSU prevention, 304
   message strength, 314
   meta-cognitive model, 308–309
   middle-range theory, 308
   motivation, 311
   objective, 312
   principles, 316
   processes, 305, 306
   PSU prevention, 316
   research, 305
   resistance role, 305
   TPB, 304
Persuasive communications, *see* Elements, persuasive communications
Pharmaceuticals, 77
Pharmacological effects models, 83, 84
Pharmacopoeias, 209
Physiological reactivity, 42
Planned behavior (TPB), 304

Plano Operacional de Repostas Integradas (PORI), 419
Policies, 414–417, 420, 422–429, 432–435
Policies, tobacco control
    adult per capita cigarette consumption, 101
    FDA, 104
    Federal Cigarette Labeling and Advertising Act of 1965, 100
    federal involvement, 102
    federal presence, 102
    incentives, 106
    information and education policies
        counter advertising media campaigns, 107
        norm changes, 108
        school health education, 108
        tobacco experience, 107
    laws and regulations, 102, 107
    legal requirement, 107
    novel products, 105
    smoking-restriction, 102
    state and local policies, 104
Policy interventions
    alcohol, 166
    drug use, 165
    research, 171
    types, 165
Positive adolescent choices training (PACT) program, 352, 353
Posterior putamen, 336
Practical implications of theoretical model, 235, 236
Pragmatic malleability, 349–352, 361, 362
Prefrontal cortex (PFC), 6, 7, 335, 336, 338
Preparing for the Drug Free Years (PDFY), 15
Prescription drugs, 109, 110, 112, 113
Prescription monitoring programs (PMPs), 173, 174
Prevention
    communication
        Lazarsfeld's model, 315
        vulnerable nonusers, 314
    campaigns
        goal, 315
        long-standing staples, 310
        PSU, 303, 304, 312, 313
    interventions, 139
    needs, 224, 225
    science
        development of, 386
        globalisation, 385
        growth, 385
        international (*see* International prevention science)
        networks and collaborations, 386
    and systems, 386
    workforce
        EDPQS, 398–401
        services, 430, 431
        substance-use, 399, 401, 402
Price increases and taxes, 165
    alcohol, 167
    marijuana, 170
    tobacco, 168

Print media, 319
Problematic substance use
    addiction, 83
    binge drinking, 76
    clinical SUD diagnosis, 76
    costs, 75
    daily fluctuations, 82
    desistance, 84
    etiology (*see* Etiology, SUD)
    illicit drugs, 76
    limitations, 92
    maturing out (*see* Maturing out)
    problematic/risky substance involvement, 76
    psychoactive substances, 75
    research, 91
Professional cultures, 395–398, 406, 408
Professional development courses, 402
Professionalisation, 395, 399, 407
Professionalism
    in prevention, 395–398
Promoting Alternative THinking Strategies (PATHS), 342
PROmoting School–community–university Partnerships to Enhance Resilience (PROSPER), 372, 374, 375, 379
Psychoactive substance use (PSU), 147, 148
    media-based, 304
    media prevention campaigns, 316
    prevention
        argument, 309–310
        communication, 315
        efforts, messages and research, 303–305, 314
        studies, 303
    salience, 310
Psychoeducational approaches, 184
Public Health Cigarette Smoking Act of 1969, 101

Q
Quality control, 418–421

R
Random drug testing, 158
Randomized controlled trials (RCT), 122, 137
Reconceptualization, 151, 152
Reinforcement, 10
Replication, 251, 254, 255
Research, 418–421
    risks and benefits, 282–289
    substance use (*see* Substance use)
Risk and protection, 151, 152, 349, 350, 352, 356, 360
Risk, for substance misuse, 38, 39
Role of campaign exposure
    Above the Influence campaign, 323
    attention, 323
    audience activity, 324
    audience members, 323
    mass media campaigns, 323

My Anti-drug, 323
online and social media, 324
selective exposure, 323
social media messages, 324
website ads, 324

S
Sale restrictions, 165
   alcohol, 167
   marijuana, 170
   tobacco, 168
Scare tactics, 158, 159
School and general population surveys, 227
School-based prevention, 153
School bonding, 154
School culture and climate, 149, 150, 154
School health education, 108
School policies, 150, 155, 156
School prevention objectives, 152, 153
School readiness, 159, 160
School-system workforce, Czech Republic, 403
Science for Prevention Academic Network (SPAN), 405
Screening, Brief Intervention, and Referral to Treatment (SBIRT), 183
Second-hand smoke, 104, 112
Self-regulation theory, 321
Self-regulatory codes, 121, 125
Sensation Seeking Targeting Prevention Approach, 321
Sequential multiple assignment randomized trial (SMART)
   adaptive preventive intervention, 272–274
   study design, 274, 275
   Web-based BASICS intervention, 274
Serviço de Intervenção nos Comportamentos Aditivos e nas Dependências (SICAD), 418, 419
Sex differences, in brain development, 10
Short-term outcomes, 217
Single-mediator model, 235, 238, 239
Single nucleotide polymorphisms (SNPs), 39
Smoke-free workplace laws, 104, 112
Smoking
   and nicotine use, 77
Social analytics programs, 328
Social and cognitive skills, 148, 149
Social capital, 414, 427–429, 434
Social cognitive theory, 321
Social-emotional learning (SEL), 341, 342
Social inequality, 414, 427–429
Socialization, 133, 134
Social media, 46
   challenges, substance use campaigns, 327–328
   content shared, 327
   enthusiastic users, 320
   interventions
      CTC campaign, 327
      engagement and participation, assessment, 326
      Facebook, 326
      health interventions, 326
      medical and other practitioners, 326
      moderator emerged, 326
      selection of, 326
      sites, 325
      Twitter, 326
   mobile computing, 320
   mobile devices, 320
   monitoring, social networks, 329
   online media, 320
   online news services, 320
   prevention messages, 320
   web-based interventions
      (*see* Web-based interventions)
Social norms, 427–429, 434
Society for Prevention Research (SPR), 137, 388, 389
Sociologists, 210
States, tribes and jurisdictions (STJ), 376
Stigmatization, 59
Stress
   changes, in brain circuitry, 42
   description, 42
   early life stressors, 43
   exposures, 42
   family processes, 43
   heart rate and skin conductance, 42
   individual experiences, 42
   negative-affect pathway, 81, 82
   parent skill training, 44
   stressors, 42
   in substance use pathways, 42
Stress exposures, 42–44
Stressors, 42–44
Subgenual anterior cingulate cortex (saACC), 337
Subgroup analysis
   advantageous, 247
   ALL exploratory, 259
   anti-drug media campaign, adolescents, 256
   Bonferroni correction, 256
   CONSORT guideline, 257, 258
   effectiveness, 247
   EU-DAP, 248
   Food and Drug Administration, 258
   hypothesis testing, 256
   iatrogenic effects, 255
   issues, 258
   latent variables, 250–251
   LCA-strategy, 257
   manifest variables, 249–250
   mixture models and GMM, 247
   prevention interventions, 255
   pro-marijuana effects, 255
   psychometrics, 257
   replication and meta-analysis, 255–256
   research, 248
   risks and limitations, 247, 252–255
   statistical approaches, 247
   types, 248, 249
   virtual twins, 257
Substance Abuse and Mental Health Services Administration (SAMHSA), 325
Substance abuse disorder (SUD), 37

Substance dependence
  alcohol dependence, 25
  amphetamine dependence, 28
  cannabis and opioid dependence, 25
  country-level prevalence, 20
  definition, 25
  DSM-5, 25
  GBD study, 25
  geographic variation, 30, 34
  heavy episodic drinking, 21
  indicators, 25
  prevalence, 28
Substance-effect sensitivity, 83
Substance prevention, 182–184
Substance-related health burden, 28
Substance use disorder (SUD), 181, 195, 236, 237, 281, 335–338, 341, 343, 397–399
  and abuse, 282–283, 336
  addiction, 59
  burden of disease, 30
  CAPT, 376
  child assent and waiver of guardian permission, 287–288
  children and adolescents, 339, 340
  cognitive skills, 11
  comorbid mental disorders, 281, 293
  conduct disorder, 273
  confidentiality, 289–291
  cumulative levels, 12
  data collections, 20
  and delinquent behaviors, 373
  DSM-5, symptoms, 59
  during adolescence, 11
  effectiveness, 377
  epidemiology (see Epidemiology)
  ethical procedures, 294
  ethnographic and community research, 284–285, 287
  "equal environment" assumption, 61
  fair vs. coercive incentives, 293
  frontal lobe gray matter volumes, 14
  front-line staff, 285
  GBD study, 20
  general population surveys, 21
  global collections, 20
  goodness-of-fit framework, 294
  group stigmatization, 283–284
  head down pathways, 11
  heavy episodic alcohol consumption and dependence, 30
  indirect methods, prevalence estimation, 21
  informed consent, 286–289
  injecting drug use, 22, 24
  international control, 19
  long-term, 263, 264
  mindfulness practice, 337–339
  monetary incentives, participation, 291–293
  mortality, 28
  multiparameter evidence synthesis, 21
  neural region, 337
  neurochemical level, 14
  neuropsychological functioning, 12
  NPS, 24, 25
  prevalence
    alcohol, 21
    illicit substance use, 22
    and related burden, 19
    tobacco, 22
  prevention, 340–342, 369, 400–401
  risk of, 30, 32, 271, 273
  selective intervention, 268
  social-political influences, 283–284
  substance dependence, 25, 28
  workforce and researchers, 399, 401, 402
  in young adulthood, 367
Surgeon general's reports
  "appropriate remedial action", 100
  DHHS, 102
  federal policies, 103
  on smoking and health, 100
  warning labels, on cigarette, 106
Sympathetic nervous system, 10
Systems
  cohesive prevention systems, 388
  'events in systems, 392
  information and identify, 389
  international prevention system, 386
  and prevention science, 385, 386
  public health, 388
  web-based/videoconference meeting, 390
  whilst telephone conferencing, 390
Systems approach, 414, 415, 433, 435

T
Technical assistance, 418, 419
Teen Intervene (TI), 267
Theoretical mediation model, 234, 235
Theories of behavior change, 151
Theory of Reasoned Action, 321
Tobacco, 216, 227
  absolute burden, 30
  advertising restrictions, 169
  age restrictions, 168
  bans, 168
  epidemiological data, 21
  GBD study, 28
  global age-standardised prevalence, 22
  health burden, 34
  mortality rates, 30
  price, 168
  research, 172
  sales, 168
  smoking prevalence, 22
  substance dependence, 30
  tax, 168